Charles P. Hughes

St. Louis 1982

AF769905

ADVANCES IN NEUROLOGY
VOLUME 32

Advances in Neurology

INTERNATIONAL ADVISORY BOARD

Konrad Akert, *Zurich*
Julius Axelrod, *Bethesda*
André Barbeau, *Montreal*
Günter Baumgartner, *Zurich*
Donald B. Calne, *Bethesda*
Macdonald Critchley, *London*
Roger C. Duvoisin, *New Jersey*
Stanley Fahn, *New York*
Robert A. Fishman, *San Francisco*
Gilbert H. Glaser, *New Haven*
Rolf Hassler, *Frankfurt*
Herbert H. Jasper, *Montreal*
Bryan Jennett, *Glasgow*
Richard T. Johnson, *Baltimore*
Harold L. Klawans, *Chicago*
C. David Marsden, *London*
J. Kiffin Penry, *Winston-Salem*
Alfred Pope, *Boston*
Dominick P. Purpura, *New York*
Derek Richter, *London*
Lewis P. Rowland, *New York*
Arnold B. Scheibel, *Los Angeles*
Peritz Scheinberg, *Miami*
Richard P. Schmidt, *Syracuse*
Donald B. Tower, *Bethesda*
T. Tsubaki, *Tokyo*
John N. Walton, *Newcastle upon Tyne*
Arthur A. Ward, Jr., *Seattle*
Melvin D. Yahr, *New York*

Advances in Neurology
Volume 32

Clinical Applications of Evoked Potentials in Neurology

Editors

Jean Courjon, M.D.
Professor
EEG and Clinical
Neurophysiology Department
Neurological Hospital
Lyon, France

Francois Mauguière, M.D.
EEG and Clinical
Neurophysiology Department
Neurological Hospital
Lyon, France

Michel Revol, M.D.
EEG and Clinical
Neurophysiology Department
Sainte-Eugenie Hospital
Lyon, France

Raven Press ▪ New York

Raven Press, 1140 Avenue of the Americas, New York, New York 10036

© 1982 by Raven Press Books, Ltd. All rights reserved. This book is protected by copyright. No part of it may be reproduced, stored in a retrieval system, or transmitted, in any form or by any means, electronic, mechanical, photocopying, recording, or otherwise, without the prior written permission of the publisher.

Made in the United States of America

International Standard Book Number 0–89004–619–0
Library of Congress Catalog Card Number 80–5549

Great care has been taken to maintain the accuracy of the information contained in the volume. However, Raven Press cannot be held responsible for errors or for any consequences arising from the use of the information contained herein.

Materials appearing in this book prepared by individuals as part of their official duties as U.S. Government employees are not covered by the above-mentioned copyright.

Advances in Neurology Series

Vol. 33: Headache: Physiopathological and Clinical Concepts
M. Critchley, A. Friedman, S. Gorini, and F. Sicuteri, editors. 437 pp., 1982.

Vol. 32: Clinical Applications of Evoked Potentials in Neurology
J. Courjon, F. Mauguière, and M. Revol, editors. 596 pp., 1982.

Vol. 31: Demyelinating Diseases: Basic and Clinical Electrophysiology
S. Waxman and J. Murdoch Ritchie, editors. 532 pp., 1981.

Vol. 30: Diagnosis and Treatment of Brain Ischemia
A. L. Carney and E. M. Anderson, editors. 424 pp., 1981.

Vol. 29: Neurofibromatosis
V. M. Riccardi and J. J. Mulvihill, editors. 282 pp., 1981.

Vol. 28: Brain Edema
J. Cervós-Navarro and R. Ferszt, editors. 539 pp., 1980.

Vol. 27: Antiepileptic Drugs: Mechanisms of Action
G. H. Glaser, J. K. Penry, and D. M. Woodbury, editors. 728 pp., 1980.

Vol. 26: Cerebral Hypoxia and Its Consequences
S. Fahn, J. N. Davis, and L. P. Rowland, editors. 454 pp., 1979.

Vol. 25: Cerebrovascular Disorders and Stroke
M. Goldstein, L. Bolis, C. Fieschi, S. Gorini, and C. H. Millikan, editors. 412 pp., 1979.

Vol. 24: The Extrapyramidal System and Its Disorders
L. J. Poirier, T. L. Sourkes, and P. Bédard, editors. 552 pp., 1979.

Vol. 23: Huntington's Chorea
T. N. Chase, N. S. Wexler, and A. Barbeau, editors. 864 pp., 1979.

Vol. 22: Complications of Nervous System Trauma
R. A. Thompson and J. R. Green, editors. 454 pp., 1979.

Vol. 21: The Inherited Ataxias: Biochemical, Viral, and Pathological Studies
R. A. Kark, R. Rosenberg, and L. Schut, editors. 450 pp., 1978.

Vol. 20: Pathology of Cerebrospinal Microcirculation
J. Cervós-Navarro, E. Betz, G. Ebhardt, R. Ferszt, and R. Wüllenweber, editors. 636 pp., 1978.

Vol. 19: Neurological Epidemiology: Principles and Clinical Applications
Bruce S. Schoenberg, editor. 672 pp., 1978.

Vol. 18: Hemi-Inattention and Hemisphere Specialization
E. A. Weinstein and R. P. Friedland, editors. 176 pp., 1977.

Vol. 17: Treatment of Neuromuscular Diseases
R. C. Griggs and R. T. Moxley, editors. 370 pp., 1977.

Vol. 16: Stroke
R. A. Thompson and J. R. Green, editors. 250 pp., 1977.

Preface

The recording of evoked potentials (EPs) has, over the past 25 years, become an extremely useful means of investigating the electrophysiological correlates of sensory processing, movement programming, and decision-making in humans. In spite of a large amount of published data, clinical applications of this noninvasive technique in neurology have yet to be firmly established. It was with this purpose in mind that this volume was developed.

The topics discussed in detail in this volume are those which will probably become the focus of future EP studies in clinical neurology and they include: the pathophysiological interpretation of abnormal somatosensory EPs, applications of EPs to the study of pain, correlations between BAEP abnormalities and the sites of lesions in the brainstem or posterior fossa, results of multimodal EP studies in the detection of subclinical lesions of the sensory pathways in multiple sclerosis, and the usefulness of serial recordings of EPs for followup studies in MS. It is the conclusion of these studies that EPs have definite diagnostic value in such neurological disorders provided that the clinical context is taken into account for the interpretation of results; in the absence of such electroclinical correlations, misleading conclusions may certainly result.

This volume will be of interest to clinical neurologists, neuroscientists, electroencephalographers, and others interested in correlations between the electrical activity of the nervous system and disease or behavioral processes.

Contents

VISUAL EVOKED POTENTIALS (VEPs)

Introduction

Lesions of the Optic Nerve

Visual Field Defects Due to Chiasmatic and Retrochiasmatic Lesions

Clinical Applications of VEPs in Neuropaediatry

Encephalopathies Dementia Heredodegenerative Diseases

BRAINSTEM AUDITORY EVOKED POTENTIALS (BAEPs)

Introduction

Acoustic Neurinomas

AUDITORY EVOKED POTENTIALS (AEPs) AND LATE COMPONENTS OF EVENT-RELATED POTENTIALS

Application of AEPs in Neuropsychology

Aging and Dementia

SOMATOSENSORY EVOKED POTENTIALS (SEPs)

Introduction

Lesions of Central Somatosensory Pathways

Lesions of Nerves, Roots, and Spinal Cord

Pain

Neuropaediatry

CLINICAL APPLICATIONS OF EVOKED POTENTIALS IN MULTIPLE SCLEROSIS

Techniques of Visual Stimulation in Multiple Sclerosis

Contributors

Clinical Applications of Evoked Potentials in Neurology,
edited by J. Courjon, F. Mauguiere, and M. Revol.
Raven Press, New York © 1982.

Problems in Defining the Normal Limits of the Visual Evoked Potential

A. M. Halliday, G. Barrett,* W. M. Carroll, and A. Kriss

Medical Research Council, Institute of Neurology, National Hospital, London WC1, England

In studying the P100 latency of the pattern-reversal evoked potential (EP) in demyelinating disease of the optic nerve, the delays are usually so marked that there is little overlap of the response from the affected patients and the healthy population (12,13,14,15). Under these circumstances, a precise definition of the upper limit of normal is not very critical and makes relatively little difference to the overall detection rate. However, attention is now being directed to the use of the pattern EP in many other neurological conditions in which latency changes are not so marked. In assessing the significance of the relatively small differences in P100 latency reported in some of these studies, one has to look much more carefully and accurately at the way the upper limit of normal is defined and to identify the important sources of variability in the normal response that may invalidate the comparison if an unmatched control group is used.

Two important variables significantly affecting P100 latency by a few milliseconds (msec) are age and sex. Stockard et al. (24) first drew attention to the fact that the mean latency of the P100 component of the checkerboard reversal response was some 2.69 msec shorter in a group of 50 healthy women than in 50 healthy age-matched men, the difference being statistically significant ($p = 0.03$). Our own data on comparison groups of 65 men and 69 women confirm the shorter latency of the response in women at a much higher level of significance (Table 1). With our particular stimulus (a mirror projector system providing a 32° field of 50′ checks with luminance levels of 8.2 cd/m^2 and 227 cd/m^2 for the black and white pattern elements, respectively), which is about twice the field and check size and brightness of the TV-generated checkerboard used by Stockard et al. (24), the mean latency of the female group was between 3.5 and 3.9 msec shorter than the corresponding mean for the same eye, the difference being significant at the $p < 0.001$ level. An even more striking sex difference in the amplitude of the response emerged from this study, with

* *Present address:* Sir Charles Gairdner Hospital, Queen Elizabeth II Medical Centre, Nedlands, Western Australia 6009, Australia.

TABLE 1. *Differences in the mean latency and amplitude of the P100 component of the checkerboard reversal response in the two sexes*

		Latency (msec)		Amplitude (μV)	
	N	Left eye	Right eye	Left eye	Right eye
Men	65	107.7 ± 4.55	108.2 ± 4.95	11.5 ± 4.28	10.9 ± 4.52
Women	69	103.8 ± 4.19	104.7 ± 4.95	16.1 ± 5.71	15.8 ± 5.85
Difference		−3.9	−3.5	+4.6	+4.9
Significance		$p < 0.001$	$p < 0.001$	$p < 0.001$	$p < 0.001$

the mean amplitude of the P100 for the female group being between 4 and 5 μV greater than for the male group ($p < 0.001$).

There have been a number of published studies of the effect of age on P100 latency (1,2,8,10,16,22,24). Most have reported an increase in the P100 latency in the elderly, but there is disagreement over the overall form of the age–latency relationship. Celesia and Daly (8) noted a linear increase in latency with age with a slope of approximately 0.18 msec/year over the age range from 15 to 70 years, whereas the data collected in other studies have suggested that there is little or no increase in latency until the age of 50 to 65, with a progressive increase thereafter (1,2,10,14,25). Shaw and Cant (22) found an increase in latency from the fifth decade onward, but this was only significant for lower intensities of the checkerboard stimulus, the brightness having an important influence on the slope of the age–latency function in the elderly subjects. One of the few studies to report amplitude differences with age found significantly higher P1 amplitudes in individuals under 25 years and over 55 (10). Stockard et al. (24), who separated out the sex differences in latency, concluded that there was no significant age effect on latency between 20 and 55 years of age. In the sixth decade, they found the P100 latency increases in variance but not in mean latency, requiring about a 5-msec increase in the upper limit of normal (defined in their study as a P100 latency beyond the entire range of appropriate normal controls, encompassing approximately 3 SD above the mean). The study also reported an increase in the mean latency as well as the variance in the over-60s, although no data are presented for this age group.

The age and sex differences for the left and right eyes of our control group are separated out in Fig. 1 for P100 latency and in Fig. 2 for P100 amplitude. As can be seen, the large sex differences in amplitude are seen throughout the age range 15 to 70, and there is no significant effect of age on P100 amplitude revealed by these data (Fig. 2). In contrast to this, there is a significant age–latency effect for the female group but not for the males, almost entirely because of an increase in mean latency between the ages of 50 and 70. This effect is significant on a one-way analysis of variance at the $p = 0.006$ level for the left eye latency and $p = 0.036$ for the right eye latency. Tests of the reality of the between-age group differences of the mean latency by the Tukey honestly signifi-

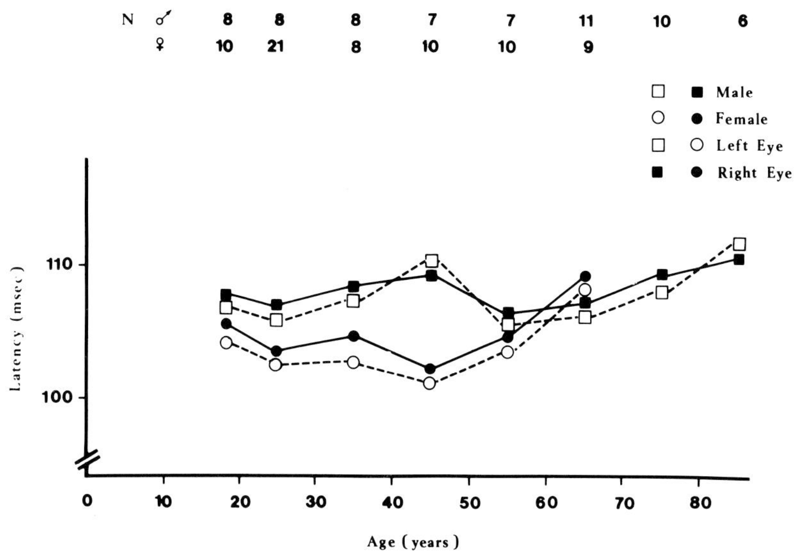

FIG. 1. Mean latency for the P100 component of the pattern-reversal response, plotted separately for the left and right eyes of the men and women in different age groups (decades), for a group of 134 healthy individuals. The *N*s for each group are given at the top of the figure. There was no significant effect of age on latency for the male group, but there was a significant effect in the female group for both left ($p = 0.006$) and right ($p = 0.036$) eye latency. As can be seen, there is a significant increase in latency in the female group between the fifth and seventh decade for the response from both eyes.

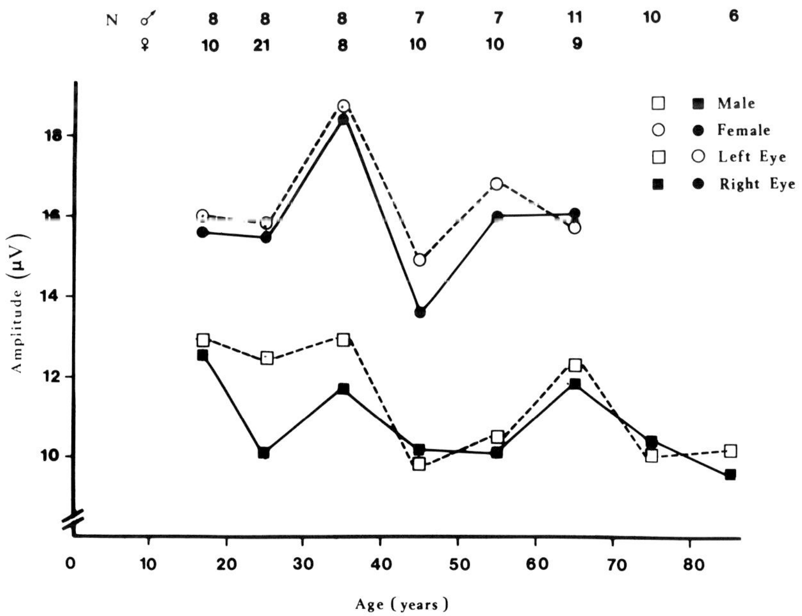

FIG. 2. Mean amplitude for the P100 component from each eye in the male and female subjects, plotted separately for each decade. Same population as for Fig. 1. There is a highly significant difference in the mean amplitude of the response for the two sexes, but no significant age–amplitude effect.

cant difference multiple-range test show that for each eye there are significant differences at the $p < 0.05$ level between the latency for the 40 to 49 age group and the 60 to 69 age group.

The explanation of these sex and age differences in mean latency and amplitude is not altogether clear, but it may be related to the smaller average head size and skull thickness in women (17,20) and possibly also to the higher deep body temperature in women (24). Shorter latencies in women have also been reported for the BAEP (19,25) and for the SEP (21). Marshall and Donchin (18) have also recently demonstrated circadian variation in the latency of the BAEP related to changes in deep body temperature. Clearly, the very large differences in the P100 amplitude of the pattern EP in women revealed by the present study are likely to be related to anatomical factors such as skull thickness, but the increase in mean latency observed in the female group between 50 and 70 might be related to structural, metabolic, or temperature changes occurring in association with the menopause. On the present data, there is no significant effect of age on either latency or amplitude for the male group. It is worth pointing out, however, that elderly patients need very careful screening for minor visual defects. Slight opacities, discoloration of the lens, and retinal lesions become more frequent in the elderly, and if adequate control data are to be collected, it is essential to carry out a careful neuroophthalmological examination to distinguish minor degrees of pathological change from other causes of normal variation. Some of these patients may be eliminated by excluding all those with interocular latency differences clearly beyond the normal limit, and this was done in the case of our own control group.

Some other easily overlooked sources of variability arise from interaction between the choice of stimulus parameters and the patient's vision. An example of this is the influence of check size and field size on the effect of refractive errors. With a checkerboard made of large checks (greater than 50′), P100 amplitude is sensitive to refractive errors and their correction, but P100 latency is relatively unaffected. With small check sizes (e.g., 12′), however, particularly if presented foveally, P100 latency may be significantly lengthened by defocusing of the image and will be reduced in latency by correction (7,9). Figure 3, which is taken from the paper by Carroll and Kriss (7), illustrates this effect in a 30-year-old patient with myopia. Uncorrected vision in the left eye was 6/60, whereas corrected vision in the same eye was 6/6. The upper two records show the checkerboard pattern responses to a 4° radius stimulus field of small 20′ checks. Removing the patient's glasses causes a very slight broadening of the P100 but only alters the latency from 103 to 105 msec. Reducing both the field size and the check size by half (lower records) increases the sensitivity of the P100 latency to the refractive error so that the mean latency increases from 108 msec to 124 msec.

Both the latency and the amplitude of the P100 component are also sensitive to the brightness levels of the checkerboard stimulus (15) and to the contrast when this is below saturation level (23). Under certain circumstances, the effec-

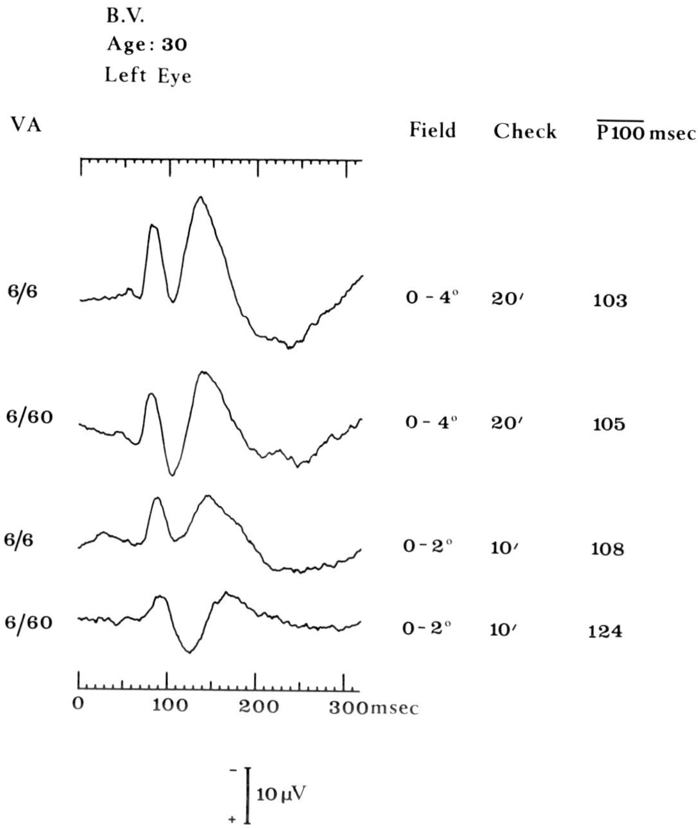

FIG. 3. Midline pattern EPs, recorded from an electrode 5 cm above the inion referred to F_z, from the left eye of a 30-year-old subject with myopia. The figure shows the responses for corrected and uncorrected vision (see visual acuities on the left) to a checkerboard stimulus of 4° radius and 20′ checks *(upper two records)* and of 2° radius and 10′ checks *(lower two records)*. Note that the latency of the response is little altered by the refractive error with the 4° field and larger checks but is significantly delayed when recorded uncorrected with the smaller field and check size. (From Carroll and Kriss, ref. 7, with permission.)

tiveness of the stimulus may therefore be altered by physiological factors that affect the sharpness, brightness, and contrast of the image (e.g., changes in the pupil size or drooping of the lids because of weakness or drowsiness), and this, too, may lead to small but significant changes in the amplitude and latency of the response (7,24). The sharpness, brightness, and contrast of the image may, of course, also be altered by minor opacities in the eye itself.

Figure 4, also from Carroll and Kriss (7), illustrates the complex interaction between the effect of minor opacities and varying stimulus parameters, such as field size, check size, and brightness, in a 31-year-old patient with a slight cataract of the right eye. Acuity in this eye was only reduced to 6/9, compared with 6/5 in the left eye. With the standard 16° radius stimulus field of 50′

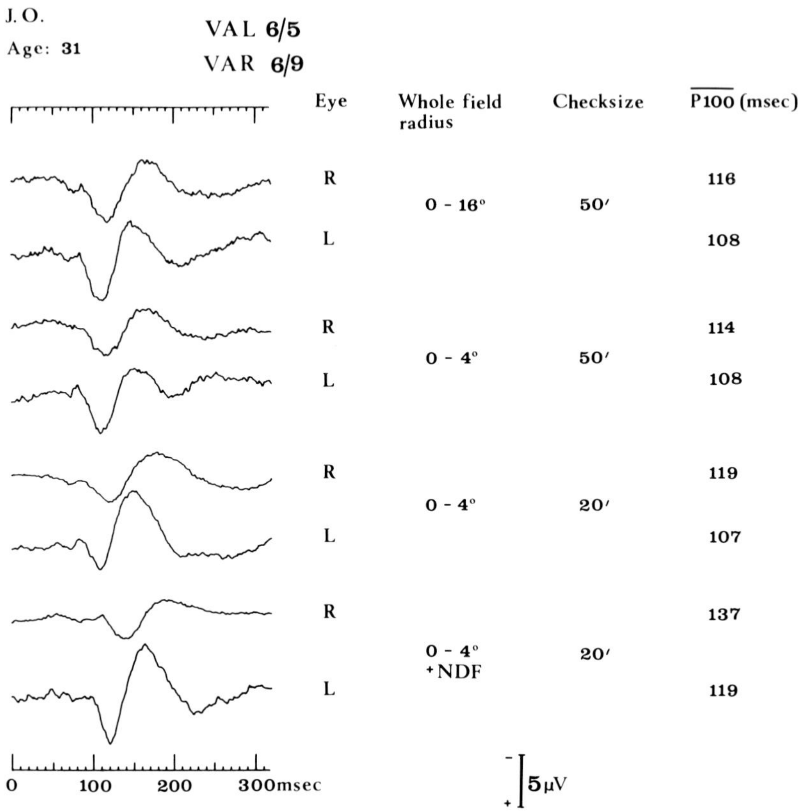

FIG. 4. Midline pattern EPs, recorded as in Fig. 3, in a 31-year-old patient with a moderate right central cataract, to a checkerboard stimulus of varying field size, check size, and brightness (as indicated on the right). Note that the latency of the response from the eye with cataract is very much more sensitive to reductions in field size, check size, and brightness than is the response from the normal eye. (From Carroll and Kriss, ref. 7, with permission.)

checks, the P100 amplitude was reduced, and the latency was at the upper limit of the normal range, 8 msec greater than in the unaffected eye. The interocular latency difference was not increased by reducing the stimulus field to 4° radius, although the amplitude of the response diminished, but with smaller 20′ checks, the P100 latency from the affected eye is delayed, with a mean latency of 119 msec and an interocular latency difference of 12 msec. The 10-fold reduction of stimulus brightness by the introduction of a one log unit neutral density filter greatly increases the interocular latency difference to 18 msec.

It is not absolutely clear which are the most important factors operating to increase the latency of the foveal response to small checks when these are defocused. Probably there is a complex interaction of the effects of brightness level and contrast. The latency of the pattern response is known to be sensitive to

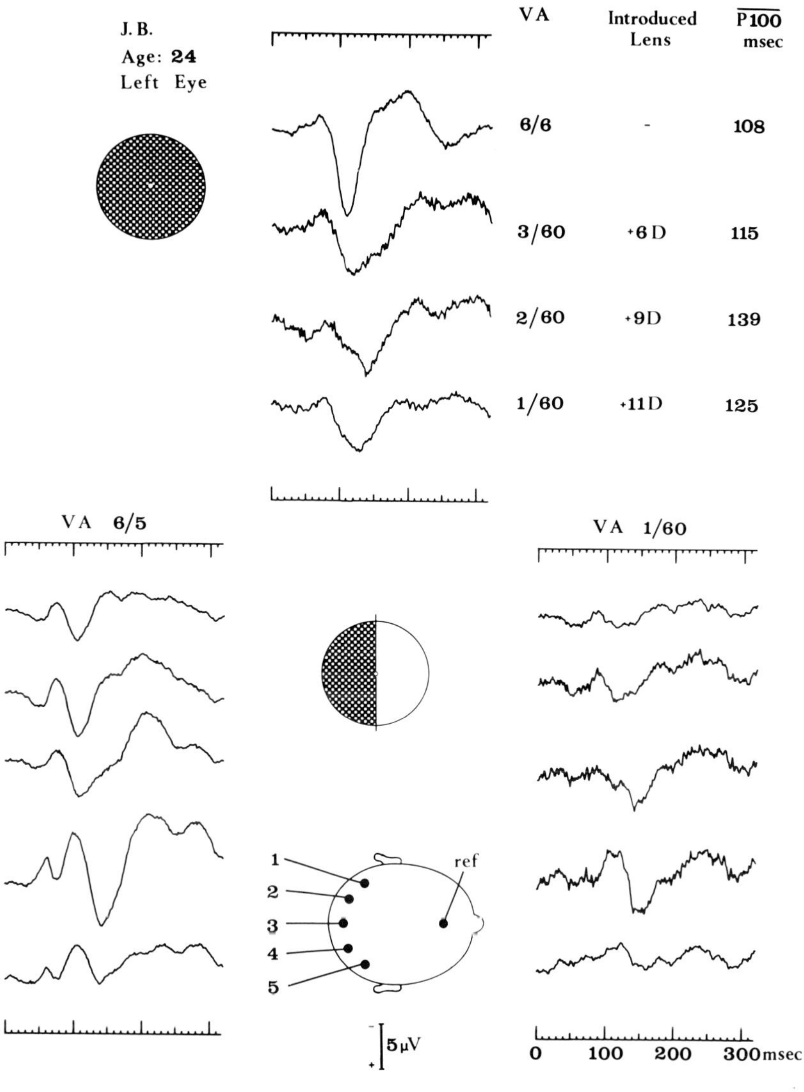

FIG. 5. Full-field pattern EPs, recorded from the midline *(upper record),* from the left eye of a healthy individual. The effect of defocusing the 16° checkerboard stimulus of 50′ checks with increasingly strong convex lenses (see indication on the right) is to alter the waveform of the response and to affect the peak latency. The lower two records of the corresponding half-field EP, recorded from a transverse row of five electrodes across the back of the head, demonstrate that the apparent increase in the latency of the midline positivity is, in fact, caused by the substitution of the macular P100 component by a paramacular P135. (From Carroll and Kriss, ref. 7, with permission.)

contrast levels when these are below saturation level, although the saturation level is quite low, and the effect of low contrast changes on response latency flattens out at levels above 20 to 40% contrast. However, low mean luminance and the presence of opacities may well operate to reduce contrast to below the critical level, as may the reduction in effective stimulus intensity by constriction in the pupil or drooping of the eyelids.

Unless the variability of the waveform and distribution of the normal pattern reversal EP is well understood, confusion can arise in the interpretation of the changes occurring in the abnormal response. The normal half-field response to a 0 to 16° stimulus of 50′ checks is made up of a macular negative-positive-negative (NPN) complex recorded ipsilaterally to the half field stimulated and a paramacular positive-negative-positive (PNP) complex recorded contralaterally (3,4,11). In central scotomata, the macular NPN complex with its P100 component is lost and is replaced by the paramacular PNP complex with its prominent P135 component following the N105 (11; see also Kriss et al., *this volume*). It is easy to confuse this P135 for a delayed P100 unless the lateralization of the component is confirmed by half-field stimulation.

Since central-field defects are not uncommon in demyelinating disease, this can be an important source of misinterpretation of EP records. It is possible to produce similar changes in the responses from the healthy individual not only by removing the stimulus from the central area with an experimental scotoma (3) but also by using extremely strong lenses to deprive the subject of fine pattern vision in the foveal area. Figure 5 illustrates the effect of introducing extremely strong lenses of up to +11 diopters while recording the monocular response from a 24-year-old healthy individual. The P100 latency undergoes an apparent increase far above the normal range for the +9 and +11 diopter lenses, but half-field stimulation with and without the lens (lower records) demonstrates that this is not an increase in the P100 latency but a substitution of the contralateral P135 component for the ipsilateral P100 component. One can easily guard against this possible source of misinterpretation of visual EP records by examining the lateralization of the component with half-field stimulation, provided that an adequate montage is used (11).

The resort to half-field stimulation to help in the interpretation of the whole-field pattern responses also markedly improves the precision with which the limits of normal asymmetry can be defined (5). This can greatly increase the detection rate of the abnormal asymmetries associated with hemianopic and quadrantanopic field defects. Similar pattern visual EP asymmetries can be seen in healthy albino subjects, associated with the anomalous crossed retinocortical projection from the temporal retina (6).

REFERENCES

1. Allison, T., Goff, W. R., and Wood, C. C. (1978): Auditory, somatosensory and visual evoked potentials in the diagnosis of neuropathology: Recording considerations and normative data.

In: *Human Evoked Potentials: Applications and Problems,* edited by D. Lehmann and E. Callaway, pp. 1–66. Plenum Press, New York.
2. Asselman, P., Chadwick, D. W., and Marsden, C. D. (1975): Visual evoked responses in the diagnosis and management of patients suspected of multiple sclerosis. *Brain,* 98:261–282.
3. Blumhardt, L. D., Barrett, G., Halliday, A. M., and Kriss, A. (1978): The effect of experimental "scotomata" on the ipsilateral and contralateral responses to pattern-reversal in one half-field. *Electroencephalogr. Clin. Neurophysiol.,* 45:376–392.
4. Blumhardt, L. D., and Halliday, A. M. (1979): Hemisphere contributions to the composition of the pattern evoked potential waveform. *Exp. Brain Res.,* 36:53–69.
5. Blumhardt, L. D., and Halliday, A. M. (1981): Cortical abnormalities and the visual evoked response. In: *Visual Pathways: Electrophysiology and Pathology. Doc. Ophthalmol. Proc. Series Vol. 27*:347–365, edited by H. Spekreijse and P. A. Apkarian. Junk, The Hague.
6. Carroll, W. M., Jay, B., McDonald, W. I., and Halliday, A. M. (1980): Pattern evoked potentials in human albinism. Evidence of two different topographical asymmetries reflecting abnormal retino-cortical projections. *J. Neurol. Sci.,* 48:265–287.
7. Carroll, W. M., and Kriss, A. (1980): Pattern visual evoked potentials in neurological and neuro-ophthalmological diagnosis: An appraisal of the nature of delayed VEPs in the absence and presence of optic nerve disease. *(In preparation.)*
8. Celesia, G. G., and Daly, R. F. (1977): Effect of ageing on visual evoked responses. *Arch. Neurol.,* 34:403–407.
9. Collins, D. W. K., Carroll, W. M., Black, J. L., and Walsh, M. (1979): Effect of refractive error on the visual evoked response. *Br. Med. J.,* 1:231–232.
10. Faust, U., Heintel, H., and Hoek, R. (1978): Altersabhängigkeit der P_2-Latenzzeiten schachbrettmusterevozierter Potentiale. *Z. EEG EMG,* 9:219–221.
11. Halliday, A. M., Barrett, G., Blumhardt, L. D., and Kriss, A. (1979): The macular and paramacular sub-components of the pattern evoked response. In: *Human Evoked Potentials: Applications and Problems,* edited by D. Lehmann and E. Callaway, pp. 135–151. Plenum Press, New York.
12. Halliday, A. M., Barrett, G., Halliday, E., and Mushin, J. (1980): A comparison of the flash and pattern-evoked potential in unilateral optic neuritis. *Wisserschaftliche Z. Ernst-Moritz-Arndt-Universität,* 28:89–95.
13. Halliday, A. M., McDonald, W. I., and Mushin, J. (1972): Delayed visual evoked response in optic neuritis. *Lancet,* 1:982–985.
14. Halliday, A. M., McDonald, W. I., and Mushin, J. (1973): The visual evoked response in the diagnosis of multiple sclerosis. *Br. Med. J.,* 4:661–664.
15. Halliday, A. M., McDonald, W. I., and Mushin, J. (1973): Delayed pattern evoked responses in optic neuritis in relation to visual acuity. *Trans. Ophthalmol. Soc. U.K.,* 93:315–324.
16. Heintel, H., Faust, U., and Faust, C. (1979): Altersabhängigkeit der P_2-Amplituden schachbrettmusterevozierter Potentiale. *Z. EEG EMG,* 10:194–196.
17. Johnston, T. B., and Whillis, J. (1938): *Gray's Anatomy: Descriptive and Applied.* Longmans, Green, London.
18. Marshall, N. K., and Donchin, E. (1980): Circadian variation in the latency of brainstem responses and its relation to body temperature. *Science,* 212:356–358.
19. Michalewski, H. J., Thompson, L. W., Patterson, J. V., Bowman, T. E., and Litzelman, D. (1980): Sex differences in the amplitudes and latencies of the human auditory brainstem potential. *Electroencephalogr. Clin. Neurophysiol.,* 48:351–356.
20. Parsons, F. G., and Keene, L. (1919): Sexual differences in the skull. *J. Anat.,* 54:58–65.
21. Shagass, C. (1972): *Evoked Brain Potentials in Psychiatry.* Plenum Press, New York.
22. Shaw, N. A., and Cant, B. R. (1980): Age dependent changes in the latency of the pattern visual evoked potential. *Electroencephalogr. Clin. Neurophysiol.,* 48:237–241.
23. Spekreijse, H., Duwaer, A. L., and Posthumus Meyjes, F. E. (1979): Contrast evoked potentials and psychophysics in multiple sclerosis. In: *Human Evoked Potentials: Applications and Problems,* edited by D. Lehmann and E. Callaway, pp. 363–381. Plenum Press, New York.
24. Stockard, J. J., Hughes, J. F., and Sharbrough, F. W. (1979): Visually evoked potentials to electronic pattern reversal: Latency variations with gender, age and technical factors. *Am. J. EEG Technol.,* 19:171–204.
25. Stockard, J. J., Stockard, J. E., and Sharbrough, F. W. (1978): Non-pathologic factors influencing brainstem auditory evoked potentials. *Am. J. EEG Technol.,* 18:177–209.

Clinical Applications of Evoked Potentials in Neurology,
edited by J. Courjon, F. Mauguiere, and M. Revol.
Raven Press, New York © 1982.

Pattern- and Flash-Evoked Potential Changes in Toxic (Nutritional) Optic Neuropathy

*A. Kriss, **W. M. Carroll, †L. D. Blumhardt, and *A. M. Halliday

**MRC External Staff, National Hospital for Nervous Diseases, London WC1N 3BG, England; **Department of Neurology, Sir Charles Gairdner Hospital, Queen Elizabeth II Medical Centre, Nedlands, Western Australia 6009, Australia; and †University Department of Neurology, Radcliffe Infirmary, Oxford OX2 6HE, England*

The cause of the visual disturbance associated with toxic optic neuropathy (so-called tobacco/alcohol amblyopia) has not been satisfactorily established. It is commonly held that a deficiency of the vitamin B complex, most importantly vitamin B_{12}, is a vital factor in this disorder, although there is controversy as to whether it is the vitamin deficiency itself that is responsible or whether toxins, such as the cyanide present in tobacco smoke, directly poison the anterior visual pathway and also lead to depletion of available B_{12} as a result of metabolic anomalies associated with the detoxification of cyanide [see Potts (7) for a review and discussion].

Ikeda et al. (6) showed that in patients with toxic optic neuropathy the corneal electroretinogram (ERG) and pattern-evoked potential, as recorded from a single midline occipital electrode, were smaller than normal. Multichannel recording and half-field stimulation have the advantage of allowing one to distinguish between macular and paramacular responses (2,3), which is particularly relevant to the assessment of toxic amblyopia because of the discrete central field defects occurring in this disorder.

METHODS

Twenty-four patients (21 males, three females; mean age 52.6 years, SD 11.2) with a diagnosis of toxic optic neuropathy were recorded, and their pattern responses were compared to those of healthy subjects of the same sex and approximately the same age (mean 53.6, SD 10.4). Flash responses from 15 of these patients were compared to those from a second group of non-age-matched controls (mean age 20.6 years; 15 females, two males). A checkerboard of 50′ squares was used to stimulate full field (0–16° radius), half field (0–16° radius), and central field (0–4° radius). Occipital potentials to both flash and pattern reversal were recorded from a transverse row of five electrodes spaced

5 cm apart on a line 5 cm above the inion; each referred to a midfrontal electrode 12 cm above the nasion. The ERG was recorded from each eye by a pair of skin electrodes, one midway along the lower eyelid, the other posterolateral to the external canthus. Further details of the recording technique may be found elsewhere (2,3).

RESULTS

Most of the patients (22/24, 92%) drank more than half a bottle of spirits or four pints of beer per day, and 71% (17/24) smoked in excess of ⅓ ounce of tobacco or 40 cigarettes per day. Sixty-three percent (15/24) both drank and smoked. Acuity from the majority of examined eyes (38/48, 79%) was worse than 6/12 at the time of the evoked potential test. All patients had color vision defects, and all showed absolute or relative central or centro–caecal scotomata. Disk pallor was present in 68% (33/48) of eyes, with 43% (21/48) having only temporal pallor. In the 13 patients who were recorded more than once, acuities were poorer than 6/12 at the first recording in 77% (20/26) of their eyes but improved considerably with B_{12} therapy, abstinence, and time, so that prior to the last recording, 85% (22/26) had acuities of 6/12 or better. There was also a general amelioration in visual field defects and color vision, although subtle residual defects were commonly found in which there was desaturation to red usually confined to the visual area between fixation point and blind spot.

The changes in the timing and general morphology of the evoked potentials showed a consistent pattern in the majority of patients. It was, therefore, considered justifiable to average the individual responses of all patients for the same stimulus condition in order to emphasize common features and to provide a representative and parsimonious means of illustrating the results.

Figure 1 shows the grand average responses to full-field (0–16° radius) pattern stimulation for 23 patients before treatment and for 13 on follow-up (upper two records) and for the control group (lower records). The full-field response of the controls is characterized by a large positivity (P100) symmetrically distributed about the midline which on average has a latency of 104 msec and an amplitude of 12 μV with no significant eye difference. The distribution of the patients' responses before treatment is different, showing a broad positivity in the midline, peaking at 130 msec. To either side of this central channel there is a positive–negative–positive (PNP) complex. A P100 component was identifiable in 15% (7/48) of the records and, on average, measured 4 μV at 111 msec, there being no significant eye difference.

On follow-up, the P100 was seen in a higher proportion of records (11/26, 38%) but showed a mean increase in amplitude of only 2 μV, remaining significantly smaller than normal ($p < 0.02$). The latency of the P100 was 10 msec later than in the controls ($p < 0.01$). The PNP complexes were seen in the remainder of records (i.e., those without P100s), and components of the complex were, on average, 1 to 2 μV larger than on the first recording.

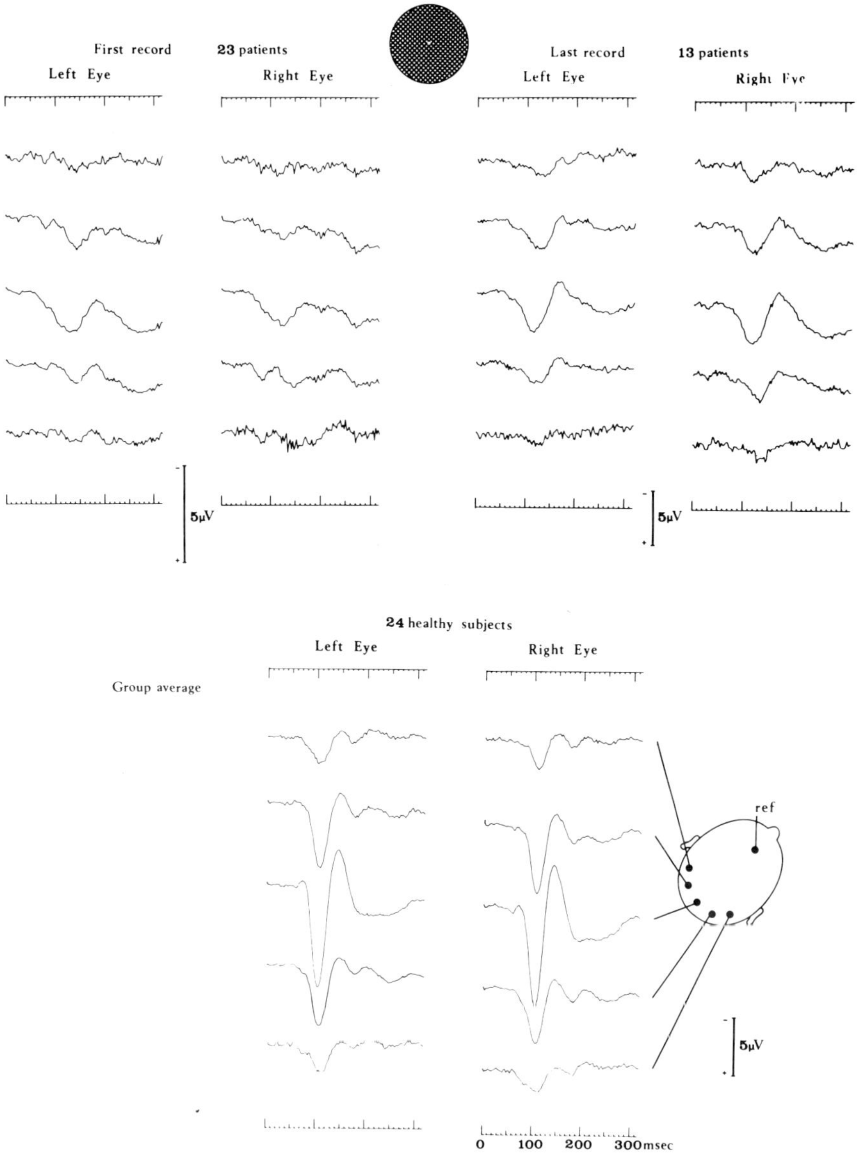

FIG. 1. Group average responses to full-field (0–16° radius) stimulation. Upper traces are those of patients before and after treatment. The mean interval between first and last recording was 2 years. The lower pair of traces are the average responses of a sex- and age-matched control group. Note differences in distribution between patients and controls before treatment and smaller responses than normal after treatment.

In order to clarify the full-field distribution, it is necessary to resort to independent stimulation of the left and right half-fields. In normals (see Figs. 2 and 3), the major positivity (P100) is seen in the midline and over the side of the head ipsilateral to the stimulated half field, measuring 6.9 μV at 105 msec, 5 cm from the midline. No significant differences in amplitude or latency were found when comparing half-field P100s. On the side contralateral to the

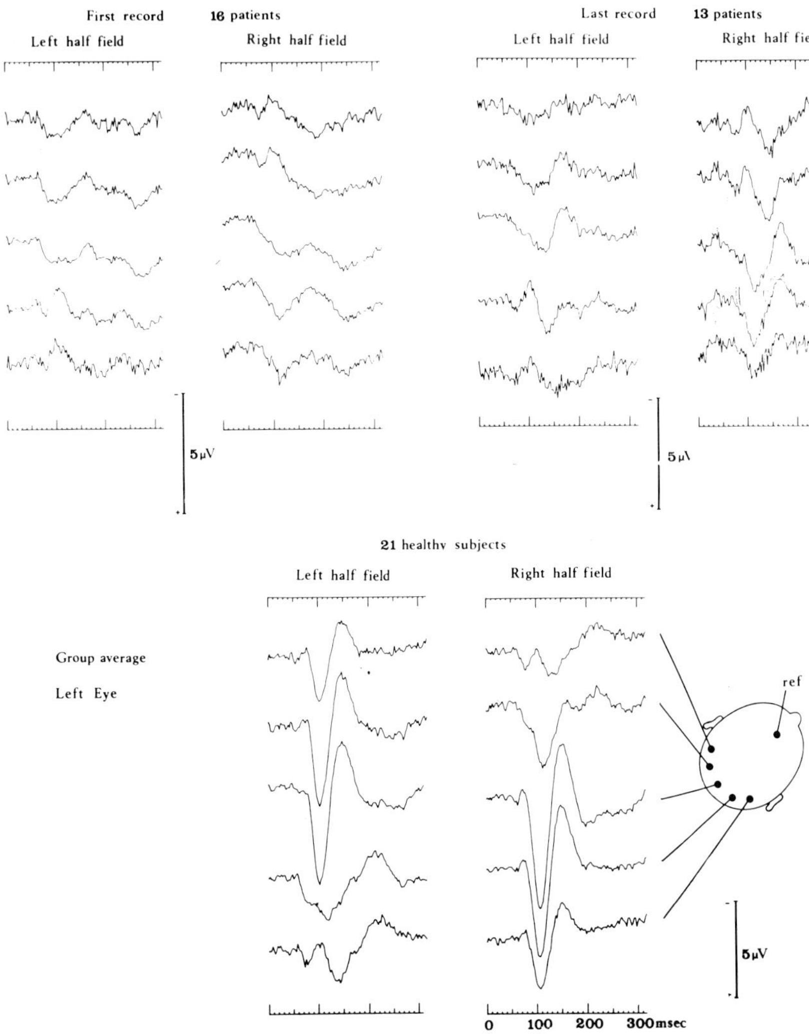

FIG. 2. Group average responses to left and right half-field stimulation of the left eye. The P100 component on the side of the head ipsilateral to the half-field stimulated is smaller in patients than in matched controls; the PNP complex on the contralateral side is seen in the channel just lateral to the midline, rather than at the 10 cm lateral electrode as in the controls.

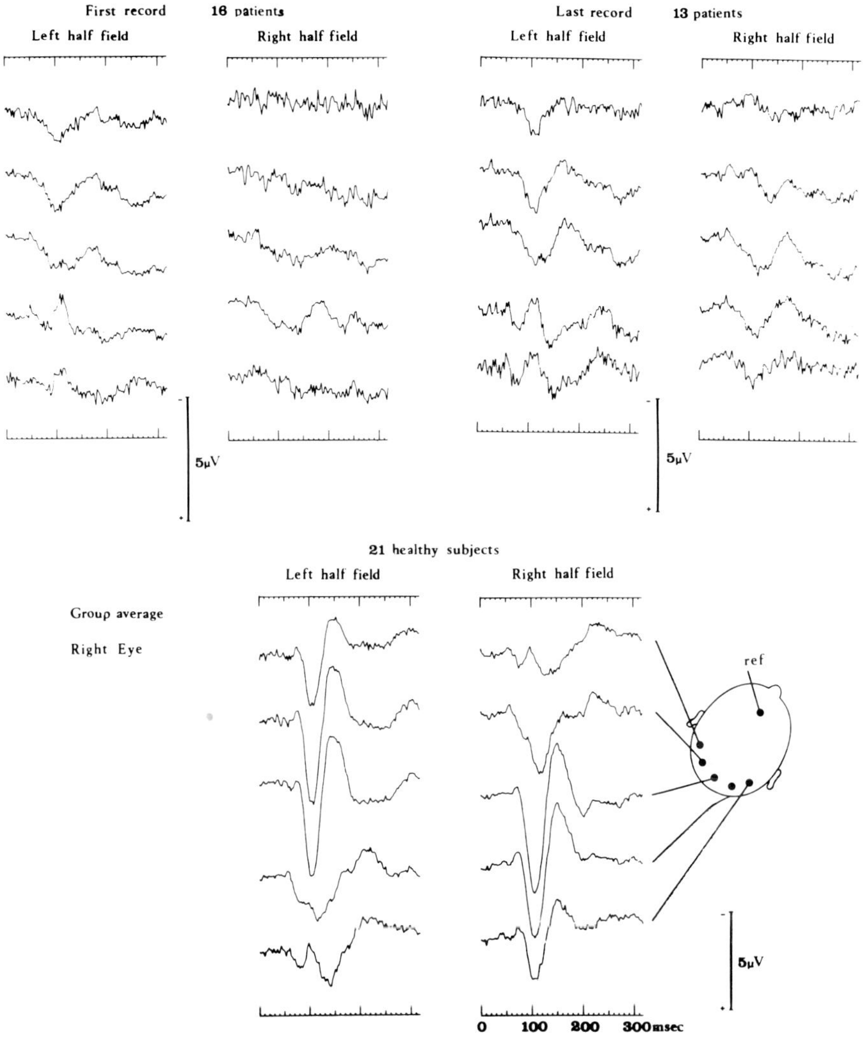

FIG. 3. Group average responses to half-field stimulation of the right eye.

stimulus field, a PNP complex (P75, N105, P135) is seen which tends to be largest 10 cm from the midline.

The pretreatment records of the patients show a much attenuated ipsilateral P100, of the order of 2 μV, and, in contrast to the healthy subjects, a conspicuous contralateral PNP complex (P80, N105, P140), best seen 5 cm from the midline, in which the negative component (N105) had a mean amplitude of 2 μV; only 41/64 (64%) of the half-field records demonstrated an ipsilateral P100. In the remainder, only the contralateral PNP complex was identifiable, and in many cases it spread over the midline to be seen in an attenuated form on the ipsilateral side. Comparison of the left and right half fields of the same eye showed a significant tendency for the P100 to be smaller ($p < 0.02$) and less well defined following temporal field stimulation. No significant differences were found for similar comparisons of the contralateral PNP complexes.

On follow-up, the incidence of P100s did not increase, but, when present, this component was on average 1 μV larger than on the first recording. There still appeared to be a tendency for the temporal half-field P100 to be smaller than its nasal field counterpart.

The central-field (0–4° radius) responses of the healthy and patient groups were strikingly different (Fig. 4). In the normals, this small field evoked a P100

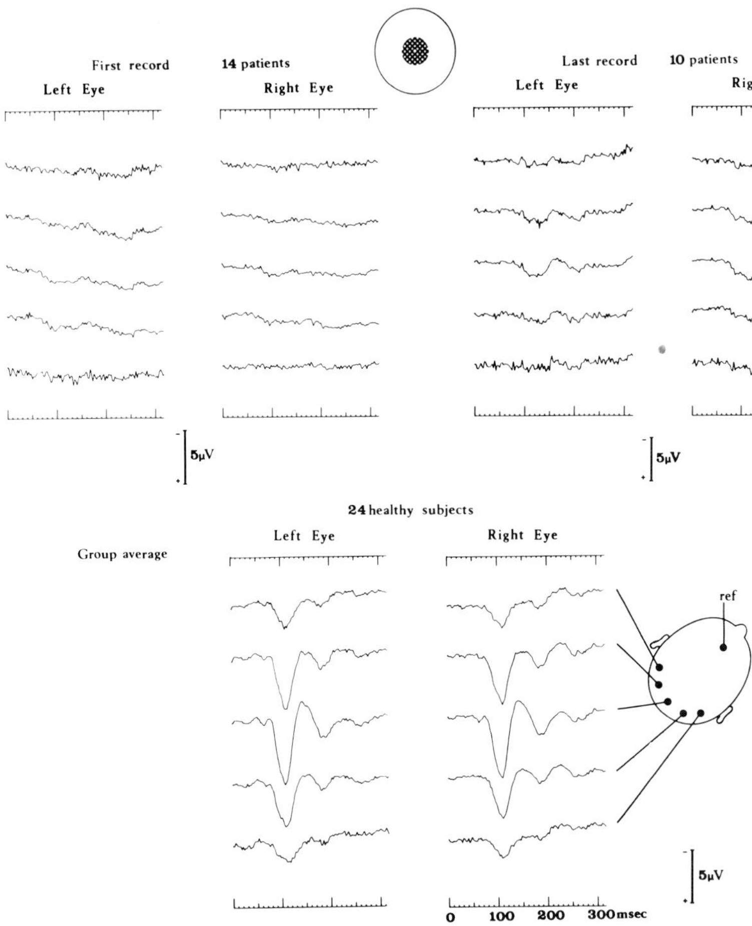

FIG. 4. Group average responses to stimulation of the central field (0–4° radius). Before treatment, patients' responses were grossly attenuated, and although, on follow-up, responses were larger, they were smaller than those of controls.

from either eye that averaged 7 μV at 106 msec. At the first recording, 11/28 (39%) of the patients' eyes' records gave P100s which, on average, measured 2.5 μV; 10/28 (36%) produced only PNP complexes, in which the N105 component had a mean amplitude of 1.5 μV; in 7/28 (25%), no response was identifiable. At the last recording, there was no increase in the incidence of P100s or in the number of records in which responses were identifiable, but on average, the P100 and N105 components were 2 μV larger.

Figure 5 illustrates the group average responses to flash stimulation. The responses from normals showed much intersubject variability in waveform, and the grand average appears as a broad postivity around 100 msec incorporating several subpeaks. In contrast, the responses from patients were remarkably consistent. In 12/15 (80%) of patients, the response comprised a bifid waveform with a positivity at about 70 msec (7 μV), a negativity at 98 msec (6 μV), and a positivity at 130 msec (6 μV). On follow-up, the bifid waveform is still evident. It has to be stated, however, that three (18%) of the controls had a bifid response similar to that seen in the patients.

There appeared to be only partial agreement between the morphology of pattern and flash waveforms when comparing individual patients. In 19/30 (63%) of the records for individual eyes, PNP waveforms were evident for both pattern and flash stimulation, and in 11/30 (36%), there was a discrepancy. The skin ERGs of the patients were within normal limits.

DISCUSSION

We have previously described (2) the effect of experimental "scotomata" of various sizes on the pattern reversal responses to half-field (0–16° radius) stimulation in healthy individuals and concluded that the P100 represented a response to central (macular) stimulation, whereas the PNP complex was associated with paramacular stimulation. On this basis, the findings from the present study suggest severe loss or dysfunction of fibers subserving central vision, and following treatment, in spite of improvement of acuity to normal levels, the pattern response only partially returns to normal. Where P100 was measurable before treatment, its average size following half-field stimulation was 2 μV, which corresponds to the average P100s obtained in normal individuals when scotomas between 4 and 6° radius are introduced into the half field. The VEP changes agreed well with the extent of the scotoma as determined by visual field testing.

The pattern of the evoked potential changes suggests that the pathological process in toxic optic neuropathy principally involves the papillomacular bundle. It is interesting to relate this inference to histological studies of optic neuropathy associated with B_{12} deficiency in the monkey (1,5). In this condition, there is a predisposition for the papillomacular bundle to degenerate in the anterior portion of the optic nerve. In the early stages of deprivation, myelin sheaths have a spongy appearance, and in long-term deficiency, there is demyelination

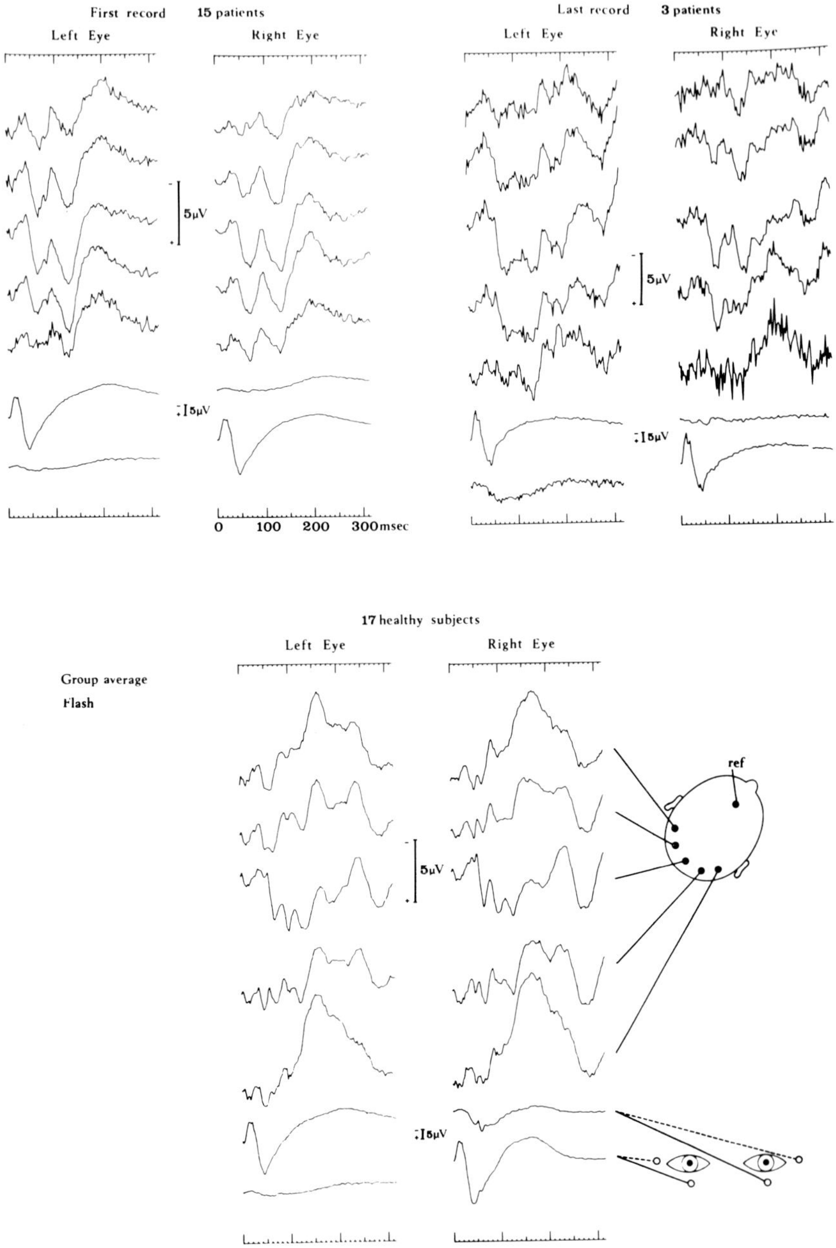

FIG. 5. Group average responses to flash stimulation. Note the simplified bifid (PNP) waveform of patients compared to the more complex waveform seen in normals.

and axonal degeneration. Treated monkeys show no evidence of repair in degenerated areas.

A bifid flash EP waveform similar to that seen in patients with toxic optic neuropathy is also seen in patients with hereditary optic atrophy and ischemic neuropathy (4). At present, however, it is not clear how closely this particular waveform change in the flash response is associated with the presence of a central scotoma.

The discrepancy between the ERG findings of the present study and those of Ikeda et al. (6) most probably reflects methodological differences, in particular the use of corneal rather than skin electrodes and the recording of low-intensity threshold values and of wavelets associated with red flicker.

ACKNOWLEDGMENTS

We would like to thank Professor Ian McDonald for allowing us to examine patients under his care and Keith Cunningham for computing assistance.

REFERENCES

1. Agamanolis, D. P., Chester, E. M., Victor, Y., Kark, J. A., Hines, J. D., and Harris, J. W. (1976): Neuropathology of experimental vitamin B_{12} deficiency in monkey. *Neurology (Minneap.),* 26:905–914.
2. Blumhardt, L. D., Barrett, G., Halliday, A. M., and Kriss, A. (1978): The effect of experimental 'scotomata' on the ipsilateral and contralateral responses to pattern-reversal in one half-field. *Electroencephalogr. Clin. Neurophysiol.,* 45:376–392.
3. Halliday, A. M., Barrett, G., Blumhardt, L. D., and Kriss, A. (1979): The macular and paramacular subcomponents of the pattern evoked response. In: *Human Evoked Potentials,* edited by D. Lehmann and E. Callaway, pp. 135–151. Plenum Press, New York.
4. Harding, G. F. A., Crews, S. J., and Good, P. A. (1980): VEP in neuro-ophthalmic disease. In: *Evoked Potentials,* edited by C. Barber, pp. 235–242. MTP Press, Lancaster.
5. Hind, V. M. D. (1972): The histology of Vitamin B_{12} deficiency optic neuropathy in monkeys. In: *The Optic Nerve,* edited by J. S. Cant, pp. 257–269. Henry Kimpton, London.
6. Ikeda, H., Tremain, K. E., and Sanders, M. D. (1978): Neurophysiological investigation in optic nerve disease: Combined assessment of the visual evoked response and electroretinogram. *Br. J. Ophthalmol.,* 62:227–239.
7. Potts, A. M. (1973): Tobacco amblyopia. *Surv. Ophthalmol.,* 17:313–339.

Clinical Applications of Evoked Potentials in Neurology,
edited by J. Courjon, F. Mauguiere, and M. Revol.
Raven Press, New York © 1982.

The Visual Evoked Potential in Hereditary Optic Atrophy

*G. F. A. Harding and **S. J. Crews

**The Clinical Neurophysiology Unit, Department of Ophthalmic Optics, University of Aston in Birmingham, Birmingham B4 7ET, England; and **Birmingham and Midland Eye Hospital, Birmingham 3, England*

Patients with hereditary optic atrophy may be divided into four groups: autosomal dominant hereditary optic atrophy; Leber's optic atrophy, which is thought to be X-sex linked (5,8,9); rare autosomal recessive hereditary optic atrophy (4); and Behr's recessive optic atrophy with central nervous system involvement (9). All these conditions are of obvious concern to the clinician, since difficulty in obtaining an accurate family history may lead to unnecessary neurological investigations. Equally, the current trend toward genetic counseling creates a need for early diagnosis of the condition so that parents may be informed of the potential sibling risk before the family group is complete. Patients with these conditions have been studied by many authors, and typical findings are summarized in Table 1.

In all these conditions, it has been reported that the electroretinogram (ERG) is normal (9), although Van Lith and Henkes (10) reported reduced photopic and scotopic ERGs in some patients with recessive inherited optic atrophy. The visual evoked potential (VEP) has, however, been found to be of some value in these conditions. Halliday (6) pointed out that patients with dense central field defects as seen in Leber's optic atrophy often showed a negative triphasic response with the peak of the negativity around 100 msec on pattern reversal stimulation. Delays in the major positive peak of the pattern reversal VEP from the affected eye have also been reported in this condition, although the abnormality was not present until the decrease in visual acuity was observed (8). Harding et al. (7) confirmed Halliday's suggestion of a marked negativity around 100 msec in patients with Leber's optic atrophy and indeed, in severely affected patients, found that the preceding and following positivities were absent, revealing an isolated negative component. In an electrophysiological study of some patients with hereditary optic atrophy, Van Lith and Henkes (10) found that patients with Behr's atrophy showed reduced ERG and VEP. Carroll and Mastaglia (1) showed a complete family with Leber's optic atrophy using the pattern reversal VEP. Fourteen members of the family were affected, and the

TABLE 1. *Symptoms and electrophysiological findings in the various types of hereditary optic atrophy*

Type	Inheritance	Onset	Symptoms	Optic	VA	Color	VEP
Autosomal dominant hereditary optic atrophy	Autosomal dominant	Insidious	Reduced vision around school age, variable expression	Temporal atrophy	6/9 to 1/60	Initial blue defect; later almost complete loss	Present study
Leber's optic atrophy	? X-linked	Acute, 10 to 30	Reduced vision, pain on eye movement	Initial disk edema, temporal or total atrophy	6/36 to 1/60	Red–green or severe	N100 response to flash; PNP to pattern
Congenital or infantile optic atrophy	Autosomal recessive (rare)	0 to 3	Severely reduced vision. Nystagmus	Total atrophy	6/60	Severe color defect	?
Behr's optic atrophy	Autosomal recessive	First 12 months	Reduced vision. Psychomotor retardation. Pyramidal tract signs	Temporal atrophy	6/18 to 6/60	Red–green or general	Reduced

remaining 40 were asymptomatic. In general, the clinical findings from the affected members correlated with the VEP which showed either absent or delayed responses. In some asymptomatic members of the family at risk, the VEP showed mildly delayed responses or a broadened, "bifid" P100.

If the VEP does show abnormalities in asymptomatic patients at risk, it might provide an early diagnostic sign that would be an attractive possibility for genetic counseling. A study of patients with dominant hereditary optic atrophy has commenced to compare the VEP to both flash and pattern reversal with the psychophysical clinical findings.

METHODS

Twenty-seven patients from six families with dominant hereditary optic atrophy, 17 of whom were affected, have been studied. Eleven members of one family were studied, and in two other families, eight and four members were investigated, respectively. In 23 of the 27 patients, all tests were completed on the same day, even though this involved a long series of tests for the patient.

Corrected visual acuity was assessed for both near and distance, but for the purpose of this analysis, if the distance vision was worse than 6/12, then the visual acuity was rated as abnormal.

The Goldmann Perimeter was initially used to record the visual fields. The scotomata were analyzed in terms of the reduction of cortical representation that would ensue, as suggested by Drasdo (2). Figure 1 shows the fields with a superimposed graticule of dots. Each dot represents an area in which a local scotoma would cause a loss of 1% of cortical and neural representation. If the loss was greater than 5%, then the fields were rated as abnormal. It will be seen that this method of scoring preferentially rates scotomata that are central, since these have greater cortical representation than those in the periphery (3). If the score from this method was within the normal range, further tests were performed using the Friedmann Visual Field Analyzer to provide more careful assessment of the central fields.

Color vision was assessed by the Farnsworth–Munsell 100-Hue test. The total error score was compared to the norms for the age, and any tritanopic tendency or defect was noted.

The VEPs were recorded from electrodes placed over the right and left occiputs and referred to the ipsilateral central electrode. Flash stimulation was given monocularly to each eye at an intensity of 1,363 candelas/m^2. A reversing checkerboard pattern, each check subtending a visual angle of 50′ of arc, was reversed at a rate of twice per second. The resulting VEPs were compared with normal age-matched controls, and the latency, amplitude, and symmetry rated as normal or abnormal. The presence of a negative response at 100 msec to either stimulus was particularly noted.

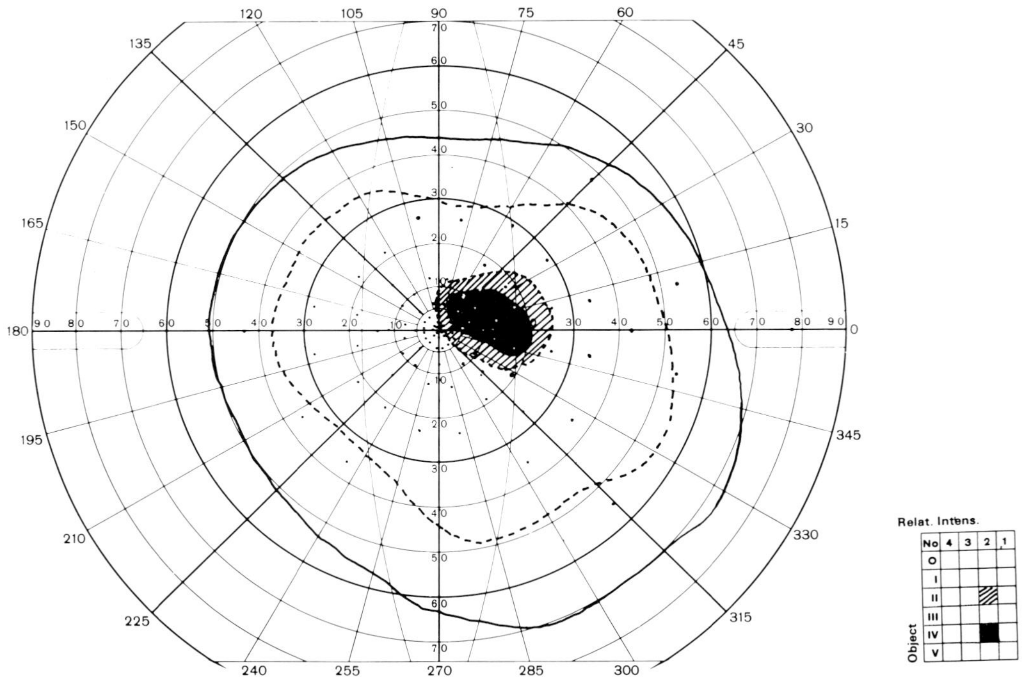

FIG. 1. The method of scoring field defects. Each dot represents a loss of 1% of neural representation. This method of scoring preferentially highlights central scotomata and is clearly the appropriate criterion for quantifying neural loss. The example given is one of the fields of an affected patient of Family W.

RESULTS

The findings of one family that we have investigated in detail are shown in Fig. 2. Affected members are shown with radial markers. Patients we have investigated are shown as enlarged symbols divided into quadrants. Abnormality of the Goldmann is shown solid in the right upper quadrant, visual acuity in the lower right, VEP in the lower left, and Farnsworth in the left upper quadrant.

The range of defects exhibited by affected members varies among individuals. It would appear that affected members over 30 years of age show all defects, whereas younger members may show a variety of defects affecting at most three of the visual acuity, field, F100, or VEP scores. This would support the suggestion of a slowly progressive condition. The VEP was abnormal in every affected patient in the entire series. The most common finding ($p < 0.01$) was a positive-negative-positive response (PNP) at about 100 msec to flash stimulation (Fig. 3). Although similar findings were sometimes seen in the pattern-reversal response, this was not significantly associated with optic atrophy, and a more common finding was a marked reduction in amplitude, particularly in patients with reduced visual acuity. Surprisingly, PNP responses to flash or pattern

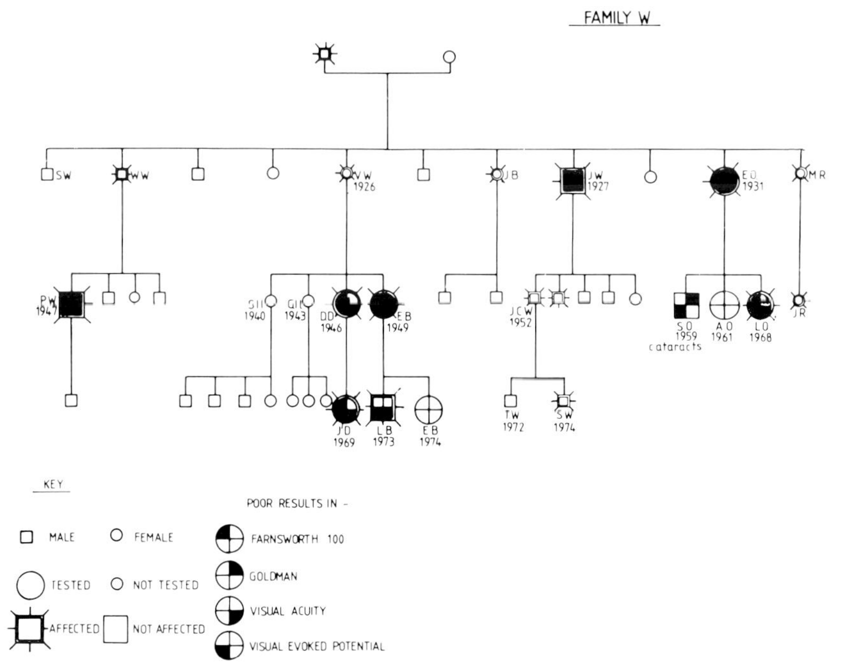

FIG. 2. Family W. The older patients show greater abnormalities, but individual variations are seen in the findings in younger affected members.

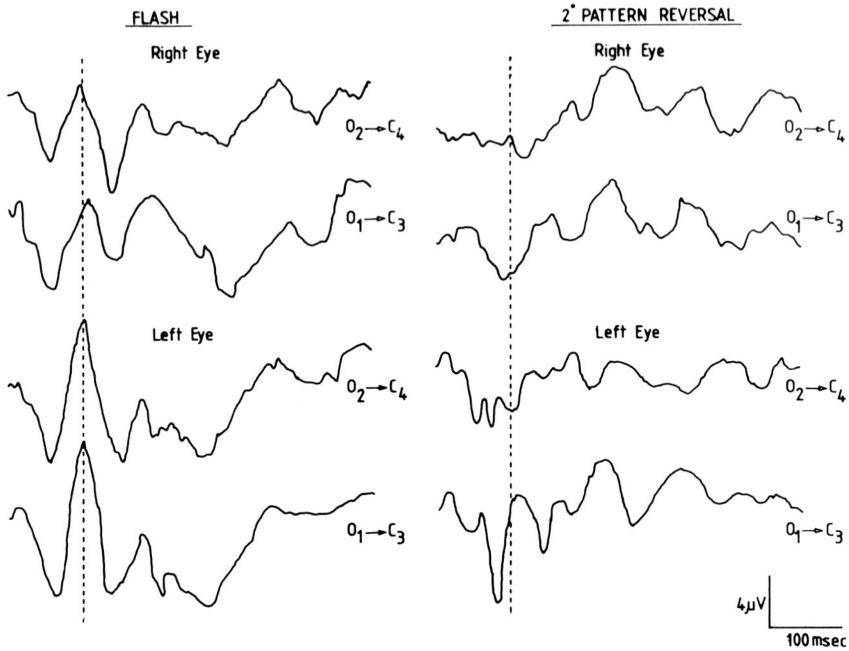

FIG. 3. Typical VEP in patients with hereditary optic atrophy of the dominant type. This patient had a normal ERG, a bilateral visual acuity of 6/36, and bilateral central scotomata. The response to flash stimulation of both the right and left eye is a classical PNP response with the negative component around 100 msec. The responses show a reduction in normal amplitude, and only the response from the left occiput on left eye stimulation shows any evidence of an N100 negativity. Polarity is negative upward.

reversal were not significantly associated with central field defects. It is difficult to know whether this peculiar triphasic PNP morphology is produced by a negative replacement of the P110 or by a marked delay in the P65, N83, and P110 components of the flash VEP.

One patient (J.Mc.) presented initially as a child with slightly reduced vision, constricted visual fields, reduced macular function on the Friedmann Visual Field Analyzer, and high Farnsworth error scores. The family history indicated a pattern of dominant hereditary optic atrophy, and indeed, when other members were investigated, they were shown to be suffering from this condition (Fig. 4). Her mother and siblings, however, did not show diagnostic signs.

On subsequent retesting, her Goldmann field, macular function, and Farnsworth score steadily improved to normal. Her VEP was consistently normal for the age and did not show a PNP response. Her two cousins were investigated. The 6-year-old child had an abnormal Farnsworth score but normal visual acuity, Goldmann Fields, and macular function. Her visual evoked potential to flash

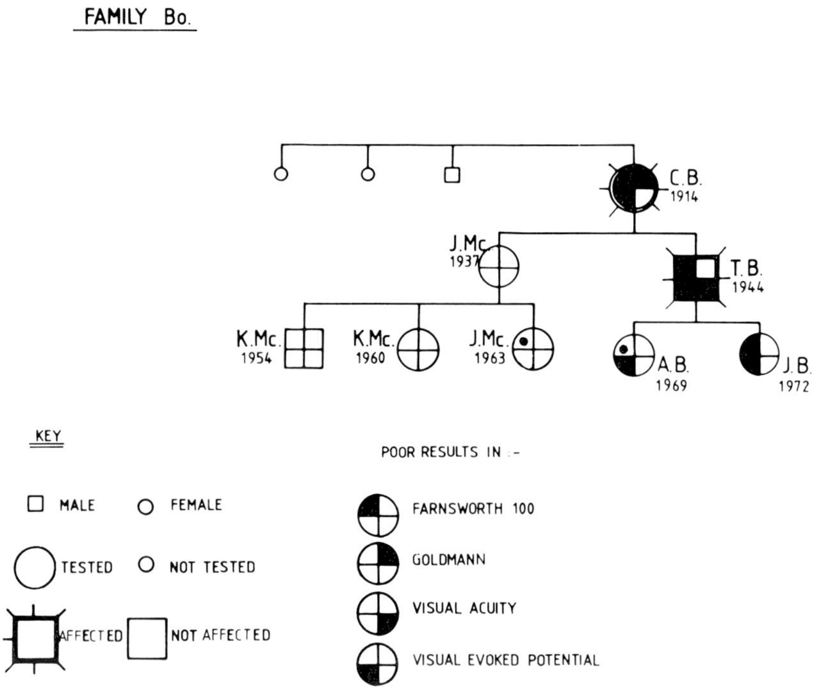

FIG. 4. Family Bo. Patient J.Mc. 1963 is the patient who presented with an initially abnormal Farnsworth–Munsell F100 Test, and since her grandmother showed evidence of hereditary optic atrophy, she and her family were thoroughly investigated. Her cousins (J.Bo. and A.Bo.) showed some abnormalities on electrophysiological and psychophysical testing.

stimulation was markedly delayed, although the pattern reversal response was within normal limits.

The elder child had a slight tritanopic defect, although her total error score on the Farnsworth–Munsell Test was within the normal range. Other tests revealed normal results except the VEP which showed marked delay to flash stimulation and a slight delay on pattern reversal (Fig. 5).

Table 2 shows a summary of the findings on the 27 patients. The families that we have studied are each collated under the family initial. It can be seen that, in general, the older the affected patient, the more defects are observed. However, in all affected patients, at least three of the results are abnormal. In certain of the unaffected patients, some of the results are abnormal, and in some cases, this is because of other ocular conditions.

In young children, the VEP proved a most useful objective diagnostic addition to psychophysical testing, since it did not require subject cooperation. In one child, the delayed VEP is the only definite abnormal finding, although the Farns-

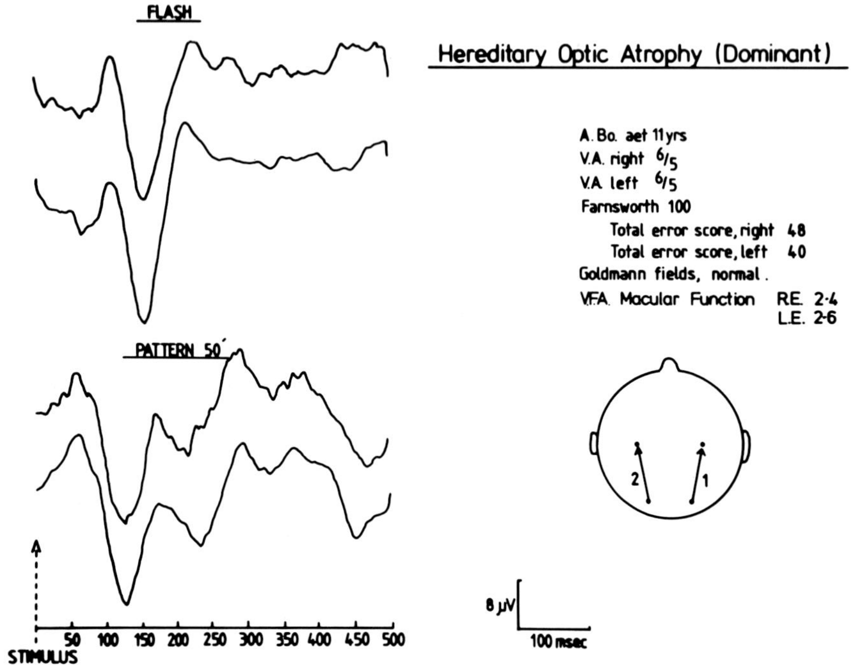

FIG. 5. Patient (A.Bo.) age 11 showed delayed flash and slightly delayed pattern responses. Polarity is negative upward. Her Farnsworth–Munsell Test revealed a slight tritanopia defect.

worth showed early tritanopic signs, and follow-up studies will be necessary to indicate the prognostic value of this finding.

The visual acuity, Farnsworth, flash VEP, and pattern-reversal VEP results are all significantly related to the presence of optic atrophy ($p < 0.01$). The abnormalities of the Goldmann Field Score were not significantly related. Further investigation using the Friedmann Visual Field Analyzer did not significantly change this finding. The visual acuity and Farnsworth scores are significantly interrelated ($p < 0.01$), an important differentiation with congenital tritanopia in which the visual acuity is not affected.

The flash VEP showed a PNP response in most of the affected patients, but unlike previous suggestions, this was not significantly associated with central field loss and cannot therefore be considered a scotomatous response. The VEP appears to offer a valuable diagnostic technique for early screening of members of the family with a view to genetic counseling.

TABLE 2. *Summary of the findings of 27 patients with dominant hereditary optic atrophy*

FAMILY	SEX	AGE	INITIALS	V.A	GOLDMANN	F 100	VEP flash	VEP pattern	OPTIC ATROPHY	COMMENTS
W										
	M	52	J.W.	X	X	X	X	X	+	
	F	44	E.O.	X	X	X	X	X	+	
	M	32	P.W.	X	X	X	X	X	+	
	F	18	A.O.							
	M	20	S.O.		X			X		CATARACTS
	F	10	L.O.	X		X	X	X	+	
	F	25	D.D.	X		X	X	X	+	
	F	34	E.B.	X	X	X	X	X	+	
	M	6	L.B.	X			X	X	+	LT CONVERGENT SQUINT
	F	4	E.B.							
	F	10	J.D.	X		X	X	X	+	
Be										
	M	60	D.B.	X	X	X	X	X	+	
	F	40	S.M.	X	X	X	X	X	+	
	F	10	J.M.				X		±	
	M	9	D.M.							
Bo										
	F	65	C.B.		X	/	X	X	+	
	M	35	T.B.	X		X		X	+	
	F	15	J.Mc		/	/				FUNCTIONAL
	M	14	Ke.Mc.	/				/		LT AMBLYOPIA
	F	12	Ka.Mc.							
	F	43	Jo.Mc.							
	F	11	A.Bo.				X	X		
	F	6	J.Bo.			X	X			
Sp										
	F	32	K.S.	X	X	X	X	X	+	
	F	37	P.B.	X	X	X	X	X	+	
F										
	F	55	F.F.	X	X	X	X	X	+	
Sh.										
	F	22	C.S.		X	X	X	X	+	

X Both eyes abnormal

\ One eye abnormal

ACKNOWLEDGMENTS

We are most grateful to Peter Good and Ann Davies for technical and secretarial assistance and to Dr. S. M. Pitts for her genetic studies.

REFERENCES

1. Carroll, W. M., and Mastaglia, S. L. (1979): Leber's optic neuropathy. A clinical and visual evoked potential study of affected asymptomatic members of a six generation family. *Brain,* 102:559–580.
2. Drasdo, N. (1977): The neural representation of visual space. *Nature,* 266:554–556.
3. Drasdo, N. (1980): Sampling system for visual field assessment and computerised perimetry. *Br. J. Ophthalmol.,* 64:705–712.
4. Francois, J. (1968): Hereditary degenerations of the optic nerve (hereditary optic atrophy) in genetic aspects of ophthalmology. In: *International Ophthalmology Clinics 8,* edited by D. M. Gordon, pp. 1016–1054. Little, Brown and Co., Boston.
5. Francois, J., Verriest, G., Francois, P., and Assessman, R. (1961): Etude comparative des dyschromatopsies acquises associees aux differents types d'atrophie optique heredo-familiale. *Ann. Oculist,* 194:217–235.
6. Halliday, A. M. (1976): Visually evoked responses in optic nerve disease. *Trans. Ophthalmol. Soc. U.K.,* 96:372–376.
7. Harding, G. F. A., Crews, S. J., and Good, P. (1979): The VEP as an aid in neuro-ophthalmic disease. In: *Evoked Potentials,* edited by C. Barber, pp. 235–241. MTP Press, Lancaster.
8. Nikoskelainen, E., Sogg, R. L., Rosenthal, A. R., Friberg, T. R., and Dorfman, L. J. (1977): The early phase in Leber's hereditary optic atrophy. *Arch. Ophthalmol.,* 95:969–978.
9. Smith, V. C., Pokorny, J., and Ernest, J. T. (1977): Primary hereditary optic atrophies. In: *Hereditary Retinal and Choroidal Diseases, Vol. 2,* edited by A. E. Krill, pp. 1109–1135. Harper & Row, New York.
10. Van Lith, G. H. M., and Henkes, H. E. (1969): Visually evoked cortical potentials and optic nerve disease. *Doc. Ophthalmol. Proc. Ser.,* 17:159–164.

Clinical Applications of Evoked Potentials in Neurology,
edited by J. Courjon, F. Mauguiere, and M. Revol.
Raven Press, New York © 1982.

The Visually Evoked Subcortical Potential to Flash Stimulation in Normal Subjects and Patients with Lesions of the Visual Pathway

G. F. A. Harding and M. P. Rubinstein

The Clinical Neurophysiology Unit, Department of Ophthalmic Optics, University of Aston in Birmingham, Birmingham B4 7ET, England

Although short-latency components of the visual evoked potential (VEP) are often described by early workers and can be seen in their records (2–4), they have received relatively little attention. Early workers used high-intensity flashes, and the later trend toward the use of structured stimuli without overall luminance change may well have contributed to this neglect. The early components of the VEP, that is, components before 50 msec latency, are poorly documented because of their minute amplitude, intersubject variability, and poor repeatability under the standardized experimental conditions used for eliciting the visual evoked cortical potential (VECP) (6).

The earliest specific description of short-latency VEP was that of Van Hasselt (10) who recorded a potential occurring at 10 msec latency of maximal amplitude around the ear and mastoid and only obtainable in 40% of subjects. Cracco and Cracco (5) described oscillatory potentials at around 100 Hz recorded from a wide distribution of scalp electrodes referred to the earlobes. The latencies were between 9 and 24 msec and of maximal amplitude in the midline and parasagittal locations.

In 1978, we carried out a pilot study on a small group of normal volunteer controls. By increasing the number of responses averaged to bright stroboscopic flashes and by multichannel recording from a variety of cephalic sites, we identified a small, less than 3-μV complex recorded by far-field techniques. This complex consisted of a positive wave at 22 msec, a negative wave at 27 msec, and a positive wave at 35 msec (8) and appeared to be located around the midtemporal region.

MATERIALS AND METHODS

Observations were made on 45 normal young university volunteers, 22 male and 23 female, mean age 23.1 years. All had visual acuities of 6/6 or better. The subjects were seated in a dimly lit room and flash stimulation delivered by a Grass PS22 photostimulator at 3,939 cd/m^2, that is, intensity 8, placed 25 cm from the eyes. A PDP8E computer was used to simultaneously average eight channels of responses to 500 stimuli which were usually presented at a rate of 6/sec, although slower presentations have been used. The band pass of the equipment was 66 to 700 Hz.

Cephalic reference sites revealed that sites anterior to the vertex were contaminated by flash-evoked ERG, and both the earlobe and mastoid were highly active at latencies around 20 to 40 msec. We found that the vertex electrode C_z was relatively inactive at early latencies. It is, of course, well known that the vertex site is highly active at later latencies. The vertex site has the added advantage of being approximately equidistant from a temporal chain of active recording sites. Since the anterior–posterior location of the source of the signal would be determined from this chain, and since the amplitude of the signal is partially proportional to the interelectrode distance, this constituted a major advantage in using the vertex reference. Electrode positions were determined according to the International 10–20 System, using additional half-distance electrodes. In the anterior–posterior study, half-distance electrodes were placed at $F_{8½}$ and $T_{4½}$. For the study of the transverse distribution, additional electrodes were placed at C_6, CP_4, and CP_6, that is, midway between the central and parietal positions, at $T_{4½}$ and $T_{8½}$.

RESULTS

The distribution of the visually evoked subcortical potentials (VESP) is shown in Fig. 1. The activity at the frontal pole is dominated by the electroretinogram (ERG) which is widely distributed, but which decreased in amplitude to a trough around the Rolandic–Sylvian fissure. At a point just behind the ear, at electrode $T_{4½}$, a triphasic wave is seen. The mean latencies of this wave are positive 20.61 ± 2.14, negative 26.22 ± 2.16, positive 33.80 ± 1.98 msec, and its mean amplitudes are positive to negative 1.32 ± 0.71, and negative to positive 2.33 ± 0.98 μV. It does not occur at similar latencies to any components of the VECP recorded at the occiput (O_z).

In the transverse direction, the amplitude of the VESP was maximal at sites below the temporal electrode chain and at a point level with but behind the pinna, that is, around the mastoid process at electrodes $T_{4½}$ and $T_{8½}$. This finding was irrespective of whether the vertex reference or a neck electrode reference site was used. This would indicate that interelectrode distance was not a confounding factor.

Since the photostimulator produces an audible click, control trials were performed both with the lamp occluded and with white noise delivered through earphones. When the lamp was occluded, similar potentials could not be recorded. When trials were performed with white noise delivered through earphones, a clear response to the photic stimulus was elicited.

Although the VESP is of a latency different from that of known myogenic

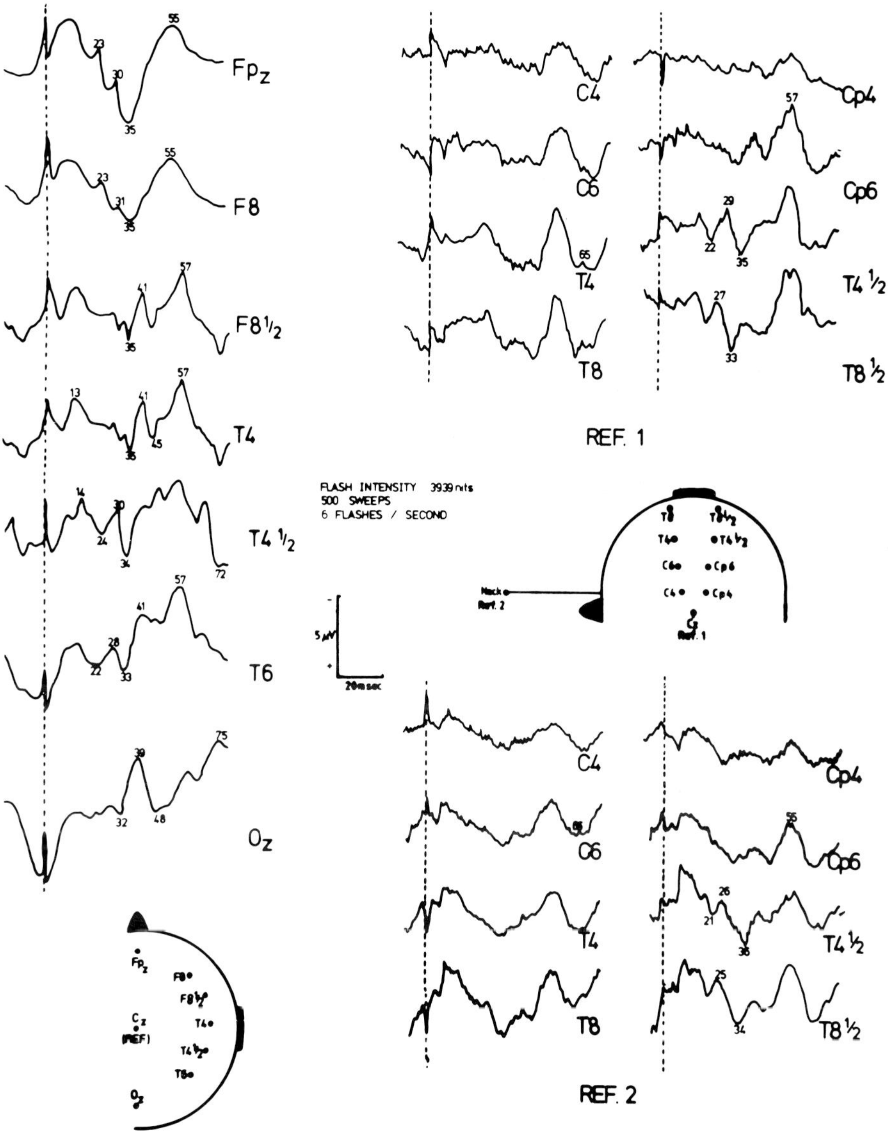

FIG. 1. Scalp topographical distribution of VESP. In the anterior–posterior direction, the ERG is shown to dominate frontal sites (FP_z, F_8), and the VECP at posterior site (O_z). At electrode $T_{4½}$ a trough develops, with triphasic complex P24–N30–P34 being generated independently of ERG or VECP. In the transverse direction, using either C_z or neck reference the VESP is shown to be of maximal amplitude around the upper mastoid area, at electrodes $T_{4½}$ and $T_{8½}$.

components, control trials were performed with subjects relaxed and also maintaining high muscular tension as monitored by the ongoing EEG. Neither of these actions altered the amplitude or latency of the VESP. The VESP was successfully recorded in 43 of the 45 subjects. Unlike auditory brainstem evoked potentials, there was no significant difference in latency between males and females. In 15 subjects, the trial–retrial repeatability was tested over a period of between 1 and 12 months. The mean variability in latency over time is relatively small, being 1.06 msec for the P20.6 wave, 1.64 msec for the N26.2 wave, and 1.43 msec for the P33.8 wave. The variation in amplitude is greater, although peak-to-peak measures of amplitude are more liable to variation, and variation in background noise will also affect the averaged amplitude and reduce its reliability.

RESULTS ON PATIENTS

Although we have only recently begun to use these techniques in patient investigations, it has been possible to study patients with lesions at various levels of the visual pathway.

Three patients with optic nerve lesions have been examined; for example, a patient presented with a fracture of the left orbit and zygoma following a fall. The visual acuity of the left eye was reduced to no light perception, and the optic disk was pale and atrophic. Electroretinograms were found to be of normal and equal amplitude in both eyes (Fig. 2). The VECP from the right eye was of normal latency and amplitude, as was the VESP. However, no VECP or VESP could be elicited on stimulation of the left eye. No significant abnormality was seen in the monitoring EEG to suggest cerebral damage. Similar results have also been seen in a case of optic nerve tumor and in macular trauma caused by a metallic intraocular foreign body.

Patients with bitemporal hemianopia arising from chiasmal compression would be expected to show a reduction in both the VESP and VECP contralateral to the eye stimulated by flash stimuli. A 66-year-old patient with bitemporal hemianopia presented for investigation. The CAT scan showed a large suprasellar cystic space-occupying lesion with expanded pituitary fossa and erosion of the floor and posterior clinoids. The VESP was reduced over the right cerebral hemisphere on left eye stimulation with flash. On right eye stimulation, the converse was observed, with reduction over the left hemisphere (Fig. 3).

We have compared the VESP to VECP responses obtained by pattern reversal of half the visual field using a 26′ checkerboard. When the left half field of the left eye was stimulated, no response was obtained. Stimulation of the nasal field, however, produced a clear response of higher amplitude over the left hemisphere. When the temporal half field of the right eye was stimulated, no cortical response was seen, whereas the nasal field produced a clear response. Similar results have been produced in one other patient we have studied with bitemporal hemianopia.

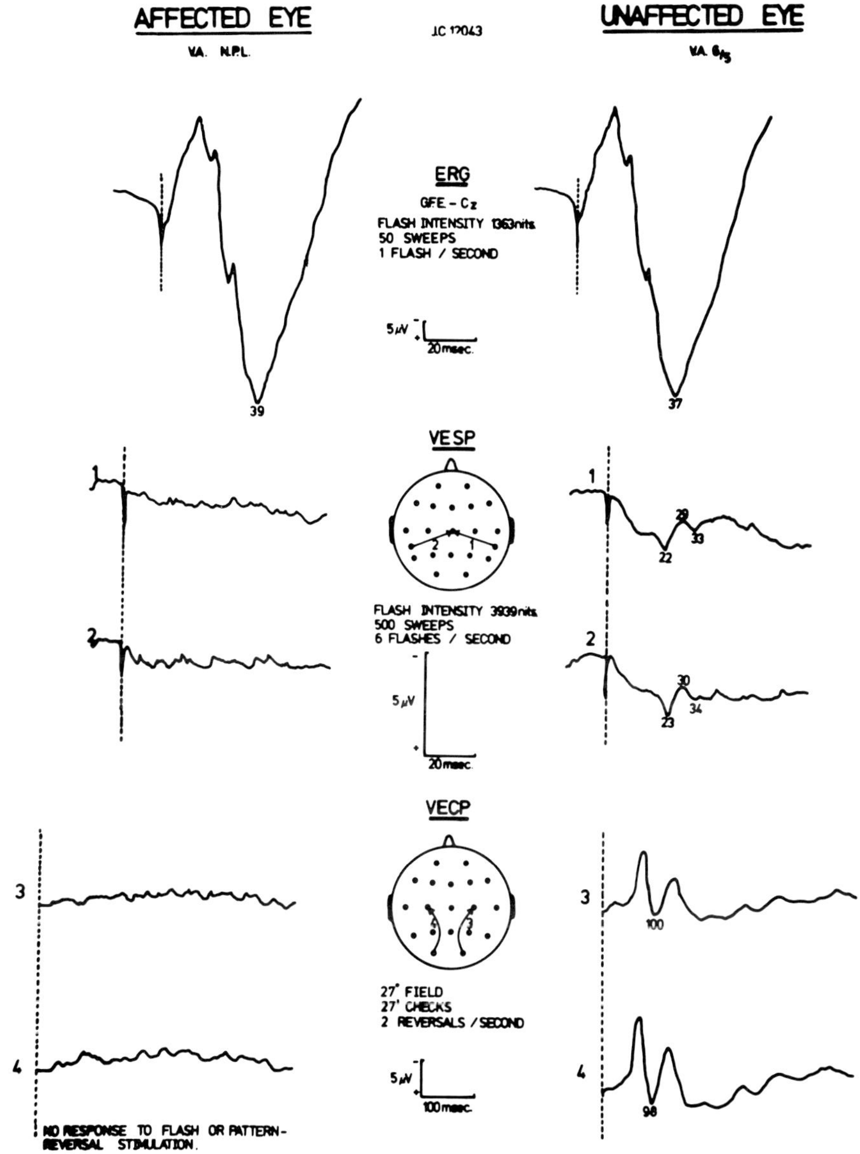

FIG. 2. Patient with left optic nerve trauma exhibiting bilaterally intact ERG (FP_1, FP_2). On stimulation of the affected eye, no VESP or VECP could be elicited, although stimulation of the unaffected eye showed normal VESP and VECP, thus contradicting the ERG origin of the VESP.

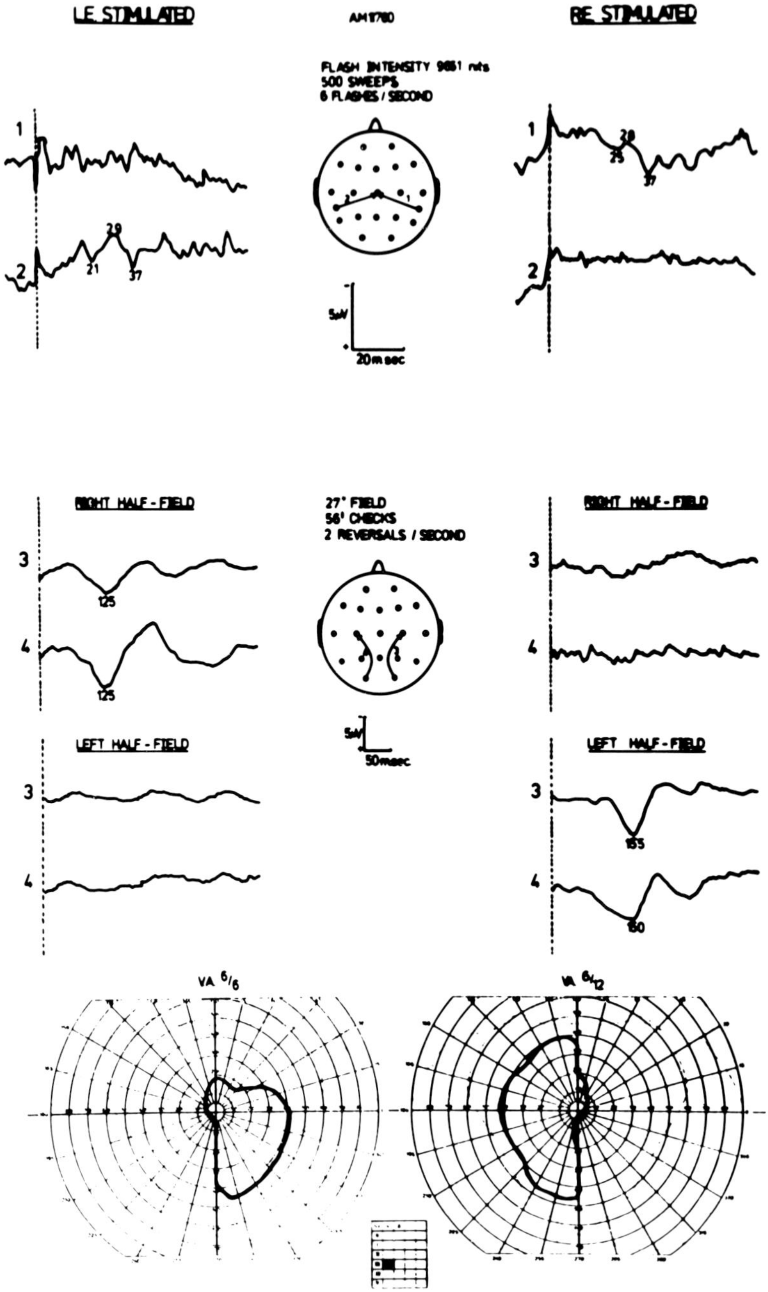

FIG. 3. Patient with pituitary adenoma and associated bitemporal hemianopia. The VESP technique on stimulation of the right eye showed a P25, N28, P37 complex on the right *(Channel 1)* but no response on the left *(Channel 2)*. On stimulation of the left eye, no response was seen on the right *(Channel 1)*, but a P21, N29, P37 complex was seen on the left *(Channel 2)*. Pattern reversal stimulation of the right half field shows no response, but a major positive at 150 to 155 msec was seen when the left half field was stimulated. Stimulation of the right half field of the left eye showed a major positive at 125 msec but no response on left half field stimulation.

In patients with a postchiasmal lesion, if the VESP does arise from a thalamic or postthalamic site, it should be reduced on the side of the head contralateral to the field defect. Six patients with such lesions have been studied. A recent patient presented with a right homonymous hemianopia following a vascular disturbance of the basilar and posterior cerebral arteries. The patient was fully conscious and was dysarthric. There was a clear right homonymous hemianopia, horizontal nystagmus on lateral gaze to either side, and a mild right-sided facial weakness. There was bilateral ataxia of all four limbs which was more evident on the right than the left; the tendon reflexes were brisk, and the plantars were flexor. A CAT scan showed global atrophy involving the left cerebral hemisphere and also the cerebellum. The visual fields are shown in Fig. 4 together with the VECP. Using flash stimulation and our standard montage, it can be

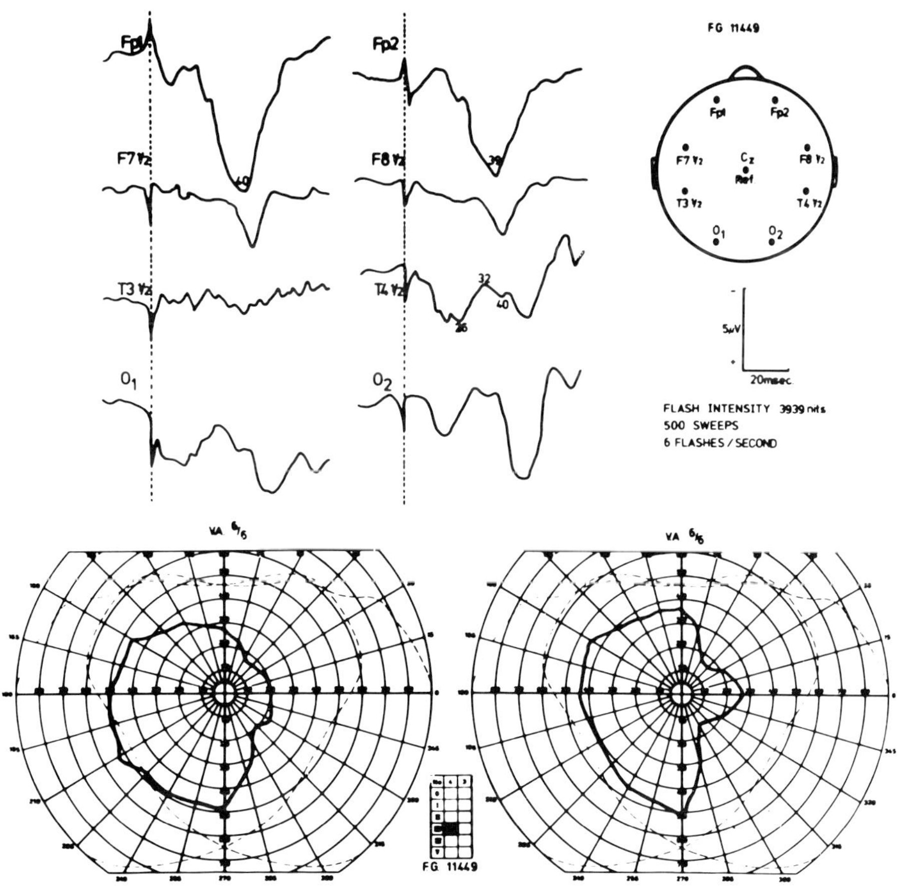

FIG. 4. Patient with brainstem vascular disturbance showing a clear VESP complex on the right ($T_{4½}$) at latencies P26, N32, P40 but which is absent on the left ($T_{3½}$). The visual fields show a well-defined right homonymous hemianopia with macular sparing.

seen that the VESP is reduced contralateral to the field defect. In the four other patients, similar findings were obtained, but one patient with a hemianopia caused by a recent cortical trauma showed preservation of the VESP coexisting with reduced flash VECP contralateral to the field defect.

Initial investigations have been carried out in six patients with unilateral retrobulbar neuritis. We have failed to show any significant increase in latency of the VESP, even though the VEP shows clear evidence of a delay of the P100 component when the affected eye is stimulated.

DISCUSSION

The visual evoked subcortical potential elicited under our standardized conditions appears to be a relatively stable phenomenon recorded in 96% of normal subjects. The potential is of low amplitude, but the confidence limits for test–retest reliability over months show remarkably little variation in latency, the P34 component only varying in latency by a mean of 1.43 msec.

The topographical distribution of the component indicates that it is maximal around the mastoid process, and indeed, it may constitute the explanation for some of the so-called early components of the visual evoked cortical potential where this site was used as an "inactive" reference (1,2,5,7,9).

Since the VESP as described in this chapter is unrelated to the amplitude of the ERG and its oscillatory potentials, it is unlikely that it arises from this source. The findings from normals and patients support the suggestion that the origin of the signal is postchiasmal and is not of visual cortex origin. The most likely explanation is that this potential arises from a thalamic or optic radiation site, and such an origin would be entirely consistent with all of our findings. It is possible that this technique may supplement the ERG and the VECP in ophthalmic electrodiagnosis of lesions of the visual pathway.

ACKNOWLEDGMENTS

We are grateful to Mr. Bernard Williams and Dr. Milne Anderson of the Midland Centre for Neurosurgery and Neurology for allowing us to study their patients.

REFERENCES

1. Allison, T., Matsumiya, Y., Goff, G. D., and Goff, W. R. (1977): The scalp topography of the human visual evoked potentials. *Electroencephalogr. Clin. Neurophysiol.*, 42:185–197.
2. Ciganek, L. (1961): The EEG response, (evoked potential) to light stimulus in man. *Electroencephalogr. Clin. Neurophysiol.*, 13:165–172.
3. Cobb, W. A., and Dawson, G. D. (1960): The latency and form in man of the occipital potentials evoked by bright flashes. *J. Physiol. (Lond.)*, 152:108–121.
4. Cobb, W. A., and Morton, H. B. (1952): The human retinogram in response to high intensity flashes. *Electroencephalogr. Clin. Neurophysiol.*, 4:547–556.

5. Cracco, R. Q., and Cracco, J. B. (1978): Visual evoked potentials in man: Early oscillatory potentials. *Electroencephalogr. Clin. Neurophysiol.*, 45:731–739.
6. Desmedt, J. E. (1977): *Visual Evoked Potentials in Man: New Developments.* Clarendon Press, Oxford.
7. Gastaut, H., Regis, H., Lyagoubi, S., Memo, T., and Simon, L. (1967): Comparison of the potentials recorded from the occipital, temporal and central regions of the human scalp, evoked by visual, auditory and somatosensory stimuli. *Electroencephalogr. Clin. Neurophysiol.*, 26:19–28.
8. Harding, G. F. A., and Rubinstein, M. P. (1980): Components of the visually evoked subcortical potential (VESP) to flash stimulation in man. In: *International Congress Series, Vol. 526, EEG and Clinical Neurophysiology,* edited by H. Lechner and A. Aranibar, pp. 464–474. Excerpta Medica, Amsterdam.
9. Kooi, K. A., and Bagchi, B. K. (1964): Observations on the early components of the visual evoked response and occipital rhythms. *Electroencephalogr. Clin. Neurophysiol.*, 17:638–643.
10. Van Hasselt, P. (1972): A short latency visual evoked potential recorded from the human mastoid process and auricle. *Electroencephalogr. Clin. Neurophysiol.*, 33:517–519.

Clinical Applications of Evoked Potentials in Neurology,
edited by J. Courjon, F. Mauguiere, and M. Revol.
Raven Press, New York © 1982.

Intracerebral and Scalp Fields Evoked by Hemiretinal Checkerboard Reversal, and Modeling of Their Dipole Generators

D. Lehmann, T. M. Darcey, and W. Skrandies

Department of Neurology, University Hospitals, 8091 Zurich, Switzerland

One of the reasons for the study of scalp topography of evoked and spontaneous EEG potentials (see 9) is to obtain information on the geometry of their generators, since the instantaneous distribution of voltages in and on the head is determined by the instantaneous distribution of its generators in the head (18). Several reports have dealt with the scalp topography of visual evoked potentials to pattern-reversal stimuli (e.g., 2,10–12,14–17). In the present chapter, we address the question of relating the scalp topography of checkerboard-reversal-evoked reponses to the generator process that produces it.

To study scalp response topography, we record average visually evoked potentials in the usual way. That is, we determine average stimulus-evoked voltages on each electrode as a function of time. We then replot these waveforms as equipotential contour maps, which show the landscape or distribution of voltages over the scalp. These maps are formed by laying out voltages on the head and drawing curves through points of the same voltage (equipotential lines). Figure 1 shows 45-channel contour maps of scalp responses to six different hemiretinal pattern-reversal stimuli (2/sec, 55′ checks). Seven maps are plotted for each stimulus, illustrating the dynamics of the distributions between 87 and 135 msec latency. Also shown are "relative field power" plots, which objectively indicate the overall level of scalp activity as a function of time, and which are used to determine the times at which this level is maximum (13). Considering the responses to upper and lower hemiretinal stimuli, it can be seen that the dominant occipitally positive component of the response around 100 msec latency peaks in the midline but more anteriorly and with shorter latency for upper than for lower hemiretinal stimulation. The dominant occipitally positive component of the left and right hemiretinal responses peaks over the hemisphere contralateral to the stimulated hemiretina for large (26°) targets but nearer the midline (ipsilateral in some subjects) for small (13°) targets. These features have been studied in detail and occur in almost all subjects (11,12).

Since the head acts as a volume conductor, it is reasonable to assume that

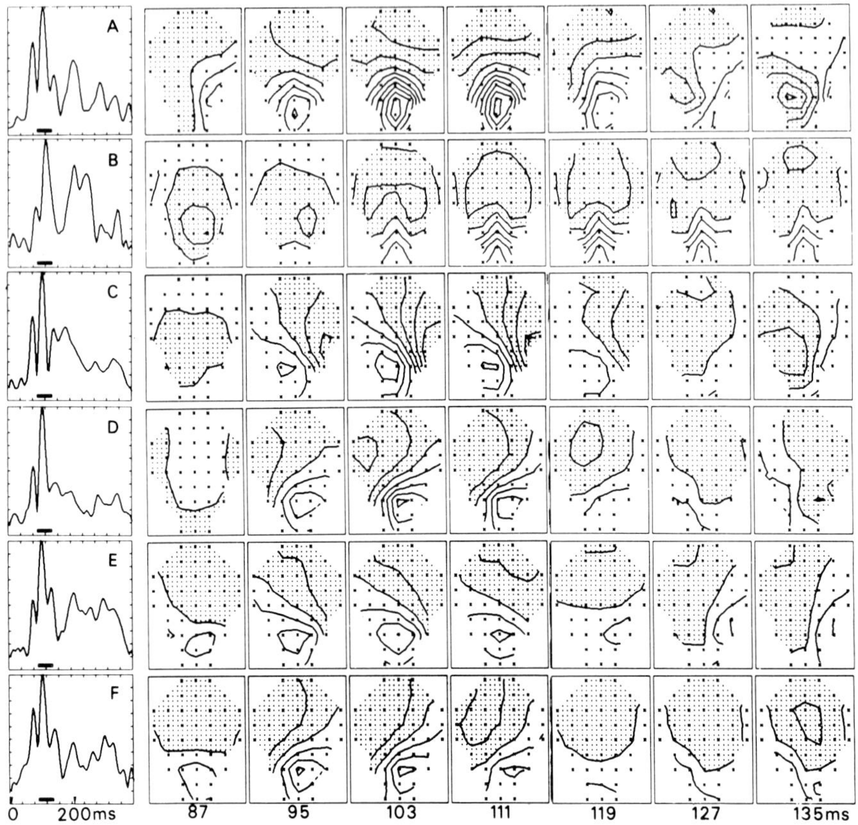

FIG. 1. Relative field power **(leftmost column)** as a function of time, and time series of equipotential contour maps of scalp fields evoked by checkerboard-reversal stimuli to **(A)** upper, **(B)** lower, **(C)** right, and **(D)** left hemiretinae using 26° targets, and **(E)** right and **(F)** left hemiretinae using 13° targets. Map series cover the times indicated by *bars* in the field power plots. Each map shows the scalp distribution at the indicated latency, head seen from above, nose up; *heavy dots* show the 45 electrode sites extending from 30% nasion–inion to 3 cm below inion; *stippled areas* indicate relative negativity; *contour lines* in 1 μV intervals.

such responses are generated in appropriate cortical areas but are conducted to the scalp as a field effect depending on the net orientation of the tissues producing them. We tested this notion by subjecting our data to a modeling procedure aimed at determining equivalent electrical generators of scalp potential data (3,4,7). Within a model head, we embedded simple generators of current. These are current dipoles, which are the first approximation to any given three-dimensional current source distribution. The approximation improves with increasing distance from the generator. Based on this model, a computer program was developed to determine equivalent sources of scalp data (3). This procedure finds the dipole or dipoles whose positions, orientations, and magnitudes generate fields that optimally fit the measured data in the least-squares sense, minimizing the squared difference between actual and model-generated data.

Figure 2 shows the results of this procedure when applied at the time of maximal response for the pattern-reversal data shown in Fig. 1. It can be seen that the best-fit dipoles are located fairly near the midline in the back of the head. For upper and lower hemiretinal stimulation, the dipoles are located in the midline and are oriented so that they point towards the occiput but more anteriorly for upper than for lower stimulation. For lateralized stimulation, the best-fit dipoles are located in the hemisphere ipsilateral to the stimulated hemiretina but are oriented so that their positive ends point toward the contralateral hemisphere. The results differ systematically for large (26°) and small (13°) targets, the dipoles being oriented more toward the midline (i.e., more radially directed when viewed from above) in the latter case. This example is representative of six subjects whom we have studied in detail (Darcey, Skrandies, and Lehmann, *in preparation*).

In carrying this work further, we had the opportunity to verify these results by measuring evoked potentials in the human brain directly. We have done this in two subjects, long-term epileptic patients in whom diagnostic stereotactic EEG examinations were performed. The positioning of electrodes was done for the diagnosis of the epilepsy and not for our evoked potential experiment. The patients volunteered on invitation to be subjects for evoked potential experiments, knowing that this was not expected to contribute to their diagnosis.

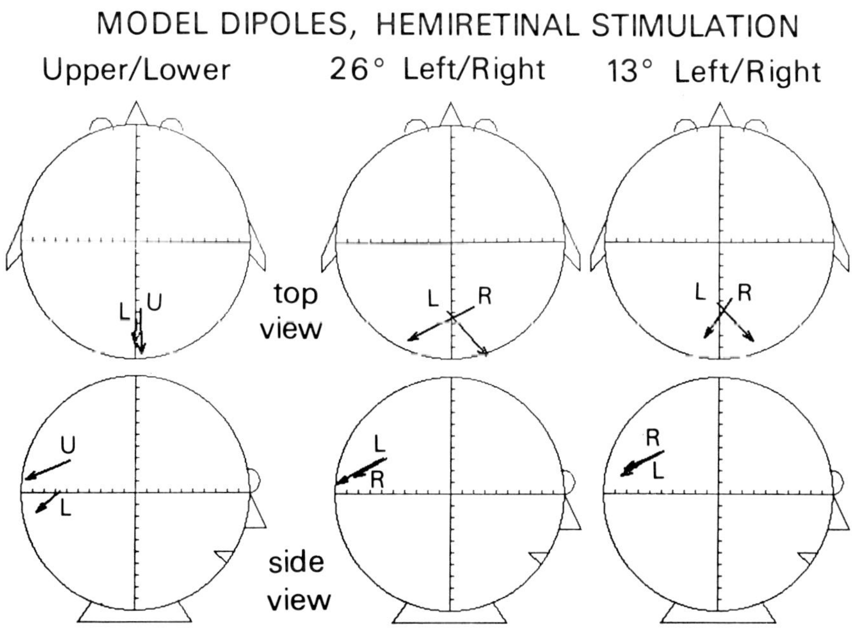

FIG. 2. Equivalent dipole model generators *(arrows)* computed for best fit at times of maximal relative field power of the fields of Fig. 1 in the six stimulus conditions. *Origins of arrows* give locations of dipoles; *lengths of arrows* indicate dipole magnitudes, *arrowheads* indicate positive side of dipoles.

We recorded visual evoked potentials in these patients from 48 locations simultaneously: in patient A, 28 intracerebral and 20 scalp; in patient B, 32 intracerebral and 16 scalp. The relationship of the electrodes to brain structures, including the calcarine fissure, was fairly well defined by the stereotactic procedure used (19). Both patients had normal and repeatable scalp responses to pattern reversal as shown in Figs. 3 and 4 for the major component (maximal field power) at approximately 100 msec latency. The intracerebral responses were repeatable, and their time behavior was highly correlated with that of the scalp responses.

We wished to compare scalp and intracerebral data in terms of their topography. Since a voltage distribution in three dimensions would be difficult to visualize, we decided to display the data in two dimensions by "cutting" the head in an imaginary way and plotting equipotential contour maps in profile for each slice. Figure 3 shows an example of such a "cut" in the right hemisphere parallel to the midline (parasagittal plane) and its contour maps for upper and lower hemiretinal stimulation of patient A at the same time as the corresponding scalp maps. It is obvious that the distributions are distinctly different for the two modes of stimulation. On the one hand, upper and lower hemiretinal stimulation evoke distributions that appear to be rotated with respect to each other by more than 90° about an axis near the middle of the calcarine fissure level, the position of which was established by the stereotactic procedure (see ref.

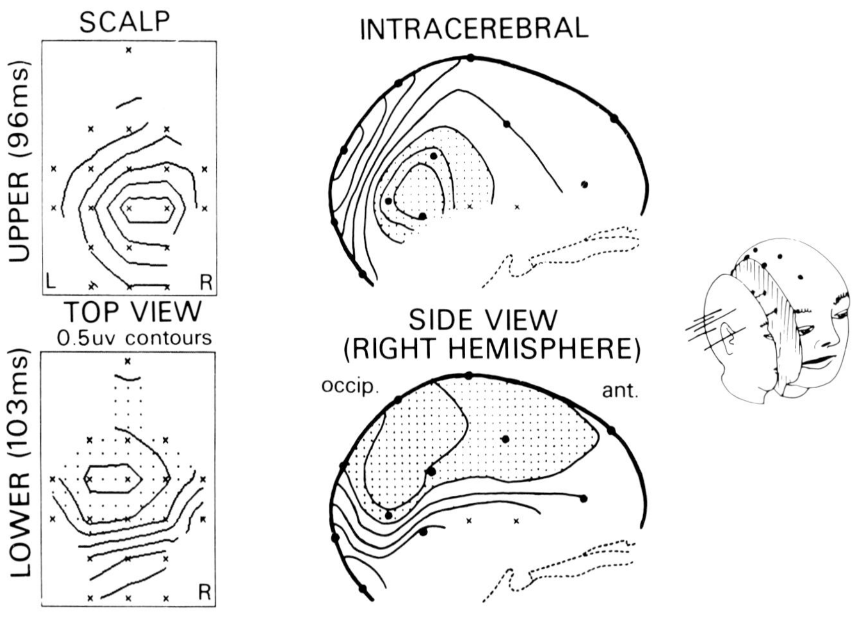

FIG. 3. Simultaneously recorded scalp and intracerebral field distributions evoked by upper and lower hemiretinal stimuli at times of maximal field power in patient A. Same plotting conventions as in Fig. 1. Intracerebral electrode sites marked by *dots;* intracerebral plane vertical, 3 cm parasagittally as shown in inset.

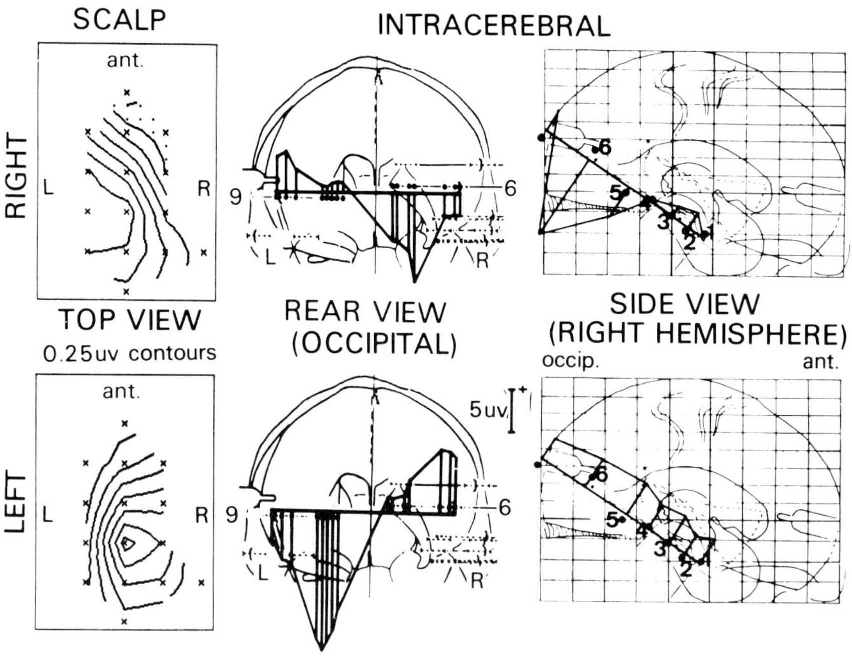

FIG. 4. Simultaneously recorded scalp field distributions and intracerebral voltage profiles evoked by right and left hemiretinal stimuli at times of maximal field power around 100 msec in patient B. **Top view** shows scalp field. Intracerebral electrodes are marked by *dots* and numbers. **Rear view** shows instantaneous voltage profiles along electrodes 6 and 9 (posterior right to left, slightly above the calcarine fissure), relative negativity down. Note polarity reversal between conditions. **Side view** shows profiles from scalp to electrode 2 in a plane 3 cm parasagittally.

19, p. 211) to be situated slightly above the most posterior intracerebral electrode. The maps also differ in the region where the highest potential gradients are, i.e., where current densities are highest. In the upper hemiretinal map, this region is above, and in the lower hemiretinal map below, the level of the calcarine fissure. Similar results were seen in different "cuts" and also at times shortly before and after the time shown.

Figure 4 shows, in rear view, transverse voltage profiles in patient B as determined from 17 locations for large-target (26°) left and right hemiretinal stimulation. The voltage distributions are fairly symmetrical, ipsilaterally negative and contralaterally positive. A surface-positive generator near the midline in the ipsilateral hemisphere but directed toward the contralateral hemisphere could give such voltage distributions (8). In addition, Fig. 4 shows, in lateral view, voltage profiles as approximated from one scalp and six intracerebral electrodes, these electrodes all being in the right hemisphere. A relatively flat voltage distribution arises from left hemiretinal stimulation, and a sharp occipitally negative distribution results from right hemiretinal stimulation.

These data strongly support the concept of an occipital generator process for the dominant occipitally positive components of the responses to pattern reversal. This process appears to consist of closely spaced surface-positive generators near the midline, and it is ipsilateral for lateralized hemiretinal stimulation (see Fig. 2). Although the locations of these generators tend to be near to each other, their net orientations vary greatly with stimulus locus. These orientations and positions might be compatible with extrastriate visual cortical origins such as those illustrated in Fig. 5. Related models based on scalp data were proposed earlier (1,6). The net field and model dipole behaviors conform reasonably well to the geometry of the suggested extrastriate generator areas if one assumes a normal dipole layer model of active cortex and cancellation of responses from closely spaced opposed surfaces (3,5). We have also considered the striate area as an alternative model generator, but we have tentatively rejected it because it fails to account for our results with upper/lower hemiretinal stimuli. The striate model with surface-positive activation predicts fields that peak over more posterior areas for upper than for lower hemiretinal stimuli, contrary to the data. Both the striate and extrastriate model correctly predict the "wrong hemisphere" peak for right/left stimuli. Both models also predict a peak location closer to the midline for smaller right/left targets (i.e., more radially directed fields), since small targets activate a proportionally larger portion of tissue on the occipital pole. Our results also support the belief that visually evoked reponses

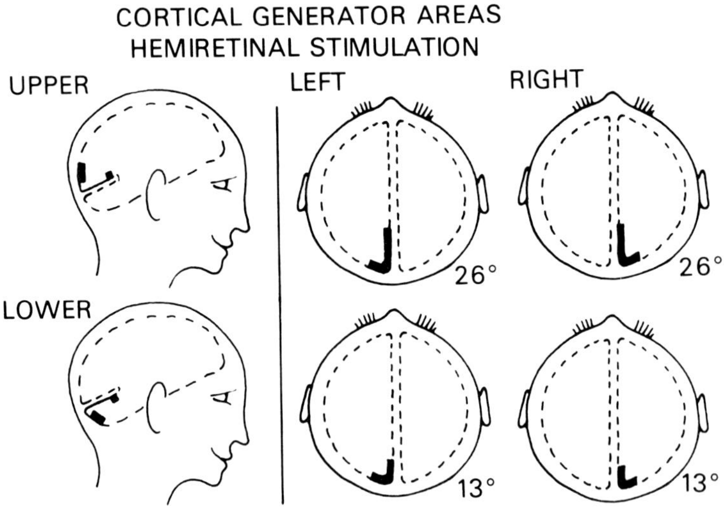

FIG. 5. Schematic illustration of the geometry of the extrastriate visual cortical areas *(darkened)* which are the hypothesized generator areas activated by the various hemiretinal stimuli, as a most plausible model to account for the data. *Lines* between darkened cortex in side views indicate striate areas which are less likely generators (see text). Side views are slightly parasagittal cross sections. Top views are cross sections slightly above (or below) calcarine fissure.

are generated at some depth in the brain and that their electrical effects propagate elsewhere in the brain and to the scalp via volume conduction.

ACKNOWLEDGMENT

This research was supported in part by grants from the Swiss National Science Foundation, EMDO, Hartmann-Mueller Foundation, and the Swiss Fund for the Treatment and Prevention of Blindness. We wish to thank Dr. H. G. Wieser for the patients with depth electrodes and Mr. H. P. Meles and Mr. A. Kaeppeli for technical assistance.

REFERENCES

1. Barrett, G., Blumhardt, L., Halliday, A. M., Halliday, E., and Kriss, A. (1976): A paradox in the lateralisation of the visual evoked response. *Nature,* 261:253–255.
2. Blumhardt, L. D., and Halliday, A. M. (1979): Hemisphere contributions to the composition of the pattern-evoked potential waveform. *Exp. Brain Res.,* 36:53–69.
3. Darcey, T. M. (1979): *Methods for Localization of Electrical Sources in the Human Brain and Applications to the Visual System.* Ph.D. Dissertation, California Institute of Technology, Pasadena (University Microfilms Order No. 7920351).
4. Darcey, T. M., Ary, J. P., and Fender, D. H. (1980): Methods for the localization of electrical sources in the human brain. *Prog. Brain Res.,* 54:128–134.
5. Freeman. W. J. (1975): *Mass Action of the Nervous System.* Academic Press, New York.
6. Jeffreys, D. A., and Axford, J. G. (1972): Source locations of pattern specific components of human visual evoked potentials. I. Component of striate cortical origin. *Exp. Brain Res.,* 16:1–21.
7. Kavanagh, R. N., Darcey, T. M., Lehmann, D., and Fender, D. H. (1978): Evaluation of methods for three-dimensional localization of electrical sources in the human brain. *IEEE Trans. Biomed. Eng.,* 25:421–429.
8. Klee, M., and Rall, W. (1977): Computed potentials of cortically arranged populations of neurons. *J. Neurophysiol.,* 403:647–666.
9. Lehmann, D. (1972): Human scalp EEG fields: Evoked, alpha, sleep and spike-wave patterns. In: *Synchronization of EEG Activity in Epilepsies,* edited by H. Petsche and M. A. B. Brazier, pp. 307–326. Springer, Berlin.
10. Lehmann, D., Meles, H. P., and Mir, Z. (1977): Average multichannel EEG potential fields evoked from upper and lower hemi-retinae: Latency differences. *Electroencephalogr. Clin. Neurophysiol.,* 43:725–731.
11. Lehmann, D., and Skrandies, W. (1979): Multichannel evoked potential fields show different properties of human upper and lower hemiretinal systems. *Exp. Brain Res.,* 35:151 159.
12. Lehmann, D., and Skrandies, W. (1979): Multichannel mapping of spatial distributions of scalp potential fields evoked by checkerboard reversal to different retinal areas. In: *Human Evoked Potentials: Applications and Problems,* edited by D. Lehmann and E. Callaway, pp. 201–214. Plenum Press, London.
13. Lehmann, D., and Skrandies, W. (1980): Reference-free identification of components of checkerboard-evoked multichannel potential fields. *Electroencephalogr. Clin. Neurophysiol.,* 48:609–621.
14. Lesevre, N., and Joseph, J. P. (1979): Modification of the pattern-evoked potential (PEP) in relation to the stimulated part of the visual field. *Electroencephalogr. Clin. Neurophysiol.,* 47:183–203.
15. Michael, W. F., and Halliday, A. M. (1971): Differences between the occipital distribution of upper and lower field pattern-evoked responses in man. *Brain Res.,* 32:311–324.
16. Ragot, R. A., and Rémond, A. (1978): EEG field mapping. *Electroencephalogr. Clin. Neurophysiol.,* 45:417–421.

17. Shagass, C., Amadeo, M., and Roemer, R. A. (1976): Spatial distribution of potentials evoked by half-field pattern-reversal and pattern-onset stimuli. *Electroencephalogr. Clin. Neurophysiol.*, 41:609–622.
18. Shaw, C., and Roth, M. (1955): Potential distribution analysis. II: A theoretical consideration of its significance in terms of electrical field theory. *Electroencephalogr. Clin. Neurophysiol.*, 7:285–292.
19. Talairach, J., and Szikla, G. (1967): *Atlas of Stereotaxic Anatomy of the Telencephalon.* Masson, Paris.

Clinical Applications of Evoked Potentials in Neurology,
edited by J. Courjon, F. Mauguière, and M. Revol.
Raven Press, New York © 1982.

The Pattern-Reversal Visual Evoked Potential in the Clinical Study of Lesions of the Optic Chiasm and Visual Pathway

L. M. Camacho, W. Wenzel, and J. C. Aschoff

Department of Neurology, University of Ulm, Ulm, West Germany

Increasing technological advances in averaging techniques and development of appropriate visual stimuli give a better understanding of the visual system in relation to clinical symptoms.

The introduction of contrast stimulation (1) together with observations by different investigators allows an early detection of lesions of the optic nerve (2,12), optic chiasm (3,18,19), and visual pathway (23,24). Diseases that tend to involve the visual system (i.e., glaucoma, pernicious anemia, migraine) can be studied by VEP according to recent publications (6,17,22).

The general approach of our study was to correlate clinical findings with results of VEP in a group of patients with different lesions of the visual system (as revealed by CT, angiography, or surgery).

MATERIAL AND METHODS

Three groups of subjects were tested. Group I (control) consisted of 23 volunteer students and members of our clinical staff. The ages ranged from 19 to 58 years, 16 males and 17 females. Group II included patients with chiasmal lesions (N = 9), four males and five females. Group III consisted of patients with parieto–occipital lesions (N = 9), four males and five females.

All 3 groups were checked for visual symptoms, fundoscopy, visual acuity, and visual field defects. Cerebral angiography and CT were performed on groups II and III. Some patients were followed up during surgery.

The averaged VEPs were recorded by midline leads, 5 cm above the inion and vertex, using silver/silver chloride electrodes with the ground electrode placed at the right mastoid. The electrode impedance was maintained under 1 kΩ over the entire study. The patient looked at the center of the commercial television checkerboard pattern from a distance of 1.3 m. The entire screen subtended a visual angle of 22°, and each square 58′.

Responses to 128 reversals were averaged on line with a Nicolet CA-1117 averager. A bandpass width of HF 1.6 Hz to LF 3.2 kHz was used. Mono and binocular stimulation of the half and full visual fields were done with a pattern-reversal frequency of 2 Hz. Analysis times were 200 and 250 msec.

The latencies of responses were determined at the first point of maximal negativity ($N_{\overline{70}}$) and positivity ($P_{\overline{98}}$) after the pattern reversal. The median values and 95% confidence interval were calculated for statistical analysis.

RESULTS

Control Group

In Table 1 we have summarized the values of the major negativity ($N_{\overline{70}}$) and positivity ($P_{\overline{98}}$) as well as the median amplitudes.

While stimulating the temporal half fields, we observed somewhat faster latencies than when stimulating nasal half fields. However, this was not statistically significant.

Chiasmal Lesions

We studied nine patients, seven of whom complained of visual symptoms. Only two had an abnormal fundoscopy (pallor and atrophy of the optic nerve). Five had diminished visual acuity together with bitemporal hemianopia. The pattern-reversal responses (see Table 2) were abnormal in eight patients. In general, they had prolonged latencies and small amplitudes. This phenomenon was enhanced by selective monocular stimulation of the temporal half fields but could also be elicited by stimulating the nasal half fields in some cases. In each of these cases, the nerve compression was verified at surgery.

Figure 1 shows the results in a 54-year-old patient. She was admitted because of headaches; she had no history of visual symptoms, no abnormalities in the visual fields. The CT showed an intrasuprasellar mass (suspected craniopharyngioma). Abnormal responses as described above were registered with VEP (note the abnormal nasal half-field response).

Parieto–Occipital Lesions

All cases ($N = 9$) complained of visual symptoms. Visual acuity was slightly diminished in only two patients. Perimetry revealed a homonymous hemianopia in seven. The VEP results are summarized in Table 3. The characteristic abnormalities were prolonged latencies and small amplitudes ($N = 4$) or absent responses ($N = 4$) by stimulation of the half fields opposite to the location of the lesion.

Figures 2 and 3 are illustrative examples. The first example (Fig. 2a) is a 55-year-old female with a left homonymous quadrantanopia and papilloedema. A cystic parieto–occipital astrocytoma of the right hemisphere was found (note the abnormal responses by left half-field stimulation). The malignant astrocytoma

TABLE 1. *Normal controls: latencies and amplitudes (median values with 95% confidence interval)*

	Monocular						Binocular		
	Full-field		Temporal		Nasal				
	Right eye	Left eye	Right eye	Left eye	Right eye	Left eye	full field	Right field	Left field
$N_{\overline{70}}$ (msec)	−68 < 71 < +73	−68 < 73 < +76	−63 < 65 < +72	−63 < 70 < +77	−67 < 73 < +75	−67 < 72 < +74	−65 < 68 < +75	−63 < 67 < +70	−64 < 68 < +72
$P_{\overline{98}}$ (msec)	−96 < 98 < +100	−95 < 101 < −102	−90 < 94 < +99	−93 < 95 < +100	−96 < 98 < +100	−98 < 100 < +103	−97 < 99 < +102	−91 < 96.5 < +99	−94 < 97.5 < +100
Amplitude (μV)	−6.3 < 9.7 < +12	−6.3 < 9.65 < +10.8	−4.6 < 6.1 < +6.5	−3 < 5.6 < +6.5	−3.8 < 4.9 < +6.2	−3.7 < 5.2 < +6.3	−11 < 12.5 < +14	−5 < 7.4 < +9.7	−5.8 < 7.1 < +8.6

TABLE 2. *Median latencies and amplitudes in patients with chiasmal lesions*

	Monocular			Binocular	
	Full field	Temporal	Nasal	Full field	Right/left
$N_{\overline{70}}$ (msec)	−78 < 85 < +87	−77 < 88 < +93	−80 < 83 < +91	−72 < 77 < +86	−74 < 87 < +101
$P_{\overline{98}}$ (msec)	−104 < 110 < +113	−103 < 118 < +148	−104 < 109 < +113	−97 < 107 < +116	−97 < 109 < +112
Amplitude (μV)	−3.0 < 3.9 < 4.4	−0.9 < 3.0 < +3.5	−2.7 < 3.8 < 4.2	−1.3 < 7.0 < +8.2	−2.0 < 3.6 < +5.6

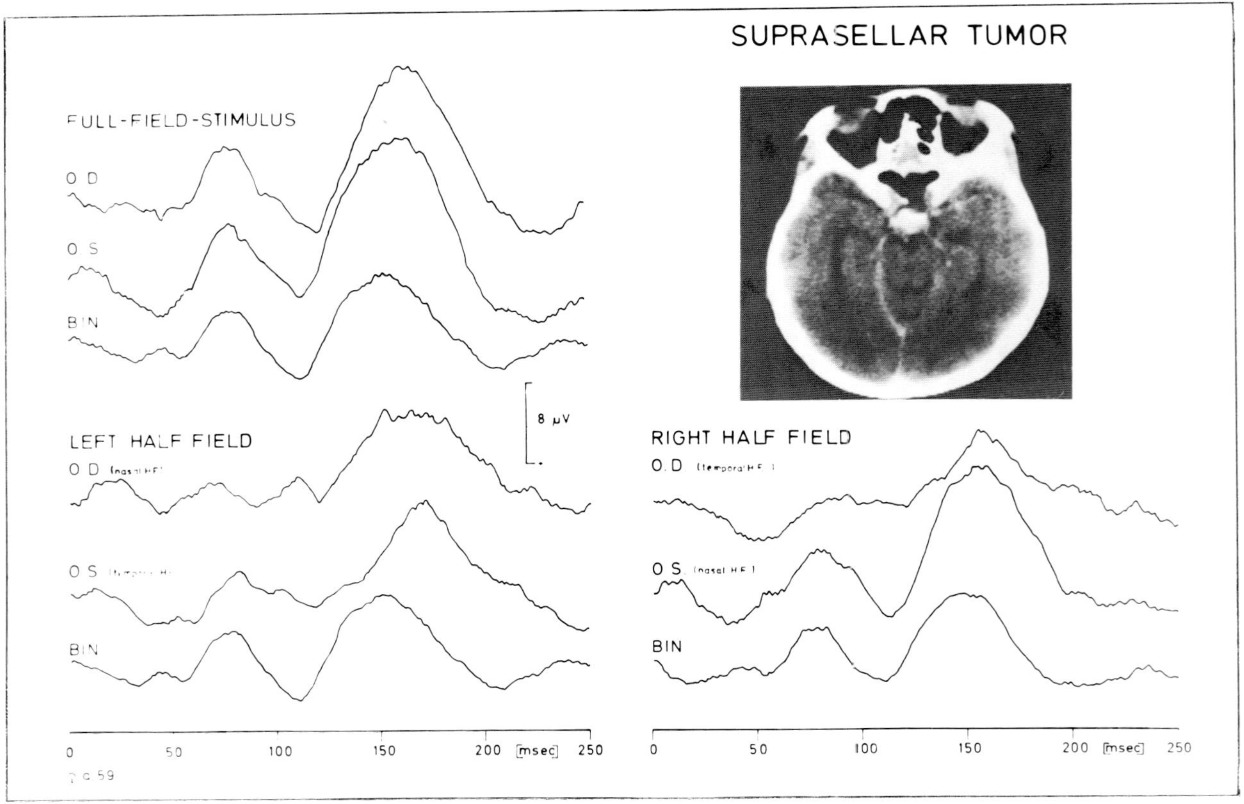

FIG. 1. Chiasmal lesion.

TABLE 3. *Median latencies and amplitudes in patients with parieto–occipital lesions*

	Monocular			Binocular		
	Full field	Contralateral[a] half field	Ipsilateral half field	Full field	Contralateral[a] half field	Ipsilateral half field
$N_{\overline{70}}$ (msec)	$-72 < 77 < +83$	$-72 < 81 < +89$	$-74 < 76 < +81$	$-60 < 74 < +76$	$-75 < 77 < +82$	$-65 < 77 < +80$
$P_{\overline{98}}$ (msec)	$-98 < 104 < +113$	$-96 < 108 < +112$	$-100 < 101 < +110$	$-91 < 106 < +109$	$-98 < 104 < +107$	$-95 < 102 < +108$
Amplitude (μV)	$-1.4 < 8.2 < +11.1$	$-1.3 < 4.7 < +6.0$	$-2.0 < 3.8 < +6.0$	$-4.1 < 9.1 < +10.8$	$-2.0 < 5.2 < +5.9$	$-2.1 < 6.1 < +9.5$

[a] Contralateral half field is the visual field opposite the location of the lesion.

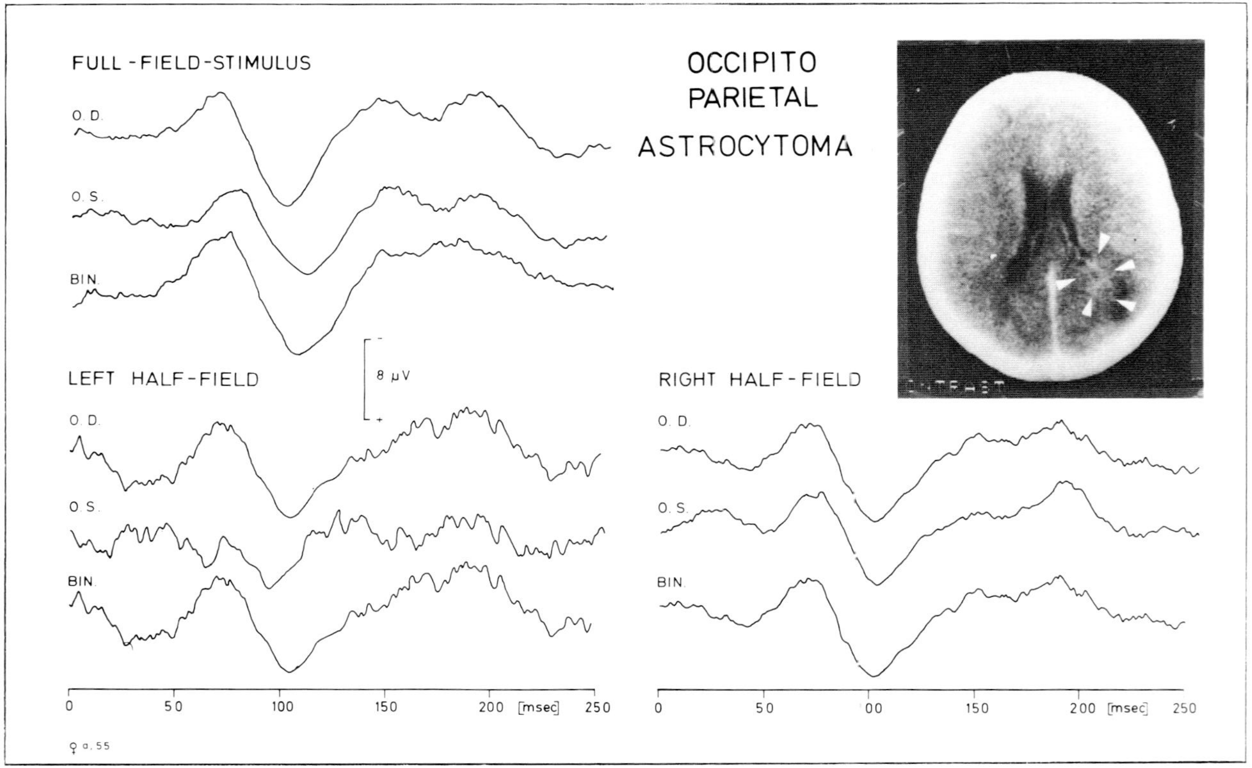

FIG. 2a. Parieto-occipital lesion preoperatory.

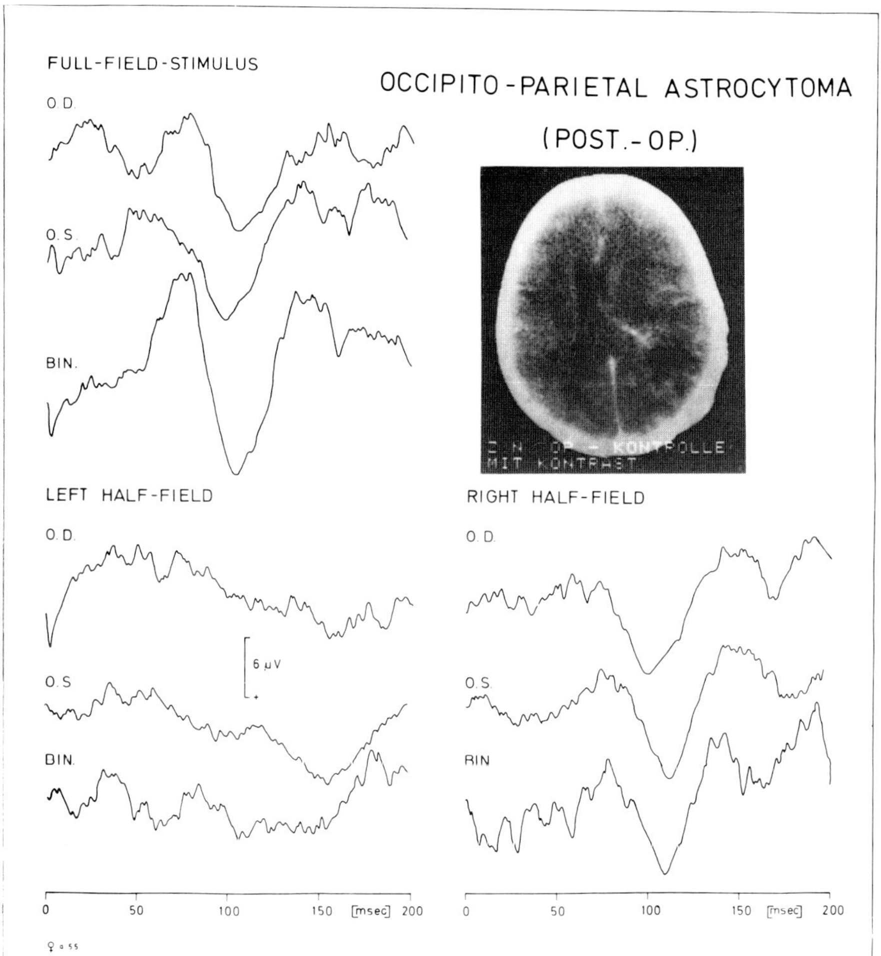

FIG. 2b. Parieto-occipital lesion postoperatory, 4 months later.

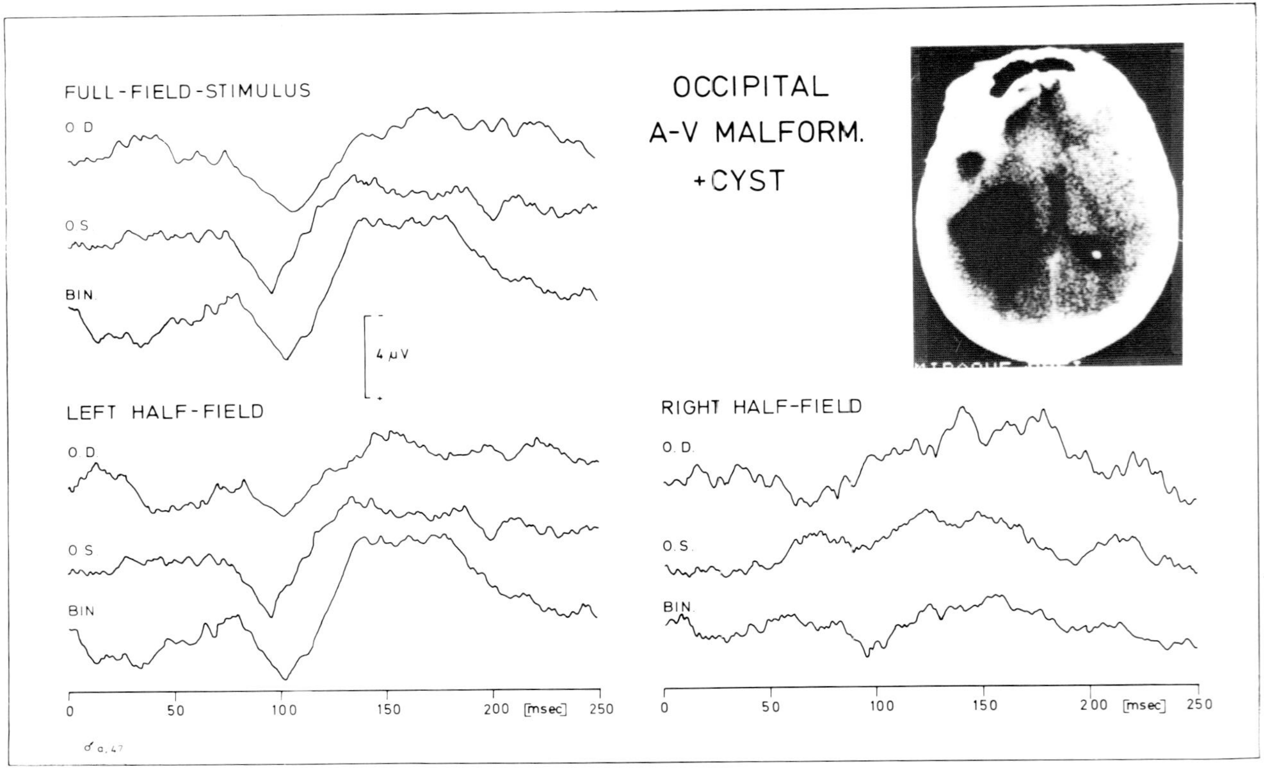

FIG. 3. Parieto-occipital lesion.

was only removed partially. Four months later, she developed a left homonymous hemianopia. No pattern-reversal responses could be obtained (see left half-field registration in Fig. 2b).

The second example is a 47-year-old male with a previously embolized A–V malformation. He was admitted because of acute headaches. The CT and angiography showed the persistence of a left occipital A–V angioma with a large cystic formation. A right homonymous hemianopia was found. The right half-field responses were absent (see Fig. 3).

DISCUSSION

The hemispheric distribution of the VEP has been studied with an array of multiple electrodes (7,10,11). However, the publications of Jeffreys and Axford (15,16), Blumhardt and Halliday (4,5), and Lesevre and Joseph (20) convinced us that hemisphere studies could also be done with midline leads.

Because our equipment did not allow us a multichannel registration, we performed our study with the simplified electrode positions mentioned above. The method was previously standardized in the control group, following international criteria (8).

Differences between nasal and temporal conduction velocities were also found by Eason et al. (9) in normal subjects. In our study, the selective stimulation of the nasal retina confirmed the perimetric findings in group II. In this group, the observation of abnormal responses to stimulation of the temporal retina in the absence of visual field alterations was interesting. These abnormal responses can be explained as being secondary to demyelination caused by compression (21).

The abnormal responses (group II) correlated well with the lesions as demonstrated by CT and surgery. The amplitude was diminished at the beginning of the disease, whereas in more advanced stages a delayed or absent response was measured.

Our findings are in agreement with recent publications by Halliday (13), Lehmann et al. (19), Korol (18), Wildberger et al. (24), and Holder (14) in relation to VEP changes in chiasmal lesions.

The abnormal pattern-reversal responses in group III were observed by selective stimulation of the visual fields corresponding to the injured hemispheres (prolonged latencies and small amplitudes or absent responses.) The abnormalities were more pronounced in the presence of visual field defects, although they sometimes occurred without perimetric defects. There were no differences between tumors and cerebrovascular diseases.

Similar results were published by Vaughan et al. (23) with flash stimulation. Blumhardt et al. (5) studied a patient with an homonymous hemianopia and made similar findings. Wildberger et al. (24) reported diminished amplitudes in a group of six hemianopic patients. Ashworth et al. (3) published bilateral abnormal VEPs in a patient with bilateral tumoral involvement of the corpus callosum and optic radiations as established postmortem.

The method allows a functional differentiation between chiasmatic and postchiasmatic lesions. In some cases, an early detection of clinically occult lesions is possible. A follow-up study, as in postoperative patients, can be helpful.

REFERENCES

1. Arden, G. B. (1972): The visual system. Neurophysiology, biophysics and their clinical applications. In: *Advances in Experimental Medicine and Biology, Vol. 24.* Plenum Press, London.
2. Arden, G. B., and Gucukoghn, A. G. (1978): Grating test of contrast sensitivity in patients with retrobulbar neuritis. *Arch. Ophthalmol.,* 96:1626–29.
3. Ashworth, B., Maloney, A., and Townsend, H. (1978): Delayed visual evoked potentials with bilateral disease of posterior visual pathway. *J. Neurol. Psychiatry,* 41:449–451.
4. Blumhardt, L. D., and Halliday, A. M. (1979): Hemisphere contributions to the composition of the pattern-evoked potentials waveform. *Exp. Brain Res.,* 36:55–59.
5. Blumhardt, L. D., Barrett, G., Halliday, A. (1977): The asymmetrical visual evoked potentials to pattern reversal in one half field and its significance for the analysis of visual field defects. *Br. J. Opthalmol.,* 61:454–61.
6. Cappin, J., Nissim, S. (1977): Visual evoked responses in the assessment of field defects in glaucoma. *Arch. Ophthalmol.,* 93:55–69.
7. Cobb, W., and Morton, H. (1970): Evoked potentials from the human scalp to visual half-field stimulation. *J. Physiol., (Lond.),* 208:39–40.
8. Donchin, E., Callaway, E., Cooper, R., Desmedt, J. E., Goff, W. R., Hillyard, S. A., and Sutton, S. (1977): Publication criteria for studies of evoked potentials in man. In: *Progress in Clinical Neurophysiology, Vol. 1,* edited by J. E. Desmedt, pp. 1–11. Karger, Basel.
9. Eason, R., Groves, P., White, C., and Oden, E. (1967): Evoked cortical potentials: Relation to visual field and handedness. *Science,* 156:1643–1646.
10. Emrich, H. (1969): Topographische Verteilung optisch evozierter Potentiale über die Hirnrinde des Menschen bei unterschiedlichen Reizen. *Vision Res.,* 9:365–76.
11. Halliday, A. M. (1970): Changes in the pattern-evoked responses in man associated with vertical and horizontal meridians of the visual field. *J. Physiol., (Lond.),* 208:499–513.
12. Halliday, A. M. (1973): Visual evoked response in diagnosis of multiple sclerosis. *Br. Med. J.,* 4:661–64.
13. Halliday, A. M. (1976): The pattern-evoked potentials in compression of the anterior visual pathways. *Brain,* 99:367–374.
14. Holder, G. E. (1978): The effect of chiasmal compression on the pattern-evoked potential. *Electroencephalogr. Clin. Neurophysiol.,* 45:278–280.
15. Jeffreys, D., and Axford, J. (1972): Source locations of pattern-specific components of human visual evoked potentials. I. Components of striate cortical origin. *Exp. Brain Res.,* 16:1–21.
16. Jeffreys, D., and Axford, J. (1972): Source locations of pattern-specific components of human visual evoked potentials. II. Components of extrastriate cortical origin. *Exp. Brain Res.,* 16:22–40.
17. Kennard, C., Gawel, M., Rudolph, N. de M., Clifford, R. F. (1978): Visual evoked potentials in migraine subjects. *Res. Clin. Stud. Headache,* 6:73–80.
18. Korol, S. (1977): Le syndrome chiasmatique—l'intéret des potentials evoqués visuels pour le diagnostic. *Klin. Monatsbl. Augenheilkd.,* 170:312–320.

19. Lehmann, D., Kavanagh, R. N., and Fender, D. H. (1969): Field studies of averaged visually evoked potentials in a patient with a split chiasm. *Electroencephalogr. Clin. Neurophysiol.*, 26:193–199.
20. Lesevre, N., and Joseph, J. (1979): Modifications of the pattern-evoked potential in relation to the stimulated part of the visual field. *Electroencephalogr. Clin. Neurophysiol.*, 47:183–203.
21. McDonald, W. (1977): Pathophysiology of conduction in central nerve fibers. In: *Visual Evoked Potentials in Man: New Developments,* edited by J. E. Desmedt, pp. 427–37. Clarendon Press, Oxford.
22. Troncoso, J., Moncall, E., and Schatz, N. (1979): Visual evoked responses in pernicious anemia. *Arch. Neurol.*, 36:168–69.
23. Vaughan, H., Katzman, N., and Taylor, J. (1963): Alteration of visual evoked response in the presence of homonymous field defects. *Electroencephalogr. Clin. Neurophysiol.*, 15:731–46.
24. Wildberger, H., Van Lith, G., Wijngaarde, R., and Mak, G. (1976): Visually evoked cortical potentials in the evaluation of homonymous and bitemporal visual field defects. *Br. J. Ophthalmol.*, 60:273–278.

Clinical Applications of Evoked Potentials in Neurology,
edited by J. Courjon, F. Mauguiere, and M. Revol.
Raven Press, New York © 1982.

Spatio-Temporal Study of Visual Evoked Potentials in Patients with Homonymous Hemianopia

*F. Chain, **N. Lesevre, *J. F. Pinel, and *M. Leblanc

*Unité de Recherche de Neurophysiologie, INSERM U 84, Hôpital de la Salpetrière, Paris, France; and **Laboratoire d'Electrophysiologie et Neurophysiologie Appliquée, Hôpital de la Salpétrière, Paris, France*

The question of whether there is a reliable correlation between visual evoked potential (VEP) characteristics and the elementary perceptive defect that constitutes hemianopia is still far from being solved given the contradictory results obtained not only by the earlier works utilizing flashes as stimuli (10,13,17,18) but even by the most recent studies analyzing the pattern-reversal response (1,3,4,8,9,19). There are indeed a great variety of factors that might influence the VEP organization of patients with visual field defects, such as the nature, site, and extent of the lesion, the presence or absence of a macular sparing, the time elapsed since the onset of the first clinical sign, etc. In the following study, the amplitude and chronotopographical characteristics of the first major positive component (the so-called $\overline{\text{P100}}$) of the pattern-reversal response recorded from 20 patients suffering from homonymous hemianopia were analyzed with respect to these various factors and compared to those of a control group in order to try to shed some light on the physiopathological mechanisms involved in the visual field defect.

POPULATION

The 20 patients (16 males, four females; age range 22 to 80 years with a mean of 59) coming from various neurological departments of the Salpétrière Hospital, were chosen according to the following criteria: (a) presence of homonymous hemianopia confirmed by ophthalmologic examination (Goldmann perimetry, Amsler table); (b) absence of a macular sparing of more than 5°; (c) a visual acuity of more than 6/10; (d) lesions well defined by scan as regards their site and nature. The nature of the lesion was: infarction (eight cases), hematoma (five cases), tumors or contusions (seven cases). The time elapsed between the moment of the first clinical sign to the VEP recording varied from 2 weeks to 390 weeks. Macula-splitting hemianopia was present in 15 cases.

A control group of 20 subjects (11 males, nine females; age range 19–55 years with a mean of 33) was recorded and studied under the same conditions.

METHOD

The montage consisted of a transverse chain of five equidistant electrodes (4 cm), the midline electrode being placed 3 cm above the inion. All electrodes were referred to a common linked-earlobes reference (in order to evaluate the influence of the common reference, for five control subjects, recordings were obtained in addition with a common midfrontal electrode placed 12 cm above the nasion). Horizontal eye movements were recorded simultaneously.

The stimulus was a black-and-white checkerboard made up of 20′ squares. The pattern was projected onto a circular field which, in the casc of full-field stimulation, was seen under a 13° angle when viewed at a distance of 1 m. For half-field stimulations, the screen was masked to produce a semicircular pattern of 6°30′ angle, the fixation point being placed ½° away from the vertical margin. The overall brightness level was 900 cd/m². Pattern reversals were produced at the regular frequency of 2/sec by a horizontal displacement (29 msec duration) of the pattern through one square's width. For each subject (controls and patients), the experiment consisted of seven different runs of 60 stimuli each: full-field, left-field, and right-field stimulations (two runs per situation) followed by a no-stimulus situation in order to evaluate the noise level in the same averaging conditions.

The VEPs were averaged by computer (Data General, Eclipse S 230) after automatic removal of events occurring during or just after eye movements exceeding a threshold value chosen after a calibration trial at the beginning of each recording. The averaged data were presented in the form of normalized conventional curves and spatiotemporal maps (14) for which amplitude values are represented as isopotential lines, the values between two successive electrodes being obtained by mathematical interpolation.

RESULTS

The following results will chiefly consist in comparing, for each subject, the $\overline{P100}$ characteristics obtained for half-field stimulation. The topography and latency values are those of the $\overline{P100}$ peaks. As regards amplitude values, they have been calculated from peak to peak between $\overline{P100}$ and $\overline{N150}$. Given the well-known interindividual amplitude variety, in order to enable interindividual comparisons, the amplitude values have been normalized and given in the form of the following amplitude index: AI $= (a - b)/(a + b)$, a and b being, respectively, the values in μV of the positive and the negative peak.

Control Group

The response to the stimulation of either the left or right half field was of smaller amplitude than that of the full-field stimulation but was usually made up of the same three main components: the first one, negative, of low amplitude, peaking around 60 msec (wave 0, N$\overline{60}$); the second one, positive, peaking toward 100 msec (wave 1, P$\overline{100}$); followed by a third wave, negative, approximately at 150 msec (wave 2, N$\overline{150}$) (Fig. 1).

The group average amplitude, latency, and topography characteristics of component 1 (P$\overline{100}$) are depicted in Table 1.

As regards topography, in most cases, whichever half-field was stimulated, P$\overline{100}$ peaked on the hemisphere contralateral to the stimulated field, approximately 4 cm away from the midline (Fig. 1 and Table 1).

Concerning latency and amplitude values, slight group average differences were observed between the responses obtained from the left and the right half-field stimulations. The importance of these differences varied markedly from one subject to another in such a way that the greatest latency difference could reach 20 msec and that an amplitude difference as high as 65% could be found.

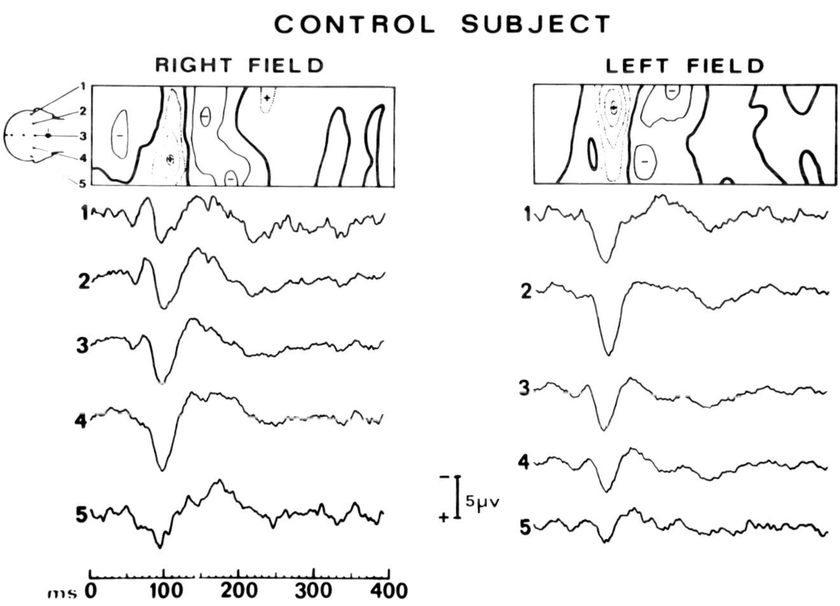

FIG. 1. Average pattern reversal-evoked response obtained from a control subject for right and left half field stimulation. On the maps, the positions of the peaks are marked by the sign + or − according to polarity. *Thick plain lines* indicate zero potential; 2 μV between successive isopotential lines positive *(broken lines)* or negative *(thin plain lines).* Whichever half field is stimulated, P$\overline{100}$ peaks on the contralateral hemisphere.

TABLE 1. *Results from the control group*[a]

CONTROL SUBJECTS

(20)

TOPOGRAPHY P 100		Contro	Ipsi	Median
	R V F	15	1	4
	L V F	15	1	4
LATENCY P 100		Mean	s.d.	Ext
	R V F + L V F	96.2	6.4	83, 112
	Diff. R V F − L V F	8.2	6	0, 22
INDEX AMPLITUDE P 100 − N 150		Mean	s.d.	Ext
	Max	53.9	29.8	21, 123
	Min	39.5	24.7	11, 87
	Diff. Max − Min	14.4 (30%)	11.3	0, 36 (65%)

[a] RVF, right visual field stimulated; LVF, left visual field stimulated. Diff RVF − LVF is the difference of P100 latency between the two half fields, calculated for each subject; the mean (8.2) is not significant.

Index amplitude max and min are the value maxima or minima of the index amplitude, whichever field was stimulated.

However, the important result was that no significant group tendency was observed in favor of one or the other half-field stimulation.

Patients with Half-Field Defects

The stimulation of the normal visual field of the patients (Figs. 2 and 3) elicited a VEP very similar to that seen for the controls, especially regarding topography, latency, and amplitude characteristics of component P100 (Table 2). Indeed, the slight group average increase in latency and decrease in amplitude noted in Table 2 were not statistically significant when compared to the average values of the control group (*t*-test).

The most striking result concerning the hemianopic field response as seen in the patient group considered as a whole was its topographical organization: indeed, when a P100 could be seen in this condition (17 cases out of 20), this component was often ipsilateral (seven cases out of 17), whereas it was contralateral, as in the control group, when the normal field of these patients was stimulated. But, in fact, the response to the hemianopic field stimulation differed in its various characteristics from one patient to another to such an extent that the average group values noted in Table 2 have little significance.

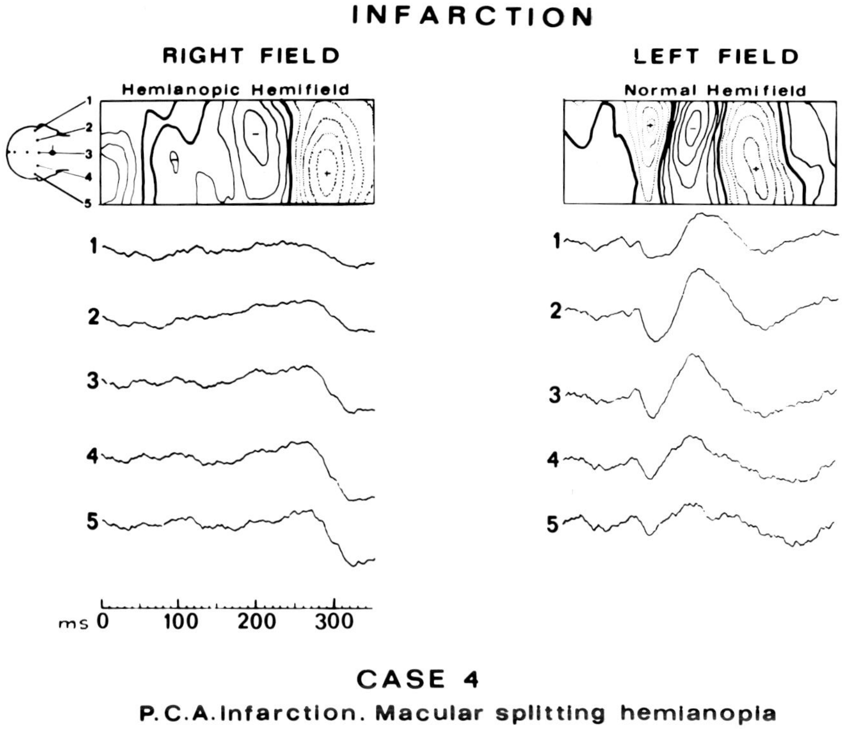

FIG. 2. Average pattern reversal response obtained from a patient with a macula-splitting right hemianopia caused by infarction. A normal response can be seen when the normal half field is stimulated, with P$\overline{100}$ and N$\overline{150}$ peaking on the contralateral hemisphere, whereas no response can be detected before 200 msec when the hemianopic field is stimulated, in particular, no positive wave.

Therefore, a case-by-case study was undertaken (Table 3). In 19 cases out of 20, the hemianopic field response could be considered as "abnormal": in three cases (two infarctions, one hematoma), no positive wave could be seen within a time window of 80 to 200 msec (the negative waves N$\overline{60}$ and N$\overline{150}$ also being absent); in the 16 other cases, a positive component could be detected, but this wave appeared quite "abnormal" regarding at least one of the three component characteristics (that is with values of latency or amplitude exceeding twice the standard deviation seen in the control group or with an "abnormal" topography).

As seen in Table 3, the characteristics of this "abnormal" hemianopic field response varied above all according to the nature of the lesion. Indeed, there was a marked tendency for patients with infarctions and, to a lesser extent, with hematoma to show hemianopic field responses made up of a very low amplitude P$\overline{100}$ only slightly delayed, peaking on the contralateral hemisphere (Fig. 2), whereas patients with tumors or contusions usually presented a delayed

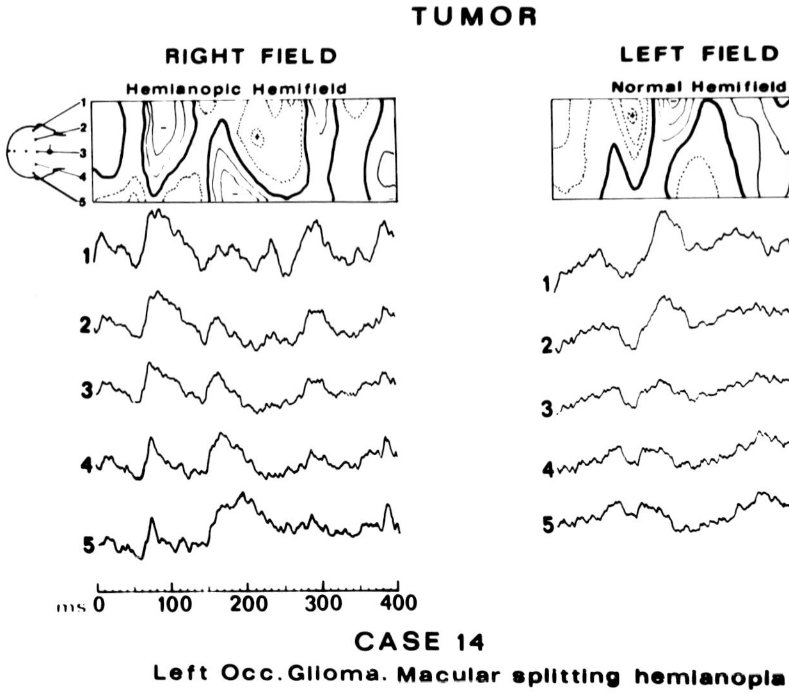

FIG. 3. Average pattern reversal response obtained from a patient with a mascula-splitting hemianopia caused by an unoperated left occipital glioma. When the normal half field is stimulated, a contralateral response made up of two contralateral waves, $\overline{\text{P100}}$ and $\overline{\text{N150}}$, is seen. The stimulation of the right hemianopic half field shows an "abnormal" response of delayed latency and high amplitude peaking on the ipsilateral hemisphere.

TABLE 2. *Results from the patients group*[a]

HOMONYMOUS VISUAL FIELD DEFECT (20 PATIENTS)

	TOPOGRAPHY P 100				LATENCY P 100			AMPLITUDE P 100-N 150		
	Contro	Ipsi	Median	No Res.	Mean	s.d.	Ext	Mean	s.d.	Ext
NORMAL HALF-FIELD	16	1	3	0	102.9	11.2	85 132	36.3	23.2	11 103
HEMIANOPIC HALF-FIELD	6	7	4	3	111.05	13.8	95 150	32	25.2	10 97

[a]The characteristics of $\overline{\text{P100}}$ are similar to those of the controls when the normal half field is stimulated. When the hemianopic half field is stimulated, the most striking result is the number of ipsilateral $\overline{\text{P100}}$ responses. Average group values of latency and amplitude have little signification because of the large differences observed from one patient to another.

TABLE 3. *Results of the 20 patients case by case*[a]

	Cases	TOPOGRAPHY P 100	LATENCY P 100 Diff. HVF-NVF	AMPLITUDE P 100 - N150 Diff. HVF-NVF
INFARCTION (8)	1	Median	+ 7 ms	- 4
	2	Contro	+ 3 ms	- 1
	3	Contro	+ 16 ms	- 12
	4	Contro	+ 17 ms	- 45
	5	Contro	+ 1 ms	+ 24
	6			
	7			
	8	Median	+ 23 ms	- 11
HEMATOMA (8)	9			
	10	Ipsi	+ 6 ms	- 18
	11	Ipsi	+ 1 ms	- 4
	12	Median	- 1 ms	+ 3
	13	Contro	+ 1 ms	- 39
TUMOR and CONTUSION (7)	14	Contro	+ 20 ms	- 10
	15	Ipsi	+ 32 ms	+ 16
	16	Median	+ 10 ms	- 3
	17	Ipsi	+ 10 ms	+ 17
	18	Ipsi	+ 30 ms	+ 1
	19	Ipsi	+ 3 ms	+ 7
	20	Ipsi	+ 18 ms	- 11

HEMIANOPIC HALF-FIELD (20 Patients)

[a] In each group the great variability of the results can be seen. However, the tendency of ischemic lesions to produce contralateral $\overline{P100}$s of low amplitude can be observed, whereas tumors and contusions produce "abnormal" responses, mostly ipsilateral, of delayed latency and high amplitude.

$\overline{P100}$ of high amplitude—often higher than that seen for the normal field stimulation—and chiefly peaking on the ipsilateral hemisphere (Fig. 3).

DISCUSSION

Given the complexity of the results which raise a number of different problems concerning methodology as well as clinicopathological correlations, only a few main points will be discussed in this chapter.

The first concerns the topography of $\overline{P100}$ which is obviously a major point for the diagnosis of hemianopia. The $\overline{P100}$ was contralateral to the half field stimulated for the majority of the controls. This finding, which has already been emphasized by a member of our team studying other control groups is in agreement with that of several other authors [Cobb and Morton (5), who showed with bipolar recordings a phase reversal of gradients on the contralateral hemisphere; Biersdorf (2); Shagass et al. (16)] but in disagreement with that of others [in particular, Barret et al. (1); Halliday et al. (6)]. Various stimulus parameters as well as the locations of both the active and the reference electrodes have been said to influence the lateralization of the pattern-reversal response (7). In fact, five of our controls were seen successively with our own conditions of stimulation and montage and with those of Halliday and co-workers: the contralateral $\overline{P100}$ of the five subjects then became ipsilateral.

The second point concerns the variability of the visual evoked response in our series of hemianopic patients and, in relation to this, the value of VEP recording for visual field defect diagnosis. In spite of pattern-reversal responses being much more reliable than flash responses—allowing the recognition of homonymous hemianopia 19 times out of 20—it must be emphasized that the differences observed in the VEP abnormalities from one patient to another, even in cases of a similar macula-splitting hemianopia, show that there is no simple correlation between the elementary perceptual defect and the VEP abnormal response. On the other hand, VEP recordings by pattern-reversal stimulation demand excellent cooperation from the patient. Given these various considerations, it seems to us that, at least in the present state of technical development and knowledge concerning the VEP generators, VEP recording cannot currently be utilized as a technique for visual field defect diagnosis.

The third and most important point concerns the interpretation of the VEP differences observed in the 20 hemianopic patients. In spite of as precise as possible a topographical study of the lesion, including a thorough clinical examination and CT scan in each case, we did not find any significant correlation between the site of the lesion and the VEP modifications. However, to give a definite answer to the question of the influence of the site of the lesion, in particular of its more or less posterior localization, a more complete VEP topographical study would be necessary (by recording simultaneously a midline longitudinal chain of electrodes and several transverse chains crossing the midline at various levels). On the other hand, with regard to the influence of the nature of the lesion, two groups of patients can be distinguished: cerebrovascular accidents, and tumors and contusions. It is interesting to note that ischemic lesions give way, when the damaged half-field is stimulated, to a VEP the salient features of which were not grossly different from those of the VEP obtained when the normal half-field was stimulated. In fact, $\overline{P100}$ was in most cases contralateral, as it was in healthy subjects, and only slightly delayed, the main abnormality being its low amplitude. These findings are in agreement with what could be expected in light of the nature of ischemic lesions, which more or less destroy the cerebral cells.

The results of the five cases of hematomas are more difficult to interpret, since hematomas are usually considered to be space-occupying lesions, and it might have been expected to find gross abnormalities as reported by Holder (8). That was not the case in our series, in which hematoma VEPs were very similar to those of ischemic cases. However, it must be recalled that our five hematoma cases were old lesions, hypodense at the scan, and therefore, very close to ischemic lesions.

In contrast to vascular lesions which showed defective half-field responses of lower amplitude but not grossly different from those of the normal half-field, tumors and contusions led to defective half-field responses that were grossly "abnormal." In most cases, patients with tumors showed a trend towards delayed $\overline{P100}$s of high amplitude. In some cases, the amplitude of the positive component was much higher than that of the normal field response and delayed to such an extent that it became difficult to tell if this wave could be considered part of an evoked response (cases 15 and 18). But the most remarkable abnormality was the lateralization of $\overline{P100}$, which was ipsilateral in five out of seven cases. The reasons why tumors and contusions more often produce ipsilateral $\overline{P100}$s remain unclear. It must be recalled that in cases of occipital lobectomy, the presence of an "ipsilateral" response—that is, of a response peaking on the side of the absent lobe—obtained when stimulating the normal half field, has been pointed out (4), this response being discussed in terms of passive electrical transmission. However, the ipsilateral $\overline{P100}$ of the patients with tumors seen in the present study was recorded from the hemianopic field, and its significance is certainly different.

Whatever may be the factors responsible for this ipsilateral lateralization, our results on the whole confirm the conclusions of Samson-Dollfus and Pouliquen (15) who found in a series of 30 hemianopic patients a tendency for "defective PEV" in ischemic lesions and "hyperactive PEV" in tumors. In a recent study of 19 hemianopic patients, Holder (8) made the same statement.

Given the complexity of the results and their variability from one patient to another, our conclusion will be that in order to better understand the pathological mechanisms underlying each case of visual field defect, this spatiotemporal study must be extended by using more electrodes, seeing more patients, and, above all, by taking into account all of the different factors that might influence the defective field VEP organization.

REFERENCES

1. Barret, G., Blumhardt, L. D., Halliday, E., and Kriss, A. (1976): A paradox in the lateralization of the visual evoked response. *Nature,* 261:253–255.
2. Biersdorf, W. R. (1974): Cortical evoked responses from stimulation of various regions of the visual field. *Doc. Ophthalmol.,* 4:249–259.
3. Blumhardt, L. D., Barret, G., and Halliday, A. M. (1977): The asymmetrical visual evoked potential to pattern reversal in one half field and its significance for the analysis of visual field defects. *Br. J. Ophthalmol.,* 61:454–461.
4. Chain, F., Lesevre, N., Leblanc, M., Remond, A., and Lhermitte, F. (1972): Etude topographique des réponses évoquées visuelles dans un cas de lobectomie occipitale. *Rev. Neurol.,* 126:372–378.
5. Cobb, W. A., and Morton, H. B. (1970): Evoked potentials from the human scalp to visual half field stimulation. *J. Physiol. (Lond.),* 208:39–40.
6. Halliday, A. M., Barret, G., Halliday, E., and Michael, W. F. (1977): The topography of the pattern evoked potential. In: *Visual Evoked Potentials in Man: New Developments,* edited by J. E. Desmedt, pp. 121–133. Clarendon, Oxford.
7. Harding, G. F. A., Smith, G. F., and Smith, P. A. (1980): The effect of various stimulus parameters on the lateralization of the VEP. In: *Evoked Potentials,* edited by C. Barber, pp. 213–218. MTP Press, Lancaster.

8. Holder, G. E. (1980): Abnormalities of the pattern visual evoked potential in patients with homonymous visual field defects. In *Evoked Potentials*, edited by C. Barber, pp. 285–291. MTP Press, Lancaster.
9. Howe, J. W., and Mitchell, K. W. (1980): Visual evoked potentials from quadrantic field stimulation in the investigation of homonymous field defects. In *Evoked Potentials*, edited by C. Barber, pp. 279–284. MTP Press, Lancaster.
10. Kooi, K. A., Guvener, A. M., and Bogghi, B. K. (1965): Visual evoked responses in lesions of the higher optic pathways. *Neurology (Minneap.)*, 15:841–854.
11. Lesevre, N., and Joseph, J. P. (1979): Modifications of the pattern evoked potential (PEP) in relation to the stimulated part of the visual field (clues for the most probable origin of each component). *Electroencephalogr. Clin. Neurophysiol.*, 27:23–34.
12. Lesevre, N., and Remond, A. (1972): Potentiels évoqués par l'apparition de patterns: Effets de la dimension du pattern et de la densité des contrastes. *Electroencephalogr. Clin. Neurophysiol.*, 32:593–604.
13. Oosterhuis, H. J., Ponsen, L., Jonkman, E. J., and Magnus, O. (1969): The average visual response in patients with cerebro-vascular disease. *Electroencephalogr. Clin. Neurophysiol.*, 27:23–24.
14. Remond, A. (1961): Integrated and topographical analysis of the EEG. *Electroencephalogr. Clin. Neurophysiol.*, 20:64–67.
15. Samson-Dollfus, D., and Pouliquen, A. (1976): Application des PEV à l'étude des hémianopsies latérales homonymes. *Rev. Electroencephalogr. Neurophysiol. Clin.*, 6:179–180.
16. Shagass, C., Amadeo, M., and Roemer, R. A. (1976): Spatial distribution of potentials evoked by half field pattern reversal and pattern onset stimuli. *Electroencephalogr. Clin. Neurophysiol.*, 41:609–622.
17. Vaughan, H. G., and Katzman, R. (1964): Evoked responses in visual disorders. *Ann. N.Y. Acad. Sci.*, 112:305–319.
18. Vaughan, H. G., Katzman, R., and Taylor, T. (1963): Alterations of visual evoked response in the presence of homonymous visual defects. *Electroencephalogr. Clin. Neurophysiol.*, 15:737–746.
19. Wildberger, H. G. H., Van Lith, G. H. M., Winjgaarde, R., and Mak, G. T. M. (1976): Visually evoked cortical potentials in the evaluation of homonymous and bitemporal visual field defects. *Br. J. Ophthalmol.*, 60:272–278.

Clinical Applications of Evoked Potentials in Neurology,
edited by J. Courjon, F. Mauguiere, and M. Revol.
Raven Press, New York © 1982.

The Visually Evoked Potential in Retrochiasmatic Lesions of the Optic Pathways: An Attempt to Interpret the Responses Obtained by Flash Pattern Stimulation and the Results of the Calculation of the Correlation Coefficient Between Visually Evoked Potentials

*D. Samson-Dollfus, *D. Parain, *J. Weber, *J. F. Menard, **B. Mihout, and †B. Vachon

**Explorations Neurologiques, Centre Hospitalier Universitaire, Rouen, France; **Clinique Neurologique, Centre Hospitalier Universitaire, Rouen, France; and †Division Contrôle des Systèmes, Université Technologique, Compiegne, France*

Comparisons of the visual evoked potentials (VEP) between different leads in the same subject or between similar leads recorded on different subjects are normally based on values of the amplitude and latency of the wave peaks. The calculation of the correlation coefficient appears to be a satisfactory method for measuring the similarities or differences between two signals or parts of signals.

This chapter is essentially concerned with the measurement of the latencies of the different peaks and with the determination of (a) interhemispheric (between the left and right central and occipital leads) and (b) intrahemispheric (between the left or right and central and occipital leads) correlation coefficients. These were calculated in control subjects and in subjects suffering from hemispheric lesions affecting the retrochiasmatic portion of the optic pathways.

METHODS AND SUBJECTS

Thirty-eight healthy young adults, 21 to 24 years of age, students or members of the laboratory staff, served as control subjects and were full-field stimulated. Eleven of these subjects were half-field stimulated, successively, on their right and then left visual half fields.

Seventeen patients suffering from visual disturbances caused by retrochiasmatic lesions verified by CT scan or through surgery were studied. Eight lesions were strictly occipital, whereas nine extended into the central, parietal, or temporal areas. Of these 17 subjects, four were suffering from cortical blindness; the 13 others had unilateral loss of vision.

The stimulus used was a square checkerboard placed 35 cm from the subject and seen from an angle of 20°; each square was seen from an angle of 30′. The pattern was illuminated approximately once every second by a flash of white light. Eighty successive stimulations were used. The duration of the flash was short (1 to 3 msec), and at the peak of the curve, the luminance of the pattern was 125 cd/m^2. It is possible to use full- or half-field stimulation.

The common reference was a linked-ears electrode. The active electrodes were placed in the right and left central regions and on the vertex, and in the right, left, and midline occipital regions according to the 10–20 system.

The first 256 to 512 msec of the responses were analyzed. The peak latencies and their amplitudes were calculated automatically through a program of peak recognition.

The interhemispheric correlation function was obtained from 150 pairs of points (300 msec) between two homologous responses: right and left occipital, then right and left central. The intrahemispheric correlation function was calculated between the right, then left, central and occipital derivations. Then the correlation coefficient was calculated for successive sets of 40 to 150 points, enabling us to evaluate the similarities of the two functions under study in successive stages: 10 to 90 msec; 40 to 120 msec; 120 to 200 msec; 200 to 500 msec. We thus obtained correlation coefficients corresponding to the different parts of the evoked potential.

All of these calculations were performed off-line with a PDP 11/40 with 32K words in its central memory, and the results were printed or shown on a visual screen. The tests used were the nonparametric Mann–Whitney or Wilcoxon tests for comparison of means. The statistical calculations concerning the correlation functions were done after Fischer transformation.

RESULTS

Control Subjects—Total-Field Stimulation

Occipital and central responses were obtained from all normal subjects. It was therefore possible to average the VEP (Fig. 1) recorded in these control subjects and calculate or observe the average latencies of the different waves and their standard deviations. We therefore observed not only occipital (Table 1) but also central responses (Table 2). The waves appearing prior to 70 msec are highly inconstant, whereas waves appearing after 70 msec are found in almost all of the subjects (Tables 1 and 2). It should be noted that the peaks of the waves obtained from the central and occipital regions are not in phase.

In order to test the similarities of the different waves with respect to each other, we calculated the correlation coefficients for the central and for the occipital leads; these values were high, and the standard deviation small, whatever

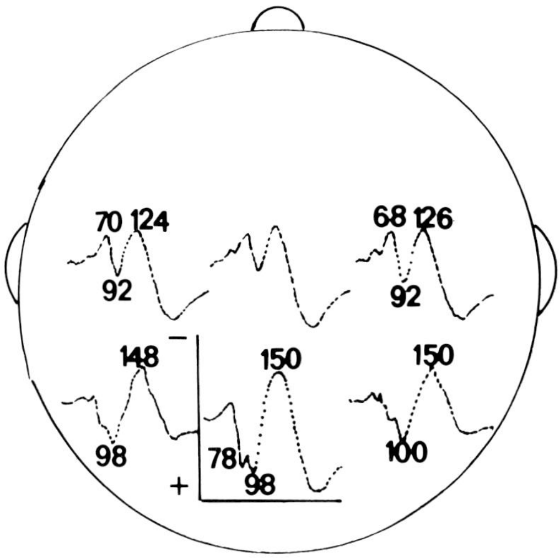

Fig. 1. Normal average VEP (38 subjects) stimulated by a full-field flash pattern. Linked-ear common reference; scale of time, 256 msec; scale of amplitude, 20 μV. An upward deflection is a negative potential.

part of the function was analyzed (Table 3). However, we noted that the values of the correlation coefficients were higher for the central than for the occipital regions; this difference was significant ($p \leq 0.01$) for the graph as a whole and for the following parts of the curve: 10 to 90 msec, 120 to 200 msec, 200 to 500 msec. The difference is significant at $p \leq 0.05$ for the 40 to 120 msec section (Table 3). However, the values are low, and we found great intersubject variability when we correlated occipital and central responses in the same hemisphere.

TABLE 1. *Average calculated latencies (L) of the different waves appearing in occipital leads and their standard deviation (σ)*

	N[a]	14	11	24	20	35	38	36
01	L	N 45	P 58	N 63	P 76	P 105	N 145	P 201
	(σ)	(4)	(3)	(6)	(5)	(10)	(15)	(16)
	N[a]			31	38		38	35
0Z	L			N 60	P 92		N 139	P 206
	(σ)			(10)	(12)		(14)	(16)
	N[a]	19	9	16	17	35	38	38
02	L	N 42	P 57	N 66	P 78	P 105	N 147	P 206
	(σ)	(8)	(6)	(9)	(4)	(12)	(14)	(17)

[a] *N* is the number of control subjects in whom the wave has been observed.

TABLE 2. *Average calculated latencies (L) of the different waves appearing in central leads and their standard deviations (σ)*

	N[a]	5	3	18	13	32	34	37	37
C3	L	N 28	P 35	N 45	P 53	N 74	P 95	N 127	P 191
	(σ)			(8)	(5)	(10)	(8)	(11)	(17)
	N[a]					29	31	37	37
CZ	L					N 67	P 95	N 124	P 184
	(σ)					(4)	(7)	(15)	(18)
	N[a]	6	2	9	10	30	32	35	38
C4	L	N 27	P 34	N 47	P 53	N 72	P 95	N 132	P 196
	(σ)			(5)	(5)	(9)	(6)	(15)	(19)

[a] *N* is the number of control subjects in whom the wave has been observed.

TABLE 3. *Average correlation coefficient (38 subjects) between C_4 and C_3 and between 0_2 and 0_1 (it is higher in the central than in the occipital areas)*

		0–500 msec	10–90 msec	40–120 msec	120–200 msec	200–500 msec
	CO	0.94	0.87	0.84	0.95	0.91
C_4–C_3	(σ)	(0.01)	(0.12)	(0.19)	(0.07)	(0.15)
		**	**	*	**	**
	CO	0.81	0.69	0.75	0.78	0.83
0_2–0_1	(σ)	(0.14)	(0.27)	(0.20)	(0.28)	(0.12)

* $p \leq 0.05$; ** $p \leq 0.01$.

Control Subjects—Half-Field Stimulation

With half-field stimulation, we observed, in the central region, almost the same response in the two hemispheres. The correlation coefficient of these two responses was high, and the responses were in phase.

However, in the occipital region, the responses of the two hemispheres differed: in the contralateral hemisphere, we observed a positive response, $\overline{\text{P100}}$, followed by a $\overline{\text{N150}}$ wave. This $\overline{\text{P100}}$ wave was sometimes out of phase, for it was occasionally preceded by a negative wave, $\overline{\text{N80–90}}$ of very low amplitude. In the ipsilateral hemisphere, we noted essentially the $\overline{\text{N120}}$ wave, sometimes preceded by a positive wave of variable amplitude, but always peaking earlier than $\overline{\text{P100}}$ (i.e., 70 msec). The calculation of the correlation coefficient for successive sections confirmed that it was in the 80 to 140 msec section that the two parts of the functions differed the most.

The stimulation of the two half fields successively did not change the central response (Fig. 2), the principal peaks of which continued to be highly correlated and in phase when superimposed.

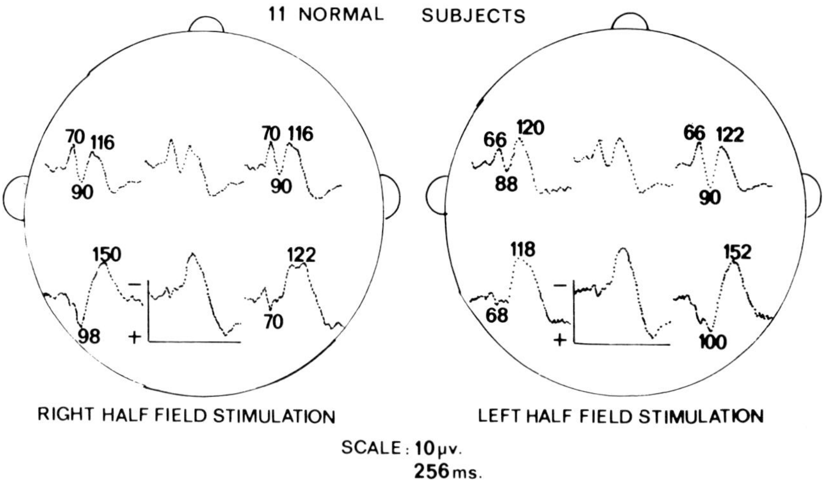

FIG. 2. Left half-field stimulation and right half-field stimulation. Average of 11 control subjects. One can see: the $P\overline{100}$ on the right occipital and the $P\overline{70}$ on the left occipital leads when the left half-field is stimulated; the $P\overline{100}$ on the left occipital and the $P\overline{70}$ on the right occipital leads when the right half field is stimulated; and no difference in the central leads.

Pathological Subjects

Bilateral Lesions

Three of these four subjects had extended parieto–occipital lesions; the responses were all pathological both in the central and occipital regions.

One patient presented a cortical blindness that regressed in 48 hr, leaving only a very limited right occipital ischemia. The central responses were symmetrical, whereas the occipital responses showed a greatly simplified and asymmetric diphasic response.

Unilateral Lesions

The anomalies of the occipital VEP were indeed manifest after whole-field stimulation, but they can be interpreted only by comparison to the data obtained from normal subjects after whole- and half-field stimulation.

In three cases of apparently unilateral lesions, the occipital responses were symmetrical, but the latencies of the various PNP waves were very abnormal on both sides with, in particular, a much delayed P wave (138 to 152 msec).

In the 10 other cases, we noted on the affected side the absence of the $P\overline{100}$ wave (Fig. 3) or its diminution of amplitude or early appearance compared to the healthy side. In contrast, 9 times out of 10, the $P\overline{100}$ of the healthy side appeared later than what remained of this wave on the affected side.

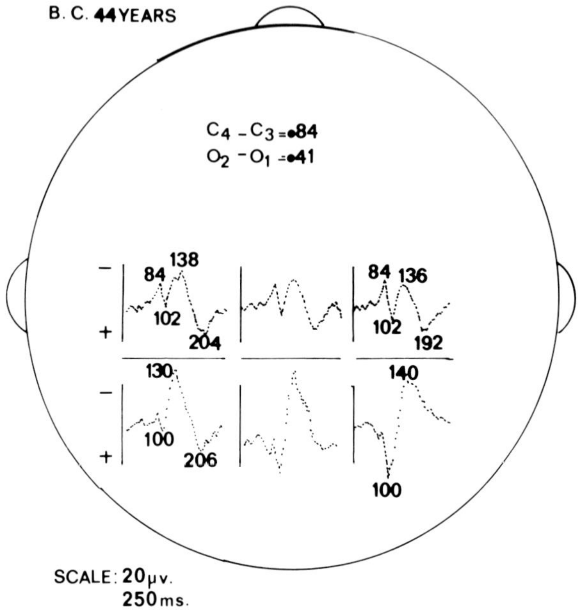

FIG. 3. This patient had left occipital ischemia, and the $\overline{P100}$ is of very low amplitude on the left occipital side. However, the central VEP are normal, and the correlation coefficient is high (0.84).

Finally, we noted on four occasions on the healthy side an "$\overline{N100}$" wave (between 88 to 110 msec) of large amplitude (Fig. 4).

Central Responses

In seven cases of unilateral lesions strictly limited to the occipital region (CT scan), the central responses were absolutely normal in six cases. In contrast, in six more extensive lesions affecting the temporal section of the visual pathways or the central regions, they were affected five times (Fig. 5).

Correlation Function

The traditional study of latency times showed an asymmetry only 8 times out of 13; the study of the correlation function of the whole graph and of the correlation coefficients of the successive segments of the visual evoked potentials showed in 11 cases values differing by more than 2 SD from the average value calculated in control subjects. Thus, in four cases, this method enabled us to note anomalies in the VEP that would have passed unnoticed in a traditional examination.

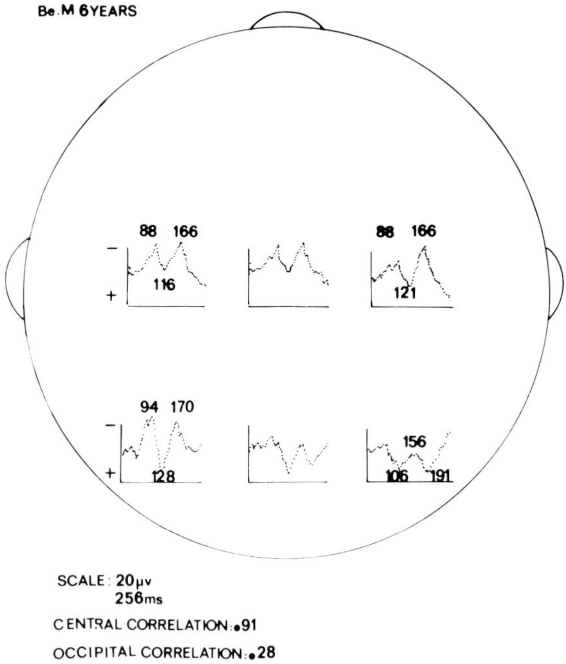

FIG. 4. P106 is of very low amplitude in the right occipital VEP (right occipital lesion), but a high-amplitude N94 is seen in the normal occipital lobe.

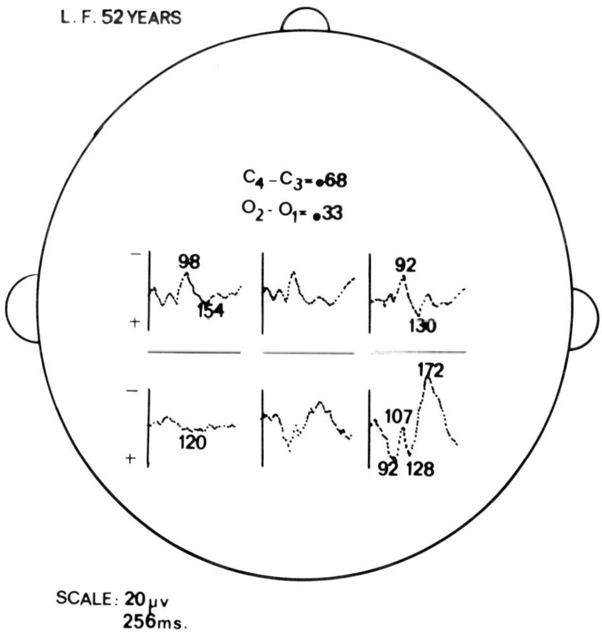

FIG. 5. Patient with a parieto–occipital tumor; the occipital VEP and the central VEP are affected. The correlation coefficient is low in the central (0.68) and the occipital leads (0.33).

DISCUSSION

Total-field stimulation (flashed pattern) produces occipital responses that are very similar to those obtained by the pattern-onset or pattern-reversal methods stimulating the whole visual field (7) or the lower half of the visual field (6). But, in addition, we noted in the sample studied here vertex and central responses that were of clear and large amplitude. The majority of authors using the pattern–reversal or pattern-onset techniques (1,3,7,12) do not seem to obtain central responses, with the exception of Lehmann and Skrandies (6) who studied their topographical distribution, but whose data show that in the central region the responses are low amplitude. In contrast, in the sample studied here, we observed a very distinct vertex response after flash stimulation (Fig. 1).

This kind of VEP has also been observed by Borda (4). This marked central response may be caused by the intensity of the stimulation or by the very rapid changes of luminance of the flash. These two factors may create a particularly effective stimulus that is able to produce a perceptive activity in the whole of the pathways carrying visual information (retino-geniculo-striate pathway, retino-tectal pathway, and retino-cerebellar pathway). The information leaving the retina may travel by the second of these pathways (9), projecting itself onto the superficial layer of the superior colliculus, to end in the thalamus via internal medullary lamina (11) or pulvinar (2). The activation may be diffused through the thalamocortical pathways to the parietal cortex, eliciting activity in the "visual fixation neurons." Mountcastle et al. (8) identified these neurons using stimuli differing considerably from ours (complex visual motor behavior). Nevertheless, Sakata et al. (10) confirm their activity in the case of unelaborated stimulation comparable with our experimental situation. In the sample of normal subjects studied here, we noted, therefore, not only a very clear central response (Fig. 1) but also a correlation coefficient that was significantly higher for central responses than in the occipital area. Finally, the correlation coefficient for the central responses evoked by half-field stimulation remains high, whereas it decreases dramatically around the occipital $\overline{\text{P100}}$ wave. Furthermore, in the majority of purely occipital lesions, the central VEP was not affected, whereas in more extensive lesions, we commonly observed an altered central response.

When we studied the interhemispheric correlation coefficient for the different segments of the occipital response in pathological subjects, we noted, depending on the segment of the function studied, values that are located more or less than 2 SD away from the average values of the control subjects. It should be noted that Jeffreys (5) and Lesevre and Joseph (7) have shown that in normal subjects the visual evoked potential is made up of components resulting from the activation of generators in different locations. The results provided by the correlation coefficients clearly show that waves are asymmetrical only in certain cases, while the rest of the function shows good correlation between the two hemispheres.

When the total field of a patient with lateral homonymous hemianopia is stimulated, it is possible to postulate that the VEP would be almost the same as that of a normal subject after half-field stimulation.

It is thus possible to explain the absence of the $P\overline{100}$ wave in the affected occipital region (Fig. 3) although the rest of the response exists and all the waves are found on the healthy side: this kind of anomaly in the VEP by total-field stimulation corresponds to the normal response observed in healthy subjects after half-field stimulation by a flashed pattern (as in this study) or pattern onset (7). It is also necessary to explain the $N\overline{80}$–$\overline{100}$ wave that was found in four cases on the healthy hemisphere in subjects suffering from unilateral occipital lesions: this $N\overline{100}$ wave does not exist in the normal subject after total-field stimulation but has been described by Blumhardt et al. (3) in the contralateral hemisphere in normal subjects after hemireversal pattern stimulation.

In conclusion, the flashed pattern is easy to use and has the advantage of evoking central response; the interpretation may aid in topographical diagnosis. The study of the correlation functions improves the sensitivity of the method.

ACKNOWLEDGMENTS

This work was supported in part by a grant from the Rouen University Scientific Council. The authors would like to express their gratitude to Eric Dreano and Françoise Suard for their invaluable technical assistance.

REFERENCES

1. Arruga, J., Feldon, S. E., Hoyt, W. F., and Aminoff, M. J. (1980): Monocular and binocular evoked visual responses to pattern half-field stimulation. *Sci.*, 46:281–290.
2. Baleydier, C., and Mauguiere, F. (1977): Pulvinar latero–posterior afferents to cortical area 7 in monkeys demonstrated by horseradish peroxidase tracing technique. *Exp. Brain Res.*, 27:501–507.
3. Blumhardt, L. D., Barret, G., and Halliday, A. M. (1977): The asymmetrical visual evoked potential to pattern reversal in one half-field and its significance for the analysis of visual field defects. *Br. J. Ophthalmol.*, 6:454–461.
4. Borda, R. P. (1977): Visual evoked potentials to flash in the clinical evaluation of the optic pathways. In: *Visual Evoked Potentials in Man: New Developments*, edited by J. E. Desmedt, pp. 481–489. Clarendon Press, Oxford.
5. Jeffreys, D. (1977): The physiological significance of pattern visual evoked potentials. In: *Visual Evoked Potentials in Man: New Developments*, edited by J. E. Desmedt, pp. 134–167. Clarendon Press, Oxford.
6. Lehmann, D., and Skrandies, W. (1980): Reference-free identification of components of checkerboard-evoked multichannel potential fields. *Electroencephalogr. Clin. Neurophysiol.*, 48:609–621.
7. Lesevre, N., and Joseph, J. P. (1979): Modifications of the pattern-evoked potential in relation to the stimulated part of the visual field (clues for the most probable origin of each component). *Electroencephalogr. Clin. Neurophysiol.*, 47:183–203.
8. Mountcastle, V. B., Lynch, J. C., Georgopoulos, A., Sakata, H., and Acuna, C. (1975): Posterior parietal association cortex of the monkey: Command functions for operations within extrapersonal space. *J. Neurophysiol.*, 38:871–908.
9. Perenin, M. T., and Jeannerod, M. (1979): Subcortical vision in man. *Trends Neurosci.*, 2:204–207.

10. Sakata, H., Shibutani, H., and Kawano, K. (1980): Spatial properties of visual fixation neurons in posterior parietal association cortex of the monkey. *J. Neurophysiol.,* 43:1654–1672.
11. Schlag-Rey, M., and Schlag, J. (1974): Visual responsiveness of eye movement neurons in thalamic internal medullary lamina of cat. *Brain Res.,* 91:311–314.
12. Shagass, C., Amadeo, M., and Roemer, R. A. (1976): Spatial distribution of potentials evoked by half-field pattern reversal and pattern on-set stimuli. *Electroencephalogr. Clin. Neurophysiol.,* 41:609–622.

Clinical Applications of Evoked Potentials in Neurology,
edited by J. Courjon, F. Mauguiere, and M. Revol.
Raven Press, New York © 1982.

Correlations Between Visual Evoked Potential Parameters of 5-Year-Old Children and Their Neonatal Neurological Condition

*K. Poortinga, *C. J. Njiokiktjien, and **S. L. Visser

*Departments of *Child Neurology and **Clinical Neurophysiology, Free University and Valeriuskliniek, 1075 BG Amsterdam, The Netherlands*

A high percentage (30–65%) of abnormal EEGs is reported (3,8,9,11,14) in the literature on the subject of minimal brain dysfunction (MBD) syndrome or hyperkinesia.

Birth trauma is presumed to be an important cause of MBD. Nevertheless, there are only few papers on the relation between the neurological condition at birth and the neurological condition and EEG data in childhood. Moreover, such studies with clinically normal children are not known to us.

More specific clinical neurophysiological techniques such as visual evoked potentials (VEPs) can provide additional evidence of cerebral organic disturbances (4,10,13,14,18). Probably, the VEP is an even more sensitive parameter of cerebral disturbances in MBD than is the EEG, but this hypothesis (10) needs confirmation. Auditory evoked potentials (AEPs) (15,16,19) and somatosensory evoked potentials (SEPs) (7) may also be disturbed, but again, there is a lack of data on the relation between evoked response at childhood and the neurological condition at birth.

Hrbek et al. (7) found abnormal VEPs in 85% of neonates with postnatal asphyxia. Sometimes the abnormalities disappeared in a few days. Gambi et al. (6) investigated 60 neonates with perinatal problems—respiratory distress and hypoglycemia. They performed a longitudinal study over a period of 9 months. The VEP was often abnormal with increased latencies. These abnormalities had not completely disappeared at the age of 9 months.

In this chapter, an investigation is presented concerning the relation between neurological condition at birth [Prechtl's neurological score, (12)] and VEP data at the age of 5 in clinically normal children. Data on the relation between the neurological condition at birth and the neuropsychological, neurological, and EEG data at the age of 5 will be published elsewhere.

METHODS

In 1975, the Obstetric Department of the Free University (Amsterdam) started a longitudinal study (17): About 150 clinically normal children were followed from birth up to the age of 5. Obstetrical and delivery conditions were assessed, as was the neurological condition of the neonates immediately after birth. At the age of 5, the developmental processes of the children were scored by clinical neurological and electrophysiological methods.

For a number of reasons, not all 150 children could be evaluated at the age of 5 (long-range removals, refusals, excess of artifacts in the EEG records). Ultimately, 89 clinically normal children (38 boys and 51 girls) were evaluated at the age of 5. All examinations were performed within 1 month before to 2 months after the fifth birthday.

Neurological Condition at Birth

Prechtl (12) developed a neurological examination procedure for neonates, resulting in a semiquantitative score which is claimed to be a reliable and valid index of the optimality of CNS function at birth and, in addition, to have some prognostic value for later neurobehavioral development. The score ranges to 42. A score >36 is supposed to be an optimal one; a score ≤36 is a sign of a nonoptimal neurological condition of the neonate.

Visual Evoked Potentials

Visual evoked potentials were recorded by surface electrodes from the leads 01–APR[1] and 02–APR[1]. Signals were amplified and recorded by means of an EEG apparatus (high-pass filter 0.3 sec, low-pass filter 70 Hz, −3 db). The signals were stored on magnetic tape for off-line processing. Light stimulus was delivered by a photostimulator (Elema-Schönander type EMT 722) at intervals randomized by hand, avoiding epochs with artifacts. Minimal flash interval was 2 sec; flash duration was 10 msec. The subjects' eyes were closed. Signals were analyzed by a small general purpose computer (PDP 11/34). From the parallel arriving signals, 60 sweeps were averaged. The sampling interval was 1.98 msec. For each channel, the total length of one analysis epoch was 450 msec. The averaged VEP was displayed by a Versatec D1100A printer/plotter. All peaks were identified by the computer program and indicated on the curve. The latency and absolute amplitude values (to mean level of the averaged signal) of all identified peaks were printed. In each VEP, six main peaks were distinguished (Fig. 1) according to generally accepted classification schemes (1,2,5). Latency and amplitude values of these peaks were used for calculation of the mean and standard

[1] APR = average potential reference.

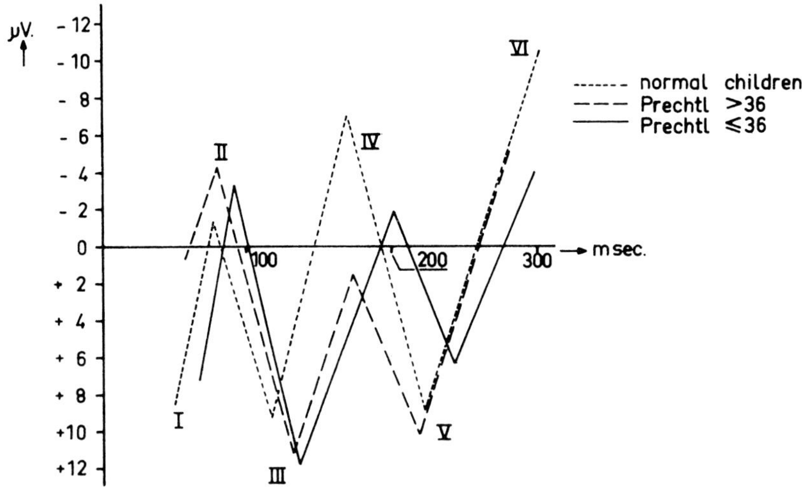

FIG 1. Comparison of the calculated mean peak I through VI latencies and amplitudes for the two Prechtl subgroups and the normal reference group.

deviation. For normal data of our laboratory, we refer to an earlier publication (2). These data for the age groups 4 to 5 and 5 to 6 years are presented in Table 1 but have not yet been statistically compared to the group under study.

RESULTS

The mean neurological score at birth for the whole group was 38.1 (SD 2.9, range 30–42); for the boys 38.4, and for the girls 38.0. This difference is not statistically significant (*t*-test).

From our own experience and from literature, it is well known that not every peak can be identified in every subject. Peak III, often called P100, is the most stable one. The number of peaks that could be identified in our material are presented in Table 2. There are no significant differences in number of peaks identified in the two subgroups (*t*-test, χ^2 test). For the whole group and the subgroups with optimal and nonoptimal neurological score, the latency and amplitude values are presented in Tables 3 and 4 and in Fig. 1, respectively.

There is a significant rank correlation (Kendall test) between Prechtl's neurological score at birth and the latency values of the VEP at the age of 5. A low neurological score (nonoptimal), as a rule, correlates with increased VEP latencies, a high score (optimal) with shorter latencies. This is true for all peaks except for peak III left and right and peak I left. The correlations for the early components are not as high as those for the late ones. For the amplitude values, the results are contradictory. In many peaks there were no significant

TABLE 1. *Latency and amplitude values of normal children 4 to 5 and 5 to 6 years old*

	Latency (msec)				Amplitude (μv)			
	Left		Right		Left		Right	
Peak	4–5 yr	5–6 yr	4–5 yr	5–6 yr	4–5 yr	5–6 yr	4–5 yr	5–6 yr
I	46 ± 5	54 ± 11	42 ± 7	58 ± 6	+4.9 ± 2.2	+13.0 ± 3.9	+3.7 ± 1.8	+12.2 ± 4.5
II	76 ± 9	80 ± 27	79 ± 15	73 ± 22	−1.6 ± 1.6	−1.3 ± 5.0	−2.4 ± 2.4	−0.1 ± 5.8
III	126 ± 29	109 ± 28	120 ± 21	113 ± 28	+7.7 ± 4.1	+9.8 ± 7.6	+7.7 ± 5.7	+11.8 ± 4.8
IV	165 ± 25	169 ± 36	173 ± 30	166 ± 35	−3.5 ± 6.2	−9.4 ± 3.8	−5.5 ± 7.2	−9.7 ± 7.8
V	217 ± 40	216 ± 30	242 ± 10	221 ± 30	+6.0 ± 2.6	+9.8 ± 7.7	+10.1 ± 1.8	+10.1 ± 10.1
VI	295 ± 35	306 ± 39	317 ± 9	299 ± 35	−6.8 ± 4.5	−14.1 ± 5.7	−5.9 ± 4.9	−15.3 ± 4.0

TABLE 2. *Number of peaks that can be identified in the total group* (N = *89*) *and subgroups with Prechtl scores* >*36* (N = *76*) and ⩽36 (N = *13*)

	Total group		Prechtl > 36		Prechtl ⩽ 36	
Peak	Left	Right	Left	Right	Left	Right
I	46	35	39	30	7	5
II	82	73	70	63	12	10
III	82	73	70	70	12	13
IV	69	68	57	57	12	11
V	67	61	55	50	12	11
VI	66	61	55	50	11	11

TABLE 3. *Latency values (msec ± SD) of total group and of subgroups based on Prechtl scores*

	total group		Pechtl > 36		Prechtl ⩽ 36	
Peak	Left	Right	Left	Right	Left	Right
I	60 ± 12	59 ± 15	58 ± 12	58 ± 15	66 ± 11	68 ± 17
II	81 ± 14	81 ± 16	80 ± 12	80 ± 15	90 ± 20	92 ± 24
III	131 ± 21	135 ± 22	130 ± 20	135 ± 21	137 ± 27	135 ± 27
IV	177 ± 38	180 ± 37	171 ± 36	175 ± 37	202 ± 40[a]	199 ± 36[a]
V	222 ± 42	224 ± 42	218 ± 41	219 ± 41	244 ± 41[a]	243 ± 43[a]
VI	282 ± 41	285 ± 42	279 ± 40	282 ± 42	300 ± 42	297 ± 42

[a] Statistically proven difference between the two subgroups (*t*-test, level of significance $p \leqslant 0.05$).

correlations; in a few cases, increased amplitudes; in other cases, decreased amplitudes. So the amplitude values are not of much worth.

CONCLUSION

Our study proves that relations exist between the neurological condition at birth, quantified by Prechtl's neurological score, and latency values for the flash-evoked VEP at the age of 5. The more optimal the neurological condition at birth, the shorter the VEP latencies at 5 years of age. This means that Prechtl's neurological score has a prognostic value and that increased VEP latencies may follow a nonoptimal neurological condition at birth. Whether, in this group, VEP latencies and EEG data correlate with clinical phenomena is under study.

TABLE 4. *Amplitude values ($\mu V \pm SD$) of total group and of subgroups based on Prechtl scores*

Peak	Total group		Prechtl > 36		Prechtl ≤ 36	
	Left	Right	Left	Right	Left	Right
I	+4.0 ± 15.1	+3.0 ± 4.5	+3.6 ± 16.2	−2.3 ± 3.8	+6.6 ± 7.5	+7.8 ± 6.1
II	−5.0 ± 3.8	−4.3 ± 4.3	−4.2 ± 5.4	−4.4 ± 4.1	−2.3 ± 5.8	−4.3 ± 6.1
III	+10.5 ± 7.4	+11.8 ± 7.2	+10.2 ± 7.3	+12.0 ± 7.4	+12.3 ± 8.3	+11.2 ± 7.8
IV	+1.2 ± 7.6	+0.8 ± 7.8	+1.6 ± 7.9	+1.4 ± 8.1	−1.8 ± 6.1	−2.1 ± 6.1
V	+9.7 ± 7.2	+9.5 ± 8.3	+10.2 ± 7.4	+10.1 ± 8.8	+6.1 ± 4.5[a]	+6.4 ± 4.2[a]
VI	−3.7 ± 13.9	−6.0 ± 5.7	−3.4 ± 15.3	−6.8 ± 5.7	−5.5 ± 5.0	−2.7 ± 5.4[a]

[a] Statistically proven difference between the two sugroups (*t*-test, level of significance $p \leq 0.05$)

REFERENCES

1. Bennett, J. S., MacDonald, J. S., Drance, S. M., and Nenoyame, K. (1971): Some statistical properties of the visual evoked potential in man and their application as a criteria of normality. *IEEE Trans. Biomed. Eng.*, 1:23–34.
2. Blom, J. L., Barth, P. G., and Visser, S. L. (1980): The visual evoked potential in the first six years of life. *Electroencephalogr. Clin. Neurophysiol.*, 48:395–405.
3. Capute, A. J., Niedermeyer, E. F. L., and Richardson, F. (1968): The electroencephalogram in children with minimal cerebral dysfunction. *Pediatrics*, 41:1104–1114.
4. Conners, C. K. (1970): Cortical visual evoked response in children with learning disorders. *Psychophysiology*, 7:418–428.
5. Dustman, R. E., and Beck, E. C. (1969): The effects of maturation and aging on the wave form of visually evoked potentials. *Electroencephalogr. Clin. Neurophysiol.*, 26:2–11.
6. Gambi, D., Rossini, P. M., Albertini, G., Sollazzo, D., Torrioli, M. G., and Polidori, G. C. (1980): Follow-up of visual evoked potential in full-term and pre-term control newborns and in subjects who suffered from perinatal respiratory distress. *Electroencephalogr. Clin. Neurophysiol.*, 48:509–516.
7. Hrbek, A., Karlberg, P., Kjellmer, I., Olsson, T., and Riha, M. (1977): Clinical application of evoked electroencephalographic responses in newborn infants. I. Perinatal asphyxia. *Dev. Med. Child Neurol.*, 19:34–44.
8. Hughes, J. R. (1971): Electroencephalography and learning disabilities. In: *Progress in learning disabilities, Vol. II*, edited by H. R. Myckleburst, pp. 18–55. Grune & Stratton, New York.
9. Klinkerfuss, G. H., Lange, P. H., Weinberg, W. A., and O'Leary, J. L. (1965): Electroencephalographic abnormalities of children with hyperkinetic behavior. *Neurology (Minneap.)*, 15:883–891.
10. Njiokiktjien, C. J., Visser, S. L., and De Rijke, W. (1977): EEG and visual evoked responses in children with learning disorders. *Neuropaediatrie*, 8:134–147.
11. Paine, R. S., Werry, J. S., and Quay, H. C. (1968): A study of minimal cerebral dysfunction. *Dev. Med. Child Neurol.*, 10:505–520.
12. Prechtl, H. F. R. (1977): The neurological examination of the full-term newborn infant. In: *Clinics in Developmental Medicine, Second Edition, Vol. 63*, pp. 1–68. Heinemann, London.
13. Preston, M. S., Guthrie, J. T., and Childs, B. (1974): Visual evoked responses (VERs) in normal and disabled readers. *Psychophysiology*, 11:452–457.
14. Satterfield, J. H. (1973): EEG issues in children with minimal brain dysfunction. *Semin. Psychiatry*, 5(1):35–46.
15. Satterfield, J. H., and Braley, B. W. (1977): Evoked potentials and brain maturation in hyperactive and normal children. *Electroencephalogr. Clin. Neurophysiol.*, 43:43–51.
16. Sohmer, H., and Student, M. (1978): Auditory nerve and brain-stem evoked responses in normal, autistic, minimal brain dysfunction and psychomotor retarded children. *Electroencephalogr. Clin. Neurophysiol.*, 44:380–388.
17. Stolte, L. A. M., Van den Berg, A. F., Bouw, G. M., De Jong, P. A., Van Kessel, H., Kurver, P. H. J., Njiokiktjien, Ch. J., and Voorhorst, F. J. (1980): Neurological status of the newborn infant as an endpoint of fetal well-being. In: *Fetal Monitoring. Current Concepts and Controversies*, edited by T. K. A. B. Eskes, H. P. van Gijn, and G. W. M. Theunissen, pp. 151–169. University of Nijmegen, The Netherlands.
18. Symann-Louett, N., Gascon, G. G., Matsumiya, Y., and Lombroso, C. T. (1977): Wave form difference in visual evoked responses between normal and reading disabled children. *Neurology (Minneap.)*, 27:156–159.
19. Zambelli, A. J., Stamm, J. S., Maitinsky, S., and Loiselle, D. L. (1977): Auditory evoked potentials and selective attention in formerly hyperactive adolescent boys. *Am. J. Psychiatry*, 134:742–747.

Clinical Applications of Evoked Potentials in Neurology,
edited by J. Courjon, F. Mauguiere, and M. Revol.
Raven Press, New York © 1982.

Evaluation of Cerebral Function in Newborn Infants with Fetal Growth Retardation

*Antonin Hrbek, *Knut Iversen, and **Torsten Olsson

**Department of Pediatrics, University of Göteborg, S-416 85 Göteborg, Sweden; and **Research Laboratory of Medical Electronics, Chalmers University of Technology, S-412 96 Göteborg, Sweden*

Fetal growth retardation (FGR) is an important risk factor. Follow-up studies have shown that children born too small have a greater disadvantage and are more likely to present further neurodevelopmental problems than children born too soon. More sophisticated methods of EEG processing and polygraphic recordings have shown during the last 10 years some disturbances of nervous function in at least a part of small-for-gestational-age (SGA) newborns. The sleep–wakefulness cycle may be disorganized and EEG maturation often retarded or abnormal (9,11,12). Experiments on effects of malnutrition in growing rats resulted in decreased numbers of nerve cells and synapses, impaired myelinization, and retarded development of enzymes (1–5,13,14).

The purpose of this study was to get more information about CNS function in SGA newborns by means of the evoked potential (EP) technique which is very useful for assessment of maturity (8) and risk for cerebral damage (6,7). Human FGR is caused not only by undernutrition but also by other factors such as genetic, toxic, and social influences, infections, drugs, etc. Recent studies have shown that alcohol abuse during pregnancy often results in FGR. These infants also have an increased incidence of neurodevelopmental abnormalities, e.g., fetal alcohol syndrome (10). Therefore a group of newborns and infants of mothers with maternal alcohol abuse syndrome (MAA) was also examined.

MATERIAL AND METHOD

This report is based on examinations of 37 SGA newborns, 25 newborns and infants of MAA, and 25 normal newborns appropriate for gestational age (AGA). Most of the newborns were examined during the first week of life. Eleven SGA newborns and 10 infants born to MAA were reexamined later. The study was performed in a separate room in the neonatal unit of the Department of Pediatrics. In almost all infants, EPs were recorded during sleep. Electrodes were placed according to the International 10–20 System; bipolar derivations were used, and the responses were averaged on a PDP-12 digital computer. Visual EPs to flashes (three different interstimulus intervals, ISI, were used: 10, 3, and 1 sec) and SEPs to electrical stimulation of the median nerve were recorded in all infants, and BAEPs in 27 SGA and 15 MAA infants. The recording and stimulation technique for SEPs has been described in detail previously (6). For more quantitative evaluation of EP abnormalities, a scoring system was used which was originally devised for examinations of newborns with perinatal asphyxia (6). Previously unpublished results on the follow-up of these children showed a high incidence of brain damage when EP risk score exceeded 40% of the highest possible number of risk points.

RESULTS

Development of EPs during the early period of life is characterized by increasing complexity, diminution and disappearance of slow waves, increasing number of fast deflections, and decreasing latencies. In full-term newborn infants (37 to 42 weeks' gestation), the morphology of a VEP differs widely from that of adults. Most characteristic is the constant positive–negative complex I and II (Fig. 1). The latency of these components is closely related to gestational age (Table 1). Their amplitudes show extreme interindividual variations but are rather stable intraindividually and dependent on stimulation frequency. The positive–negative complex is usually followed by two slower waves (III, IV), which are much more variable in shape, latency, and amplitude. Often, small deflections preceding the whole response can be seen, but they are not constant.

The response pattern of VEPs in SGA newborns generally corresponded to

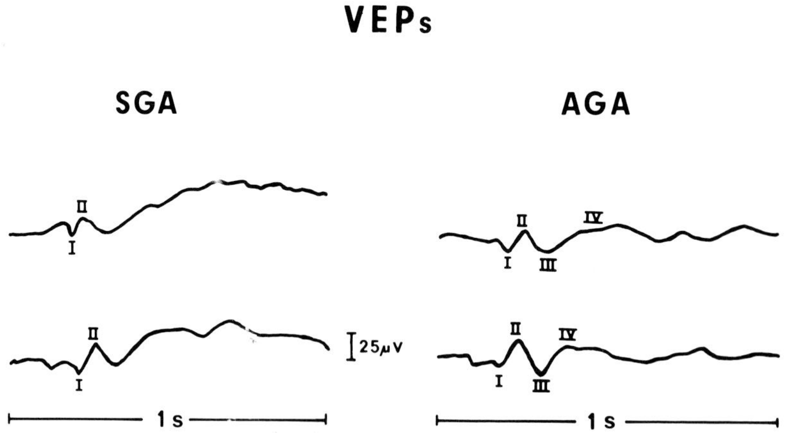

FIG. 1. Visual EPs in two SGA newborns **(left)** and AGA newborns **(right).** In SGA newborns, the characteristic initial fast components I and II are followed by a slow wave. Deviations O_z–P_z; 30 responses averaged. In this and all following figures, upward deflections represent negativity.

TABLE 1. *Latencies (msec) of deflections I and II*[a]

Gestational age (weeks)	I	II
37	197	244
38	192	239
39	187	234
40	182	228
41	176	223
42	171	218

[a]Standard deviation of peak I is 12 msec, that of peak II, 10 msec. The values are based on examination of more than 1,000 infants in laboratories in Prague, Groningen, and Gothenburg.

gestational age, but in 57% of cases, a very slow negative wave following the initial complex (positive–negative deflection) was present (Fig. 1) as a symptom of some immaturity. Similar waves dominate the response pattern in the preterm newborn. Latency distribution of VEPs around the mean (for age) was not symmetrical in SGA newborns (Fig. 2). There was a clear shift towards longer values, and in 16.6% of cases, the latency shift exceeded +2 SD. When shorter ISIs than 10 sec were used, latencies increased even more (Fig. 3), and VEPs diminished or disappeared. Both immature characteristics and increased exhaustibility seemed to be transient; the rate of normalization was different. Distinct abnormalities of VEPs responsible for a high risk score exceeding 40% of the highest possible number of risk points was present only in one case (2.7%).

Immature characteristics of VEPs were also present in MAA infants (40%), but in 25% of cases, quite abnormal response patterns were observed (Fig. 4), and a risk score higher than 40% was present in 17% of these infants.

Somatosensory EPs showed immature characteristics in 25.6% of SGA newborns, and the latency distribution was similar to that of VEPs. Surprising was the finding of distinct side differences in 37.1% of SGA newborns. There was only one case with similar differences in the control group (a monozygotic twin to a SGA sibling). Infants of MAA showed a high incidence of distinct SEP abnormalities (56%) including very bad, flat responses and absence of early or late components (Fig. 5). In 52% the changes were unilateral. In 32% of cases in this group, the SEP risk score was above 40%.

The morphology of BAEPs in normal newborns is similar to that in adults, but the transmission time (I–V difference) is longer, 5.3 msec (SD, 0.28) in our data on 150 infants. A bad response with very low amplitude and hardly identifiable components following peak I was observed in only one case among the SGA newborns. It was a dizygotic twin who later developed psychomotor retardation. In the group of MAA infants, three had a prolonged brainstem

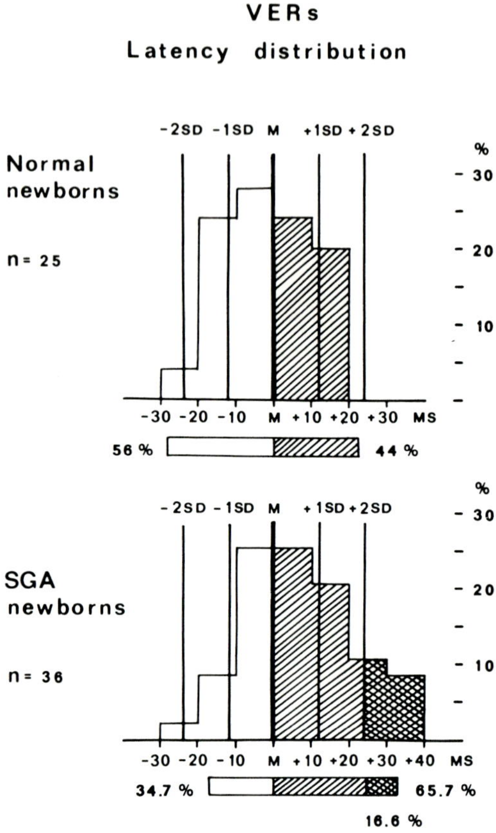

FIG. 2. Latency distribution of VEPs around the mean for gestational age in AGA **(above)** and SGA **(below)** newborns. ISI, 10 sec.

transmission time; this was not discovered during the neonatal period but only at the age of 7 months to 2½ years.

CONCLUSIONS

The development of cerebral functions assessed by means of EPs generally follows gestational age, even during FGR, and there is no direct relationship to birth weight. Nevertheless, in many SGA newborns, EPs had some immature characteristics, mostly in the form of late slow waves. Increased exhaustibility observed in VEP examinations may be a sign of increased vulnerability. Longer latencies could be explained by impaired myelinization, but further prolongation with shorter intervals between stimuli gives evidence that the metabolism of transmitter substances is affected. For evident abnormalities such as side differences in SEPs, other factors besides undernutrition may be responsible. The

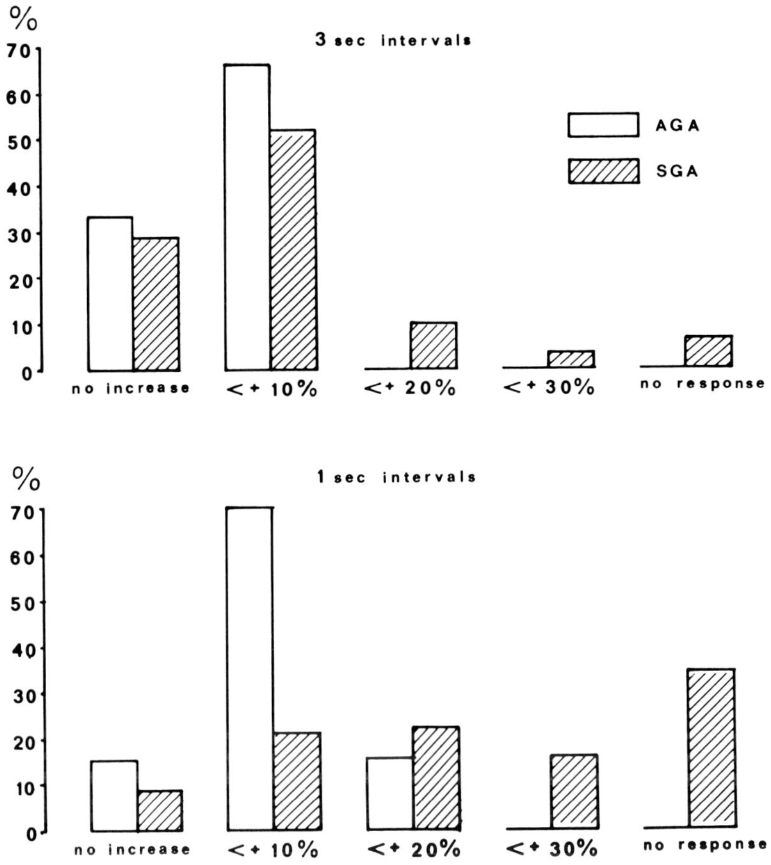

FIG. 3. Increase of latencies of VEPs with shorter ISIs in AGA and SGA newborns.

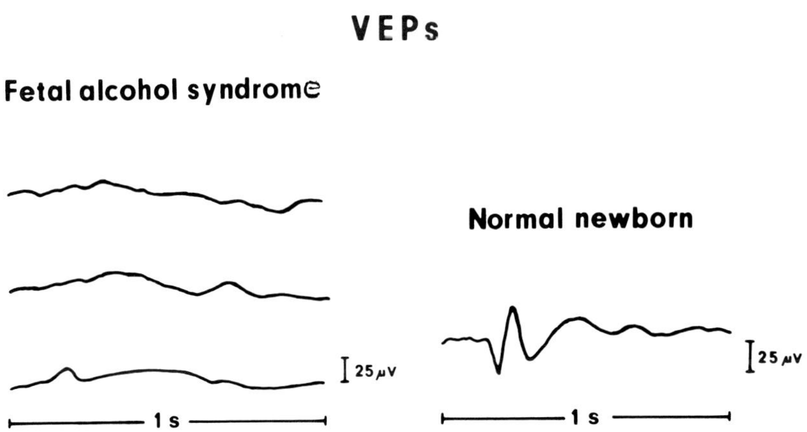

FIG. 4. Quite abnormal VEPs in three newborns with fetal alcohol syndrome **(left)** in comparison with a typical normal response pattern **(right)**. Deviations, O_z–P_z; 30 responses averaged.

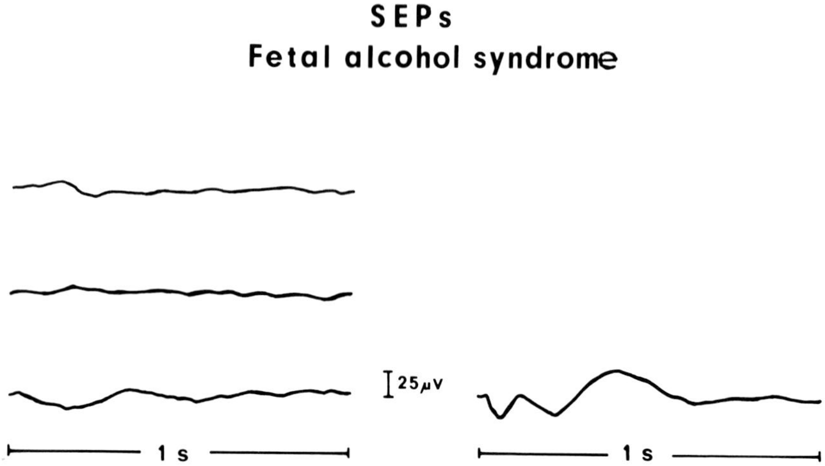

FIG. 5. Abnormal SEPS in three newborns with fetal alcohol syndrome **(left)** in comparison with a normal response pattern **(right).** Deviations, C_3– or C_4–F_z; 50 responses averaged.

role of these factors is well demonstrated in the group of MAA infants in whom the incidence of distinctly abnormal EPs was significantly enlarged. We can conclude that, as in previous studies in newborns with perinatal asphyxia or respiratory distress, recording of EPs is a very valuable objective method for studies of brain function in the very early period of life, at a time where no or very few neurological symptoms are present.

REFERENCES

1. Adlard, B. P. F., and Dobbings, J. (1972): Vulnerability of developing brain. V. Effects of fetal and postnatal undernutrition on regional brain enzyme activities in three-week-old rats. *Pediatr. Res.,* 6:38–42.
2. Adlard, B. P. F., and Dobbing, J. (1972): Vulnerability of developing brain. 8. Regional acetylcholinesterase activity in the brains of adult rats undernourished in early life. *Br. J. Nutr.,* 28:139–143.
3. Bass, N. H., Netsky, M. G., and Younge, E. (1970): Effect of neonatal malnutrition on developing cerebrum. I. Michrochemical and histologic study of cellular differentiation in the rat. *Arch. Neurol.,* 23:289–302.
4. Bass, N. H., Netsky, M. G., and Younge, E. (1970): Effect of neonatal malnutrition on developing cerebrum. II. Michrochemical and histologic study of myelin formation in the rat. *Arch. Neurol.,* 23:303–313.
5. Coyle, J. T., and Enna, S. J. (1976): Neurochemical aspects of the ontogenesis of gabaergic neuron in the rat brain. *Brain Res.,* 111:119–133.
6. Hrbek, A., Karlberg, P., Kjellmer, I., Olsson, T., and Riha, M. (1977): Clinical application of evoked response EEG in newborn infants. I. Perinatal asphyxia. *Dev. Med. Child Neurol.,* 19:34–44.
7. Hrbek, A., Karlberg, P., Kjellmer, I., Olsson, T., Riha, M. (1978): Clinical application of evoked EEG responses in newborn infants. II: Idiopathic respiratory distress syndrome. *Dev. Med. Child Neurol.,* 20:619–626.
8. Hrbek, A., Karlberg, P., and Olsson, T. (1973): Development of visual and somatosensory

evoked response in preterm newborn infants. *Electrocephalogr. Clin. Neurophysiol.,* 34:225–232.
9. Kazuyoshi, W., Katsuhoko, I., and Kimiko, H. (1974): Development of slow-wave sleep in low-birthweight infants. *Dev. Med. Child Neurol.,* 16:23–31.
10. Olegård, R., Sabel, K. G., Aronsson, M., Sandin, B., Johansson, P. R., Carlsson, C., Kyllerman, M., Iversen, K., and Hrbek, A. (1979): Effects on the child of alcohol abuse during pregnancy. *Acta Paediatr. Scand.* [*Suppl.*], 275:112–121.
11. Prechtl, H. F. R., Vos, J. E., Akiyama, Y., and Casaer, P. (1973): Neonatal EEG: Age, codes and coherence functions in relation to intra-uterine growth and oestrogen levels. In: *Ontogenesis of the Brain,* Vol. II, edited by L. Jílek and S. Trojan, pp. 201–210. Universita Karlova, Praha.
12. Schulte, F. J., Hinze, G., and Schrempf, G. (1971): Maternal toxemia, fetal malnutrition and bioelectric brain activity of the newborn. *Neuropaediatrie,* 2:439–460.
13. Sereni, F., Principe, N., and Pinceni Sereni, L., (1966): Undernutrition and the developing brain. I. Influence of acetylcholinesterase and succinic acid dehydrogenase activities and on norepinephrine and 5-OH tryptamine tissue concentrations. *Biol. Neonatol.,* 10:254–265.
14. Smart, J. L., and Dobbing, J. (1971): Vulnerability of developing brain. II. Effects of early nutritional deprivation on reflex ontogeny and development of behaviour in the rat. *Brain Res.,* 28:85–95.

Clinical Applications of Evoked Potentials in Neurology, edited by J. Courjon, F. Mauguiere, and M. Revol. Raven Press, New York © 1982.

Visual Evoked Potentials in Children with Nonhemiplegic Cerebral Palsy

P. Laget, L. Gagnard, C. Ostre, and A. M. d'Allest

Laboratoire d'Electroencéphalographie et de Neurophysiologie, Clinique de l'Enfant, Hôpital Trousseau, Paris 75012, France; and Institut National de Réadaptation, St. Maurice 94410, France

Much study and care has been devoted to the purely locomotor disabilities of children with cerebral palsy; only relatively recently has attention been turned to the perceptuomotor dysfunctions that also occur (1). These poorly understood disorders frequently impair the childrens' abilities to learn, leading to problems that are often more disabling than their motor handicaps. Until now, few possibilities were afforded for appreciating by objective methods the presence and extent of these perceptive, especially visual, defects. The results obtained in a previous study on the modifications of the somesthetic evoked potentials (SEP) and the good correlation existing between the lateralization of the clinical signs and the alterations of the responses (5) prompted us to explore cortical visual potentials in children suffering from other forms of cerebral palsy (spasticity, choreoathetosis, and so forth) in which the presence of cortical lesions is less obvious than in hemiplegy but in which the perceptuomotor disorders are very common and represent a heavy handicap.

MATERIAL AND METHODS

We studied 69 pathological children between 3 and 15 years of age and 50 normal subjects of the same age group. In all children VEP were recorded, and in pathological patients one or more EEG examinations were performed.

Clinical Features

Table 1 summarizes the main neurological signs of the subjects, the existence of convulsive fits, and EEG findings at the moment when the VEP were performed.

The ophthalmological features are reported in Table 2. Unfortunately, a complete set of data could not be obtained from all patients, for a number of them were poorly cooperative.

TABLE 1. *Major neurological signs of subjects*

Main pathological motor symptom	Convulsive seizure	Paroxysmal anomalies in EEG
Spasticity, 49	14 (28.6%)	21 (42.9%)
Spastic tetraplegy, 15	4	7
Spastic triplegy, 8	3	5
Spastic diplegy, 26	7	9
Athetosis, 16	5 } (25%)	4 } (25%)
Cerebellar symptoms, 4	0 }	1 }

TABLE 2. *Ophthalmological features of subjects*

Eye examination finding	
Normal	44
Alterations	11
Unknown	14
Strabism	
Normal	43
Strabic	26
Unknown	0
Visual acuity	
Normal	7
Low remote acuity	25
Unknown	37
Refractory defects	
Absent	20
Present	15
Unknown	34

In Table 3 are collected the obstetrical antecedents, the term and weight at birth, and the mental level, whenever possible.[1]

The 50 normal subjects were emmetropic, free from neurological defects or convulsive fits, and normal with respect to mental and psychomotor development.

Visual Evoked Potential Recordings

An electrode was placed on each occipital scalp 2 cm from the midline, and the VEP derived between each occipital electrode and a frontal or sometimes earlobe reference electrode in order to avoid the artifact caused by eye blinking.

Two types of stimuli were used. The first was a conventional blue–white

[1] The main nonverbal tests used were: Brunet-Lésine, (nonverbal) Borel-Maissony, (nonverbal) WISC, Leiter, Columbia.

TABLE 3. *Obstetrical antecedents and mental level*

Birth weight	
Over 2,500 g	23
Under 2,500 g	30
Unknown	16
Term	
More than 8 months	31
Less than 8 months	24
Unknown	14
Reanimation	
Unnecessary	30
Necessary	22
Unknown	17
IQ (nonverbal performance)	
Higher than 90	6
Between 60 and 90	11
Lower than 60	32
Unknown	20

flash of a 20 μsec duration and an energy of 0.3 joules. The flash lamp was set in front of the subject's eye at a distance of 20 cm. The stimulus frequency was 0.5/sec. Fifty flashes were used for each recording. The second stimulus was produced by a television screen which could deliver two different frames: the first was only the white diffuse field of the illuminated screen; the second was a rectangular checkboard of 24 white and black squares. The screen was set 1.50 m in front of the subject, and the shapes of the squares were chosen so that the subtended square edge was 1° between the center of each square and those of the adjacent ones. The luminance of both stimuli was the same and equal to 2.5 lux. The white screen or the checkboard was presented during 750 msec and followed by an extinction of 1,250 msec. The duration of each full cycle was 2 sec. Fifty presentations were used for the recording of the evoked potentials. All recordings were made in a dark room with a background illumination of 0.25 lux.

The cortical signals, after appropriate amplification, were fed into a four-channel computer of average transients and projected on an X–Y plotter.

Electroencephalogram Recordings

Routine EEG recordings were obtained on a 10-channel electroencephalograph with bipolar leads. Recordings were taken from children awake but with eyes closed. When the mental development of the subject permitted, we used a 4-min hyperventilation. In all cases, an intermittent light stimulation was performed.

Selected Parameters in the Analysis of Responses

VEPS Obtained by Flashes

In each response in normal and pathological subjects, we considered number, signs, and latencies to peak of the various deflections and compared the peak-to-peak amplitudes between right and left occipital VEP to determine casual asymmetry.

VEPS Obtained by Diffuse or Patterned Light Stimulation

In each "on" and "off" response we considered number, signs, and latencies to peak of various deflections and compared the peak-to-peak amplitudes between right and left occipital responses.

In addition, in each normal or pathological subject, we compared the "on" and "off" responses produced by diffuse or patterened light stimulation. Four criteria of intraindividual comparison were used: (a) number and signs of deflections; (b) latencies to peak; (c) peak-to-peak amplitudes; and (d) presence or absence of an afterdischarge.

An "on" or "off" afterdischarge was considered present if two or more deflections were observed 350 msec after the beginning or the end of the stimulus presentation.

The difference in the (a) criterion was considered significant (+) if the responses differed in at least two deflections. For the criterion (b), the difference was considered significant (+) if the difference between latencies to peak in at least two deflections was equal to or greater than 20%. For the criterion (c), the differences were significant (+) if the difference between the peak-to-peak amplitudes was equal to or greater than 15%.

For the criterion (d), the only quoted difference (+) was between absence or presence of an afterdischarge.

In each subject, responses evoked by diffuse and patterned light stimulation, respectively, and taken as a whole were estimated significantly different (+) if they differed by the criterion (a) plus one of the three other criteria or by the three criteria (b), (c), and (d) in "on" and/or "off" responses and were not significantly different in all other cases.

RESULTS

Visual Evoked Potentials in Normal Subjects

Visual evoked potentials produced by flashes are comparable to those described in a previous work (3) and recorded in normal children in the same age range. The diagrams of Fig. 1 summarize the main features of the responses: mean values and standard deviations of latencies to peak and presence percentages

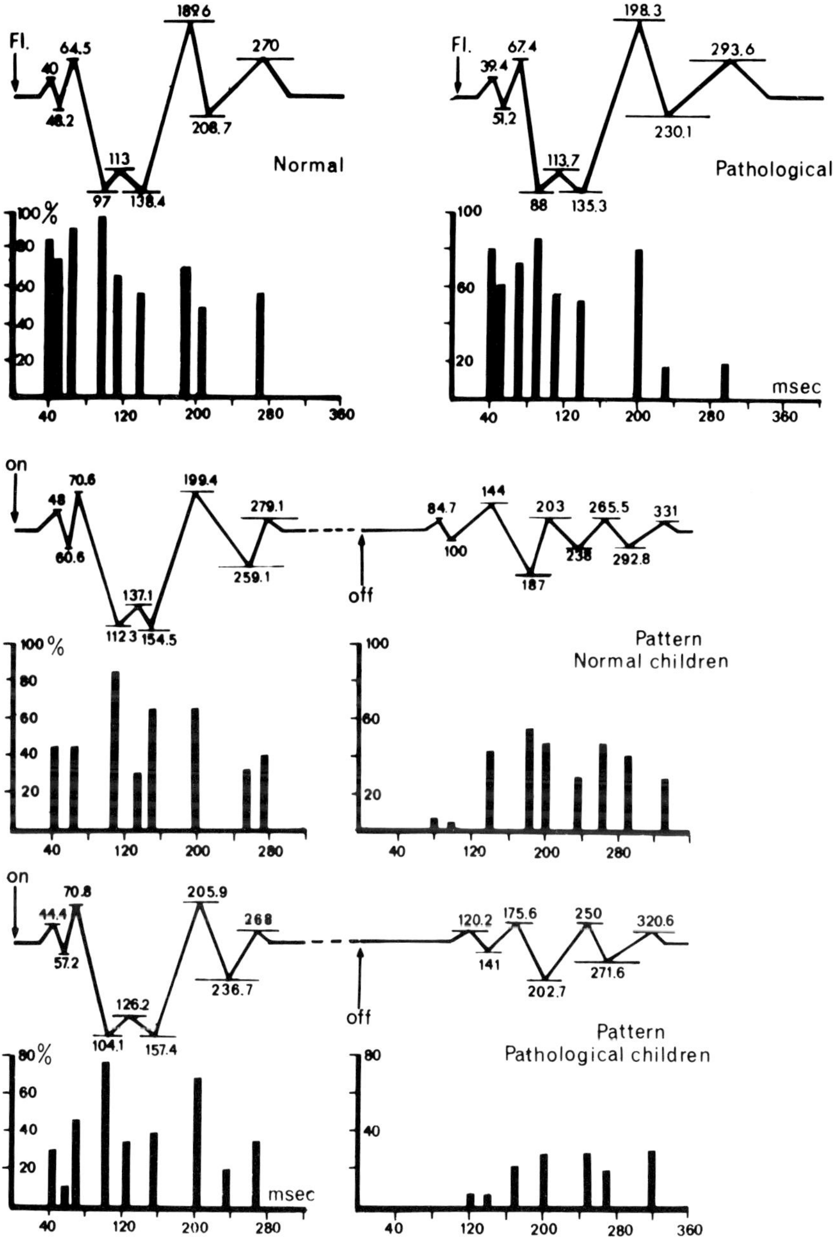

FIG. 1. Diagrams of the mean responses obtained by flash (Fl) and patterned stimuli in normal and pathological children. The standard deviations of the latencies to peak are indicated by *horizontal lines*. The *vertical bars* represent the presence percentages of each deflection. The only marked differences are observed in the "off" responses (especially in the presence percentages).

of each deflection. These values are the same in right and left occipital VEP, and the differences in peak-to-peak amplitudes are between 20 and 30% in five subjects (10%), between 10 and 20% in 16 (32%), and less than 10% in 29 (58%).

The VEP produced by patterned or diffuse light stimuli are shown in diagrams of Figs. 1 and 2. In the "on" responses, P_2 (100) is the most constant and conspicuous deflection. The general morphology is very similar to that of responses produced by flash, but mean values of latencies to peak are larger, and presence percentages of each deflection have lower values because of the differences in the stimulation intensity.

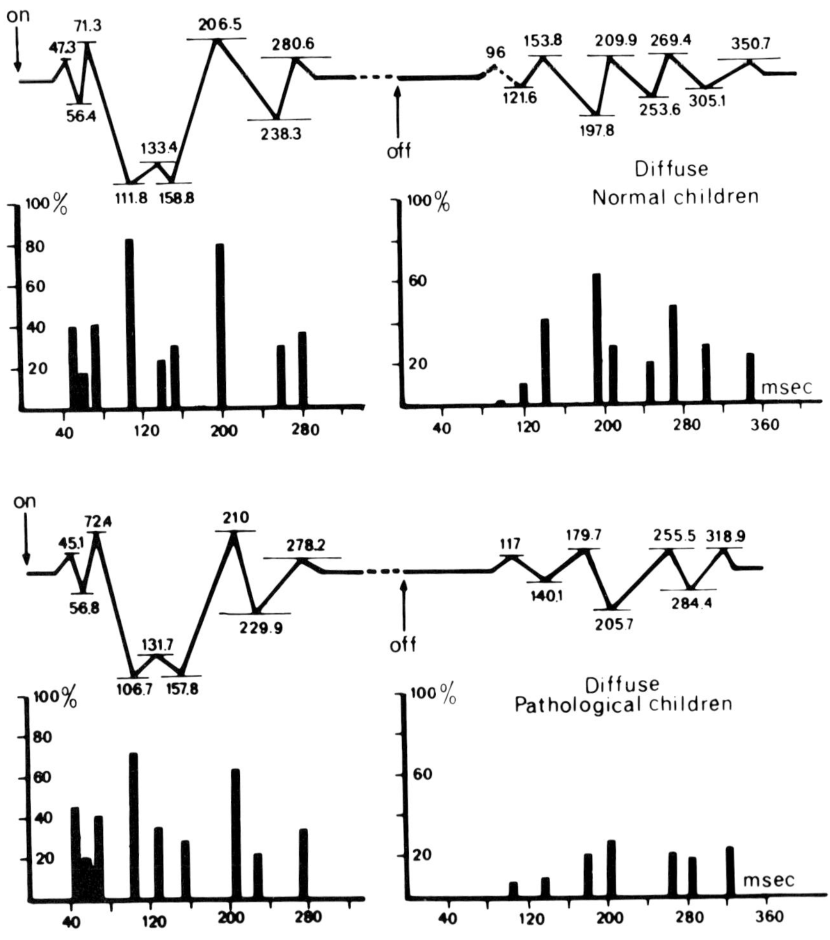

FIG. 2. Diagrams of the mean responses obtained by diffuse stimulus in normal and pathological subjects. The only marked differences are in the "off" responses. Display as in Fig. 1.

The "off" responses are present in every subject. Their morphology is complex. Their amplitude is usually lower than that of the "on" responses, and latency to peak of the main positive deflection is important. In the whole group, the mean values of the latencies and the presence percentages of deflections are not significantly different in VEP produced by patterned or diffuse light stimulation, but comparison of the intraindividual responses gives a quite different result. Indeed, the use of the criteria previously reported shows that intraindividual differences are present in every child of the normal group (Fig. 3).

Visual Evoked Potentials in Pathological Subjects

The VEP produced by flash were not significantly different from normal and exhibited a degree of asymmetry in the same range of variations. Indeed, the differences of peak-to-peak amplitudes in right and left occipital responses were between 20 and 30% in nine subjects (13.1%), between 10 and 20% in 17 (24.6%), and less than 10% in 43 (62.3%).

In the VEP produced by patterned or diffuse stimulation, the "on" response did not exhibit significant differences with respect to that of normal subjects (see diagrams of Figs. 1 and 2), but the "off" responses were absent in 17 patients (27.1%), and in the other children, the latencies to peak and presence percentages of the main deflections were different.

But the most interesting observation consisted in the intraindividual comparison between the VEP produced by patterned and diffuse light stimulation. Indeed, in 22 patients (31.9%), there was no observed intraindividual difference between VEP produced by both stimuli, whereas this situation was never encountered in normal subjects (Fig. 4).

This puzzling result about VEP recorded in pathological subjects suggested a search for a possible correlation with various clinical and electroencephalographical signs or antecedents.

Electroencephalographical Correlations

Table 1 summarized the main features of the EEG recordings. The results confirm those of previous authors (2). Indeed, the proportion of paroxysmal alterations in spastic subjects (21/49, 42.9%) is higher than in choreoathetotic and cerebellar ones (5/20, 25%), but there was no significant correlation between the presence of paroxysmal anomalies and presence or absence of intraindividual differences in VEP produced by diffuse or patterned stimuli ($\chi^2 = 1.4$, $p = 0.76$).

Electroclinical Correlations

No correlation was encountered between subjects exhibiting presence or absence of intraindividual differences in VEP produced by patterened or diffuse

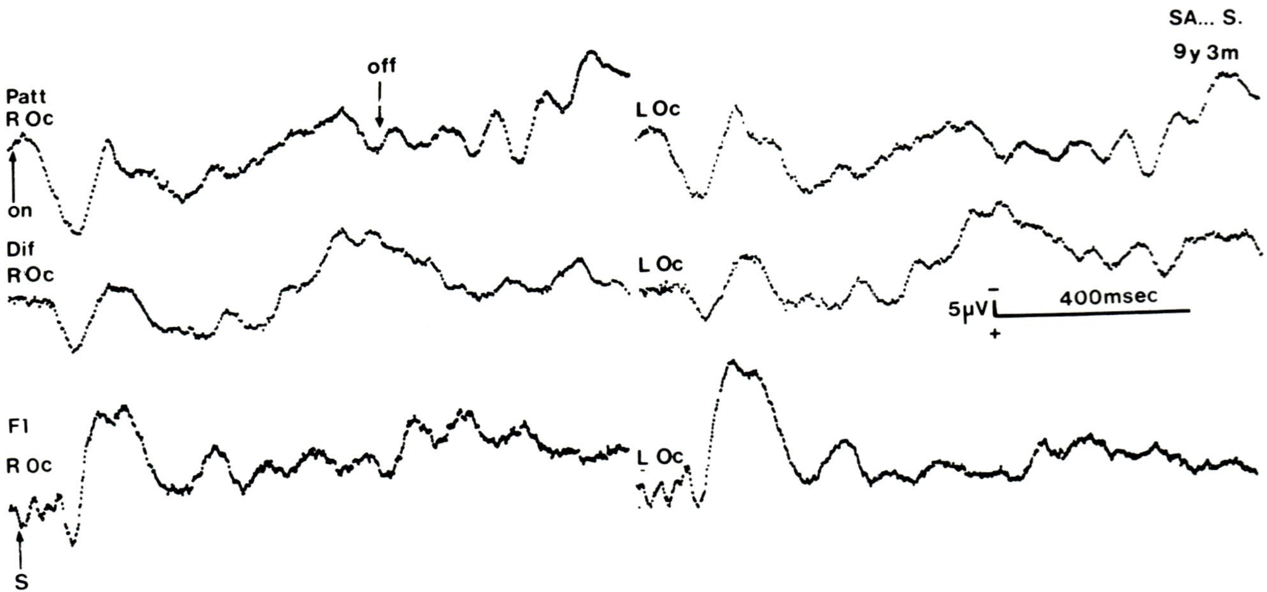

FIG. 3. Visual evoked potentials recorded in a normal child. The differences in morphology, latencies, and amplitudes between the responses obtained by patterned and diffuse stimuli are clearly marked.

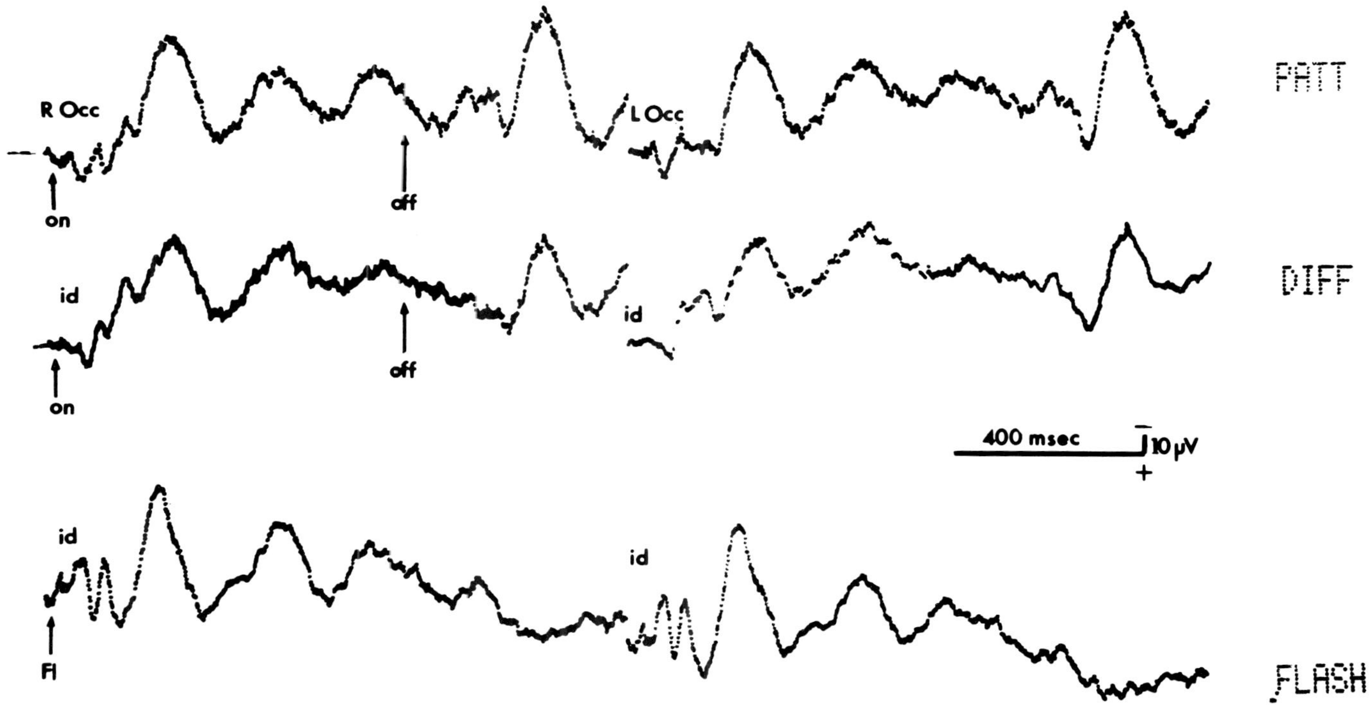

FIG. 4 Visual evoked potentials recorded in a spastic child of the same age as in Fig. 3. The differences between the responses produced by patterned and diffuse stimuli are negligible.

light stimulation and clinical data concerning (a) ophthalmological signs, (b) presence or absence of spasticity, (c) birth weight, or (d) neonatal reanimation.

A good correlation was found with mental level. Indeed, if the set of pathological subjects was divided into three groups—IQ < 60, IQ between 60 and 90, and IQ > 90—patients of the highest level exhibited more intraindividual differences in VEP, and the correlation was statistically significant ($\chi^2 = 8.30$, $p = 0.98$).

There was also a correlation with presence of prematurity (pregnancy shorter than 8 months). Indeed, in this case, $\chi^2 = 5.83$, and $p = 0.98$.

DISCUSSION AND CONCLUSION

Our first comment is that, in pathologic subjects, stimulation by flash cannot always be sufficient to bring out alterations of the VEP, and stimulation by patterned stimulus is necessary. However, this method reveals its limitations when it involves both a noticeable lengthening of the examination time and increased cooperation of the patient. Together, these can raise obstacles to correct recordings in awake encephalopathic children, and in our group of pathologic subjects, we think that we have approached the limit of the possibilities.

If we consider the presence or absence of electroclinical correlations, some points deserve attention. It was somewhat puzzling to observe no significant correlation between the various ophthalmological troubles of the patients and the presence or absence of differences in the VEP produced by both types of stimulus (pattern versus diffuse). Indeed, it is known that the use of a patterned stimulus is a good objective method for determination of low visual acuity and various refractive troubles (7). We think that the choice of a pattern in which the differences in contrast (black and white squares) subtended a large visual angle (1°) permitted partial elimination of the disturbing influences of the trivial ametropies.

The absence of a positive correlation among EEG alterations, convulsive fits, and the VEP could be thought of as a confirmation of the results that we obtained in epileptic children in the same age range (4) who exhibited paroxysmal responses (spikes, spike waves) to intermittent light stimulation (ILS). Indeed, in these subjects, no significant differences in the VEP produced by various stimulation frequencies could be observed relative to reference groups of normal or pathological children who were insensitive to the ILS.

Our results also show that the type of the predominant neurological signs (spasticity or choreoathetosis) could not be positively correlated with alterations of the VEP. We do not think this situation very surprising, for many subjects (see Table 1) showed a large diffusion of neurological symptoms, especially in spastics. Therefore, it was possible to assume a similar diversity in localization and extent of the cerebral lesions and, therefore, privileged relations between visual cortical areas and the nervous structures of autonomic or voluntary control of movement and muscular tonus should be ruled out.

The significant statistical correlation between the nonverbal mental level of the children and the alterations of the VEP seems a valuable justification of the method. It is possible that the use of more sophisticated and discriminative patterned stimuli in which the cognitive visual factors would be more important would permit the objective measurement of discrete perturbations of visual perception in children suffering from less massive neurological troubles than our patients.

The positive and significant correlation observed between the alterations of the VEP and the birth term could be related to some anatomic–pathological data. Indeed, various publications (e.g., 6) have clearly established that ischemic ante- or perinatal lesions accountable for neurologic problems (especially motor) are followed by an infarction of the white matter, producing a periventricular leucomalacia. This alteration related to peculiarities of the fetal brain vascularization predominates in the white matter of the occipital lobe, especially in the optic radiations. This model could support an anatomic–functional justification of the observed correlation.

REFERENCES

1. Abercrombie, M. L. J. (1964): *Little Club Clinics in Developmental Medicine. 11. Perceptual and Visuo-Motor Disorders in Cerebral Palsy.* Spastics Society Medical Education and Information Unit in association with William Heinemann, London.
2. Gibbs, F. A., Gibbs, E. Z., Perlstein, M. A., and Rich, C. L. (1963): Electroencephalographic and clinical aspects of cerebral palsy. *Pediatrics,* 32:73–84.
3. Laget, P., Flores-Guevara, R., d'Allest, A. M., Ostre, C., Raimbault, J., and Mariani, J. (1977): La maturation des réponses évoquées visuelles chez l'enfant normal. *Electroencephalogr. Clin. Neurophysiol.,* 43:732–744.
4. Laget, P., Flores-Guevara, R., Mariani, J., and Raimbault, J. (1978): Etude des réponses évoquées visuelles chez le grand enfant normal ou présentant des réponses paroxystiques à la stimulation lumineuse intermittente. *Electroencephalogr. Clin. Neurophysiol.,* 44:626–640.
5. Laget, P., Salbreux, R., Raimbault, J., and d'Allest, A. M. (1976): Relationship between changes in somesthetic evoked responses and electroencephalographic findings in the child with hemiplegia. *Dev. Med. Child Neurol.,* 18:620–631.
6. Pape, E. K., and Wigglesworth, J. S. (1979): *Haemorrhage, ischaemia and the perinatal brain.* Spastics International Medical Publications and Williams Heinemann, London, and J. B. Lippincott, Philadelphia.
7. Sokol, S. (1977): Visual evoked potentials to checkboard pattern stimuli in strabismic amblyopia. In: *Visual Evoked Potentials in Man: New Developments,* edited by J. E. Desmedt, pp. 410–417. Clarendon Press, Oxford.

Clinical Applications of Evoked Potentials in Neurology,
edited by J. Courjon, F. Mauguiere, and M. Revol.
Raven Press, New York © 1982.

Visual Evoked Potentials in Aging of the Brain

V. Cosi, E. Vitelli, L. Gozzoli, A. Corona, M. Ceroni, R. Callieco

Institute of Neurology, University of Pavia, 27100, Pavia, Italy

There have been a number of contributions to the literature that have addressed the EP modifications that occur both in normal subjects with age (e.g., 2) and in elderly demented people (6). At present, computerized tomography (CT) supplies us with morphometric data that can be usefully related to EP. Our research aims at defining the possible modifications of VEP according to age both in subjects without atrophy visible at CT (elderly normals) and in people with cerebral atrophy at CT (elderly persons with or without dementia).

MATERIAL AND METHOD

The investigation was carried out on 78 hospitalized patients (44 males, 34 females) aged between 41 and 80 (mean age 61.2). All of the subjects were examined from neurological and neuropsychological points of view and were submitted to EEG, skull X-ray, CT, and to the study of VEPs. For our purpose, the subjects were divided into two groups on a CT basis: group I (30 cases) included those subjects without any sign of cerebral atrophy; group II (48 cases) including those subjects with cerebral atrophy. This second group was further divided into two subgroups: group II-A (30 cases), subjects with cerebral atrophy without dementia, and group II-B (18 cases), subjects with cerebral atrophy and dementia. The 18 cases of group II-B (atrophy and dementia, mean age 62.6, range 41–80) were labeled as senile and presenile dementia. The 30 cases of group II-A (atrophy without dementia, mean age 62.2, range 41–80) and the 30 cases of group I (no CT atrophy, mean age 59.3, range 41–75) were labeled in quite a different way: they were hospitalized for mild psychiatric disorders, headache, arterial hypertension, and cerebral arteriosclerosis.

For the evaluation of the presence and severity of the ventricular atrophy, we employed Huckman's (5) relative number, determined by the sum, in millimeters, of the opening and of the width of frontal horns at the level of the head of nucleus caudatus (ventricular number). For the evaluation of cortical atrophy, we considered the sum of the four wider cortical sulci visible in the three higher slices of the cortex as suggested by Huckman (cortical number). We classified the ventricular and cortical atrophies according to three severity levels, evaluating them separately and simplifying the classification proposed by Huckman.

We considered as normal a ventricular number up to 15, as an expression of moderate atrophy the values 16 to 20, and as an expression of severe atrophy the values higher than 20; we considered as normal the cases with cortical number up to 5, as sign of moderate atrophy the values 6 to 9, and as a sign of severe atrophy the values higher than 9. In order to correlate VEPs and CT data, our atrophic cases, because of their small number, were divided into three groups: cortical atrophy (moderate or severe), three subjects; ventricular atrophy (moderate or severe), 24 subjects; diffuse atrophy (cortical and ventricular, moderate or severe), 21 cases. All patients were examined at least 1 week after admission, no drugs active on the CNS having beeen administered. They were comfortably seated in a semidark room far from noise sources; midriatic eyedrops were used.

Evoked potentials were recorded from leads O_1–O_2 (International 10–20 System) with bilateral ear reference by means of surface electrodes (silver disks, 9 mm in diameter) fixed by collodion, with care taken that the impedance was less than 3 kΩ. Signals were amplified and averaged on-line by means of the Neuroaverager OTE Biomedica® (512 words), band width 1.6 to 70 Hz, bin width 0.97 msec, time base 500 msec, with a prestimulus sample of 50 msec. Visual evoked potentials were recorded by an *X–Y* plotter (Philips 8120); for each subject three averages of 80 responses each were recorded. Ocular artifacts were recorded and averaged before and/or after the VEP; on the basis of this recording, some cases with unclear VEP were excluded from our study.

The light stimulus was binocularly delivered by a stimulator (Alvar Pluristim IV®) at intervals randomized by hand (flash interval 1–3 sec, flash duration 0.1 msec, 0.7 joule); the lamp was placed 30 cm from the open eyes. The VEP peaks were identified visually and labeled according to Cigànek (1); the amplitudes were measured peak to peak.

For our correlation, the values previously obtained in 30 younger normal adults were also considered.

RESULTS

The VEPs obtained from normal elderly subjects and from the atrophic ones were quite similar with regard to wave form, but their latencies differed significantly from those recorded in young normal adults. Some VEPs obtained in the different groups are shown in Fig. 1. The average values of the latencies obtained in our cases are shown in Table 1; the average values of the amplitudes are shown in Table 2. As can be noticed, the latencies of the VEPs in the 30 subjects aged 41 to 75 (average age 59.3) and with normal CT significantly exceeded those of the group of 30 normal subjects aged 19 to 40 (average age 30.7); moreover, the late waves (IV, V, VI) in elderly subjects exhibited a higher and significant variability of latencies. Also, the amplitudes increased with age, such increase being higher for the first waves: amplitude I–II and II–III ($p < 0.01$), amplitude III–IV and IV–V ($p < 0.05$). The trend to such latency

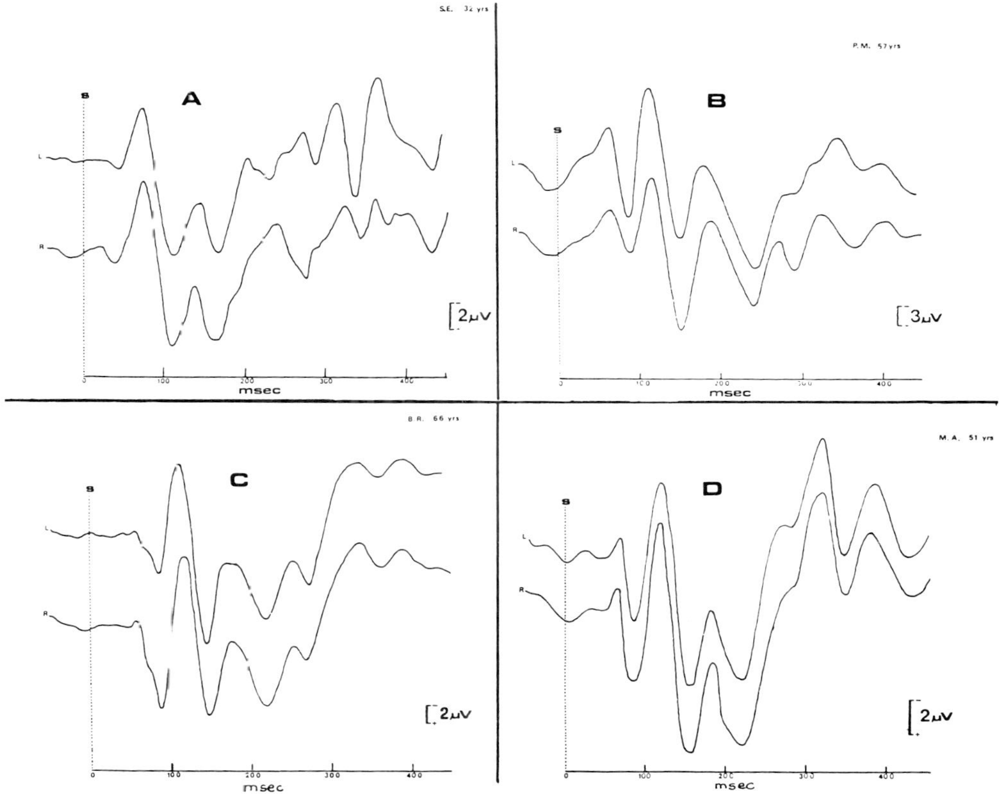

FIG. 1. Examples of VEPs. **A:** Normal adult, 32 years old. **B:** Elderly subject, 57 years old, without cerebral atrophy. **C:** Elderly subject, 66 years old, with moderate cerebral atrophy. **D:** Elderly subject, 51 years old, with severe cerebral atrophy. (For technical details see text.)

TABLE 1. *Mean latencies (msec ± SD) of VEPs in 78 elderly subjects and in 30 younger normal adults*

Peak	Normal adults 19–40 years (N = 30)	I Without atrophy (N = 30)	II With atrophy (N = 48)	II-A Without dementia (N = 30)	II-B With dementia (N = 18)
I	56.6 ± 3.2	54.1 ± 6.1	57.7 ± 9.0	57.5 ± 9.0	58.0 ± 9.2
II	67.1 ± 10.6	76.3 ± 11.9	86.1 ± 9.0	85.0 ± 10.3	88.0 ± 6.1
III	77.9 ± 12.9	96.7 ± 14.1	114.6 ± 15.3	110.9 ± 15.2	120.6 ± 13.9
IV	117.5 ± 13.3	139.4 ± 27.0	157.9 ± 23.9	150.0 ± 22.0	171.7 ± 21.1
V	154.3 ± 18.9	172.2 ± 31.7	198.4 ± 32.6	193.3 ± 33.7	208.7 ± 28.7
VI	200.4 ± 25.0	212.2 ± 41.0	237.0 ± 41.3	229.9 ± 41.6	251.8 ± 37.9
VII	285.0 ± 35.8	304.1 ± 46.9	325.1 ± 53.3	308.0 ± 54.4	350.8 ± 41.7

increase with aging could be noticed, despite the small number of cases, even by dividing the elderly subjects without atrophy at the CT by decade. That increase was significant only for some waves: III and IV ($p < 0.01$) and V ($p < 0.05$). Also, when the VEP latencies of the 48 atrophic patients were divided according to decades, no significant differences existed with regard to age. The VEP amplitudes of the atrophic patients were significantly greater than those of younger controls.

This increase was similar to that observed in the elderly subjects without atrophy. No differences in amplitude were observed among atrophic patients in relation to severity of the atrophy, the presence of dementia, or age. We must underline that the VEPs of atrophic patients had increased latencies in comparison with nonatrophic ones; this increase was statistically significant for all waves II to VI ($p < 0.01$). In contrast, the amplitudes did not differ. If we divide the cases with cerebral atrophy into "dement" and "nondement" patients, we can notice that the latencies of the dement group were higher than those of the nondement group; this increase was statistically significant for waves III ($p < 0.05$) and IV($p < 0.01$). The latencies of both subgroups differed signifi-

TABLE 2. *Mean amplitudes (μV ± SD) of VEPs in 78 elderly subjects and in 30 younger normal adults*

Wave	Normal adults 19–40 years (N = 30)	I Without atrophy (N = 30)	II With atrophy (N = 48)	II-A Without dementia (N = 30)	II-B With dementia (N = 18)
II	2.9 ± 1.3	7.2 ± 4.2	8.7 ± 5.4	9.2 ± 4.8	8.4 ± 4.2
III	5.4 ± 2.5	9.9 ± 4.9	12.1 ± 9.7	13.6 ± 6.5	11.1 ± 5.7
IV	10.8 ± 3.9	14.2 ± 6.4	13.5 ± 6.3	13.8 ± 5.9	13.3 ± 5.2
V	5.5 ± 3.2	8.0 ± 4.9	8.1 ± 5.1	9.3 ± 5.2	7.6 ± 3.8
VI	6.8 ± 4.2	9.6 ± 6.5	6.0 ± 4.1	6.5 ± 5.3	5.7 ± 4.4
VII	8.4 ± 5.5	13.7 ± 5.3	11.6 ± 5.4	13.1 ± 6.1	11.3 ± 5.5

cantly from those of the nonatrophic group, but this difference was more evident in the subgroup of atrophic dements.

Visual evoked potentials of the atrophic subjects were also divided according to the localization and the severity of the atrophy. The group of cases with both ventricular and cortical atrophy, i.e., the most severely atrophic ones, exhibited average latencies higher than the group of cases with ventricular atrophy only, but such differences were not significant. The increased latencies of the atrophic patients in comparison with the nonatrophic ones were significantly higher for the subgroup with more severe atrophy (cortical and ventricular).

As pointed out before with regard to the group of atrophic cases, the dement patients presented a higher increase of latencies than did the nondement ones, and the subjects with diffuse atrophy showed a higher increase of latencies than did those with only ventricular or cortical atrophy. This observation cannot be accounted for by a single explanation; in fact, the cases with diffuse atrophy were present in a similar percentage in both groups of dement and nondement atrophic patients.

DISCUSSION

On the basis of our results, some observations can be pointed out. The VEPs obtained from elderly subjects (mean age 59.3) without cerebral atrophy at CT present a significant increase of latencies over those of a group of younger subjects (mean age 30.7). Also, the amplitudes of all peaks increase, this increase being significant for the earlier waves (I to IV). These results are partially in agreement with those in the literature; in our opinion, however, there are some differences to be pointed out. First, the increase of latencies seems to be much more evident than previously reported (2,3,7). Moreover, we found an increase of the latencies as far as almost all the waves were concerned; in contrast, latency increases of only the earlier waves have usually been reported. The increase of the amplitudes concerns the wave form as a whole and is more evident in the earlier peaks (2,3); therefore, we fail to confirm the previously reported progressive diminution of the later waves in elderly subjects (3).

The VEPs obtained in patients with cerebral atrophy at CT are modified in the same way as those obtained in the elderly subjects: there is an increase of both latencies and amplitudes in comparison with younger subjects. The increase of amplitudes is quite similar in both elderly groups, whereas that of the latencies is more divergent in that they are significantly increased in patients with atrophy, not only in comparison with the younger subjects, but even with the elderly patients without cerebral atrophy. As previously noted, such increases in the latencies may partially be related to the severity of cerebral atrophy, because it is higher in patients with diffuse atrophy than in those with only ventricular or cortical atrophy.

Within the group of the atrophic patients, those with dementia present clearer alterations of VEPs than do those without dementia; as we indicated above, these results cannot be related to the severity of cerebral atrophy.

The VEP alterations in our dement atrophic patients are similar to those noticed by Visser et al. (10) who studied the VEPs in 19 patients suffering from senile or presenile dementia. When compared with the group of normal subjects, the latencies of waves II through VI were increased or markedly increased; the amplitudes of waves III and VI, and less consistently those of waves II and IV, were increased. In contrast, Squires et al. (9) noticed an increase of latency of P300 in 80% of a group of dement patients, whereas there was no difference in the latencies of the earlier stimulus-related waves in comparison with those of control subjects. Also, Laurian et al. (8) did not find any modified VEPs from occipital leads, but only alterations of the vertex responses in a group of patients suffering from senile or presenile dementia.

No greater differences of latencies and amplitudes than in normal subjects were found in the occipital leads from the right and left hemispheres of our patients with or without dementia. Thus, our results cannot support the opinion of Gerson et al. (4) who suggest, on the basis of described asymmetries of the responses of the two hemispheres to both visual and auditory stimuli, that the dementia brain is less well coordinated than is the brain of a normal elderly person.

Finally, a comparison between the VEPs obtained in patients with cerebral atrophy at CT and those obtained in age-matched patients without atrophy allowed us to trace a pattern of the alterations of VEPs in normal aging of the brain. The alterations of VEPs noted in atrophic patients are similar to those observed in elderly subjects without cerebral atrophy, but the increase in the latencies is much more evident.

Computerized tomography is surely quite useful in investigating the morphology of the brain, but it is not the only means of investigation of the boundaries between the normal and the pathological brain. The presence of cerebral atrophy is not the only explanation for the VEP alterations found in atrophic patients, as was suggested from the observation that in dement atrophic patients the previously described alterations of VEP are more evident, even if the severity of cerebral atrophy is superimposable. Metabolic, biochemical, and circulatory factors cannot be disregarded, even if these last may not have yet overtly affected the brain. Such factors seem to be more meaningful if we consider that alterations of the VEP were noted in elderly patients without cerebral atrophy at CT. In our opinion, one should not yet rule out the possibility that future improvements in the CT criteria used to evaluate the severity of cerebral atrophy will allow us to ascribe the VEP alterations found in our "normal" elderly subjects to a mild level of atrophy.

REFERENCES

1. Cigànek, L. (1961): The EEG response (evoked potential) to light stimulus in man. *Electroencephalogr. Clin. Neurophysiol.,* 13:165–172.

2. Dustman, R. E., and Beck, E. C. (1969): The effects of maturation and aging on the waveform of visually evoked potentials. *Electroencephalogr. Clin. Neurophysiol.,* 26:2–11.
3. Dustman, R. E., Schenkenberg, T., Lewis, E. G., and Beck, E. C. (1977): The cerebral evoked potential: Life-span changes and twin studies. In: *Visual Evoked Potentials in Man,* edited by J. E. Desmedt, pp. 363–377. Clarendon Press, Oxford.
4. Gerson, I. M., Roy, J. E., Bartlett, F., and Koenig, V. (1976): Average evoked response (AER) in the electroencephalographic diagnosis of the normally aging brain: A practical application. *Clin. Electroencephalogr.* 7:77–91.
5. Huckman, M. S., Fox, J., and Topel, J. (1975): The validity of criteria for the evaluation of cerebral atrophy by CT. *Radiology,* 116:85–92.
6. Klorman, R., Thompson, L. W., and Ellingson, R. J. (1978): Event related brain potentials across the life span. In: *Event Related Brain Potentials in Man,* edited by E. Callaway, P. Tueting, and S. H. Koslow, pp. 511–570. Academic Press, New York.
7. Kooi, K. A., and Bagchi, B. K. (1964): Observations on early components of the visual evoked response and occipital rhythms. *Electroencephalogr. Clin. Neurophysiol.,* 17:638–643.
8. Laurian, S., Gaillard, J. M., Gruber, G., Heiman, H., Lobrinus, A., and Wertheimer, J. (1979): Evoked potentials in senile dementia. In: *Human Evoked Potentials: Application and Problems,* edited by D. Lehmann and E. Callaway, p. 460. Plenum Press, New York and London.
9. Squires, K., Goodin, D., and Starr, A. (1979): Event related potentials in development, aging and dementia. In: *Human Evoked Potentials. Applications and Problems,* edited by D. Lehmann and E. Callaway, pp. 383–396. Plenum Press, New York and London.
10. Visser, S. L., Stam, F. C., Van Tilburg, W., Op Den Velde, W., Blom, J. L., and De Rijke, W. (1976): Visual evoked response in senile and presenile dementia. *Electroencephalogr. Clin. Neurophysiol.,* 40:385–392.

Clinical Applications of Evoked Potentials in Neurology,
edited by J. Courjon, F. Mauguiere, and M. Revol.
Raven Press, New York © 1982.

Evoked Brain Potential Differentiation Between Geriatric Subjects and Chronic Alcoholics with Brain Dysfunction

B. Porjesz and H. Begleiter

Downstate Medical Center, Department of Psychiatry, Brooklyn, New York 11203

It has been hypothesized that alcoholism accelerates the aging process, as similarities in cognitive dysfunction between young alcoholics and old people have been reported (e.g., abstraction and adaptive abilities) (4,5,7,8,20). Although alcoholics may exhibit similar behavioral deficits to old people (e.g., perseverative tendencies), these behavioral deficits may well reflect the endpoints of different complex neurophysiological processes.

For the past several years, we have systematically examined electrophysiological aberrations in various patient populations with the use of event-related potentials (ERPs) (1,2,12,13). These ERP techniques require the subject to be actively engaged in a task, usually an information-processing task. In the present study, we investigated the P3 or P300 component of the ERP in alcoholics and elderly people. A P300 wave can only be elicited under rather specific conditions relating to stimulus significance; namely, task relevance, unpredictability, and infrequency (17–19).

We were interested in investigating the ability of these subjects to differentiate between relevant and irrelevant inputs and their ability to probability-match stimuli in terms of their frequency of occurrence. Therefore, we designed a visuospatial P300 task that both groups of subjects would find somewhat difficult, as it required them to change sets; stimuli that were relevant in one block were no longer relevant in another block.

METHODS

Subjects

Three groups of education-matched, right-handed male subjects were studied: 30 alcoholics, 10 geriatrics, and 30 controls. All subjects (Ss) were otherwise healthy and medication-free for a minimum of 3 weeks. The alcoholics (mean age 36) had been drinking an average of 10 years and had been abstinent from alcohol a minimum of 1 month. The geriatric subjects were elderly people who were all over 65 years of age (mean age 72). They ranged from nondrinkers to occasional "social drinkers," and none had ever had a drinking problem. The control group consisted of young males who were age-matched to the alcoholic group (mean age 34). Their drinking histories were similar to those of the geriatric group.

Procedure

The subject sat in a sound-attenuated room with his head resting on a chin rest so that he was looking directly at the center of a computer-generated display located 50 cm from his eyes. All stimuli were presented in the center of the screen at a random rate of every 2 to 5 sec. The stimuli consisted of two regular geometric shapes (square and triangle) and irregular geometric forms, all equated for size and intensity.

The subject's task was to press a button only to the target stimulus which was either a square or triangle. When the square was the target (T), the triangle was the nontarget (NT), and vice-versa, so that ERPs could be obtained to the same stimulus when it served as a T or NT. The T stimuli occurred rarely (8.3%), as did the novel stimuli (irregular shapes), whereas the NTs made up the remaining 83.3% of the stimuli. Each novel (N) stimulus was presented only once. The T and NT stimuli were alternated every other block, with a tone indicating the beginning of a new block; the subject had to keep track of which stimulus was T and which was NT.

Monopolar recordings were obtained from midline occipital (O_z), parietal (P_z), central (C_z), and frontal (F_z) scalp locations in accordance with the 10–20 International System, using the linked ears as reference and the nasion as ground; vertical eye leads recorded electrooculograms (EOG). The ERPs were amplified by Grass amplifiers (bandwidth 0.3–60 Hz) and were sampled by a PDP 11/40 computer for a 500-msec epoch (200 points/sec).

In order to do the data analysis on an equal number of ERPs in each stimulus category, ERPs were averaged to all the novels (N) together, targets (T) together, and only the nontargets immediately preceding the target stimuli. These stimuli were named preceding nontargets (PNT) and are labeled as such in all figures. Results from peak-to-peak amplitude and latency measures of N2–P3 recorded at P_z only will be reported here; the other results will be reported elsewhere.

RESULTS

A two-way analysis of variance with repeated measures on one factor was performed (21).

As indicated in Fig. 1, the amplitude of N2–P3 was found to be significantly smaller in the alcoholic subjects to the T stimuli only, both in comparison with the control group ($p < 0.001$) and the geriatric group ($p < 0.02$). No significant amplitude difference existed between groups for PNT and N stimuli. The

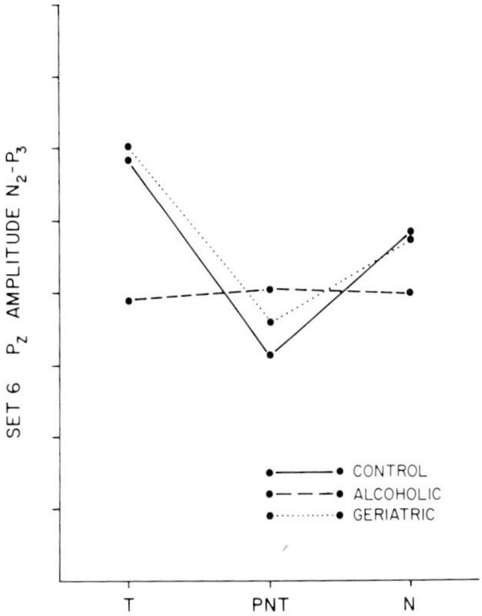

FIG. 1. Mean amplitude of N2–P3 for the three stimulus categories (target, nontarget, and novel) in the three subject groups: control *(solid line)*, alcoholic *(dashed line)*, and geriatric *(dotted line)*. Each division on the *ordinate* is equal to 1.5 μV. Standard deviations are as follows: T (1.69, 1.83, 2.36), PNT (1.45, 1.56, 1.54), N (1.69, 1.37, 2.1) for the control, alcoholic, and geriatric groups, respectively, for each stimulus category.

amplitude of N2–P3 was not statistically different between old people and normal controls.

The amplitude of N2–P3 differed significantly across the three classes of stimuli in both the control and the geriatric groups (Fig. 1); it was largest for T, next largest for N, and smallest for PNT ($p < 0.001$, controls; $p < 0.02$, geriatrics). As indicated in Fig. 1, this was not the case for the alcoholic group who maintained the same low-level P3 amplitude regardless of task.

As Fig. 2 indicates, P3 amplitude was significantly larger when the same stimulus served as T or NT in the control group ($p < 0.001$) and the geriatric group ($p < 0.005$). There was no significant difference in P3 amplitude between T and NT in the alcoholic group.

The difference in waveform (P3 amplitude) to T or NT stimuli in the control group is illustrated in Fig. 3. As Fig. 3 indicates, the P3 component was significantly larger to the T than the NT. In addition, there is a latency shift in P3 that occurs significantly earlier when the stimulus is a NT than when it is a T in both the control and geriatric groups ($p < 0.001$, control; $p < 0.001$, geriatric); the difference in P3 latency between T and NT in the alcoholic group was negligible.

In contrast to the control group, the alcoholic grand mean waveform did not differ significantly in any respect between T and NT stimuli (Fig. 4). The magnitude of the P3 component to T stimuli was significantly depressed in alcoholics in comparison to controls (Fig. 3).

As is indicated in Fig. 5, P3 occurred significantly later in the geriatric group than in each of the other two groups ($p < 0.001$) for all stimulus categories. On the other hand, the latency of P3 fell within the normal range for the chronic alcoholics.

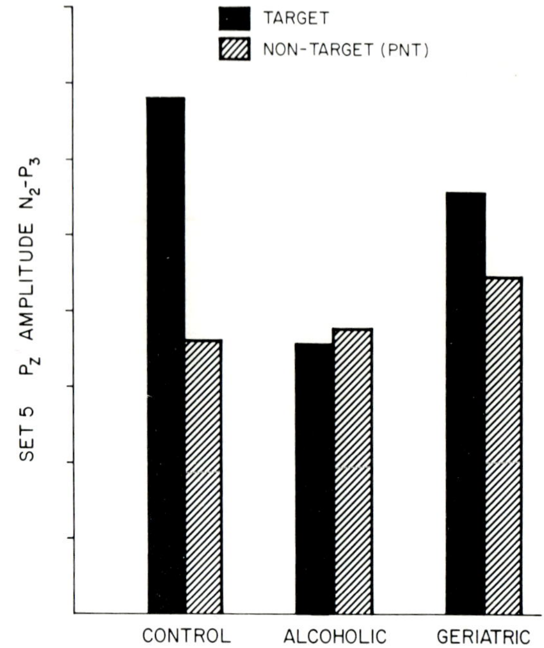

FIG. 2. Mean VERP amplitude N2–P3 to target *(solid bars)* and nontarget *(hatched bars)* stimuli for the three groups of subjects: control, alcoholic, and geriatric. Each division on the ordinate is equal to 1.5 μV. See Fig. 1. for SDs.

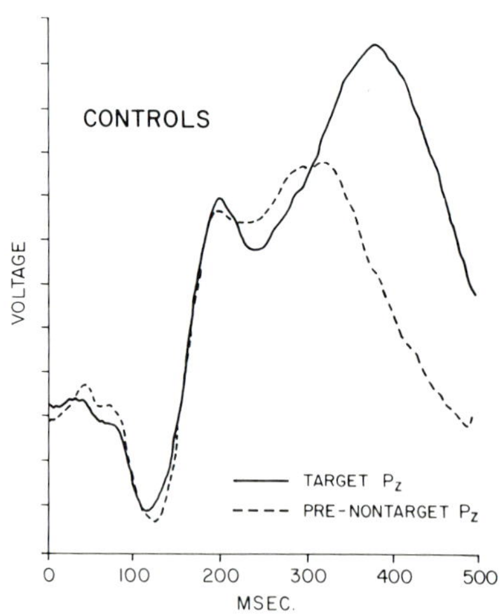

FIG. 3. Grand mean ERP waveforms recorded at P_z to the target stimulus *(solid line)* and nontarget stimulus *(dashed line)* in the control group. Each division on the ordinate is equal to 2 μV.

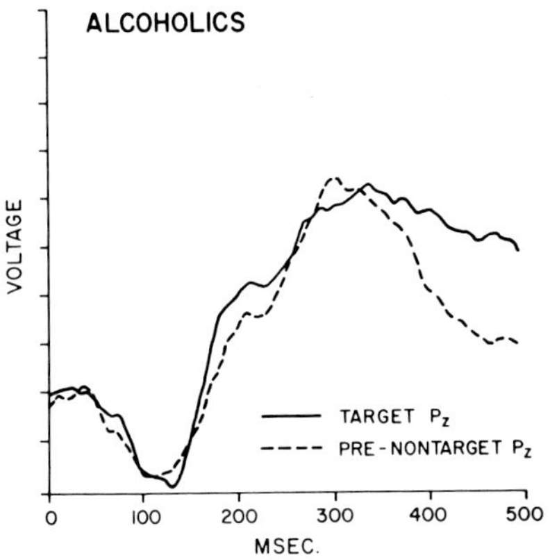

FIG. 4. Grand mean ERP waveforms recorded at P_z to the target stimulus *(solid line)* and nontarget stimulus *(dashed line)* in the alcoholic group. Each division on the ordinate is equal to 2 μV.

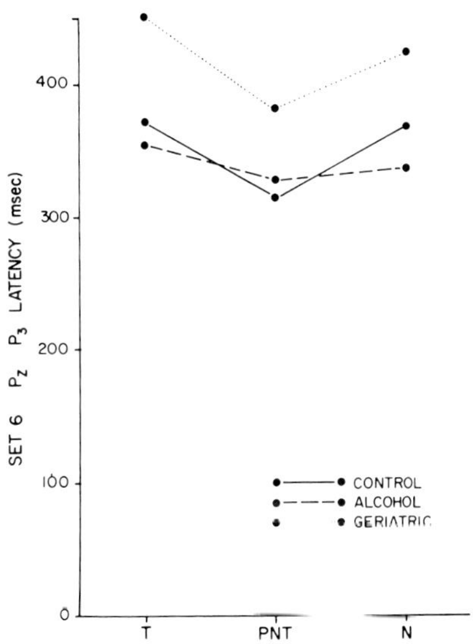

FIG. 5. Mean latency of P3 to the target (T), nontarget (PNT), and novel (N) stimuli in the control, alcoholic, and geriatric groups of subjects. Standard deviations are as follows: T (41.11, 42.35, 36.6), PNT (30.13, 40.39, 43.39), N (47.05, 39.74, 54.18), for the control, alcoholic, and geriatric groups, respectively, for each stimulus category.

The latency of N2 also occurred significantly later in the geriatric group than in the other two groups ($p < 0.001$ for T and N; $p < 0.02$, PNT), whereas latencies of N2 were virtually identical between the alcoholic and the control group.

DISCUSSION

The results of this study indicate that the P3 component was significantly reduced in chronic alcoholics. This component is of normal amplitude in elderly subjects but occurs significantly later. Thus, it appears that although ERPs in both groups differ from those of young healthy controls, the nature of their aberration is different.

The finding that P3 amplitudes are similar in old people and normal controls indicates that old people are able to probability-match as well as young people. The P3 amplitude was significantly larger and later to target than nontarget stimuli in both the control group and elderly group. This indicates that old people are able to respond to relevant target stimuli and attenuate responding to irrelevant stimuli. On the other hand, the alcoholics maintained the same low amplitude and identical latencies of P3 to both target and nontarget stimuli regardless of stimulus relevance. Thus, they seem to be unable to respond differentially to relevant and irrelevant inputs. This seems to indicate a deficit in "sensory filtering" in chronic alcoholics and an inability to utilize available information.

As P3 latency reflects the amount of time necessary to make a decision, the significantly longer P3 latency in the elderly group suggests that old people are slower in deciding whether a stimulus is target. The P3 latencies have been found to correlate with reaction time latencies (11,14,16), and both of these seem to increase with age (3). Our finding that P3 occurs later in old people without concomitant amplitude decrements has been reported in several different laboratories (6,9,15). In one normative P3 study (10), the rate of delay in latency with age was found to be 0.7 msec/year for P2, 0.8 msec/year for N2, and as high as 1.8 msec/year for P3.

It seems, therefore, that both the alcoholic and elderly groups manifest electrophysiological brain dysfunction. However, although both groups resembled each other behaviorally, they were quite different from each other electrophysiologically. The major ERP aberrations in the alcoholic group were (a) the lack of differentiation between their responses to relevant and irrelevant inputs, and (b) the low voltages of their event-related brain activity. Although the major electrophysiological aberration in the alcoholic subjects is one of voltage, the major electrophysiological dysfunction in the geriatric subjects is one of latency. The alcoholics manifest impaired "sensory-filtering" and probability-matching processes (responding identically to infrequent relevant and frequent irrelevant inputs), whereas the geriatric subjects differentiate between relevant and irrelevant inputs. The geriatric subjects, on the other hand, exhibit impaired stimulus evaluative mechanisms with regard to speed of evaluation, requiring a longer period of time to determine the relevance of a stimulus.

Thus, on the basis of this information-processing event-related-potential experiment, it was concluded that although ERPs in both alcoholic and geriatric subjects differ from those of young, healthy controls, the nature of brain dysfunction is different. Despite behavioral similarities between alcohol-related deficits and those of the aging process, the underlying neurophysiological aberrations are quite different in the two groups and suggest caution in the postulation of a common neuropathological mechanism.

ACKNOWLEDGMENTS

We would like to thank Lynda Herskovits for her invaluable assistance in all aspects of the study. We would also like to thank Dr. Joel Solomon, Dr. Israel Samuelly, Sharon Schurtz, and Maureen Meehan for their most helpful recruiting and screening of patients. This study was supported by Grant R01 AA02686.

REFERENCES

1. Begleiter, H., Porjesz, B., and Tenner, M. (1980): Neuroradiological and neurophysiological evidence of brain deficits in chronic alcoholics. *Acta Psychiatr. Scand.*, 62:(Suppl.) 286:3–13.
2. Begleiter, H., Porjesz, B., and Chou, C. L. (1981): Auditory brainstem potentials in chronic alcoholics. *Science*, 211:1064–1066.
3. Benton, A. L. (1977): Interactive effects of age and brain disease on reaction time. *Arch. Neurol.*, 34:369–370.
4. Blusewicz, M. J., Dustman, R. E., Schenkenberg, T., and Beck, E. C. (1977): Neuropsychological correlates of chronic alcoholism and aging. *J. Nerv. Ment. Dis.*, 165:348–355.
5. Blusewicz, M. J., Schenkenberg, I., Dustman, R. E., and Beck, E. C. (1977): WAIS performance in young normal, young alcoholic, and elderly normal groups: An evaluation of organicity and mental aging indices. *J. Clin. Psychol.*, 33:1148–1153.
6. Brent, G. A., Smith, D. B. D., Michalewski, H. J., and Thompson, L. W. (1976): Differences in the evoked potential in young and old subjects during habituation and dishabituation procedures. *Psychophysiology*, 14:96–97.
7. Fitzhugh, L. C., Fitzhugh, K. B., and Reitan, R. M. (1960): Adaptive abilities and intellectual functioning of hospitalized alcoholics. *Q. J. Stud. Alcohol*, 21:414–443.
8. Fitzhugh, L. C., Fitzhugh, K. B., and Reitan, R. M. (1965): Adaptive abilities and intellectual functioning of hospitalized alcoholics: Further considerations. *Q. J. Stud. Alcohol*, 26:402–411.
9. Ford, J. M., Hink, R. F., Hopkins, W. F., Roth, W. T., Pfefferbaum, A., and Kopell, B. S. (1979): Age effects on event related potentials in a selective attention task. *J. Gerontology*, 34:388–395.
10. Goodin, D. S., Squires, K. C., Henderson, B. H., and Starr, A. (1978): Age-related variations in evoked potentials to auditory stimuli in normal human subjects. *Electroencephalogr. Clin. Neurophysiol.*, 44:447–458.
11. Kutas, M., McCarthy, G., and Donchin, E. (1977): Augmenting mental chronometry: The P300 as a measure of stimulus evaluation. *Science*, 197:792–795.
12. Porjesz, B., and Begleiter, H. (1979): Visual evoked potentials and brain dysfunction in chronic alcoholics. In: *Evoked Brain Potentials and Behavior*, edited by H. Begleiter, pp. 277–302. Plenum Press, New York.
13. Porjesz, B., Begleiter, H., and Garozzo, R. (1980): Visual evoked potential correlates of information processing deficits in chronic alcoholics. In: *Biological Effects of Alcohol*, edited by H. Begleiter, pp. 603–623. Plenum Press, New York.
14. Ritter, W., Simson, R., and Vaughan, H. (1972): Association cortex potentials and reaction time in auditory discrimination. *Electroencephalogr. Clin. Neurophysiol.*, 33:547–555.
15. Smith, D. B. D., Tom, C. E., Brent, G. A., and Ohta, R. J. (1976): Attention, evoked potentials, and aging. In: *Research Directions of Psychophysiological Changes with Aging.* Symposium presented at the meeting of the Western Psychological Association, Los Angeles, California, April 8–11.
16. Squires, N. K., Donchin, E., Squires, K. C., and Grossberg, S. (1977): Bisensory stimulation: Inferring decision-related processes from the P300 component. *J. Exp. Psychol.* [*Hum. Percept.*] 3:299–315.
17. Sutton, S., Braren, M., Zubin, J., and John, E. R. (1965): Evoked-potentials correlates of stimulus uncertainty. *Science*, 150:1187–1188.
18. Sutton, S., Tueting, P., Zubin, J., and John, E. R. (1967): Information delivery and the sensory evoked potential. *Science*, 155:1436–1439.

19. Tueting, P., Sutton, S., and Zubin, J. (1971): Quantitative evoked potential correlates of the probability of events. *Psychophysiology,* 7:385–394.
20. Williams, J. D., Ray, C. G., and Overall, J. E. (1973): Mental aging and organicity in an alcohol population. *J. Consult. Clin. Psychol.,* 41:392–396.
21. Winer, B. J. (1962): *Statistical Principles in Experimental Design.* McGraw-Hill, New York.

Clinical Applications of Evoked Potentials in Neurology,
edited by J. Courjon, F. Mauguiere, and M. Revol.
Raven Press, New York © 1982.

Transient and Steady State Visual Evoked Potentials by Checkerboard Reversal Pattern in Renal Diseases

*P. M. Rossini, *L. Marchionno, *D. Gambi, **A. Albertazzi, and **B. Di Paolo

**Laboratory of Neurophysiology, Department of Neurology, and **Department of Nephrology, University G. D'Annunzio, 66100 Chieti, Italy*

Uremic encephalopathy is often a complication of chronic renal failure (CRF) (14) and has been ascribed to an unknown circulating toxin altering both synaptic and axonal membrane mechanisms (6,12). Previous papers have emphasized the reliability of the EEG in detecting uremic encephalopathy (18) even if it often becomes clearly altered only in late stages without any correlation with conventional blood chemistries (19).

A flash visual evoked potential (VEP) higher than normal with delayed latencies was also noted (6,11) without any clear correlation with any of the circulating potential toxins. Since the contrast-modulated VEP by a checkerboard reversal evokes a more cortical (7,16) and reproducible transient response characterized by a major positive deflection, we analyzed a population of uremic subjects by means of this technique.

PATIENTS AND METHODS

Twenty-three males and 11 females (47.5 ± 16 years) suffering from CRF of variable etiology and undergoing maintenance therapy for at least 8 months were admitted in this trial. Each eye was separately stimulated by square-wave checks (7.5′, 25′, 30′, 60′ of visual angle) at two contrast levels (20% and 50%), which were reversed at 2, 10, 20, or 40 times/sec in a TV monitor (20° × 18° of visual angle; mean luminance 75 cd/cm²). The pattern change was synchronized to the frame-sync signal to ensure that the pattern change occurred off screen; this was to avoid a line moving up or down the screen and giving an unwanted movement of the patient's fixation. The poststimulus time analysis was 300 msec for the transient response (average of 64 replications) and 200, 100, and 50 msec, respectively, for the steady state stimulation at 10, 20, and 40/sec (average of 256 replications). Refractory defects were corrected; an occipital midline Ag/AgCl electrode fixed 4 cm above the inion was referred to the linked earlobes or to the left one (ground on the frontal electrode). In 10 control subjects, simultaneous recordings from O_z–C_z–F_z referred to the left earlobe and O_z–C_z, O_z–F_z were also done. The following recording parameters were utilized: gain, 2×10^5; bandwidth, 0.8 to 32 Hz for the transient and 3.2 to 16, 8 to 32, and 16 to 80 respectively at 10, 20, and 40 reversals/min for the repetitive stimulation. Latencies, amplitudes, and phases were visually and automatically measured (PDP 11/10) from the FM tape recorder (Racall 4). Before each recording session, creatinine, blood urea nitrogen (BUN), parathormone (PTH), and glomerular filtration rate (GFR) were tested. The major positive deflection (P100) was considered delayed if 2.5 SD above the mean of controls. None of the examined subjects had remarkable EEG abnormalities at routine analysis.

RESULTS

The time taken for the raster to write from the top to the bottom strip in our TV monitor (625 lines, 50 fields) was 20 msec; since most of the VEP is generated from the macular region, and since our data were obtained during central fixation, a half-frame 10-msec period must be subtracted, that being the average delay between the trigger pulse and the raster reaching the screen

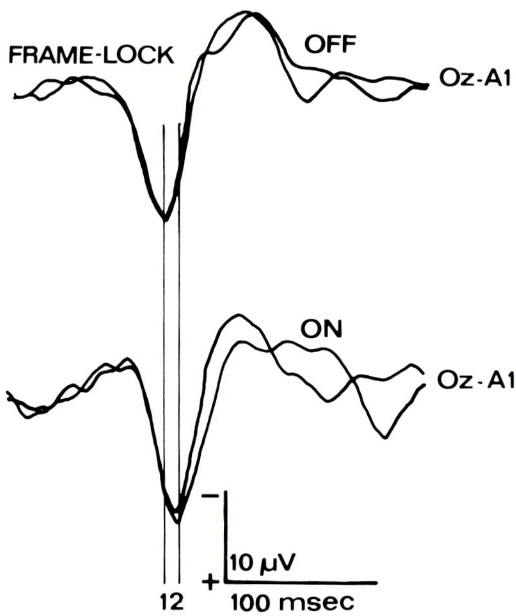

FIG. 1. Control subject (15′ checks at 50% contrast). Note the latency difference of 12 msec between the frame-locked and the frame-unlocked pattern reversal.

center. Furthermore, to obtain a pattern change off screen (frame lock on, Fig. 1), the stimulus triggering (USC 6 Medelec) the pattern-generator (video stimulator Medelec) was delayed. We calculated this delay in five control subjects to have a stable value of 12 msec. The two aforementioned factors added to the narrow filtering bandpass may account for the longer latencies we have reported compared to other workers; the earlobe and/or scalp references did not significantly vary the P100 latency.

The transient VEP was significantly delayed in 34% of the tested eyes, mainly when evoked by small and low-contrast checks (Table 1); this was also statistically correlated with the blood chemistries (Table 2). For steady state stimulation, absence of synchronization or phase lag between the sinusoidal response and the trigger were also present in 46.2% of the cases (Fig. 2). Also, the amplitudes of both transient and steady state VEPs were reduced in terms of the difference present at the two contrast levels regardless of the check size. The P100 decrease secondary to the increase of the stimulus spatial frequency (checks/°) was enhanced in some of our subjects with more prolonged latencies for small checks than for the coarse ones (Fig. 3).

TABLE 1. *P100 latencies in controls and uremic subjects (msec)*

	Spatial frequency							
	7.5′		15′		30′		60′	
Contrast	20%	50%	20%	50%	20%	50%	20%	50%
Controls	150.1	144.9	131.9	128.2	120.9	121.0	119.0	119.2
SD	6.6	6.7	5.0	5.2	5.3	4.8	7.5	4.2
Patients	160.9	156.8	148.8	143.1	129.5	126.0	126.0	124.2
SD	6.5	5.7	6.3	8.6	6.2	6.6	6.6	6.9
Difference (*p*)	<0.05	<0.05	<0.01	<0.05	ns	ns	ns	ns

TABLE 2. *Correlations*[a] *between the VEP latencies and the blood chemistries* (r *of Pearson*)

	Spatial frequency							
	7.5′		15′		30′		60′	
Contrast	20%	50%	20%	50%	20%	50%	20%	50%
Creatinine	++	++	+	−	−	−	−	−
BUN	+++	++	++	+	+	−	−	−
GFR	++	++	+	+	−	−	−	−
PTH	+++	++	+	+	−	−	−	−

[a] +, $p < 0.05$; ++, $p < 0.01$; +++, $p < 0.001$.

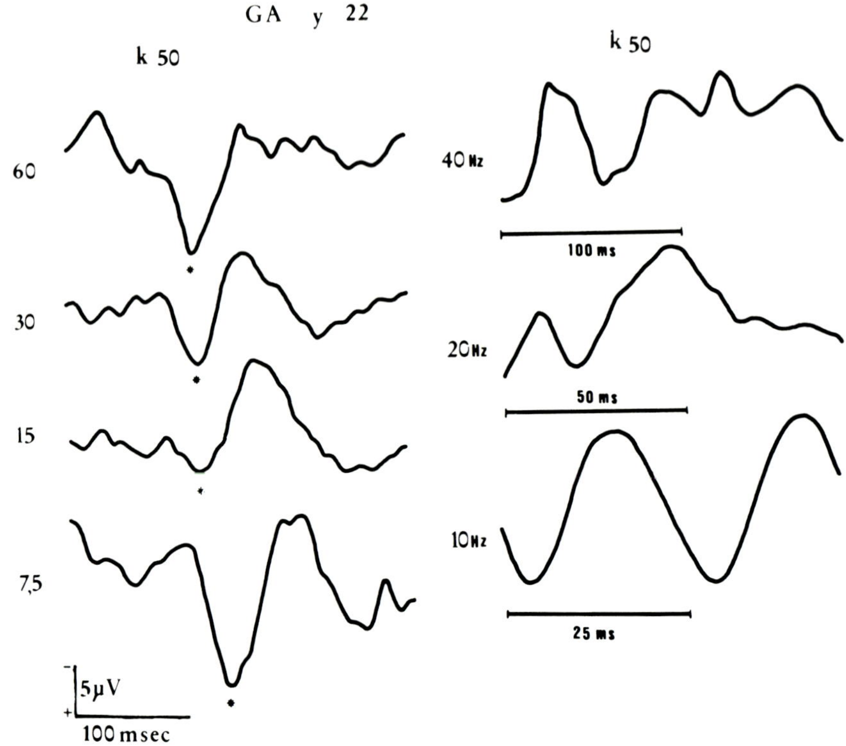

FIG. 2. Patient with CRF. On the **left** are the VEPs of the left eye at different spatial frequency stimulations elicited by a transient (2 Hz) reversal; they are normal in latencies, amplitudes, and latency difference between detailed and coarse checks (30 msec). Conversely, the steady state stimulation **(right)** evoked a sinusoidal response only at 10 Hz, but did not at 20 and 40 Hz.

DISCUSSION

It is well known that in advanced stages of CRF there appear clinical and behavioral symptoms that have been ascribed to electrolyte imbalance (1) or to the increased concentration of some circulating substances (3,6), one of which is PTH (2) which has been found to induce EEG changes typical of CRF in dogs made uremic (5). In our patients, the PTH was abnormally elevated in 37% of cases. The delayed propagation of the visual input could be attributed both to the presence of demyelinated zones sometimes encountered along the visual pathways in uremic brains and to the action of an unknown neurotoxin at any one of the optic pathway relays (retinal, geniculate, calcarine).

The progressive delay observed in normals when the spatial frequency (checks/°) of the patterned stimulus is increased was interpreted by others on the basis of a lower contrast sensitivity for small details or of an increased integration time needed with fine checkerboard (13,17) or of a transition of

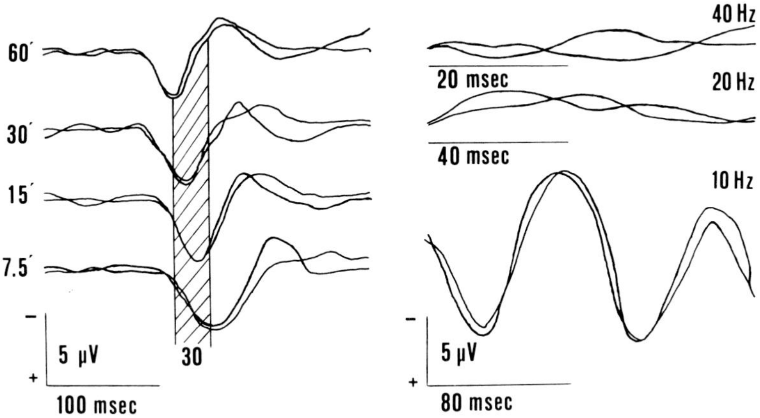

FIG. 3. Amplitude histograms of the transient VEPs. Note the decrease in the subjects with CRF, showing a less delineated difference at the two contrast levels. K = contrast.

operation from slow channels (detailed vision) to fast channels (coarse vision or movement vision) (4,9,15). Based on our findings, it is hard to say which of the above mentioned mechanisms could be involved in those patients showing a large difference between the VEP latencies elicited by fine and coarse checks. Since the VEPs depending on coarse checks engage different visual mechanisms because of their high content of luminance variation (conversely, fine checks when reversing, produce a pure contrast modulation) (17), one may suggest that the "potential" neurotoxins, among which the BUN seems to play a particular role (8), act differently on the pathways underlying the two responses. This could also account for the lack of statistical correlation between the renal blood chemistries and the VEP dependence on wide check reversal.

In conclusion, the pattern reversal method can engage the human visual channels devoted to the vision of moving or steady, coarse and detailed targets as already reported by others (10). This technique can further disclose at an early stage any anomalous propagation of the neural impulse started in the receptor retinal layers and reaching the calcarine cortex in patients suffering from chronic renal failure.

ACKNOWLEDMENTS

This work was partly supported by C.N.R., Special Project on Biomedical Engineering.

REFERENCES

1. Arieff, H. I., and Guisado, R. (1976): Effects on the central nervous system of hypernatremic and hyponatremic states. *Kidney Int.*, 10:104–116.

2. Avram, M. M., Feingold, D. A., and Huatuco, A. M. (1978): Search for uremic toxin. Decreased motor-nerve conduction velocity and elevated parathyroid hormone in uremia. *N. Engl. J. Med.,* 298:1000–1003.
3. Bourne, J. R., Ward, J. W., Teschan, P. E., Musso, M., Johnston, H. B., Jr., and Ginn, H. E. (1975): Quantitative assessment of the electroencephalogram. *Electroencephalogr. Clin. Neurophysiol.,* 39:377–388.
4. Gambi, D., Rossini, P. M., Onofrj, M., Marchionno, L. (1980): Visual evoked cortical potentials (V.E.C.P.) by television presentation of different patterned stimuli to patients with multiple sclerosis. *Ital. J. Neurol. Sci.,* 2:101–106.
5. Hagstam, K. E. (1971): EEG frequency content related to chemical blood parameters in chronic uremia. *Scand. J. Urol. Nephrol.,* 7(Suppl.): 1–56.
6. Hamel, B., Bourne, J. B., Ward, J. W., and Teschan, P. E. (1978): Visually evoked cortical potentials in renal failure: Transient potentials. *Electroencephalogr. Clin. Neurophysiol.,* 44:606–611.
7. Hubel, D. H., and Wiesel, T. N. (1977): Functional architecture of macaque monkey visual cortex. *Proc. R. Soc. Lond.* [*Biol.*], 198:1–59.
8. Hughes, J. R. (1980): Correlation between EEG and chemical changes in uremia. *Electroencephalogr. Clin. Neurophysiol.,* 48:583–594.
9. Jones, R., and Keck, M. J. (1979): Visual evoked responses as a function of grating spatial frequency. *Invest. Ophthalmol.,* 17:652–659.
10. Kulikowski, J. (1977): Separation of occipital potentials related to the detection of pattern and movement. In: *Visual Evoked Potentials in Man,* edited by J. E. Desmedt, pp. 184–196. Clarendon Press, Oxford.
11. Lewis, E. G., Dustman, R. E., and Beck, E. C. (1978): Visual and somatosensory evoked potentials characteristics of patients undergoing hemodialysis and kidney transplantation. *Electroencephalogr. Clin. Neurophysiol.,* 44:223–231.
12. Nielsen, V. K. (1974): The peripheral nerve function in chronic renal failure. X. Decremental nerve conduction in uremia. *Acta Med. Scand.,* 196:83–86.
13. Parker, D. M., and Salzen, E. A. (1977): Latency changes in the human visual evoked response to sinusoidal gratings. *Vision Res.,* 17:1,201–1,204.
14. Raskin, N. H., and Fishman, R. A. (1976): Neurologic disorders and renal failure. *N. Engl. J. Med.,* 294:143–147, 204–210.
15. Rossini, P. M., Pirchio, M., Sollazzo, D., and Caltagirone, C. (1979): Foveal vs peripheral retinal responses: A new analysis for early diagnosis of multiple sclerosis. *Electroencephalogr. Clin. Neurophysiol.,* 47:515–523.
16. Sokol, S. (1976): Visual evoked potentials: Theory, techniques and clinical application. *Surv. Ophthalmol.,* 21:18–44.
17. Vassilev, A., and Strashimirov, D. (1979): On the latency of the human visually evoked response to sinusoidal gratings. *Vision Res.,* 19:843–845.
18. Yano, M., and Hirata, K. (1970): Uremia: Evaluation by EEG. *IRYO,* 24:961–967.
19. Zysno, E., Durr, F., Reichenmiller, H. E., and Nieth, H. (1967): EEG examination in uraemic encephalopathy during intermittent peritoneal dialysis. *Electroencephalogr. Clin. Neurophysiol.,* 22:193.

Clinical Applications of Evoked Potentials in Neurology,
edited by J. Courjon, F. Mauguiere, and M. Revol.
Raven Press, New York © 1982.

Visually Evoked Potentials in Friedreich's Ataxia

W. Wenzel, L. Camacho, D. Claus, and J. Aschoff

Abteilung für Neurologie, Universität Ulm, Klinik Dietenbronn, D-7959 Schwendi, West Germany

Since Halliday (10), in 1972, found pathological VEP results in patients suffering from multiple sclerosis even if they had never had visual symptoms, this test has become a valuable tool in MS diagnosis. But VEP changes are not specific for MS: they have also been demonstrated in glaucoma (7), migraine (12), and chiasmal processes (11). Few reports exist about optic neuropathy in Friedreich's ataxia; however, visual evoked potentials have recently been recorded in a great number of these patients by Carroll et al. (8). In this chapter we shall present the results of VEP testing in 45 patients with Friedreich's ataxia.

PATIENTS AND METHODS

The group examined consisted of 45 patients with a confirmed diagnosis of Friedreich's ataxia based on the criteria of Andermann (1), Barbeau (2), Becker (4), Bodechtel (6), and Refsum and Skre (13,15). The patients belonged to 33 families; the mode of inheritance was autosomal recessive. For patients' data, see Table 1.

Before VEP recording, visual acuity was tested and corrected by glasses if necessary; patients wore these glasses during VEP recording. Ophthalmoscopy was performed to assess the degree of decoloration of the optic disks. The VEP was recorded with Beckman silver chloride cup electrodes between C_z and O_z; the mastoid served as ground. Electrode impedance was always maintained below 1 kΩ. The patient looked at a small white fixation mark in the

TABLE 1. *Friedreich's ataxia: Patients' data:* (N = *45*)

	Mean values and SD
Male	28
Female	17
Age at investigation (years)	32.9 ± 13.8
Age at onset of illness (years)	11.7 ± 5.5
Duration of illness (years)	21.2 ± 10.1

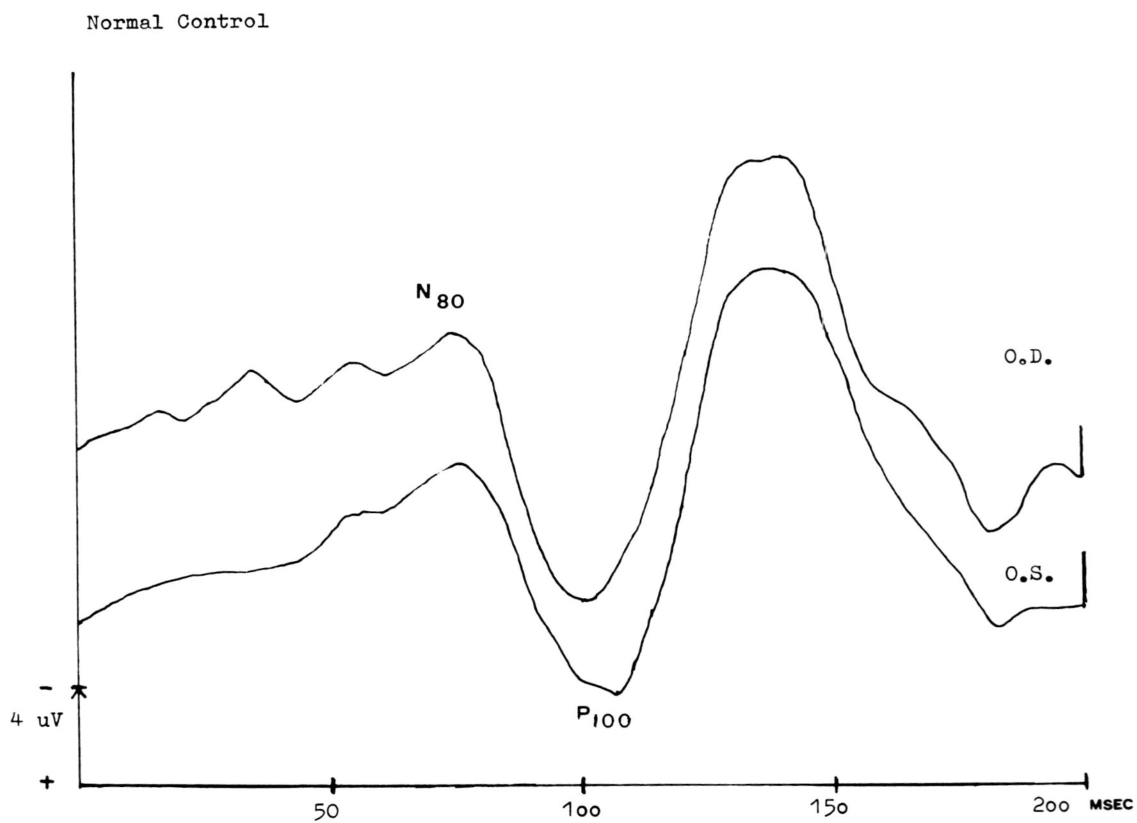

FIG. 1. Visual evoked potential of a normal control. Latencies of N80 and P100 peaks are, respectively, 75 and 102 msec for the right eye and 76 and 107 msec for the left eye. Amplitudes for the two eyes are, respectively, 11.2 and 9.2 μV.

middle of a commercial TV screen on which a checkerboard pattern was presented. We used monocular stimulation, and the other eye was covered. The entire screen subtended a visual angle of 22°, each square 58′. Overall luminance was 100 cd/m^2, and contrast between black and white checks 90%. Pattern reversal frequency was 2 Hz; the reversal was desynchronized from the TV frame period. Responses to 128 or 256 reversals were averaged on line with a Nicolet Ca 1117 averager. Filters were set at 1.6 (HF) and 320 Hz (LF). Analysis times were 200 and 250 msec. A normal VEP is shown in Fig. 1.

Latency times were measured at the first major positive component P100. Amplitudes were measured between N80 and P100 if both peaks were clearly discernible. A VEP was classified as pathological if the latency of P100 was higher than our laboratory standard (97.5 ± 6.6 msec) plus 3 SD, i.e., higher than 118 msec, or the difference between both eyes was more than 8 msec.

RESULTS

A survey of our results is given in Table 2. We found normal VEPs in 20 cases; ophthalmological examination also revealed no abnormalities. In six cases, there had been no response because of optic atrophy; five of these showed pearly white disks, and one severe decoloration. In all six cases, the visual acuity was below 0.3. Temporal decoloration of the optic disks of a mild to moderate degree could be observed in 12 of the remaining 19 patients with a pathological VEP. Nine of these had visual acuity scores between 0.5 and 0.8; the remaining 10 patients had full vision. Funduscopy was normal in seven cases of those with pathological VEPs.

Altogether, the VEP was pathological in 55.5% of our cases, ophthalmoscopy in 40%; visual acuity was reduced in 33%. Significant differences between right and left eye could not be observed.

For exact latency times see Table 3. The P100 latency was 115.3 ± 18.2 msec in the patient group, and interocular difference 6.2 ± 6.7 msec. The difference from the values of normal subjects is significant at the 1% level.

The amplitudes in Friedrcich's ataxia patients are reduced in comparison with normal controls (Table 4). Compared with the pathological VEP group,

TABLE 2. *Friedreich's Ataxia: Results of VEP examination* (N = 45)

Results	No. of patients
Normal VEP	20
Pathological VEP (total)	25
No reaction	6
Symmetrical increase of P100 latency	7
Pathological interocular difference only	1
Increased latencies and pathological interocular difference	11

TABLE 3. *Friedreich's ataxia: Latencies of P100, interocular difference*

	Mean values and SD
P100	
Normal controls	97.5 ± 6.9 msec
Friedreich's ataxia (all, N = 39)	115.3 ± 18.2 msec
Friedreich's ataxia (normal VEP)	104.5 ± 6.5 msec
Friedreich's ataxia (pathological VEP)	126.6 ± 19.3 msec
Interocular difference	
Normal controls	1.9 ± 1.3 msec
Friedreich's ataxia (all, N = 39)	6.2 ± 6.7 msec
Friedreich's ataxia (normal VEP)	2.7 ± 1.9 msec
Friedreich's ataxia (pathological VEP)	9.7 ± 8.1 msec

TABLE 4. *Friedreich's Ataxia: Amplitudes*

	Mean values and SD
Normal controls	9.7 ± 3.4 μV
Friedreich's ataxia (all, N = 36)	5.6 ± 3.2 μV
Friedreich's ataxia (normal VEP)	6.8 ± 3.8 μV
Friedreich's ataxia (pathological VEP)	4.4 ± 1.8 μV

the distinction is significant on the 1% level. That means that a pathological VEP in Friedreich's ataxia is statistically connected with a reduced amplitude. This inverse amplitude–latency relationship is shown in Fig. 2.

An example of a pathological VEP is given in Fig. 3.

No significant relation could be found between VEP latencies and either visual acuity or age of the patients. Similarly, we found no relation between VEP results and duration of illness (see Fig. 4). The distribution of results corresponds with the age distribution in our group. In the 10 families in which we examined more than one member, we found with one exception the same results, pathological or normal, in all sick members of the family.

DISCUSSION

Data on the involvement of the optic nerve in Friedreich's ataxia are rare, and figures for atrophies range from 5.2 to 12% (2,3,14). Numerous investigators reported optic atrophies or visual disturbances in some of their patients; Friedreich (9) himself, in 1876, described reading difficulties in a patient, but he referred this to the nystagmus. Van Leuuwen and van Bogaert (16) described three kinds of optic nerve involvement in patients with heredoataxias.

The first is associated with retrobulbar neuritis, significant reduction of visual acuity, pale optic disks on the temporal side, and central scotoma. Histologically, a degeneration of the maculopapillar bundle is found in these cases.

The second occurs with rapid appearance of optic atrophy, and severe visual

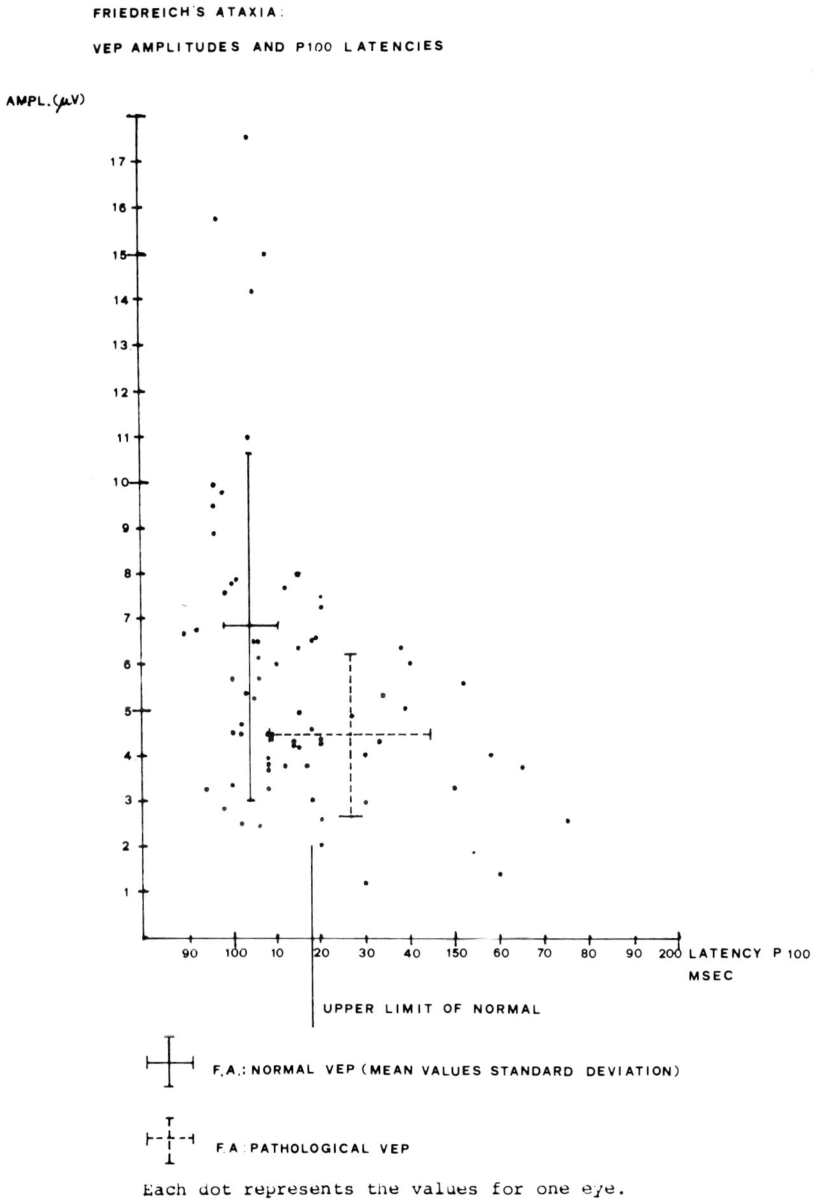

FIG. 2. Visual evoked potential amplitude–latency relationship in Friedreich's ataxia.

loss, even to complete blindness; the disks are porcelain white and totally atrophied. Histologically, total demyelinization of the optic nerves is found. The third is associated with more or less severe visual loss and concentric restriction of visual fields; its progression is slow.

According to this classification, the six patients without visual evoked response

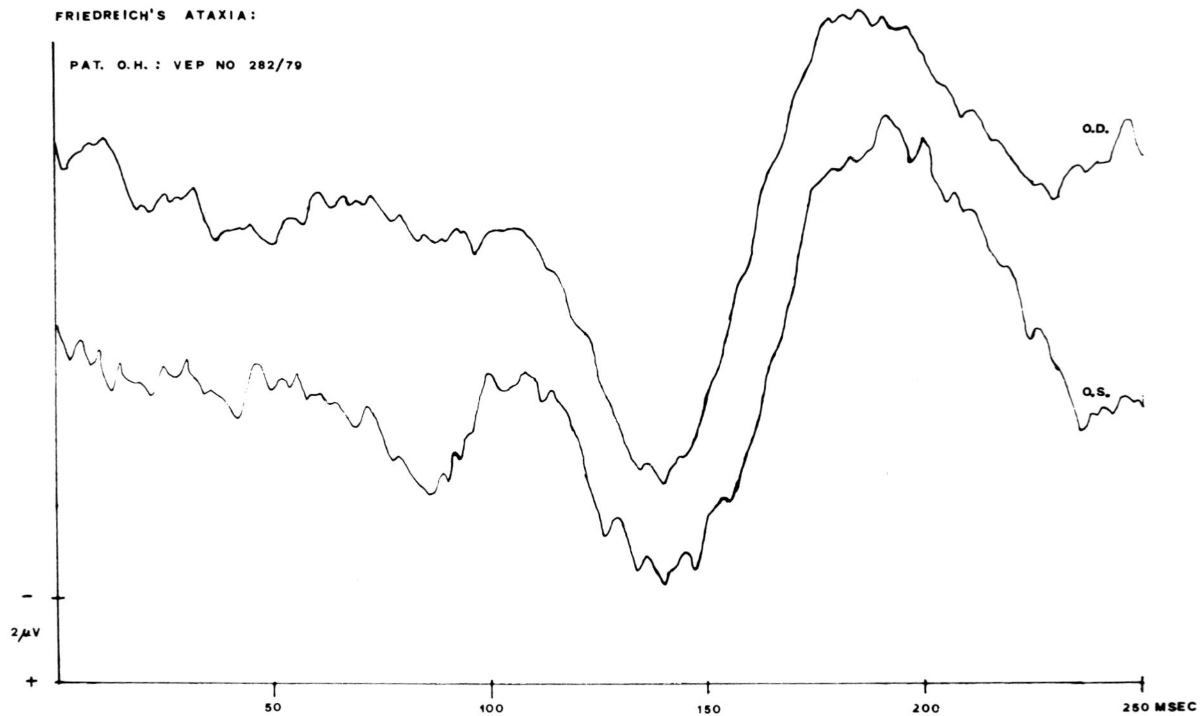

FIG. 3. Visual evoked potentials in a patient with Friedreich's ataxia. Patient showed bilateral decoloration of the disk and had visual acuity of 0.8 in each eye. Latencies of N80 and P100 peaks are, respectively, 108 and 141 msec for the right eye and 110 and 141 msec for the left eye. Amplitudes for the two eyes are, respectively, 6.0 and 5.7 μV.

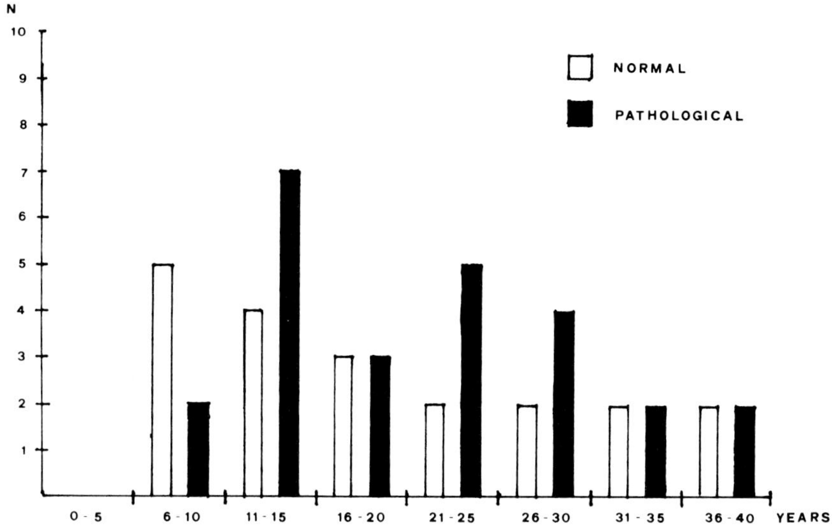

FIG. 4. Visual evoked potential results over the duration of Friedreich's ataxia.

because of optic atrophy can be assigned to the second type: they all had a rapid loss of vision in the early stage of the disease, showed severe decoloration of the optic disks, and had poor vision at investigation. The other patients with a pathological VEP correspond to the first of the above classifications. We did not find loss of vision and pale optic disks in every case; this can be attributed to the higher accuracy of the method compared to conventional ophthalmological examination. By VEP recording, optic lesions can be detected before there is any clinical manifestation or after remission, as has been shown in MS patients (10).

Pattern reversal preferentially stimulates the fovea; thus, we found no patient whom we could assign to the third group. A familiar constellation of symptoms, especially optic atrophy, has already been reported by Bell and Carmichael (5). Our figures show a high degree of conformity with the results of Sjögren (14) who found manifest optic atrophy in 12% (our group, 13%), but in 52% of his cases with a duration of sickness over 20 years, optic atrophies, or temporal decoloration of the disks. That corresponds to 55% of pathological VEP results in our patients.

Just recently, Carroll et al. (8) reported on "the incidence and nature of visual pathway involvement in Friedreich's ataxia." They found pathologies in 64% of their 22 patients suffering from Friedreich's ataxia. The major conclusions from their data were that (a) there is no temporal dispersion of the P100 potential; (b) there is an inverse relationship between latency and amplitude of P100; and (c) that these results are the reverse of what is observed in MS. From these findings, they concluded that the underlying process of visual pathway involvement in Friedreich's ataxia is different from that in other diseases with VEP changes (MS, Leber's optic atrophy, compression of the optic nerve). Although we also found an inverse amplitude–latency relationship, there were no major differences between VEPs of Friedreich's ataxia or MS patients because of the high incidence of temporal dispersion or extinguished responses in our group. For these differences there may be several reasons. The influence of unsteady fixation caused by nystagmus could be greater in a TV stimulator than in a rotating mirror arrangement. Temporal dispersion in our group may have resulted from this. In our group, we had six patients with optic atrophy, but other major group differences (age, duration of sickness) could not be observed. Thus, our data cannot support Carroll's conclusions about the nature of the visual pathway involvement in Friedreich's ataxia.

The above-mentioned and our own results show that optic nerve involvement in Friedreich's ataxia is not a rare symptom, but it is not obligatory as shown by the fact that about half of our cases who have normal VEPs despite long durations of illness and other severe disabilities. Although group differences between VEP findings in MS and Friedreich's ataxia can be found, the VEP is, unfortunately, no help in the differential diagnosis between these diseases.

SUMMARY

Visual evoked potentials to pattern-reversal stimulation have been recorded in 45 patients with Friedreich's ataxia. In six patients, no response could be obtained because of optic atrophy; altogether, pathological results were found in 25 patients (55%). Normal latencies were recorded in 20 patients (45%). No statistically significant connection could be drawn between the result of the VEP testing and visual acuity, age, or onset and duration of sickness, but there was a strikingly familiar accumulation of results.

There is a good conformity between our results and the incidence of optic atrophy in later stages of the disease as shown by pathological–anatomical and epidemiological studies. We have demonstrated that optic nerve lesions in Friedreich's ataxia are not as rare as is frequently assumed and that the VEP is a valuable tool for detecting them. On the other hand, unfortunately, the VEP is of no help in the differential diagnosis of Friedreich's ataxia versus multiple sclerosis.

REFERENCES

1. Andermann, E., Remillard, G. M., Goyer, C., Blitzer, L., Andermann, E., and Barbeau, A. (1976): Genetic and family studies in friedreich's ataxia. *J. Can. Sci. Neurol.*, 3:287–301.
2. Barbeau, A. (1976): Friedreich's ataxia 1976—An overview. *J. Can. Sci. Neurol.*, 3:389–397.
3. Barbeau, A. (1978): Friedreich's ataxia 1978—An overivew. *J. Can. Sci. Neurol.*, 5:161–165.
4. Becker, P. E. (1966): Krankheiten mit hauptsächlicher Beteiligung des spino-cerebellären Systems (Erbliche Ataxien). In: *Krankheiten des Nervensystems, Band V/1, Humangenetik,* edited by P. E. Becker and G. Koch, pp. 208–313. G. Thieme Verlag, Stuttgart.

5. Bell, J., and Carmichael, E. A. (1939): On hereditary ataxia and spastic paraplegia. *Treas. Hum. Inherit.*, 4:141–281.
6. Boechtel, G., and Schrader, A. (1953): Die Erkrankungen der Rückenmarks. In: *Handbuch der Inneren Medizin, 2. Teil,* edited by G. Bergmann, pp. 512–520. Springer Verlag, Göttingen, Berlin, Heidelberg.
7. Cappin, J. M., and Nissim, S. (1978): Visual evoked responses in the assessment of field defects in glaucoma. *Arch. Ophthalmol.,* 93:9–18.
8. Carroll, W. M., Kriss, A., Baraitser, M., Barrett, G., and Halliday, A. M. (1980): The incidence and nature of visual pathway involvement in Friedreich's ataxia. *Brain,* 103:413–434.
9. Friedreich, N. (1876): Über Ataxie mit besonderer Berücksichtigung der hereditären Formen. *Virchows Arch. Pathol. Anat.,* 68:145–245.
10. Halliday, A. M., McDonald, W. I., and Mushin, J. (1973): Visual evoked responses in diagnosis of multiple sclerosis. *Br. Med. J.,* 4:661–664.
11. Holder, G. E. (1978): The effect of chiasmal compression on the pattern-evoked potential. *Electroencephalogr. Clin. Neurophysiol.,* 45:278–280.
12. Kennard, G., Gawel, M., Rudolph, N. de M., and Clifford Rose, F. (1978): Visual evoked potentials in migraine subjects. *Res. Clin. Headache,* 6:73–80.
13. Refsum, S. and Skre, H. (1978): Neurological approaches to the inherited ataxias. *Adv. Neurol.,* 21:1–13.
14. Sjögren, T. (1943): Klinische und Erbbiologische Untersuchungen über die Heredoataxien. *Acta. Psychiatr. Scand.* [*Suppl.*], 27:1–197.
15. Skre, H. (1975): Friedreich's ataxia in western Norway. *Clin. Genet.,* 7:287–298.
16. Van Leuuwen A., and Van Bogaert, L. (1949): Hereditary ataxia with optic atrophy of the retrobulbar neuritis type and latent pallidolysian degeneration. *Brain,* 72:340–363.

Clinical Applications of Evoked Potentials in Neurology,
edited by J. Courjon, F. Mauguiere, and M. Revol.
Raven Press, New York © 1982.

Huntington's Disease: Alterations of Visual and Somatosensory Cortical Evoked Potentials in Patients and Offspring

G. Oepen, M. Doerr, and U. Thoden

Neurologische Universitätsklinik mit Abteilung für Neurophysiologie, 7800 Freiburg, West Germany

One of the tragic features of Huntington's chorea (H.Ch.) is the delayed appearance of clinical symptoms until after the reproductive age is reached (2,3). Hitherto, there have been only a few reports on methods for early detection of the disorder while still in a subclinical stage (12). Although EEG recordings showing a low-voltage fast activity, especially in the later course of the disease (7,13,17), are not appropriate for the discovery of the early signs in offspring (3), the asymmetry of cortical atrophy occurring early in the disease (2) leads to the assumption that cortical evoked potentials may be alterated in the very beginning of H.Ch. Moreover, in doubtful cases of H.Ch. without clear hereditary features, alterations of cortical evoked potentials might be helpful in discriminating the disease from other degenerative processes.

In light of the various reports on this subject (6,11,14), the aim of this study was to reexamine visual evoked potentials (VEP) and somatosensory evoked potentials (SEP) in H.Ch. in comparison to clinically asymptomatic offspring.

PATIENTS AND METHODS

Thirteen patients with manifest H.Ch. (28–65 years, seven males, six females) were compared to nine clinically asymptomatic offspring (six females, three males, 24–44 years) and to normal controls (VEP: 40 subjects, SEP: 10 subjects).

For VEP, a black-and-white checkerboard reversal pattern was produced on a television monitor, subtending 20° of the visual field. Reversal of the checkerboard was performed by a time pulse generator at intervals of 800 msec. At constant overall luminance, the luminance of the white squares was 51.3 cd/m^2; that of the black ones was 0.34 cd/m^2. The recording electrode was placed 6 cm above the inion in the midline with the reference on the left ear and ground connection on the right ear. Sixty-four responses were averaged over 500 msec, and the series was repeated twice. The filters used were 70 Hz with a time constant of 0.1 sec.

For SEP, electrical stimulation of the median nerve was performed at the wrist with pulses of 0.2-msec duration every 500 msec at intensities just at motor threshold. Electrodes were placed following our own previous studies (15) and according to Lehmann et al. (9) over the hand area at 25% of the distance between the two external acoustic meati, corresponding to the middle between T_3–C_3 and T_4–C_4 in the 10–20 System of EEG recording. Scalp recordings were performed between the electrode contralateral to the stimulation and an indifferent electrode at 30% of the nasion-inion distance in the midline (9). A time constant of 0.1 sec and filter of 30 Hz were used; 256 sweeps were averaged by a DL 102 (Data Lab, Ltd., England) and repeated two times. Recordings were performed in a supine position in a darkened room at constant temperature.

RESULTS

Visual Evoked Potentials

For controls, the mean latency of P_{100} was 98 $\pm$ 8.3 msec ($\bar{x} \pm$ SD); the mean amplitude of P_{100}/N_{120}, measured as peak-to-peak distance, was 9 $\pm$ 4μV. In manifest H.Ch., the mean latency of P_{100} was 101 $\pm$ 6.1 msec; the mean amplitude (P_{100}/N_{120}) was 6 $\pm$ 2.5 μV. The late components also seemed to be decreased in amplitude and rather irregular in shape (Fig. 1). In all offspring, the mean latency of P_{100} was 102 $\pm$ 6.6; the mean amplitude of P_{100}/N_{120} was 9.6 $\pm$ 3.9. Four of the offspring showed a flat curve with mean amplitudes (P_{100}/N_{120}) of 6.3 $\pm$ 1.6 msec, and the other five showed no obvious abnormalities. None of the patients or offspring was found outside the normal range (normal mean value $\pm$ 2 SD for latencies and amplitudes).

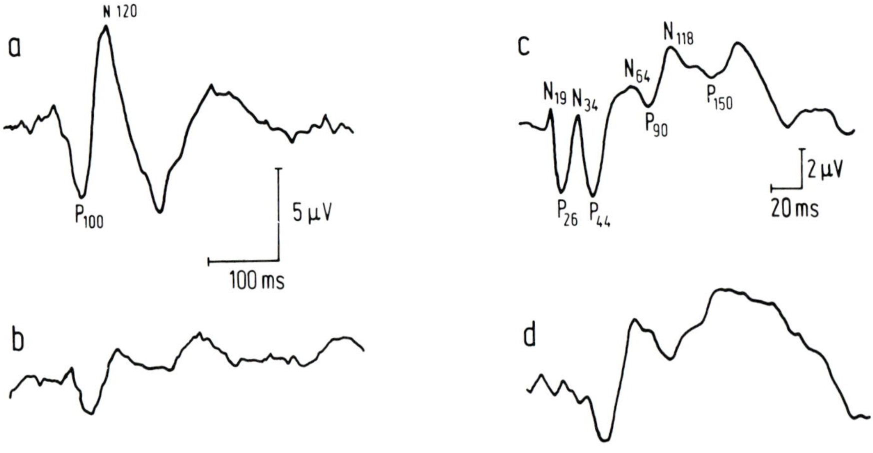

Fig. 1. Raw recordings of **(a)** normal VEP, **(b)** VEP in a patient with H.Ch., **(c)** normal SEP, and **(d)** SEP in a patient with H.Ch.

Somatosensory Evoked Potentials

When the mean latencies of the controls ($N_{19}/P_{26}/N_{34}/P_{43}/N_{64}/P_{90}/N_{120}/P_{150}$) were compared with the mean latencies of the patients ($N_{20}/P_{30}/N_{38}/P_{55}/N_{77}$), the latter seem to be slightly prolonged, less in the early peaks than in the following ones (Table 1). The prolongation of latencies of P_{44}, N_{64}, and P_{90} were significant ($p \leq 0.05$) according to Student's *t*-test; 7 of 13 patients fell out of the normal range ($\bar{x} \pm 2$ SD). The later components after 70 to 80 msec could not be evaluated in patients, as they were often attenuated or even absent (Fig. 1). The mean curves with standard deviations for amplitudes and latencies are indicated in Fig. 2. Also, the number of discriminable peaks during the first 200 msec was diminished in H.Ch. to 3 to 6 as compared to the normal group with 5 to 10. The mean peak-to-peak amplitudes N_{19}/P_{26} and P_{26}/N_{34} were also decreased (see Fig. 2). Using Student's *t*-test, only the reduction of N_{19}/P_{26} was significant ($p \leq 0.05$) in comparison to the controls.

Although SEPs over both hemispheres were rather similar in shape in normal subjects, interhemispheric asymmetries of latencies, amplitudes, and shape were marked in H.Ch. The mean interhemispheric difference for the best recognizable peak, N_{34}/P_{43}, was 1.3 μV (1.0–3.2 μV) and 4.9 msec (1–12 msec) in H.Ch. (normal controls: 0.62 μV, 0–4.1 μV; 1.6 msec, 0–5 msec). This was not significant by Student's *t*-test ($p \leq 0.05$). The later components were not accurately evaluable.

In offspring, three out of nine showed slightly altered SEPs with attenuated or absent late components, interhemispheric asymmetry of amplitudes (2–4 μV), but normal latencies of the early components. Clinically, in 9 out of 13 patients, the sense of position was severly disturbed, in another two slightly; only two patients had no sensory alteration at all. In none of the offspring could comparable symptoms be detected.

DISCUSSION

Despite the fact that electrode position is of great importance for amplitudes of evoked potentials, and VEP and SEP might be partially altered because of technical influences, this might be negligible because all subjects were investigated under the same conditions. The results described above of reduced amplitudes of VEP and SEP and a slight shift of latency in SEP confirmed the findings of Ellenberger et al. (6) and Takahashi and Okada (14). Increased amplitudes of cortical evoked potentials were reported by another author without any details (12). The prolonged latencies of SEPs might be caused by the degenerative alterations found especially in the posterior funiculi of the spinal cord (5,10) and may correlate with the clinical finding of a disturbed sense of position, not known as a usual symptom in H.Ch. This appeared in most of our patients.

As shown in various electrophysiological findings in aging and presenile dementia on the one hand (16) and H.Ch. on the other, the general reduction

TABLE 1. *Amplitudes and latencies of SEPs ($\bar{x} \pm SD$)* in Huntington's chorea

Subject	Mean latencies (msec)								Mean amplitudes (μV)				Number of recognizable peaks in first 200 ms
	N_1	P_1	N_2	P_2	N_3	P_3	N_4	P_4	N_1/P_1	P_1/N_2	N_2/P_2	P_2/N_3	
Huntington's chorea ($N = 13$)	20.2 ±2.5	30.75 ±6.9	38 ±8.7	54.6 ±11.7	77 ±17	127 ±32			1.31 ±0.63	1.13 ±0.99	2.83 ±1.41		4.5 ± 1.3
Offspring ($N = 9$)	18.9 ±2.3	26.4 ±3.5	36.8 ±3.9	48.3 ±3.8	66.9 ±7.2	92.4 ±15.8	134.9 ±16.2	153 ±8.7	2.73 ±1.48	2.72 ±1.72	2.28 ±1.26	2.56 ±1.39	7.1 ± 1.6 $N = 3$: 5.3 ± 0.8 $N = 6$: 8 ± 1,1
Normal group ($N = 10$)	19 ±1.3	26.4 ±2.4	33.9 ±2.6	43.6 ±3.1	64.4 ±8.2	88.9 ±11.7	117.8 ±13.6	150.5 ±6.4	4.37 ±1.95	2.45 ±1.56	2.60 ±1.5	7.06 ±3.21	7.8 ± 1.1

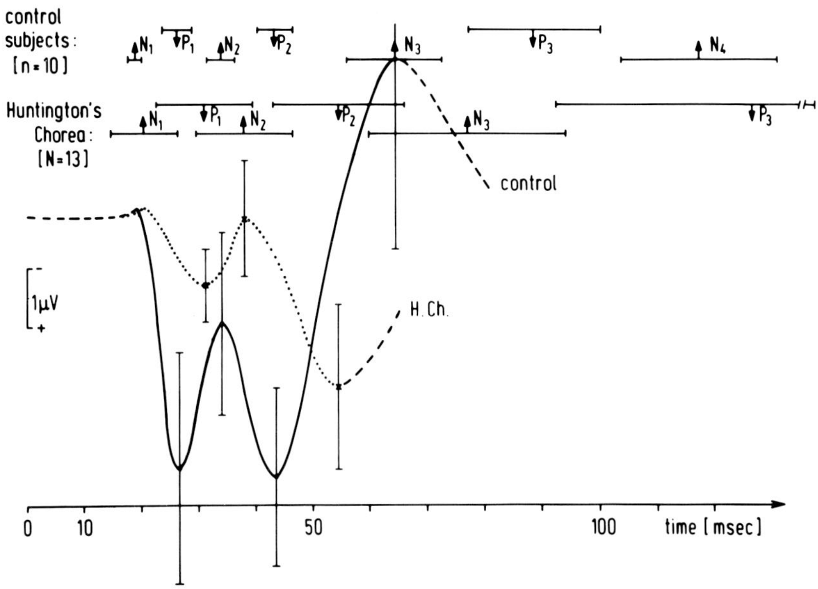

Fig. 2. Averaged SEPs calculated from mean values of patients with H.Ch. *(dotted line),* in comparison to normal controls *(continuous line).* The standard deviation (SD) is given for amplitudes with *vertical* and for latencies with *horizontal lines.*

of amplitudes in H.Ch. is not sufficiently explained when one considers cortical processes only. Therefore, the striking atrophy of the caudate nucleus in H.Ch. was regarded as responsible for the amplitude reduction by Takahashi and Okada (14). As animal experiments demonstrating an inhibition of cortical evoked potentials by caudate stimulation do not support this hypothesis (4,8), degenerative alterations of nonspecific thalamic structures with thalamic–striato–cortical loops (10) might be more appropriate to explain the electrophysiological findings.

The mean findings in offspring are a reduced number of recognizable peaks after 70 to 100 msec, a reduction of amplitudes in VEP and SEP, and, more accentuated than in manifest H.Ch., an interhemispheric asymmetry in SEP in parallel to the asymmetric neuropathological degeneration in the early disease (2). The lack of altered VEPs in offspring as reported by other authors (6) probably has technical reasons, as the flashlight technique was used, a technique not directly comparable with the checkerboard–reversal stimulation used in this study (1). The slight changes reported in offspring seem to be of interest as two of the three offspring with altered SEPs and all four offspring with altered VEPs also showed subclinical abnormalities of eye movements as detected by electrooculography (11). Nevertheless, none of the offspring fell out of the normal ranges of VEPs or SEPs. Thus, these techniques are of less value for diagnostic purposes.

SUMMARY

In 13 patients suffering from Huntington's chorea (H.Ch.), VEPs and SEPs were investigated in comparison to 9 clinically inconspicuous offspring and normal adults.

1. The mean amplitude of VEP was reduced in choreatic patients and in four out of nine offspring.
2. Latencies of P_{100} in VEP were normal in all subjects.
3. The late components were reduced in amplitude and rather irregular in shape.
4. The latencies of SEPs were slightly prolonged, less marked in the early peaks and more pronounced in the later ones.
5. The late components after 70 to 100 msec were often attenuated or even absent.
6. The mean amplitude of the first two peaks was reduced.
7. Interhemispheric asymmetries were pronounced in three out of nine offspring.

ACKNOWLEDGMENT

Supported by Sonderforschungsbereich Hirnforschung und Sinnesphysiologie (SFB 70) der Deutschen Forschungsgemeinschaft (DFG).

REFERENCES

1. Arden, G. B., Bodis-Wollner, I., Halliday, A. M., Jeffreys, A., Kulikowski, J. J., Spekrejse, H., Regan, D., (1977): Methodology of patterned visual stimulation. In: *Visual Evoked Potentials in Man: New Developments,* edited by J. E. Desmedt, pp. 3–15. Clarendon Press, Oxford.
2. Bruyn, G. W. (1969): Huntington's chorea: Historical, clinical and laboratory synopsis. In: *Handbook of Neurology, Vol. 13,* edited by P. Vinken and G. W. Bruyn, pp. 298–378. North-Holland, Amsterdam.
3. Chandler, J. H. (1966): EEG in prediction of Huntington's chorea. An eighteen year follow-up. *Electroencephalogr. Clin. Neurophysiol.,* 21:79–80.
4. Demetrescu, M., and Demetrescu, M., (1962): The inhibitory action of the caudate nucleus in the cortical primary receiving areas in the cat. *Electroencephalogr. Clin. Neurophysiol.,* 14:37–50.
5. Desmedt, J. E. (1979): Somatosensory evoked potentials in man: Maturation, cognitive parameters and clinical uses in neurological disorders. In: *Human Evoked Potentials,* edited by D. Lehmann and E. Callaway, pp. 83–103. Plenum Press, New York and London.
6. Ellenberger, C., Denis, J. P., and Ziegler, S. B., (1978): The visually evoked potential in Huntington disease. *Neurology,* 28:95–97.
7. Gibbs, F. A., and Gibbs, E. L., (1941): *Atlas of Electroencephalography.* Cummings, Cambridge, Massachusetts.
8. Krauthamer, G. M., and Albe-Fessard, D., (1964): Electrophysiologic studies of the basal ganglia and striopallidal inhibition of nonspecific afferent activity. *Neuropsychologia,* 2:73–83.
9. Lehmann, D., Gabathuler, U., and Baumgartner, G., (1979): Right/left differences of median nerve evoked scalp potentials in multiple sclerosis. *J. Neurol.,* 221:15–24.
10. McCaughy, W. T. E. (1961): The pathological spectrum of Huntington's chorea. *J. Nerv. Ment. Dis.,* 133:91–103.

11. Oepen, G., Clarenbach, P., and Thoden, U., (1981): Disturbances of eye movements in Chorea Huntington. *Arch. Psychiat. Nervenkr.,* 229:205–213.
12. Paulson, G. W. (1979): Diagnosis of Huntington's disease. In: *Advances in Neurology, Vol. 23,* edited by T. N. Chase, N. S. Wexler, and A. Barbeau, Raven Press, pp. 177–184. New York.
13. Scott, D. F., Heathfield, K. W. G., Toone, B., and Margerison, J. H., (1972): The EEG in Huntington's chorea: A clinical and neuropathological study. *J. Neurol. Neurosurg. Psychiatry,* 35:97–102.
14. Takahashi, K., and Okada, E., (1972): Somatosensory and visual evoked potentials in Huntington's chorea. *Clin. Neurol. (Tokyo),* 22:381–385.
15. Thoden, U., Doerr, M., Dieckmann, G., and Krainick, J. U., (1979): Medial thalamic permanent electrodes for pain control in man: An electrophysiological and clinical study. *Electroencephalogr. Clin. Neurophysiol.,* 47:582–591.
16. Visser, S. L., Stam, F. C., van Tilburg, W., Op den Velde, W., Blom, J. L., De Rijke, W., (1976): Visual evoked response in senile and presenile dementia. *Electroencephalogr. Clin. Neurophysiol.,* 40:385–392.
17. Vogel, F., Wendt, G. G., and Oepen, H., (1961): Das EEG und das Problem einer Frühdiagnose der Chorea Huntington. *Dtsch. Z. Nervenheilk,* 182:355–361.

Clinical Applications of Evoked Potentials in Neurology,
edited by J. Courjon, F. Mauguiere, and M. Revol.
Raven Press, New York © 1982.

Visual Evoked Potentials and Alcohol-Induced Brain Damage

*J. Posthuma and **S. L. Visser

**Department of Clinical Neurophysiology, Psychiatric Hospital, Dennenoord Zuidlaren, The Netherlands; and **Academisch Hospital, Free University and Valeriuskliniek, Amsterdam, The Netherlands*

It is well known that chronic alcoholism may lead to damage to the nervous system. Previous studies have shown that dietary factors and thiamine deficiency may be the proximate cause of the disease, whereas Haferkamp (4) supposed that ethyl alcohol and other toxic metabolites may be the cause of damage.

Electroencephalography is not very helpful in the detection of alcohol-induced brain damage. As a rule, the EEG is normal or shows slight aspecific abnormalities. Only in serious cases of the Wernicke–Korsakow syndrome is there an increase in slow and periodic delta activity in the EEG (1,6).

The effect of alcohol on visual evoked potentials (VEP) is most often studied by acute administration of alcohol to healthy subjects (7–11). The results of these studies suggest a decrease in late component EP amplitudes rather than a change of latencies. Furthermore, there is an inverse relationship between the dose and blood level of the alcohol and EP amplitude (11).

There are only a few studies on EPs in chronic alcoholics. The results again suggest a decrease in late component EP amplitudes. Alcohol withdrawal is followed by recovery of late EP components' amplitudes. In chronic alcoholics, interhemispheric asymmetries are decreased (2,8,12).

In clinical neurophysiological practice it is difficult to detect alcohol-induced brain damage in an early stage. The aim of the present study is to investigate whether it is possible to prove alcohol-induced brain damage by VEPs.

METHODS

Subjects

The study was carried out on three groups of subjects. The first consisted of 20 normal volunteers, employees of the psychiatric hospital Dennenoord. None of them were alcoholics. They included 11 males and 9 females and had a mean age of 49.0 years. The second group included 20 chronic alcoholics without clinical signs of brain damage. There were 19 males and 1 female, and they had a mean age of 46.9 years. The third group of subjects included 16 alcohol-induced Korsakow patients (deterioration of memory in clear consciousness was the most prominent intellectual defect; disorientation was frequently present). This group contained eight males and 8 females with a mean age of 55.0 years.

All patients were admitted to the mental hospital Dennenoord. At the time of examination, all subjects had been free of medication at least 7 days. None of them suffered from ophthalmological abnormalities, corrected refraction excluded.

Visual Evoked Potentials

Evoked potentials were recorded with the subjects seated in an electrically shielded and darkened room. Surface electrodes were placed at scalp locations F_z, P_z, O_z, O_1, and O_2. Recording was carried out in a bipolar manner (P_z–F_z, O_z–F_z, O_1–F_z, and O_2–F_z).

Brain potentials were amplified by a Siemens-Elema Mingograph EEG apparatus and stored on magnetic tape. Band width of the system was 0.5 to 70 Hz at 3 dB. Visual evoked potentials were evoked by checkerboard pattern reversal, according to Halliday et al. (5), and by flashes of a Siemens-Elema photo stimulator, flash duration 10 msec. In each subject, VEPs were evoked by checkerboard and flashes in one session (always in that sequence).

Subjects were asked to fixate on the center of the checkerboard and lamp. The distance from eyes to checkerboard or lamp was 43 cm. Check size was 1°20′; field size, 33°20′. The measured luminance of the total checkerboard pattern at the location of the subjects' eyes was 115 lux, and for the flashes, 50 lux. Sixty-four stimuli were delivered at random to both eyes with intervals between 1 and 2.5 sec, and artifacts in the EEG were avoided. The 64 responses were averaged for analysis by a PDP 11/34 computer, and the averaged response was plotted. Figure 1 is a graphical display of an individual VEP evoked by checkerboard and by flash. The sampling rate was 500/sec; analysis time was 450 msec.

For statistical analysis, the Wilcoxon two-sample test was used (level of significance 5%).

RESULTS

Table 1 presents the data on the number of peaks that could be identified by checkerboard reversal and flashes in the lead O_z–F_z. The results show P3 (P100) to be the most constant and easiest detectable peak. Because of this experience and data from literature, we focused our study on P3.

In healthy volunteers, P3 latency evoked by pattern reversal was shorter (95.5 msec; Table 2) than that evoked by flash (120.0 msec; Table 3). Moreover, the variability was less in pattern-evoked VEPs.

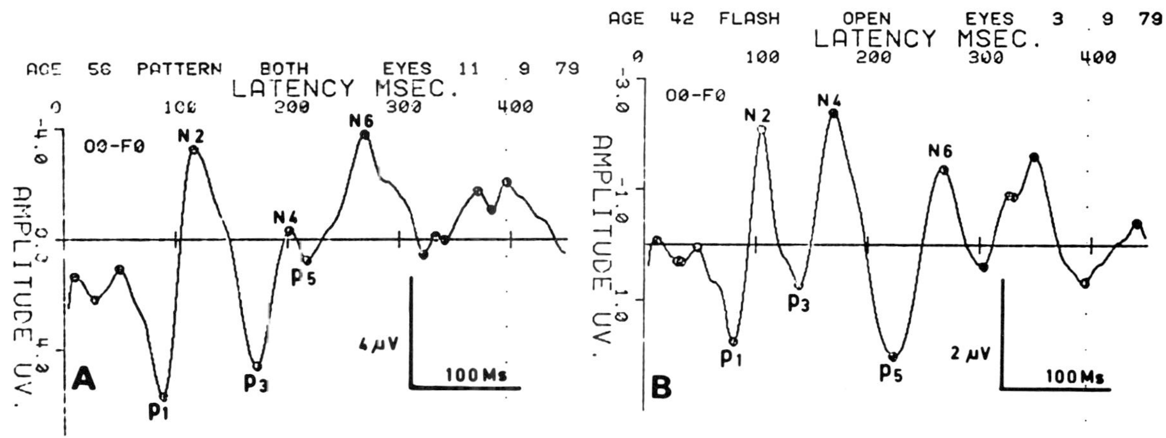

FIG. 1. Example of the graphical display of an individual VEP evoked **(A)** by checkerboard reversal and **(B)** by flash.

TABLE 1. *Number of healthy volunteers and patients in whom peaks 1 to 6 could be identified*[a]

Peak	Healthy Volunteers ($N=20$)		Chronic Alcoholics ($N=20$)		Korsakow Patients ($N=16$)	
	Checkerboard	Flash	Checkerboard	Flash	Checkerboard	Flash
P1	2	15	6	9	11	14
N2	6	18	13	12	14	15
P3	20	18	20	15	15	14
N4	19	16	18	15	13	9
P5	13	13	15	10	10	8
N6	10	12	12	10	8	8

[a] Both eyes were stimulated; recording was O_z–F_z.

TABLE 2. *Mean latency (msec ± SD) for peaks of visual evoked potentials evoked by checkerboard pattern reversal*

Peak	Healthy volunteers ($N=20$)	Chronic alcoholics ($N=20$)	Korsakow patients ($N=16$)
P1	54.2 ± 5.6	65.7 ± 26.4	71.9 ± 13.8
N2	65.7 ± 5.5	76.1 ± 19.9	85.7 ± 25.4
P3[a]	95.5 ± 4.2	103.2 ± 19.8	121.8 ± 30.1
N4	128.5 ± 7.1	140.3 ± 22.4	158.0 ± 22.8
P5	166.3 ± 12.9	178.8 ± 24.8	197.3 ± 32.2
N6	219.4 ± 27.9	211.4 ± 32.0	239.6 ± 50.0

[a] Differences between normals and chronic alcoholics are not significant ($p > 0.05$); differences between normals and Korsakow patients and between chronic alcoholics and the Korsakow group are statistically significant ($p \leq 0.05$).

TABLE 3. *Mean latency (msec ± SD) for peaks of visual evoked potentials evoked by flash*

Peak	Healthy volunteers ($N=20$)	Chronic alcoholics ($N=20$)	Korsakow patients ($N=16$)
P1	71.6 ± 15.6	69.8 ± 16.2	73.3 ± 13.8
N2	91.5 ± 17.3	98.6 ± 18.4	102.8 ± 19.4
P3[a]	120.0 ± 14.5	129.0 ± 14.4	143.9 ± 20.9
N4	153.9 ± 20.3	163.3 ± 18.4	173.9 ± 32.5
P5	199.3 ± 25.2	213.1 ± 26.9	211.9 ± 40.5
N6	249.4 ± 31.2	248.2 ± 43.9	260.0 ± 64.5

[a] Differences between normals and chronic alcoholics are not significant ($p > 0.05$); differences between normals and Korsakow patients and between chronic alcoholics and the Korsakow group are statistically significant ($p \leqslant 0.05$).

TABLE 4. *Mean amplitude (μV ± SD) for peaks in visual evoked potentials evoked by checkerboard pattern reversal and flash*

Peak	Healthy volunteers (N = 20)		Chronic alcoholics (N = 20)		Korsakow patients (N = 16)	
	Checkerboard	Flash	Checkerboard	Flash	Checkerboard	Flash
P1	+2.2 ± 1.9	+3.0 ± 3.0	+2.0 ± 2.0	+5.2 ± 4.9	+4.2 ± 5.3	+5.4 ± 5.9
N2	−2.3 ± 2.1	−1.8 ± 3.3	−0.7 ± 1.3	−2.6 ± 5.2	−1.8 ± 2.9	−1.7 ± 2.6
P3[a]	+8.7 ± 3.4	+4.0 ± 2.5	+7.8 ± 4.2	+4.6 ± 3.1	+7.1 ± 5.0	+6.2 ± 3.4
N4	−2.8 ± 3.1	−1.4 ± 2.3	−2.0 ± 2.3	−2.3 ± 2.9	−2.0 ± 1.7	−1.6 ± 3.4
P5	+2.7 ± 1.2	+4.2 ± 3.2	+1.3 ± 1.4	+2.8 ± 2.5	+2.2 ± 1.5	+5.5 ± 4.2
N6	−2.0 ± 1.6	−2.1 ± 2.1	−3.4 ± 2.9	−2.4 ± 1.9	−1.8 ± 1.2	−2.8 ± 2.6

[a] None of the amplitude differences between groups are statistically significant ($p > 0.05$).

In the patient groups, latencies were longer than those in normal volunteers and showed an increased variability. Within the patient groups, Korsakow patients showed more abnormalities than chronic alcoholics without memory deterioration.

In our study, VEP amplitudes gave smaller intergroup differences than did latencies (Table 4). In chronic alcoholics and alcohol-induced Korsakow patients, there seemed to be a decrease of amplitude in peak N2–P5 evoked by the checkerboard. In contrast, the amplitudes of peaks P1, P3, N4, and P5 seemed to be increased when evoked by flash.

DISCUSSION

We compared the VEPs of 20 chronic alcoholics and 16 alcohol-induced Korsakow patients with the VEPs of 20 healthy volunteers. The results show that in the patient groups, latencies were longer.

Our results show P3 (P100) to be the most constant and easiest detectable peak. The most delayed P100 responses were recorded in patients with Korsakow. In the patient groups, increased peak latencies were more easily detected when evoked by checkerboard reversal.

Normal ranges were defined as the mean ± 2.5 SD. We compared these values with those in the patient groups. In the Korsakow group, in nine patients P3 latencies were out of the normal range when evoked by pattern reversal; in one, P3 was not detected, and in six patients, the latencies were not delayed. There were no abnormal latencies when evoked by flash.

In chronic alcoholics, in three out of 20 patients, P3 latencies were delayed when evoked by checkerboard reversal. None of the patients showed delayed latencies when evoked by flash. Our results are in agreement with those of Dustman et al. (3) and Porjesz and Begleiter (8). In their experiments with flash-evoked VEPs in alcoholics, they found an increase of peak latencies of late components.

In our study, the amplitudes give less information in the patient groups. The amplitudes of N2 up to and including P5 evoked by checkerboard seemed to be decreased in the patient groups. This is in agreement with the experiences with flashes in other studies (2,8,12). In our experience with flash-evoked VEP, the amplitudes of P1, P3, N4, and P5 in the patient groups seemed to be increased. However, when we compare our results with mean ± 2.5 SD in normals, the amplitudes are within normal limits.

In our opinion, VEPs evoked by checkerboard pattern reversal may give diagnostic evidence of alcohol-induced brain damage in Korsakow patients. In chronic alcoholics, the diagnostic value is less. Visual evoked potentials evoked by flash have, in our opinion, no diagnostic value in this type of patient.

ACKNOWLEDGMENT

We thank Mrs. Agnes M. J. Lauxen-Bon for her dedicated support and technical assistance.

REFERENCES

1. Brewer, C., and Perrett, L. (1971): Brain damage due to alcohol consumption: An air-encephalographic, psychometric and electroencephalographic study. *Br. J. Addict.,* 66:170–182.
2. Coger, R. W., Dymond, A. M., Serafetinides, E. A., Lowenstam, I., and Pearson, D. (1976): Alcoholism: Averaged visual evoked response amplitude–intensity slope and symmetry in withdrawal. *Biol. Psychiatry,* 11:435–443.
3. Dustman, R. E., Snyder, E. W., Callner, D. A., and Beck, E. C. (1979): The evoked response as a measure of cerebral dysfunction. In: *Evoked Brain Potentials and Behavior,* edited by H. Begleiter, pp. 321–363. Plenum Press, New York and London.
4. Haferkamp, G. (1976): Neurologische Komplikationen bei chronischer Alkoholvergiftung. *Dtsch. Med. Wochenschr.,* 101:55–59.
5. Halliday, A. M., McDonald, W. I., and Mushin, J. (1972): Delayed visual evoked response in optic neuritis. *Lancet,* 1:982–985.
6. Hootsmans, W. J. M. (1961): Elektro-encefalografische bevindingen bij de ziekte van Wernicke. *Ned. Tijdschr. Geneeskd.,* 105:1722–1724.
7. Lewis, E. G., Dustman, R. E., and Beck, E. C. (1970): The effects of alcohol on visual and somato-sensory evoked responses. *Electroencephalogr. Clin. Neurophysiol.,* 28:202–205.
8. Porjesz, B., and Begleiter, H. (1979): Visual evoked potentials and brain dysfunction in chronic alcoholics. In: *Evoked Brain Potentials and Behavior,* edited by H. Begleiter, pp. 277–302. Plenum Press, New York and London.
9. Rhodes, L. E., Obitz, F. W., and Creel, D. (1975): Effects of alcohol and task on hemispheric asymmetry of visually evoked potentials in man. *Electroencephalogr. Clin. Neurophysiol.,* 38:561–568.
10. Salamy, A. (1973): The effects of alcohol on the variability of the human evoked potential. *Neuropharmacology,* 12:1103–1107.
11. Salamy, A., and Williams, H. L. (1973): The effects of alcohol on sensory evoked and spontaneous cerebral potentials in man. *Electroencephalogr. Clin. Neurophysiol.,* 35:3–11.
12. Salamy, J. G., Wright, J. R., and Faillace, L. A. (1980): Changes in average evoked responses during abstention in chronic alcoholics. *J. Nerv. Ment. Dis.,* 160:19–25.

Clinical Applications of Evoked Potentials in Neurology,
edited by J. Courjon, F. Mauguiere, and M. Revol.
Raven Press, New York © 1982.

Brainstem Auditory Evoked Potentials in Clinical Neurology

Keith H. Chiappa

Department of Neurology, Electroencephalography Laboratory, Harvard Medical School and Massachusetts General Hospital, Boston, Massachusetts 02114

In only a few years of clinical use, brainstem auditory evoked potentials (BAEPs) have become an integral part of the practice of neurology. They have direct application in the diagnosis and management of patients with acoustic neuromas, other cerebello–pontine angle tumors, intrinsic brainstem lesions such as tumors, vascular disease, degenerative diseases, trauma, and brain death, and coma as well as during surgery.

The clinical utility of BAEPs stems from their close relationship to the anatomy of brainstem auditory pathways. This anatomic specificity allows localization of conduction defects to within a centimeter or so in contrast to the more diffuse generator sources of longer latency potentials. Because of this specificity, patients with significant brainstem lesions can have normal BAEPs if the auditory tracts in the pontine tegmentum and midbrain are not involved. For example, patients with "locked-in" syndrome sometimes have normal BAEPs; this fact simply reflects the predominantly ventral pontine involvement in that disease.

For purposes of clinical interpretation, BAEPs are unaffected by the psychological state of the patient (e.g., drowsiness), general anesthesia, temperature, or even high-dose barbiturate intoxication or therapy of increased intracranial pressure. These factors of reliability and consistency in even the most difficult clinical situations are the basis for the clinical utility of BAEPs.

However, the generator sources of BAEP waveforms are presently poorly documented. Early work in cats showed a separation between the first and fifth waves of 5.3 msec, more than 1 msec greater than the I–V separation in humans. Yet, the fact that the fifth wave disappeared when the inferior colliculus was removed from the cats has been taken as evidence for a relationship in humans between wave V and the inferior colliculus (the results of those animal studies have been challenged recently). There are no published cases of clinico–pathological correlations in humans that provide good evidence on BAEP waveform generators, especially for waves IV and V.

In humans, there is little evidence that bears on the laterality of generator sources of BAEPs. Brainstem lesions usually produce BAEP abnormalities most marked following stimulation of and recording from the ear ipsilateral to the lesion. However, the majority of these lesions involve lower pontine structures; reports of pathologically proven cases with the lesion restricted unilaterally to the upper pons or midbrain have not yet been published. Thus, all of these are areas that are in great need of further observations in humans.

Proper clinical interpretation of BAEPs requires: (a) Use of a test protocol that demonstrates waveform reproducibility—one method is repetition and superimposition of separate trials (each trial consisting of the average of at least 1,000 stimuli) using the same stimulus and recording parameters; a minimum of two trials is required, and usually three or four are done. (b) Normal parameters based on results obtained from more than 35 normal subjects using all subject (e.g., age and sex), stimulus (e.g., click rate, intensity, and polarity), and recording (e.g., filter bandpass) parameters that will be used in testing patients. (c) Use of definitions of abnormality that exclude at least 98% of normals. (d) Special attention paid to recording a clear eighth nerve activation potential (wave I)—special electrodes should be used if wave I is not seen with the conventional earlobe placement. (e) Use of only interwave separation measurements except in special circumstances. (f) Attention to the important interactions between audiogram shape and stimulus parameters (e.g., click polarity and intensity) that are still being investigated. (g) Discussion of localization of a conduction defect in light of the uncertainty regarding generator sources and laterality as stated above. Publication criteria should be based on at least these points.

Clinical Applications of Evoked Potentials in Neurology,
edited by J. Courjon, F. Mauguiere, and M. Revol.
Raven Press, New York © 1982.

Correlation of Brainstem Evoked Response with Direct Acoustic Nerve Potential

J. P. Spire, G. J. Dohrmann, and P. S. Prieto

The University of Chicago, Department of Neurology, Chicago, Illinois 60637

The initial purpose of this study was to design a procedure to document electrophysiologically the effect of microvascular decompression of the trigeminal nerve for intractable tic douloureux. It was thought that we should be able to identify the fifth nerve action potential, pre- and postmicrovascular decompression. However, as the eighth nerve is more readily accessible at posterior fossa craniotomy, we thought to devise the fifth nerve methodology by approaching the eighth nerve first. No human data of the direct acoustic nerve action potential has yet been published to our knowledge. Moreover, it seemed interesting to correlate the eighth nerve action potential (NAP) with brainstem auditory evoked response (BAER) as the first peak of that response is purported to be the eighth NAP recorded from a far field.

MATERIALS

Twenty patients (18 women, 2 men) ranging from 19 to 74 years of age (mean, 53.5 years) were studied. All patients carried a diagnosis of intractable trigeminal neuralgia unresponsive to conventional medical management. Five patients proved unsatisfactory for study because of either severe presbyacusis or technical difficulties. Informed consent was obtained from each patient. The recording procedure itself increased anesthesia time (mean, 2.5 hr) by 15 to 20 min only. Many patients were studied audiologically before the study, and baseline BAERs were obtained 24 hr prior to the operation. In most instances, the NAP recordings were obtained after the microvascular decompression procedure of the fifth nerve.

METHODS

An unfiltered click was delivered to the ear by a miniature hearing-aid-type transducer (Knowles ED 1912) fitted in a plastic molded earpiece placed directly into the external auditory canal. The frequency response of the transducer was from 25 to 8,000 Hz with maximum energy at 1,000 Hz. A 0.1-msec compression click generated by a Grass S8 stimulator was delivered at rates between 20/sec and 300/sec. The recording electrode, a small 1.5-mm silver ball placed in a specially designed frame, was positioned directly on the eighth nerve between the porus acousticus and the brainstem. The reference electrode was either the unilateral or linked mastoids or ears, no appreciable difference being noted for either. The BAER active electrode was the conventional C_Z site also referenced to linked ears. The signals were processed by a Nicolet 1074 averager with an amplifier bandpass of 3 to 3,000 Hz. The averaged response of 1024 clicks permitted an excellent signal-to-noise ratio for most of the NAPs.

RESULTS

Direct Nerve Action Potential

A typical NAP is shown in Fig. 1. It consists typically of a surface positive upward deflection followed by a large negative deflection and some smaller following peaks. Although the negative deflection was always clearly identifiable, the initial positive peak amplitude varied from subject to subject. The NAPs in general were stable in configuration, amplitude, and latency for a given patient, but substantial differences of the relative amplitude of the peaks were seen from patient to patient. Late peaks were not always identifiable. We have labeled the onset "ϕ" and successive peaks "1," "2," "3," "4," or positive–negative, positive–negative. The amplitude (μV) is defined as the maximum peak-to-peak deflection between peaks 1 and 2. The location of the reference electrode(s) had no effect on the configuration or amplitude of the NAP (Fig. 2).

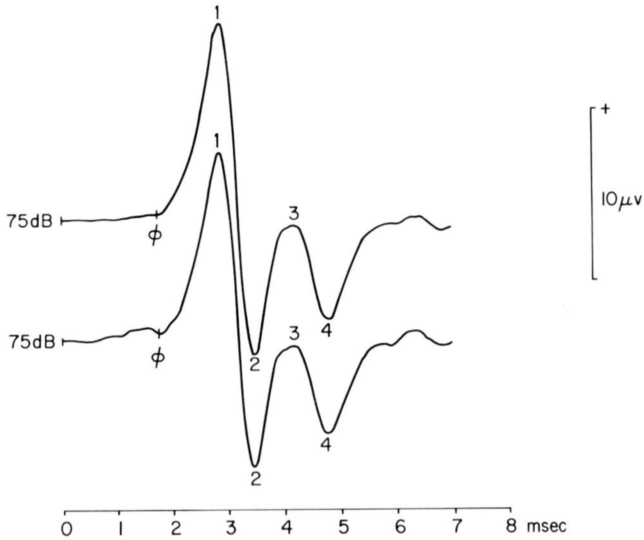

FIG. 1. Human eighth nerve action potential.

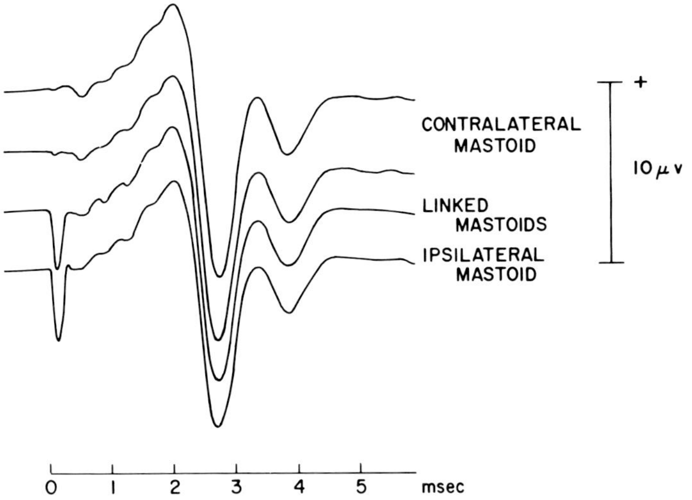

FIG. 2. Human eighth nerve action potential with various reference electrode sites evoked by 60-dB SPL.

Latency, Amplitude, and Stimulus Intensity

The latency, amplitude and configuration of the NAP changes as the click intensity is reduced in 5-dB steps. In two of the younger patients, we were able to follow the NAP down to 0 dB SPL (Fig. 3). The NAP became inapparent at stimuli levels below 45 dB as many patients presented some degree of presbyacusis and high-frequency hearing loss.

For comparative purposes, we divided our patients into younger (19–42 years; mean, 35 years) and older groups, (50–73 years; mean, 63 years) As the stimulus intensity is decreased, there is the anticipated increase of NAP latencies (Tables 1 and 2). The latency of the NAP of the older ears is slightly longer than for the younger ears (Fig. 4).

The maximum peak-to-peak (peaks 1–2) amplitude of the response of each group (younger and older) was measured and plotted in relation to decreasing stimulus intensity (Fig. 4). The older ears show that the NAP response will extinguish at approximately 48 dB (presumably reflecting high-frequency loss from presbyacusis encountered in these patients). The slopes of the lines comparing the younger- and older-ear NAP amplitudes for decreasing stimulus intensity appear to be the same.

Simultaneous Brainstem Auditory Evoked Response and Nerve Action Potential

We obtained reliable data in only four patients for click intensities between 55 and 75 dB. Failure to obtain satisfactory BAERs in the operating room

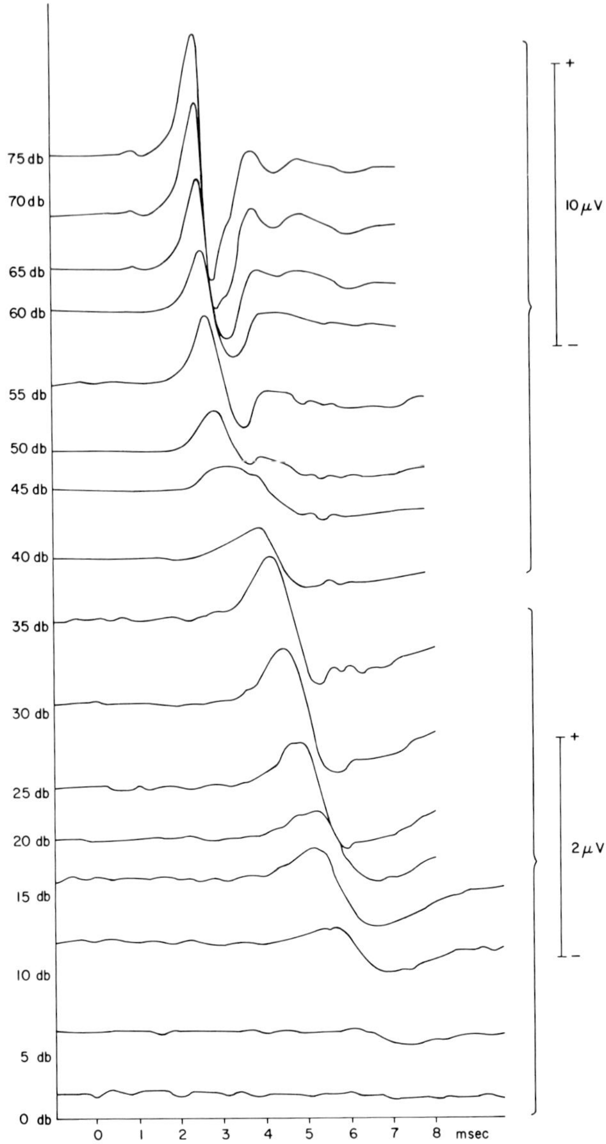

FIG. 3. Latency of human eighth nerve action potential versus intensity of stimulus (rate at 20/sec).

was attributed to electrical contamination from surrounding equipment. The typical simultaneous response may be seen in Fig. 5. Note amplitude scaling differences between the BAER and NAP. The results comparing BAER and NAP latencies are given in Table 3. It would appear that the onset of NAP and BAER are only comparable in that Peak 1 of NAP and Peak I of BAER

TABLE 1. *Latency and amplitude of eighth nerve action potentials in younger ears*[a]

Stimulus intensity	Latency of NAP (msec)					Amplitude of NAP (μV)
	Onset	1	2	3	4	
75 dB	1.5 ± 0.15	2.2 ± 0.2	2.7 ± 0.3	3.4 ± 0.4	4.2 ± 0.1	31.7 ± 1.5
70 dB	1.5 ± 0.2	2.2 ± 0.2	2.8 ± 0.3	3.5 ± 0.4	4.1 ± 0.3	27.6 ± 3.7
65 dB	1.4 ± 0.4	2.2 ± 0.4	2.8 ± 0.6	3.3 ± 0.5	4.2 ± 0.6	20.1 ± 3.4
60 dB	1.6 ± 0.4	2.2 ± 0.4	2.8 ± 0.5	3.5 ± 0.5	4.2 ± 0.6	17.3 ± 6.1
55 dB	1.8 ± 0.3	2.4 ± 0.4	3.1 ± 0.5	3.8 ± 0.5		13.8 ± 2.9
50 dB	1.8 ± 0.4	2.4 ± 0.5	3.1 ± 0.6	3.6 ± 0.6	4.3 ± 0.7	8.2 ± 2.2
45 dB	2.2 ± 0.4	2.7 ± 0.3	3.8 ± 1.3			7.20 ± 1.00

[a] Ages were 19 to 42 years (mean, 35 years); *N* ranged from 3 to 7. All values are mean ± SD.

TABLE 2. *Latency and amplitude of eighth nerve action potentials in older ears*[a]

Stimulus intensity	Latency of NAP (msec)					Amplitude of NAP (μV)
	Onset	1	2	3	4	
75 dB	1.7 ± 0.1	2.7 ± 0.5	3.4 ± 0.6			23.7 ± 4.8
70 dB	1.9 ± 0.2	2.8 ± 0.4	3.5 ± 0.5			21.6 ± 1.8
65 dB	1.8 ± 0.2	2.7 ± 0.4	3.5 ± 0.5	4.0 ± 0.2		16.5 ± 12.5
60 dB	2.0 ± 0.2	2.7 ± 0.4	3.5 ± 0.5	4.0 ± 0.2		9.3 ± 8.4
55 dB	2.0 ± 0.1	2.6 ± 1.0	3.6 ± 0.8	4.1 ± 0.2		8.9 ± 6.8
50 dB	2.7 ± 1.8	3.9 ± 1.04	5.8 ± 0.2			1.8
45 dB	2.7 ± 1.8	3.9				1.7

[a] Ages were 50 to 73 years (mean, 62 years); *N* ranged from 4 to 8. All values are mean ± SD.

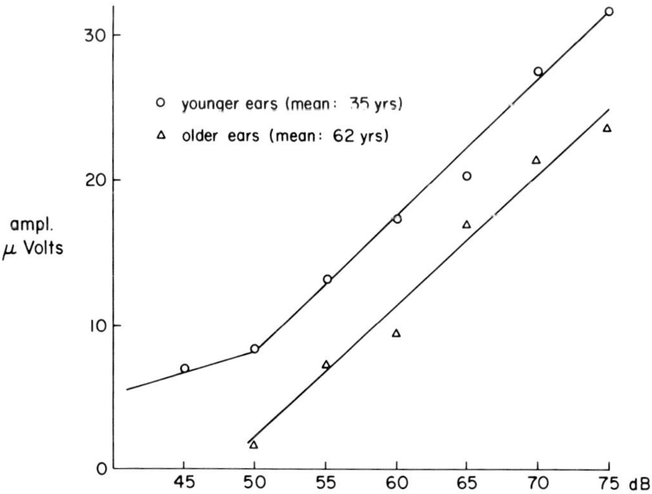

FIG. 4. Human eighth nerve action potential maximum amplitude as a function of click intensity: comparison of younger and older ears.

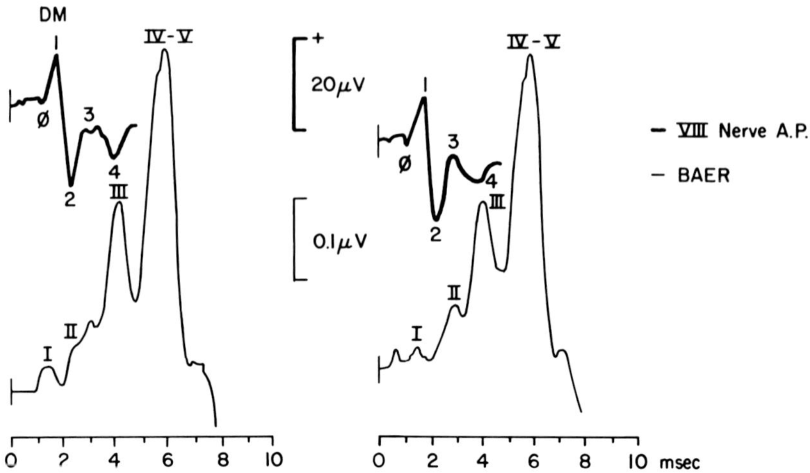

FIG. 5. Simultaneous records of eighth nerve action potential and BAER in the same subject with 75 and 70 dB SPL, 0.1-msec broad-band clicks (*N* = 1,024; rate = 20/sec).

TABLE 3. *Latencies[a] of eighth nerve action potentials and brainstem auditory evoked responses recorded simultaneously[b]*

NAP		BAER	
Peak	Latency	Peak	Latency
0	1.55 ± 0.205	0	1.43 ± 0.326
1	2.37 ± 0.462	I	1.97 ± 0.422
2	3.01 ± 0.569	II	3.53 ± 0.228
3	4.03 ± 0.634	III	4.87 ± 0.384
4	4.77 ± 0.396	IV–V	6.87 ± 0.180

[a] Means ± SD.
[b] Evoked by 75 dB SPL.

are within the same latency time frame. However, none of the NAP peaks or troughs actually fell in concordance with the BAER peaks. Because of this discrepancy, we realized that knowledge of exact position of our electrode on the nerve as well as the conduction velocity (CV) of the eighth nerve must be important factors. Therefore, in our most recent case, we determined the conduction velocity of the human acoustic nerve by careful placement of the electrode along the nerve, moving it from the porus acousticus (internal auditory meatus) laterally to its most medially accessible position (Fig. 6). The compound action potential of the acoustic nerve for this patient had a conduction velocity of approximately 12 to 25 m/sec, each peak of the NAP having a slightly different latency in relation to distance; these determinations are being validated by additional observations. Also, the latency of peak 1 of the NAP at the porus was almost the same as the latency peak I of BAER recorded simultaneously. The

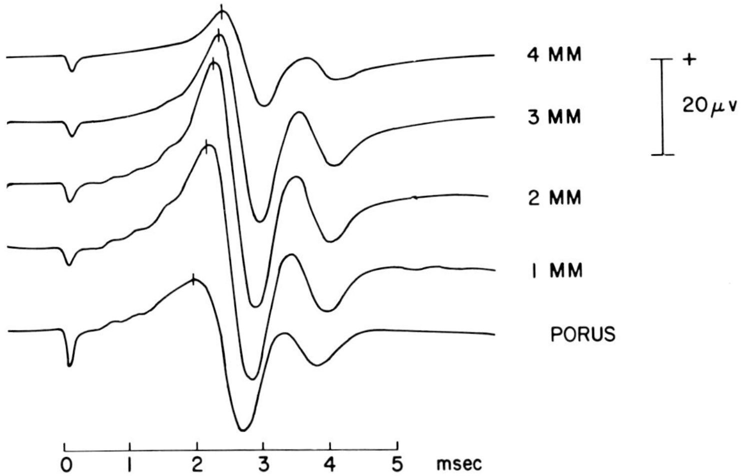

FIG. 6. Change in eighth nerve action potential relative to distance from the porus (75 dB SPL).

second positive peak of the NAP was also synchronous with peak II of the BAER (Fig. 7).

DISCUSSION

So far, there has been some general agreement on the approximate location of the neural generators of the BAER peaks: peak I, the eighth nerve; peak II, the cochlear nucleus; peak III, the superior olivary complex; peak IV, the region of the lateral lemniscus and/or inferior colliculus. Recent lesion studies in cats by Buchwald and Huang (3) suggest that the first two components are generated prior to any decussation of the auditory pathway. More recent work by Achor and Starr (1,2) suggests that, in cats, the first few components (within 2 msec) are attributed to activity in a single structure only, the eighth nerve; each of the later components had substantial contributions from more than one auditory brainstem structure. Our early NAP data with limited numbers of recordings and correlation with peak I of the BAER were clearly affected by our failure to note the exact location of the active recording electrode on the eighth nerve. Subsequent recordings prove this to be an important factor.

The length of the eighth nerve in humans from the porus to its entry into the brainstem is between approximately 10 and 14 mm when dissected at routine postmortem examination *(unpublished data).* The actual length of the total nerve must be of the order of 20 to 24 mm if one includes the intracannicular portion of the nerve (the distance from cochlea to the porus is approximately 10 mm). Since normal human data of the BAER shows an extremely narrow latency variation of the I and II peaks in matched normal controls, and the nerve

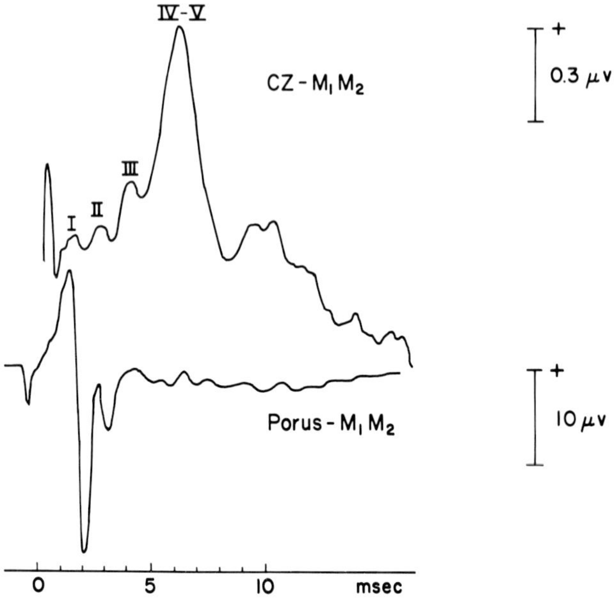

FIG. 7. Human eighth nerve action potential at porus and BAER (75 dB SPL).

has a conduction velocity between 12 and 25 m/sec, the I peak of the BAER must reflect an extremely early NAP, unaffected by differences of eighth nerve length.

Moreover, in rhesus monkeys, cats, and guinea pigs, the average diameter of the myelinated fibers on the cochlear portion of the auditory nerve is 2 to 3.5 μm (4). In man, the diameter of the myelinated fibers is estimated to lie in the neighborhood of 2 to 5 μm (R. Hinojosa, *personal communication*). Extrapolation from the known conduction velocity changes with myelinated fiber diameter size (5) would yield a nerve conduction velocity of approximately 15 to 25 m/sec, well in agreement with our own direct measurement.

Our single case with recording of the NAP at specific intervals from the porus had given us reason to suspect that, as in cats, the II peak of the human BAER may rather reflect the eighth NAP, whereas the third peak of the human BAER will prove to correspond to the cochlear nucleus and other brainstem auditory structures.

These data are of interest for a number of reasons. First, the technique is simple and permits an *in vivo* demonstration of eighth nerve action potential with an electrode placed on the nerve itself. Second, we have determined the conduction velocity of this nerve to be approximately 10 to 25 m/sec. Third, we believe that the first peak of BAER probably reflects activity of the most distal portion of the eighth nerve. Finally, a direct clinical application of this technique is the continuous monitoring of the acoustic nerve activity during surgical procedures involving this nerve directly or indirectly.

REFERENCES

1. Achor, L. J., and Starr, A. (1980): Auditory brain stem responses in the cat. I. Intracranial and extracranial recordings. *Electroencephalogr. Clin. Neurophysiol.*, 48:154–173.
2. Achor, L. J., and Starr, A. (1980): Auditory brain stem responses in the cat. II. Effect of lesion. *Electroencephalogr. Clin. Neurophysiol.*, 48:174–190.
3. Buchwald, J. S., and Huang, C. M. (1975): Farfield acoustic responses: Origins in the cat. *Science,* 189:382–388.
4. Gacek, R. R., and Rasmussen, G. L. (1961): Giver analysis of the statoacoustic nerve of guinea pig, cat, and monkey. *Anat. Rec.,* 139:455–463.
5. Hursh, J. B. (1939): Conduction velocity and diameter of nerve fibers. *Am. J. Physiol.,* 127:131–139.

Clinical Applications of Evoked Potentials in Neurology,
edited by J. Courjon, F. Mauguiere, and M. Revol.
Raven Press, New York © 1982.

Detection of Acoustic Neuromas with Brainstem Auditory Evoked Potentials: Comparison Between Cochlear and Retrocochlear Abnormalities

*†P. Feblot and **A. Uziel

**Service ORL, Centre Hospitalier Universitaire, Strasbourg, France; and ** Laboratoire d'Explorations Neuro-sensorielles, Service ORL, Hôpital Saint-Charles, Montpellier, France*

Within the past 10 years, audiologic testing has evolved considerably after having been developed to attempt to separate cochlear from retrocochlear disorders. Conventional otoneurologic evaluation has quite often proven to be unreliable for the diagnosis of acoustic tumors. The development of auditory electrophysiological measurements has provided better accuracy in tumor detection and has led to a definite trend toward the identification of tumors at an earlier stage.

Of the electric auditory responses, electrocochleography (ECoG) and brainstem auditory evoked potentials (BAEP) have been the most widely studied. The numerous studies performed with ECoG, however, failed to prove any tumor-characteristic pattern; abnormal responses have been encountered in Meniere's disease as well as in acoustic neurinomas (1,3,6).

The use of BAEP for acoustic detection was first investigated by Selters and Brackman (11) and Clemis and Mitchell (3). The BAEP is a simple, noninvasive neurophysiologic assessment of auditory function that represents the electric activity between the eighth nerve (wave I) and the inferior colliculus (wave V). The time interval between waves I and V has been shown to be prolonged in lesions involving the auditory nerve and brainstem and may provide a reliable indicator of retrocochlear deficits. The BAEP may thus be used to identify sites of lesions within the auditory pathways.

The purpose of this chapter is to describe the efficacy of this test in a clinical setting and to evaluate its relative usefulness in establishing whether a hearing loss is of cochlear or retrocochlear origin.

METHODS

Brainstem auditory evoked potentials were recorded from 45 patients with surgically proven cerebellopontine angle tumors, 63 patients with unilateral sen-

† Present address: Service ORL, Hôpital Dupuytren, Limoges, France.

sorineural hearing loss, and 101 audiometrically normal adults. All of the patients from the tumor group underwent a full neurotologic evaluation including a pure-tone air and bone conduction audiogram, "sisi test" and tone decay tests, an acoustic reflex decay test, an electronystagmograph (ENG), petrous pyramid X-rays, CAT scans, and posterior fossa myelograms.

The BAEP recordings were performed in a special audiometric test room. Intradermic electrodes were applied to the vertex, the earlobe in the test ear, and the forehead (ground). The electrodes were connected to a Medelec AA 6 Mk 3 amplifier with a gain of 10^5 and a bandpass of 100 to 3,200 Hz (6 dB down). The output of the amplifier was led to a 1,024-point analog averager (Medelec DAV 6) which was gated on during the 20-msec period following each click. The averaged responses to 2,048 click stimuli were recorded and drawn with an X–Y plotter.

The BAEP were elicited with clicks 0.1 msec in duration and of alternating polarity which were delivered to a TDH-39 earphone shielded in Nu-metal and copper. The click repetition rate was 20/sec. The signal level was varied in 10-dB steps from 100 dB HL to threshold. Normal thresholds (0 dB HL) were determined by obtaining behavioral thresholds from 10 normal-hearing adults using the same stimuli and sound delivery system as in the BAEP procedure. Because the patients had asymmetric hearing losses, a wide-band noise masker was presented to the better ear when the poorer was tested according to the basic principles of conventional audiometry.

Latencies of vertex-positive peaks I, III, and V and the I–III, III–V, and I–V interpeak latencies were measured. Both ears were tested and compared in order to determine interaural latency differences (IT III, IT V) and interaural interval differences (IT I–III, IT III–V, and IT I–V). For example, IT I–V = (I–V interval of the affected ear) − (I–V interval of the normal ear).

RESULTS

A BAEP could be obtained in all except nine cases, all in the tumor group (Table 1). These cases corresponded to patients who had no audiologic responses above 500 Hz and whose ears failed to produce a recordable response at the highest deliverable intensity.

The major peaks, i.e., I and V, were observable in 30 cases with hearing loss less than 75 dB HL. In these cases, the brainstem responses were generally not as complete or as clearly defined as the sequence of five peaks observed in normal ears. Waves II and III could not be recorded in a large number of cases. At such times, predominance of wave V was established by reducing the stimulus level until the one peak remained.

All of the patients with acoustic tumors had a normal or nearly normal latency of wave I at high intensity but showed prolonged I–V interval (Fig. 1).

Figure 2 compares the distribution of I–V intervals, in 30 patients with acoustic

TABLE 1. *Summary of BAEP results from tumor patients*

Finding	N
Hearing threshold <75 dB HL	
IT I–V >0.3 msec	30
Wave I only	2
No response at 100 dB	2
Cophosis	
Wave I only	2
No response at 100 dB	9
Total tumor detected	36 (80%)
No conclusion	9 (20%)
Total false negatives (BAEP normal)	0
Total tested	45

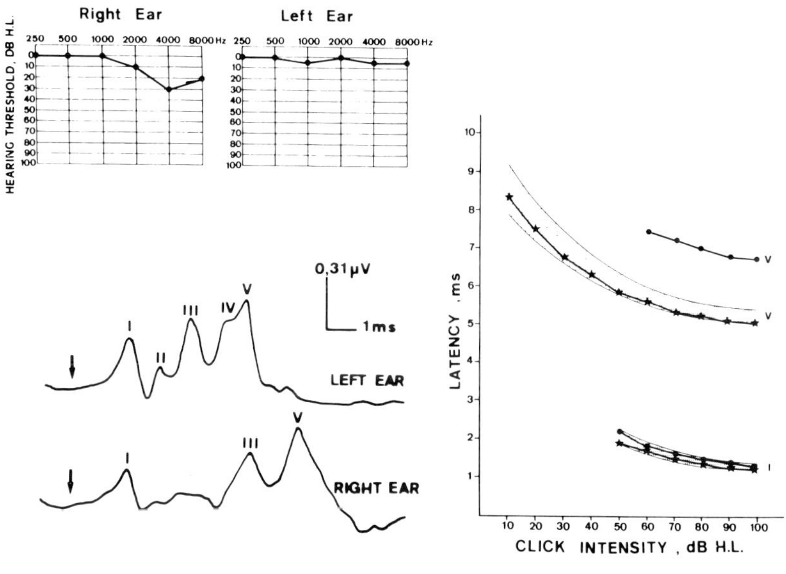

FIG. 1. Brainstem auditory evoked response from a patient with a right acoustic neuroma. The audiogram shows a mild sensorineural hearing loss. The BAEP shows an increased latency of waves III and V in the right ear in contrast with normal latencies in the left ear. The diagram on the **right** gives a comparison of wave I and V latencies from the tumor (●) and the unaffected ear (★) with normative data. Shaded area includes ±1 SD from the means.

tumors, 63 patients with unilateral sensorineural hearing loss, and 101 subjects with normal hearing. The I–V interval in cochlear disease is not significantly different from the I–V interval of normal ears. On the other hand, there is a clear separation between tumor and nontumor groups. All but two of the patients from the tumor group have I–V intervals that fall outside the upper limit of the 95% confidence interval of the normal population (4.40 msec).

Calculation of the interaural I–V interval difference (IT I–V) seems to increase the separation between retrocochlear and cochlear abnormalities (Fig. 3). In

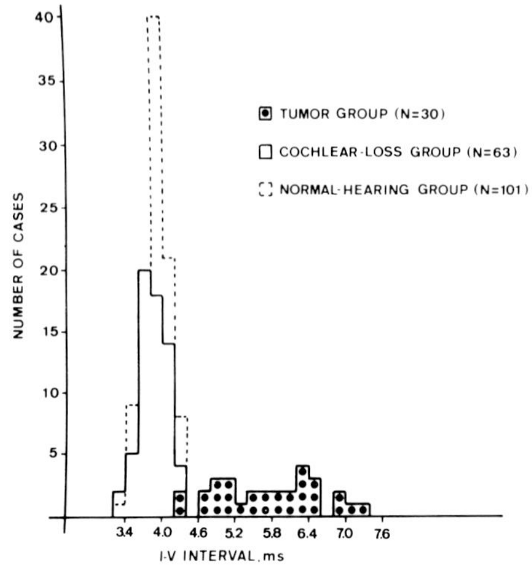

FIG. 2. Distribution of the I–V interval for tumor group, cochlear-loss group, and normal-hearing group.

normally hearing subjects, IT I–V is never greater than 0.3 msec. In patients with cochlear deficits, the I–V interval tends to decrease with high-frequency hearing loss so that the distribution of the IT I–V is slightly skewed to the negative side. The 30 tumor cases had IT I–V of 0.35 to 3.30 msec, which is highly significant.

In fact, when wave III was present, the abnormality of the I–V interval resulted mainly from a I–III interval prolongation, the III–V interval often being normal.

Wave V was absent in the other cases, so that IT I–V could not be used as an indicator of retrocochlear deficit.

In two cases with subjective click thresholds of 60 and 65 dB HL, BAEP showed only the first wave to be present in the affected side. The absence of

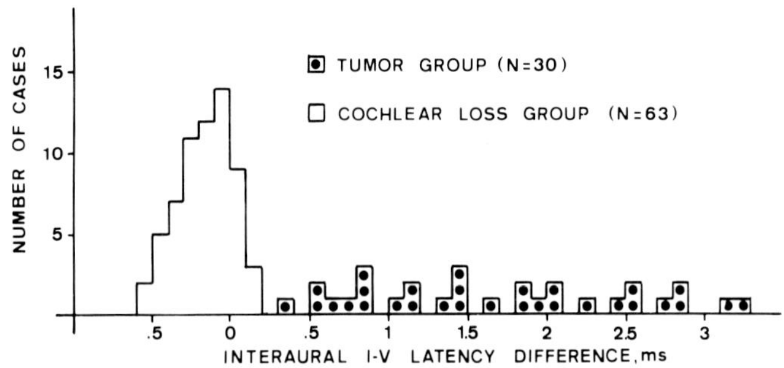

FIG. 3. Distribution of interaural I–V interval difference (IT I–V) for tumor group and cochlear-loss group.

waves III and V was consistent with a retrocochlear lesion. In two other cases, it was possible to record a well-identifiable wave I from patients with unilateral cophosis, whereas the other waves were absent. The preservation of wave I and the discrepancy between BAEP and subjective threshold was considered to be significant of retrocochlear abnormality. Finally, BAEP showed no response in two other cases, whereas the subjective threshold for clicks was 40 and 70 dB HL. Such a phenomenon was never observed in normal and cochlear loss groups and was interpreted as a loss of wave III and subsequent waves.

Figure 4 shows the correlation between tumor size and IT I–V. The IT I–V was approximately proportional to the size of the tumor: the larger the tumor, the longer the delay of the response. Our correlation of tumor size and IT I–V was significant at the 0.02 level. Nevertheless, there was a great variability among patients.

Table 2 compares the efficiency of BAEP with other tests. It is apparent that BAEP demonstrates the best true-positive rate of all of the tests (80% including the cases of cophosis).

Auditory tests, including Bekesy, tone decay, and impedance reflex decay tests, were suggestive of retrocochlear pathology in only 16 of 38 patients (42%). Electronystagmography showed vestibular areflexia in 25 cases (55%), hypofunction in 17 cases (37%), and no abnormality in three cases (8%). In these last three cases, BAEP was consistent with retrocochlear disorder. On the other hand, ENG gave a positive finding in the cases of cophosis in which BAEP was not conclusive. Nevertheless, ENG is a nonlocalizing test.

X-rays gave a positive finding in 24 patients (60%) and a false negative rate of 22%. Computed axial tomography, which is unable to detect intracanicular tumors, and myelograms are not screening tests and, therefore, were not taken into account.

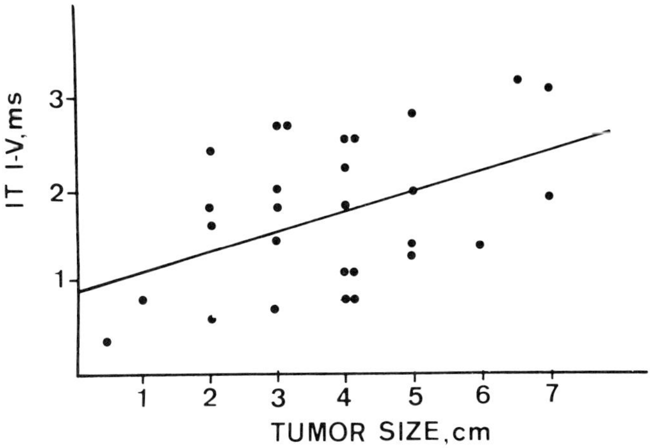

FIG. 4. The IT I–V as a function of tumor size.

TABLE 2. *Screening test failures to detect tumors*

Test	True-positive rate	False-negative rate	No conclusion
BAEP	80%	0%	20% (Cophosis)
Auditory tests	42%	22%	36%
ENG	55%	8%	37%
X-ray	60%	22%	18%

DISCUSSION

The use of BAEP for acoustic tumor detection was first investigated by Selters and Brackmann (11) and later by Clemis and Mitchell (3), Coats (4), Conraux and Feblot (5), Clemis and McGee (2), House and Brackmann (8), and Glasscock et al. (7). They found either a delay or absence of wave V and concluded that the latency value of wave V was the best way to screen for tumors affecting the auditory nerve. Wave V latencies may be assessed in two ways: either by a comparison with normative values or, in cases of unilateral disorders, by a comparison with the contralateral uninvolved ear. The latter is called interaural latency difference. Selters and Brackmann (11) demonstrated that the wave V interaural latency difference (IT V) was a more sensitive measure than absolute latency for detecting acoustic neuromas and that an IT V of greater than 0.3 msec could be considered abnormal. An abnormal IT V (or no wave V response) was reported in 100% of Selters and Brackmann's tumor-proven cases. On the other hand, further studies showed between 2 and 10% false-negative results (tumor missed) in proven tumor cases (2,3,8). Furthermore, abnormal wave V measures have been found in a great number of sensorineural hearing losses of different etiologies, such as sudden hearing loss of Meniere's disease, giving rise to a high false-positive rate (2). Any conductive loss of hearing will also result in a wave V latency increase. An abnormal IT V is not, therefore, pathognomonic of tumors affecting the auditory nerve.

Coats (4) suggested that the I–V interval could separate retrocochlear from cochlear ears with better reliability than V latency. This interval, which is believed to represent the conduction time within the auditory nerve and brainstem, is relatively insensitive to stimulus intensity changes and is unaffected by conduction hearing loss. Furthermore, this interval is increased in tumors affecting the auditory nerve, whereas it remains within normal limits in cochlear hearing losses and tends to decrease with high-frequency cochlear deficits (4). However, this interval was within normal limits in two cases of proven tumors in our study, and the choice of this parameter would have thus been responsible for two false-negative results.

Therefore, the efficiency of the test is increased if the I–V interval is compared not with normative values but with contralateral values. In normal subjects, the difference in the I–V interval between the two ears is never greater than 0.3 msec. Any prolongation of the IT I–V corresponds to a slowing of conduction on one side of the auditory pathways. The efficiency of this parameter was proven by the absence of false-negative results in our study and by the 100% true-positive rate in our patients with hearing loss less than 75 db.

However, the IT I–V measure cannot be used for all cases. A disadvantage of the IT I–V measure is its inability to detect bilateral tumors or to detect a tumor in an only hearing ear. The only way, in these cases is to compare the absolute I–V interval with normative data. On the other hand, Selters and Brackmann (11) showed that an increase in the III–V interval in the nontumor side may occur when a large tumor, pushing the brainstem toward the normal side, creates an axial shift. It is likely that in such cases, the interaural I–V interval difference (IT I–V) may not be as increased as it should be. In fact, it is reasonable to assume that these large tumors will produce such an increase of the I–V interval on the affected ear that false negative results will be improbable. Another difficulty is that the first wave of the BAEP may be difficult to recognize on the record, introducing an element of uncertainty into the measure of the I–V interval. In these cases, it can be useful to combine BAEP with electrocochleography which gives more precise information as to the latency of the auditory nerve response (9,10).

Absence of wave V appears to be another finding that is typical of acoustic tumors. In that situation, there is a preservation of wave I and a loss of subsequent waves, but the patient is able to hear the signal. This absence of wave V at suprathreshold levels has been reported in half of the patients of Selters and Brackmann (11) and 16% of the patients of Clemis and McGee (2). It has been found in 7% of our tumor cases in which the pure-tone thresholds did not exceed 75 dB HL. The absence of wave V may be caused by decreased or desynchronized nerve conduction resulting in a response that is either delayed or so smeared that it is unrecognizable. Consequently, patients may be considered to have a positive result for tumor detection when their BAEP shows one of the three characteristics: (a) an I–V interval significantly different from the normal mean; (b) an interaural I–V difference (IT I–V) greater than 0.3 msec; (c) a preservation of wave I with no wave V response at suprathreshold levels.

With these criteria, BAEP appears to be the most efficient test available in the search of acoustic tumors. The high correlation of positive results and the small percentage of false negatives are appreciated when one compares BAEP with other tests used in acoustic neuroma detection. The main limitation of the test is that BAEP can only be utilized when the hearing loss in the affected ear is less than 75 dB HL. In these cases, the accuracy of the test has been found to be 100%. It is likely that BAEP, used as an adjunct to the neurotologic evaluation, will make it possible to detect aoustic neuromas at earlier stages of development.

REFERENCES

1. Aran, J. M., and Negrevergne, M. (1973): Aspects cliniques de quelques formes pathologiques particulières des résponses du nerf auditif chez l'homme. *Audiology,* 12:488–503.

2. Clemis, J. D., and McGee, T. (1979): Brainstem electric response audiometry in the differential diagnosis of acoustic tumors. *Laryngoscope,* 89:31–42.
3. Clemis, J. D., and Mitchell, C. (1977): Electrocochleography and brainstem responses used in the diagnosis of acoustic tumors. *J. Otolaryngol.,* 6:447–458.
4. Coats, A. C. (1978): Human auditory nerve action potentials and brainstem evoked responses. *Arch. Otolaryngol.,* 104:709–717.
5. Conraux, C., and Feblot, P. (1979): Les potentiels évoqués auditifs précoces at semi-précoces dans les tumeurs de l'angle ponto-cérebelleux. *Rev. Laryngol. Otol. Rhinol. (Bord.),* 100:41–48.
6. Gibson, W. P. R., and Beagley, H. A. (1976): Trans-tympanic electrocochleography in the investigation of retrocochlear disorders. *Rev. Laryngol. Otol. Rhinol. (Bord.),* 97:507–516.
7. Glasscock, M. E., Jackson, C. G. Josey, A. F., Dickins, J. R. E., and Wiet, R. J. (1979): Brainstem evoked response audiometry in a clinical practice. *Laryngoscope,* 89:1021–1034.
8. House, J. W., and Brackmann, D. E. (1979): Brainstem audiometry in neurotologic diagnosis. *Arch. Otolaryngol.,* 105:305–309.
9. Portmann, M., Cazals, Y., Negrevergne, M., and Aran, J. M. (1980): Transtympanic and surface recordings in the diagnosis of retrocochlear disorders. *Acta Otolaryngol.,* 89:362–369.
10. Salomon, G., Elberling, C., and Tos, M. (1979): Combined use of electrocochleography and brainstem recordings in the diagnosis of acoustic neuromas. *Rev. Laryngol. Otol. Rhinol. (Bord.),* 100:697–707.
11. Selters, W. A., and Brackmann, D. E. (1977): Acoustic tumor detection with brainstem electric response audiometry. *Arch. Otolaryngol.,* 101:222–226.

Clinical Applications of Evoked Potentials in Neurology,
edited by J. Courjon, F. Mauguiere, and M. Revol.
Raven Press, New York © 1982.

Contribution of Brainstem Auditory Evoked Potentials to Diagnosis of Tumors and Vascular Diseases

*C. Fischer, *F. Mauguière, **J. F. Echallier, and *J. Courjon

**Hôpital Neurologique, 69394 Lyon, France; and **CEMI Unité INSERM, Lyon, France*

The field of practical applications of BAEP, long limited to otorhinolaringology, has recently been extended into neurology. Works published over the last 5 years have noted correlations between data from records and proven lesions of the CNS, especially at the level of the posterior fossa (5,6,10,12,13,15). This was the first glimpse of their contribution to neurological diagnosis, and Stockard and Sharbrough (14) reported three cases in which BAEP had allowed the existence of an expansive lesion in the posterior fossa to be suspected although radiological investigations were negative. In order to define specifically what BAEP can bring to neurological diagnosis, we examined and recorded 25 patients having definite vascular diseases and 66 patients suspected of or suffering from rhombencephalic or mesencephalic tumors, most of them checked by CT scan. Twenty-eight of this last group were operated on, and postmortem anatomical examination was performed on four of them. Patients with acoustic neurinomas were excluded from this study.

METHODS AND MATERIALS

We used alternate filtered clicks at 4,000 Hz at an intensity of 90 or 80 dB (90 dB SL), 10 clicks per second. Stimulation was monaural; when necessary, the contralateral ear was masked by a continuous white noise the intensity of which was determined individually for all patients. The clicks were presented through Scintrex MKIV earphones.

The bipolar EEG activity was recorded between the vertex and the ipsilateral mastoid, amplified 500,000 times by a Grass polygraph Model 7, and analyzed in 1,024 points. The band pass was 150 to 3,000 Hz. After averaging by means of a Sems-Solar computer, the evoked response was analyzed for 15 msec or 12 msec and displayed on oscilloscope and tracing table. The latency of each positive peak was measured automatically. Stimulation, recording, and control of data were facilitated by a programmable minicomputerized system (7). At least two series of 4,000 stimulations were carried out for each ear. None of

TABLE 1. *Normative latency values of BAEP*

90 dB SL clicks (msec)			Interwave latency (msec)		
Wave	Mean	SD	Waves	Mean	SD
I	1.88	0.09	I–II	1.19	0.21
II	3.07	0.17	I–III	2.14	0.19
III	4.01	0.16	I–IV/V	3.46	0.27
IV/V	5.36	0.21	I–V	4.09	0.24
IV	5.23	0.17	III–V	1.93	0.26
V	5.93	0.25	V–VI	1.60	0.28
VI	7.50	0.26			

the patients received any sedative medication before the recording session; they were tested in a supine position in a sound-shielded room. The normative data of our laboratory were established in 50 normal subjects, volunteers of both sexes (mean age 35 years), and may be found summarized in Table 1.

The latencies were classified as abnormal when they were 2 SD over the mean values for normals; a 2.5-SD range was accepted for the interpeak latency and interear wave latency. Amplitudes and amplitude ratios were not classified as abnormal except when abnormalities were unvarying on repeated trials. Finally, the morphology of BAEP and the interear asymmetry were taken into account when consistent over successive trials. Figure 1 shows the recording of a BAEP we considered normal.

The patients studied were referred by 13 neurologists and neurosurgeons of our hospital. The final diagnoses of the patients are to be seen on Table 2.

RESULTS

In some cases, especially in cases of vascular lesions, BAEP only confirmed the data of the clinical examination. No abnormalities of morphology or of

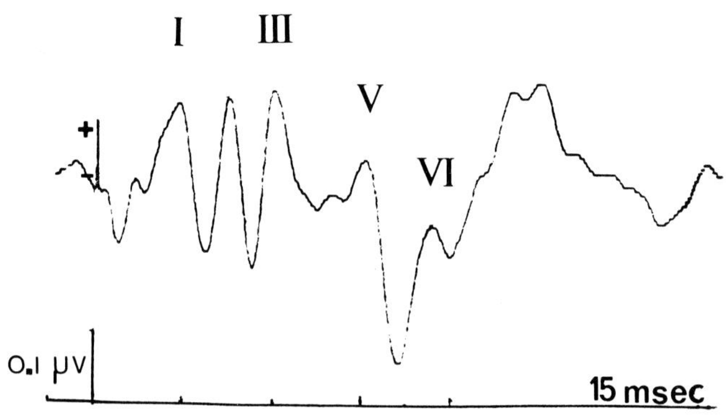

FIG. 1. A normal BAEP.

TABLE 2. *Final diagnosis of the patients*

Vascular diseases (25 patients)	
Locked-in syndrome	4
Wallenberg syndrome	4
Posterior fossa angiomas	4
Vertebrobasilar transient ischemic attacks	5
Posterior cerebral artery softening	3
Thalamic hematoma	2
Definite vertebrobasilar attack	3
Suspected and proved tumors (66 patients)	
Meningiomas	8
Cerebellar tumors	5
Bulbocervical infiltrative tumor	2
Third ventricle colloid cyst	2
Fourth ventricle ependymoma	2
Brainstem-involving tumor with positive CT scan	8
Suspected brainstem tumor with negative CT scan	33
Miscellaneous	6
(1 germinoma, 1 trigeminal neuralgia, 1 pinealoma, 1 hemispheric astrocytoma, 1 craniopharyngioma, 1 subthalamic cyst)	

latencies were observed in four patients showing a Wallenberg syndrome, in four patients with a locked-in syndrome whose clinical evolution was favorable over a few months, allowing only a neurological deficit to persist that did not cause great disability, and in five patients with transient vertebrobasilar ischemic attacks or rapidly regressing disease of the same topography. We also recorded four patients with large mesencephalic angiomas without abnormality or significant asymmetry of BAEP. The same did not hold true in three cases of vascular ischemic attack with a massive neurological deficit including homolateral palsy of the fifth to the 12th cranial nerves and, therefore, the eighth nerve with a contralateral motor defect. In these cases, abnormalities in BAEP were obvious and bilateral. On the side of the cranial nerve nuclear palsy, there was no response, and peak I was absent. On the other side, peak I was present, and response was entirely disorganized, so that peak V was hardly identifiable.

In meningiomas of the posterior fossa (eight cases) and in cerebellar tumors (5 cases), BAEP were modified to an extent dependent on the volume of the tumor and especially on its relationship to the auditory pathways. In these 13 cases, the existence of the tumor was always proven by the CT scan. Compared with the information supplied by the latter technique, the diagnostic information provided by the BAEP was negligible except in the following two particular cases.

In a 38-year-old man, a voluminous tumor of the posterior cerebral fossa had just been discovered; in order to adapt the operational strategy as well as possible, the exact relationship of the tumor with the brain stem was discussed. The BAEP were normal and symmetrical (Fig. 2). Thus, the voluminous tumor visualized by CT scan was thought to be extraparenchymatous or located in

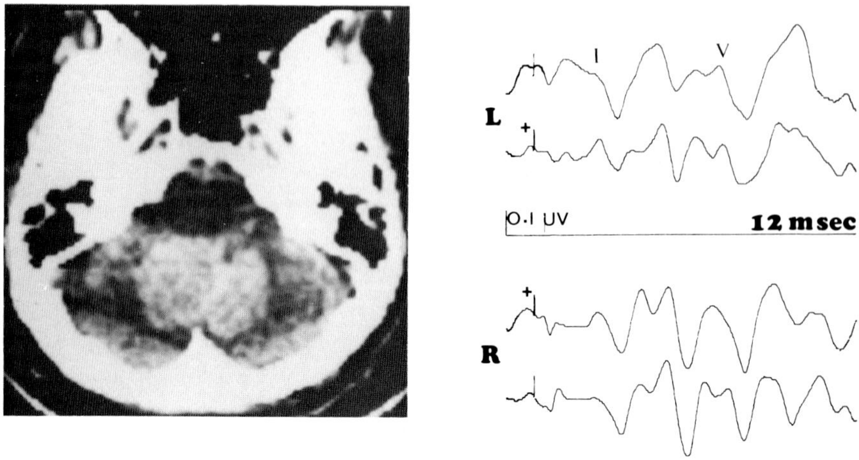

FIG. 2. Patient with a voluminous extraaxial tumor (meningoblastoma). L, left; R, right.

the fourth ventricle. On operation, a meningoblastoma located at the level of the occipital foramen was found.

The second case concerned a 64-year-old woman who had a voluminous tumor of the posterior fossa. The diagnosis of hemangioblastoma affecting the left cerebellar hemisphere, the vermis, and the brainstem seemed probable. The BAEP were not widely modified: the response on the right was normal; on the left, the amplitude of response was reduced beyond peak I. Such tenuous abnormalities were not compatible with a tumor invading the brainstem itself. On operation, it was seen to be a meningioma of the cerebellar convexity.

With 36 patients, BAEP helped the diagnosis along by providing useful information. Two patients were going to be operated on for a bulbocervical tumor and were referred for evaluation of tumor's rostral extension. In the first case (infiltrating astrocytoma), the pontine extension was diagnosed by abnormal preoperational BAEP. In the second patient whose BAEP were normal, a cystic hemangioblastoma was discovered on operation: it did not extend beyond the bulbocervical junction.

In a 52-year-old woman suffering from late onset epileptic seizure, the CT scan showed a hypodense thalamo-subthalamic image that seemed to intersect the median geniculate body (Fig. 3). Diagnosis was uncertain between glioma and nonevolutive cysts. The second hypothesis was retained since waves VI were present and latencies of right and left waves V and right and left V–VI intervals were symmetrical. Moreover, the somatosensory evoked responses were normal and perfectly symmetrical. A second CT scan performed 1 year after the first one did not reveal any modification of appearance.

Thirty-three patients were suspected of tumor in the brainstem, and the CT scan had neither confirmed nor eliminated this hypothesis when we recorded

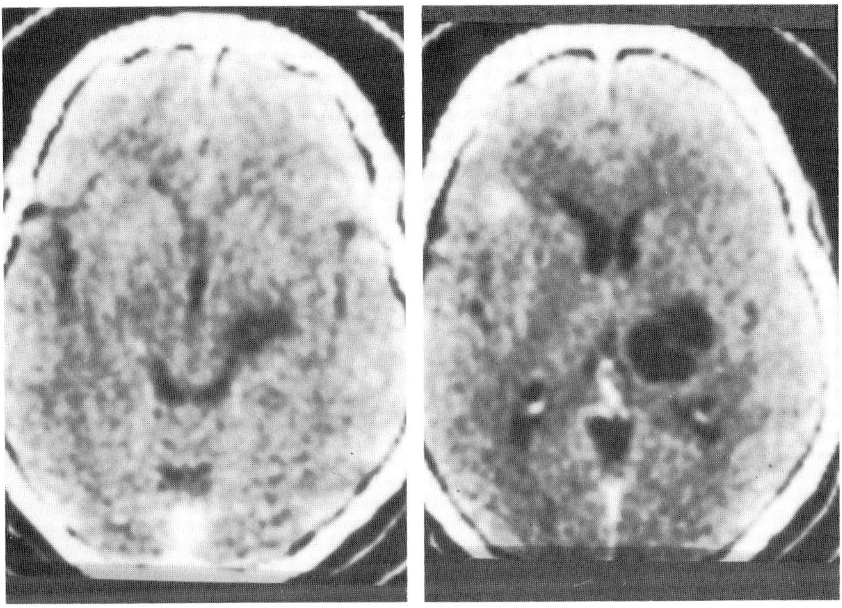

FIG. 3. Patient with a thalamo-subthalamic lesion involving the right median geniculate body. The BAEPs were normal and symmetrical for waves V and VI.

them. Four showed very large abnormalities in the BAEP that contrasted with poor clinical symptoms: for instance, disappearance of any response beyond peak II in a man with normal hearing suffering from an apparently isolated trigeminal neuralgia. The four patients did have infiltrating tumors of the brainstem, the existence of which was later on proved by postmortem anatomical examination for two and by surgery for another. In 15 of these 33 patients, the normality of BAEP caused the diagnosis of brainstem tumor to be considered highly unlikely; this assumption has not proved wrong over a follow-up period of nearly 2 years for all cases. In the other 14 patients, the diagnostic problem was between a first relapse of MS involving the brainstem and an early tumor. In this last group of patients, a normal BAEP seemed to eliminate a tumor but left the diagnostic problem of MS.

Finally, in some patients, the BAEP recording stimulated a neurophysiological discussion. What value can be attributed to wave VI, the presumed generator of which is the median geniculate body? None at all when it is absent, and a very high one when it is present. Thus, a 23-year-old male had a voluminous diencephalo–hypothalamic tumor, the posterior extension of which, on CT scan, seemed to press on or invade the rostral part of the brainstem. Waves V and VI were perfectly identifiable with strictly normal latencies and interpeak intervals and with no asymmetry whatever. This pleaded for the total integrity of the lower quadrigeminal bodies and of the median geniculate bodies, the integrity of which was verified at autopsy 1 week later.

Have waves IV and V an ipsi- or contralateral generator? We would say contralateral on the basis of the following case. A young woman showed a grade I astrocystoma in the left hemisphere extending down to the peduncle without, however, unsettling it (Fig. 4). Revealing symptoms were very active complex partial epilepsy without any deficit on neurological examination or, in particular, any brainstem symptom. Four series of stimulations were carried out at the level of each ear, and recording was performed again 1 week later. Lower amplitudes in waves IV and V as well as lengthening of the V–VII interval were consistently observed with an ipsilateral reference electrode after stimulation of the right ear (Fig. 5).

The discussion was the same for three patients with recent ischemic attacks in the region of the right posterior cerebral artery whose lesions were clearly visible on the CT scan. Two women patients had normal BAEP. The third one had a delayed left wave V (Fig. 6). However, a young man with a left third nerve palsy and a small dense peduncular lesion clearly seen on CT scan showed delayed ware V latency and morphological abnormalities after ipsilateral stimulation. This patient has not yet undergone surgery. A contralateral brainstem involvement remains possible.

DISCUSSION

The contribution of BAEP to the neurological diagnosis is well established in the evaluation of multiple sclerosis (1,9,14). What this method will bring to the diagnosis of vascular diseases and especially tumors also seems very promising for the future. Brainstem auditory EPs are most useful in the cases when the clinical examinations, the complementary examinations, and the CT scan remain uncertain, as, for instance, when there is some doubt between an infiltrating lesion and a first relapse of a demyelinating disease. In tumors of the posterior fossa visible on the scanner, the BAEP abnormalities, when they exist, depend on the volume of the tumor and especially on its relationship with the auditory pathways. And it is easily understood that brainstem tumors always produce large abnormalities (8). We also saw that for two meningeal tumors, the electrophysiological recording brought useful information for neurosurgical strategy, although BAEP were not indispensable since the tumor was voluminous on the CT scan. Stockard and Sharbrough (14) were among the

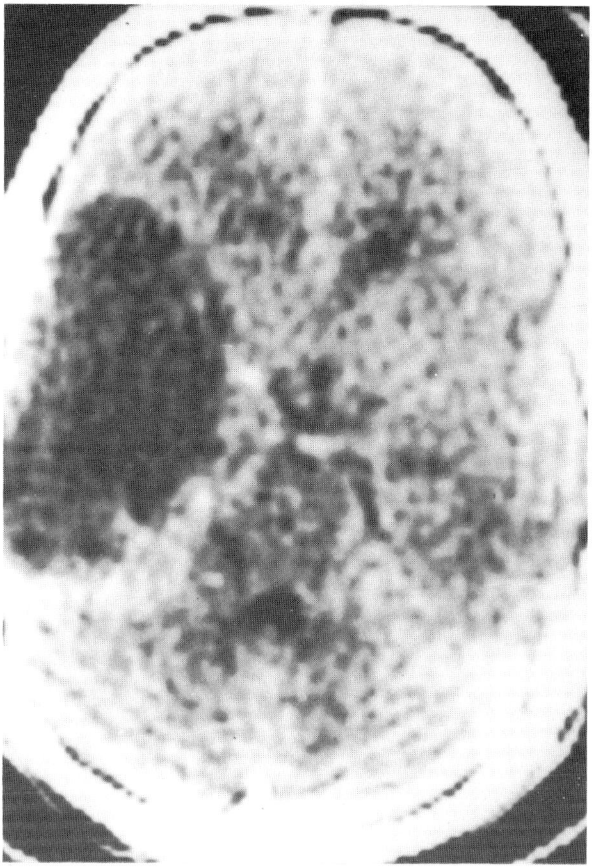

FIG. 4. Grade I astrocytoma deep in the left hemisphere.

first to have had a glimpse of the usefulness of the BAEP in the diagnosis of infraradiological expansive lesions for three out of the 15 tumors that they reported.

Vertebrobasilar vascular pathology lends itself well to establishing fine correlations between BAEP and the site of lesions. But it is rare for the vascular or topographic nature of the lesions not to be established by more precise neurological examination alone. Permanent vascular diseases produce large abnormalities of BAEP depending on the size of the lesions and on the involvement of the auditory pathways. We agree with those authors (1,14) who admit the normal character of BAEP is authentic transient ischemic attack. Moreover, contrary to some of them (4), we did not observe any significant abnormalities of BAEP in the locked-in and Wallenberg syndromes. Our cases were clinically very pure,

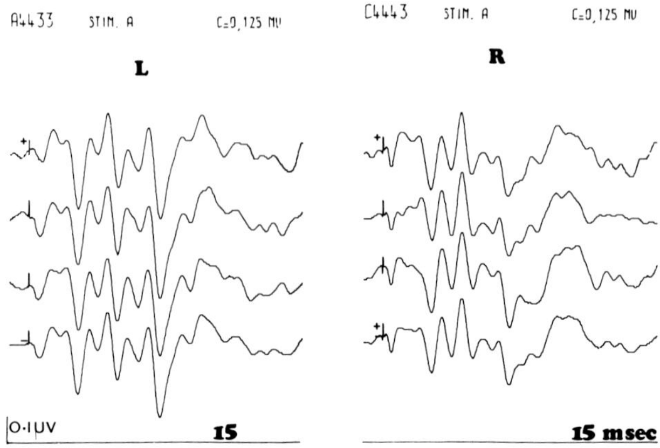

FIG. 5. Steady latency and amplitude abnormalities contralateral to the tumor. See Fig. 4 and text.

and it can be admitted that limited lesions of the ventral pons and of lateral fossa of the medulla oblongata do not cause damage to the auditory pathways and are small enough not to perturb BAEP.

As to neurological discussion, the value of wave VI remains a subject of debate, as it is absent in nearly one-half of normal subjects. Its absence is, therefore, not significant with regard to lesions, and in the case reported above, its presence coincides with the integrity of the median geniculate body but does not prove that it generates it. More interesting is the discussion of the generator of wave V, very probably the lower colliculus (11), ipsilateral for some authors (1), contralateral for others (3,16). A definite opinion will be

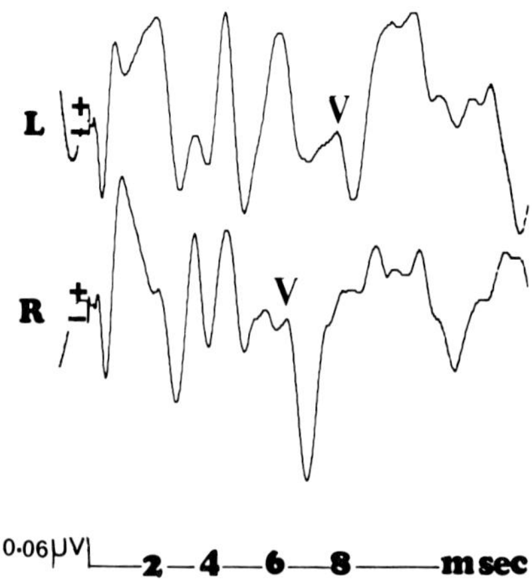

FIG. 6. Right cerebral posterior artery softening including its collicular branch with contralateral latency delay.

formed only with some documented anatomoclinical observations; however, our observations plead for the contralateral origin of wave V, and in one observation, it may be reasonably presumed that the obliteration intersected the right posterior cerebral artery at its origin, especially its collicular branch (2). With the last patient, we should think of an ipsilateral generation for wave V, but this cannot be a firm conclusion for the time being.

REFERENCES

1. Chiappa, K. (1980): Pattern shift visual, brainstem auditory, and short-latency somatosensory evoked potentials in multiple sclerosis. *Neurology (Minneap.),* 30(2):110–123.
2. Duvernoy, H. M. (1978): *Human Brainstem Vessels.* Springer, Berlin.
3. Epstein, C. M., Stappenbek, R., and Karp, H. R. (1980): Brainstem auditory evoked responses in palatal myoclonus. *Ann. Neurol.,* 7:592.
4. Gilroy, J., Lynn, E. L., Ristow, G. E., and Pellerin, R. J. (1977): Auditory evoked brainstem potentials in a case of "locked-in" syndrome. *Arch. Neurol.,* 34:492–495.
5. Hashimoto, J., Ishiyama, Y., and Tozuka, G. (1979): Bilaterally recorded brain stem auditory evoked responses. Their asymetric abnormalities and lesions of the brain stem. *Arch. Neurol.,* 36:161–167.
6. Kjaer, M. (1980): Localizing brain stem lesions with brain stem auditory evoked potentials. *Acta Neuol. Scand.,* 61:265–274.
7. Maraval, G., Pernier, J., Peronnet, F., Echallier, J. F., Gerin, P., and Mauguiere, F. (1980): Evøq.: Système configurable de stimulation automatique et d'enregistrement des potentiels évoqués moyens sur mini-ordinateur. *Int. J. Biomed. Comput.,* 11:225–239.
8. Nodar, R. H., Hahn, J., and Levine, H. L. (1980): Brain stem auditory evoked potentials in determining site of lesion of brain stem gliomas in children. *Laryngoscope,* 110:258–265.
9. Robinson, K., and Rudge, P. (1980): The use of the auditory evoked potential in the diagnosis of multiple sclerosis. *J. Neurol. Sci.,* 45:235–244.
10. Starr, A., and Achor, J. (1975): Auditory brain stem responses in neurological disease. *Arch. Neurol.,* 32:761–768.
11. Starr, A., and Achor, L. J. (1979): Anatomical and physiological origins of auditory brain stem responses (ABR). In: *Human Evoked Potentials,* edited by D. Lehmann and E. Callaway, pp. 415–429. Plenum Press, New York.
12. Starr, A., and Hamilton, A. E. (1976): Correlations between confirmed sites of neurological lesions and abnormalities of far field auditory brainstem responses. *Electroencephalogr. Clin. Neurophysiol.,* 41:595–608.
13. Stockard, J. J., and Rossiter, V. S., (1977): Clinical and pathologic correlates of brain stem auditory response abnormalities. *Neurology (Minneap.),* 27:316–325.
14. Stockard, J. J., and Sharbrough, F. W. (1980): Unique contributions of short-latency auditory and somatosensory evoked potentials to neurologic diagnosis. In: *Progress in Clinical Neurophysiology, Vol. 7,* edited by J. E. Desmedt, pp. 231–263. Karger, Basel.
15. Stockard, J. J., Stockard, J. E., and Sharbrough, F. W. (1977): Detection and localization of occult lesions with brain stem auditory lesions. *Mayo Clin. Proc.,* 52:761–769.
16. Stockard, J. J., Stockard, J. E., and Sharbrough, F. W. (1980): Brainstem auditory evoked potentials in neurology: Methodology, interpretation, clinical application. In: *Electrodiagnosis in Clinical Neurology,* edited by M. J. Aminoff, pp. 370–413. Churchill Livingstone, London.

Clinical Applications of Evoked Potentials in Neurology,
edited by J. Courjon, F. Mauguiere, and M. Revol.
Raven Press, New York © 1982.

Brainstem Auditory Evoked Potentials and Vertebral–Basilar Reversible Ischemic Attacks

*A. Ragazzoni, *A. Amantini, **L. Rossi, †P. Pagnini,
**G. Arnetoli, **P. Marini, **C. Nencioni, *A. Versari, and
**R. Zappoli

**Service of Neurophysiopathology, **Second Neurological Institute, and † Service of Audiology, University of Florence, Florence, Italy*

Many authors (1,2,5,6,9–12) have studied brainstem auditory evoked potentials (BAEPs) in various vascular brainstem disorders. Nevertheless, to our knowledge, no systematical research with this technique has been conducted on patients with reversible ischemic attacks (RIAs) in the vertebral–basilar arterial system. The present study was undertaken to define the utility of BAEP recording in the assessment of this relevant kind of cerebral vascular pathology. Moreover, EEG and otoneurological findings, together with other instrumental data (provided by brain CT, angiography, Directional C. W. Doppler) have been collected. Particular attention was given to the results obtained from BAEP recording and otoneurological examination: Both of these noninvasive procedures supply, in fact, a measure of brainstem function.

The BAEPs proved to be a sensitive electrophysiological parameter, complementing the otoneurological examination in assessing brainstem impairment in patients affected by RIAs.

MATERIAL AND METHODS

A total of 26 patients affected by RIAs in the vertebral–basilar arterial system have been studied. Fifteen patients (four females, 11 males, age range 41–68 years, mean 55 years) had presented two to five transient ischemic attacks (4,7) completely clearing in 24 hr, whereas the other 11 patients (two females, nine males, age range 33–73 years, mean 55 years) suffered from ischemic strokes in which a full recovery took place over a longer period, on the average 3 weeks from onset (strokes with full recovery: SFR) (4).

All patients underwent BAEP recording 7 to 20 days from the last RIA, when all signs and symptoms had disappeared. They received no sedation. The stimuli consisted of broad-band clicks, with a peak acoustic power of 2.0 to 4.0 kHz, critically damped within 0.35 msec of their onset. They were generated

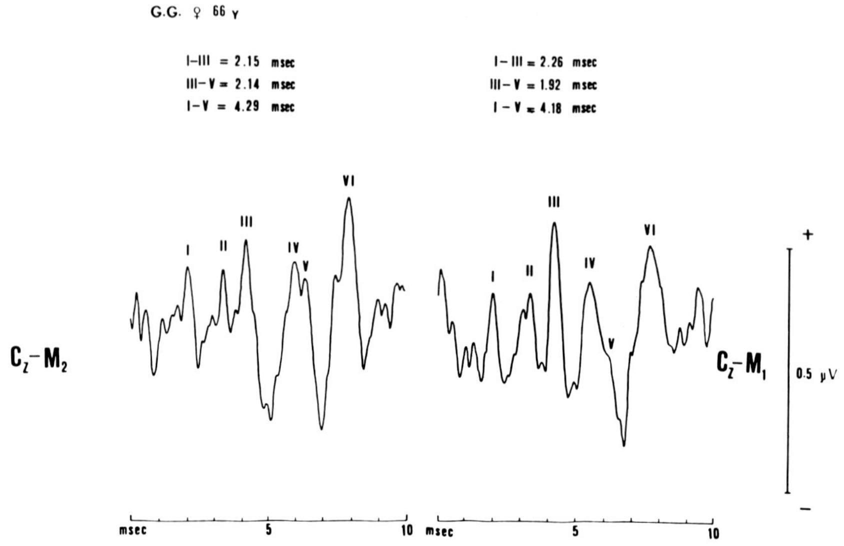

Fig. 1. The BAEPs of a patient (G.G., ♀, 66 yr) with recurrent TIAs of the vertebral–basilar arterial system showing an abnormal (>2.5 SD from normal value) I-V IPL to stimulation of the right ear and a borderline (> 2.0, < 2.5 SD from normal value) I-III IPL to stimulation of the left ear. Responses to 70-dB SPL, 10 Hz clicks were recorded from the vertex and the mastoid ipsilateral to stimulation.

by passing 0.2-msec square pulses of alternating polarity through shielded earphones. The stimuli were presented to the subjects monaurally at a rate of 10 Hz and with a 70 dB SPL intensity. Both ears were subsequently stimulated.

Nonpolarizing silver–silver chloride electrodes filled with isotonic jelly were applied to the vertex (C_z) and the mastoids (M_1, M_2), with interelectrode impedances always below 3,000 ohms. A midfrontal electrode served as ground. Bipolar EEG activity recorded from the vertex and the mastoid ipsilateral to stimulation was amplified through a differential amplifier (Hewlett Packard 1510 A) with a filter bandpass of 0.3 to 3.0 kHz (12 dB down). The output of the amplifier was monitored continuously on an oscilloscope, and averaging was discontinued whenever the EEG was contaminated with muscle or movement artifacts. Two sets of 1,500 averaged responses, in which peaks were clearly detectable, were obtained from each ear, and summated by a Neuroaverager® O.T.E. model 1172. They were written out with an X-Y plotter for measurement. Analysis time was 10 msec from stimulus onset. Peak latencies for the first five waves [labeled after Jewett and Williston (3)] and the I-III, III-V, I-V interpeak latencies (IPLs) as well as the IV-V/I amplitude ratio were measured and compared with the values obtained in a group of 15 normal subjects matched for age (Table 1). As the purpose of this study was to evaluate brainstem function, attention was focused mainly on IPLs, which allow the measurement of transmission time at different levels (8). Interpeak latencies prolonged by more than

TABLE 1. *Latencies of brainstem auditory evoked potentials in 15 normal subjects*[a]

Peak latencies (msec)			Interpeak latencies (msec)		
Wave	Mean	SD	Wave	Mean	SD
I	1.86	±0.09	I–III	1.96	±0.14
II	2.91	±0.21	III–V	1.96	±0.19
III	3.83	±0.17	I–V	3.91	±0.15
IV	4.98	±0.17	I–II	1.05	±0.16
V	5.78	±0.19	I–III	0.91	±0.12
VI	7.17	±0.26	II–V	2.86	±0.20
VII	8.87	±0.34	V–VI	1.39	±0.28
			V–VII	3.12	±0.40

[a] Potentials evoked by monaural clicks, 70 dB SPL, 10/sec.

2.0 or 2.5 SD from normal mean values were considered as "borderline" or "abnormal," respectively. A IV-V/I amplitude ratio greater than 1.0 was considered normal.

All patients were submitted, within 24 hr of BAEP recording, to routine EEG (by means of eight-channel electroencephalographs, using the standard 10–20 system of electrode placement) as well as to otoneurologic examination.

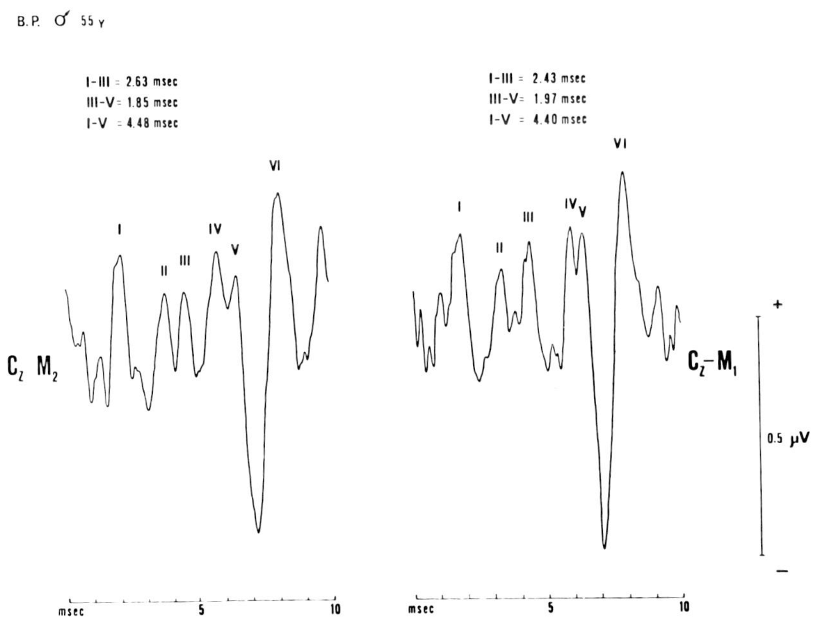

FIG. 2. The BAEPs of a patient (B.P., ♂, 55 y) affected by strokes with full recovery (SFR) revealing a bilateral abnormal increase (> 2.5 SD from normal value) of the I–III and I–V IPLs.

This included pure-tone audiometric tests, control of conjugated oculomotricity, spontaneous and evoked nystagmus detection, and labyrinthine bithermal caloric and rotoaccelleratory stimulation under ENG recording. No patient had hearing losses below 4.0 kHz. Patients were also explored by radiological examinations: brain CT (all patients) and angiography (14 patients). Directional C. W. Doppler of the vertebral arteries was performed in 19 patients.

In five patients, BAEPs were retested 3 months after the first recording.

RESULTS

Although the IV–V/I amplitude ratio always remained normal, increased IPLs were detected in transient ischemic attack (TIA) as well as in SFR patients when all signs and symptoms had disappeared.

TIA Patients

Eight patients out of 15 suffering from TIAs showed IPLs deviated from normal values: six of these were evaluated as abnormal, and two as borderline. All presented a prolonged I–V IPL in response to stimulation of the right as well as of the left ear. In Table 2 are reported the IPLs (I–III, III–V, I–V) observed in each patient for stimulation of the right and left ear. Among these eight patients, the I–III IPL was altered in two cases, and III–V IPL in five cases.

SFR Patients

Among the 11 patients with SFR, prolonged IPLs were detected in six, all of whom showed I–III and I–V IPLs 2.5 SD greater than normal values. In one of these patients, moreover, a borderline III–V IPL (i.e., >2.0, but <2.5 SD from normal values) was observed. More details on IPLs of single patients to monaural right and left ear stimulation can be obtained from Table 2.

The BAEP, otoneurological, and EEG findings in all patients are reported in Table 3. Of particular interest are the data provided by the otoneurological examination. In fact, like the BAEPs, it allows the functional exploration of different brainstem structures. This examination yielded abnormal results (i.e., showing an impairment of vestibular structures and/or of conjugated oculomotricity) in 17 out of 26 patients tested (10 in the TIA group and seven in the SFR group). These otoneurological abnormalities were in agreement with BAEP alterations in nine cases, and the combination of BAEPs and otoneurological examination gave objective evidence for brainstem dysfunction in 22 out of 26 patients.

Conventional EEG procedures documented abnormal findings in 17 cases (10 TIA patients and seven SFR patients). A moderate diffuse slowing of EEG activity associated with prominent photic driving was detected in five patients.

TABLE 2. *BAEP interpeak latencies in patients with vertebral–basilar RIAs*[a]

TIA patients							SFR patients						
	I–III		III–V		I–V			I–III		III–V		I–V	
Patient	R	L	R	L	R	L	Patient	R	L	R	L	R	L
S.V. ♂ 50 yr	−	−	−	−	−	−	R.G. ♂ 43 yr	−	−	−	−	−	−
F.M. ♂ 47 yr	−	−	−	−	−	−	B.S. ♂ 51 yr	+	+	−	−	±	+
B.E. ♂ 59 yr	−	−	−	±	−	+	G.R. ♂ 33 yr	+	+	−	−	+	+
G.W. ♂ 59 yr	−	−	−	−	−	−	B.P. ♂ 55 yr	+	+	−	−	+	+
P.E. ♂ 61 yr	−	−	−	−	−	−	P.P. ♂ 54 yr	+	−	−	±	+	±
M.A. ♂ 65 yr	−	−	−	−	+	+	G.M. ♂ 33 yr	−	−	−	−	−	−
S.A. ♂ 64 yr	−	−	−	−	−	−	D.A. ♀ 54 yr	+	+	−	−	−	±
C.A. ♂ 68 yr	−	−	−	±	±	±	F.L. ♂ 71 yr	±	±	−	−	+	+
G.G. ♀ 66 yr	−	±	−	−	+	−	R.R. ♀ 53 yr	−	−	−	−	−	−
T.F. ♂ 47 yr	±	−	−	+	+	+	F.A. ♂ 57 yr	−	−	−	−	−	−
M.M. ♂ 59 yr	−	−	+	+	+	+	P.G. ♂ 73 yr	−	−	−	−	−	−
M.A. ♀ 58 yr	−	−	−	−	+	−							
B.P. ♀ 51 yr	−	−	−	±	−	±							
N.P. ♀ 41 yr	−	−	−	−	−	−							
D.C.A. ♂ 43 yr	−	−	−	−	−	−							

[a] Abbreviations: R, stimulation to right ear; L, stimulation to left ear; −, normal IPLs; ±, borderline (>2.0, <2.5 SD from mean normal values) IPLs; +, abnormal (>2.5 SD from mean normal values) IPLs.

Mild abnormalities (transient theta activity) appeared to be predominant in the left temporal regions in three patients. Nonspecific alterations consisting of transient bisynchronous theta waves without the typical Frontal Intermittent Rhythmic Delta Activity (FIRDA) pattern occured in the other nine cases.

Data provided by other examinations can be summarized as follows: arteriography (performed in 14 patients) showed abnormalities of the vertebral–basilar system in nine cases; brain CT revealed a mild, diffuse cortical atrophy in 12 out of 26 patients; Directional C. W. Doppler demonstrated absence or reduction of blood flow in the vertebral arteries in 9 out of 19 patients.

Five patients (four of the TIA group, one of the SFR group) presenting prolonged IPLs underwent BAEP recording 3 months after the first examination;

TABLE 3. *BAEP, otoneurological, and EEG findings in patients with vertebral–basilar RIAs*[a]

TIA patients				SFR patients			
Patient	BAEP	Otoneurological examination[b]	EEG	Patient	BAEP	Otoneurological examination[b]	EEG
S.V. ♂ 50 yr	−	−	+	R.G. ♂ 43 yr	−	+	+
F.M. ♂ 47 yr	−	−	−	B.S. ♂ 51 yr	+	−	−
B.E. ♂ 59 yr	+	+	−	G.R. ♂ 33 yr	+	+	−
G.W. ♂ 59 yr	−	−	+	B.P. ♂ 55 yr	+	+	+
P.E. ♂ 61 yr	−	+	−	P.P. ♂ 54 yr	+	−	+
M.A. ♂ 65 yr	+	+	+	G.M. ♂ 33 yr	−	+	+
S.A. ♂ 64 yr	−	−	+	D.A. ♀ 54 yr	+	−	
C.A. ♂ 68 yr	±	+	−	F.L. ♂ 71 yr	+	−	+
G.G. ♀ 66 yr	+	+	+	R.R. ♀ 53 yr	−	+	+
T.F. ♂ 47 yr	+	+	+	F.A. ♂ 57 yr	−	+	−
M.M. ♂ 59 yr	+	+	+	P.G. ♂ 73 yr	−	+	+
M.A. ♀ 58 yr	+	+	+				
B.P. ♀ 51 yr	±	−	+				
N.P. ♀ 41 yr	−	+	−				
D.C.A. ♂ 43 yr	−	+	+				

[a] Symbols: −, normal; ±, borderline; +, abnormal.
[b] Considered abnormal when showing an impairment of vestibular structures and/or of conjugated oculomotricity.

no modification of the previously observed abnormalities was detected in any of them.

DISCUSSION

From the above results, it appears that BAEPs may be altered in cases of RIAs of the vertebral–basilar system even when all other symptoms have cleared and no objective abnormalities can be found on a detailed neurological examination. Even in the absence of a number of patients great enough to allow a statistical evaluation, BAEP abnormalities seemed to present a similar incidence among TIA patients as among SFR patients. An analogous distribution of abnormalities in the two groups also resulted from EEG and otoneurological findings. According to the current clinical criteria, we have differentiated TIAs and SFR exclusively on the duration of symptoms. Nevertheless, their pathogenesis is presumably identical, and both of them can be labeled under the common heading of RIAs, as suggested by Loeb (4).

The prognostic value of BAEPs can be stated only by a comparison of the results obtained in a series of follow-up recordings. Maurer et al. (6) observed in one patient with vertebral–basilar insufficiency a normalization of the altered BAEP waves recorded 6 months previously. Control recordings performed in five of our patients at a 3-month interval from the first examination did not show any changes in the previously observed abnormalities. This observation suggests that a brainstem dysfunction can still be present some months after the complete clinical recovery. However, it cannot be excluded that modifications of BAEP abnormalities could be detected in further controls.

The variety of symptoms observed in our patients seldom displayed the involvement of a definite brainstem level; therefore, a correspondence between localized BAEP abnormalities and the level of clinically suspected lesions could hardly be established.

Similarly to BAEPs, otoneurological examination showed abnormalities in a high number (17 out of 26) of RIA patients, and it is remarkable that at least one of these examinations showed impairment in as many as 22 patients. The BAEPs provide an evaluation of the brainstem auditory pathway, whereas the otoneurological examination assesses the function of central vestibular structures and of those regulating the conjugated oculomotricity. Therefore, we suggest the use of these two noninvasive procedures as complementing each other in the diagnosis and assessment of vertebral–basilar RIAs.

ACKNOWLEDGMENTS

The authors thank Mrs. C. Pietri Bosi for her valuable technical assistance.

REFERENCES

1. Green, J. B., and McLeod, S. (1979): Short latency somatosensory evoked potentials in patients with neurological lesions. *Arch. Neurol.*, 36:846–851.
2. Hashimoto, I., Ishiyama, Y., and Tozuka, G. (1979): Bilaterally recorded brainstem auditory evoked responses. *Arch. Neurol.*, 36:161–167.
3. Jewett, D. L., and Williston, J. S. (1971): Auditory-evoked far fields averaged from the scalp of humans. *Brain,* 94:681–696.
4. Loeb, C. (1978): Clinical aspects of cerebral ischemia. *Eur. Neurol.*, 17(Suppl. 1):33–41.
5. Lynn, G. E., Gilroy, J., and Maulsby, R. (1977): Auditory evoked brainstem potential (AEP) in vertebral–basilar artery disease. *Electroencephalogr. Clin. Neurophysiol.*, 43:465.
6. Maurer, K., Marneros, A., Schafer, E., and Leitner, H. (1979): Early auditory evoked potentials (EAEP) in vertebral–basilar insufficiency. *Arch. Psychiatr. Nervenkr.*, 227:367–376.
7. Ross Russell, R. W. (1976): Transient cerebral ischaemia. In: *Cerebral Arterial Disease,* edited by R. W. Ross Russell, pp. 125–145. Churchill-Livingstone, London, Edinburgh.
8. Rowe, M. J. (1978): Normal variability of brainstem auditory evoked response in young and adult subjects. *Electroencephalogr. Clin. Neurophysiol.*, 44:459–470.
9. Rowe, M. J. (1980): The brainstem auditory response (BSAER) in patients with vertigo. *Electroencephalogr. Clin. Neurophysiol.*, 49:5P.

10. Starr, A., and Achor, L. J. (1975): Auditory brainstem responses in neurological disease. *Arch. Neurol.,* 32:761–768.
11. Starr, A., and Hamilton, A. E. (1976): Correlation between confirmed sites of neurological lesions and abnormalities of far-field auditory brainstem responses. *Electroencephalogr. Clin. Neurophysiol.,* 41:595–608.
12. Stockard, J. J., and Rossiter, V. (1977): Clinical and pathological correlates of brainstem auditory response abnormalities. *Neurology (Minneap.),* 27:316—325.

Clinical Applications of Evoked Potentials in Neurology,
edited by J. Courjon, F. Mauguiere, and M. Revol.
Raven Press, New York © 1982.

Clinical Applications of Brainstem Auditory Evoked Potentials in Comatose Patients

*A. Uziel, **J. Benezech, *S. Lorenzo, **Y. Monstrey, †M. P. Duboin, and †B. Roquefeuil

**Laboratoire d'Explorations Neurosensorielles, Clinique ORL, Hôpital Saint-Charles, Montpellier, France; and **Clinique Neurochirurgicale and †Département de Neuroréanimation, Hôpital Gui-de-Chauliac, Montpellier, France*

Improved methods of evaluating central nervous system (CNS) function are needed in comatose patients to localize areas of brain dysfunction. In fact, most diagnostic studies reflect the anatomical condition much more than the functional condition of the CNS. A major contribution was made by Plum and Posner (10), who presented a series of clinical tests of cerebral hemispheric and brainstem integrity based on the clinical assessment of brainstem reflexes and posture. This logical approach has found ready application to the clinical evaluation of patients with severe head injury (1,9,20). Evidence and location of brainstem dysfunction was confirmed in certain cases of comas by the study of brainstem reflexes and histopathological findings (9,10). It was thus possible to define "levels of coma" corresponding to either a specific anatomical brain lesion or a functional disturbance of the nervous pathways.

Brainstem auditory evoked potentials (BAEPs) permit a noninvasive neurophysiological test that provides an objective measure of brainstem function and has proven to be clinically useful in evaluating the condition of patients with neurological diseases. In particular, structural or functional damage of the auditory pathways caused by tumor, demyelination, or diminished circulation in the brainstem can be reflected in abnormalities of the amplitude and latency of the various components (13,16). Measurement of BAEPs has also proven to be relevant in evaluating brainstem function in acute traumatic comas (3–5, 11, 22). The procedure is eminently suitable for clinical application in that technical improvements have made it possible for portable equipment and recording devices to be brought to the bedside of acutely ill individuals.

Our investigations were directed at (a) defining the relationship that exists between areas of brain dysfunction as defined by BAEPs and posttraumatic neurological conditions such as posture and brainstem reflexes and (b) evaluating clinical applicability and prognostic value of BAEPs in posttraumatic comas.

MATERIAL AND METHODS

Brainstem auditory evoked potentials were recorded from 60 comatose patients following severe head trauma (48 cases) or vascular (eight cases), anoxic (one case), or tumoral (three cases) damage to the CNS. Thirty-seven patients were tested during the acute phases of the coma. The other 23 patients were chronically comatose patients (apallic state, long vegetative state, akinetic mutism). Twenty of these 60 patients, taken from a previous report (22), were studied in an electrically shielded, sound-attenuated room. The other patients were recorded at the bedside in the neurosurgical intensive care unit with a portable stimulating and recording system (Racia EP 3).

Click signals (0.1-msec square wave pulses of alternating polarity) were presented monaurally through an electromagnetically shielded TDH 39 earphone at an intensity of 100 dB HL and a rate of 20/sec. A white noise masking of 60 dB HL was presented to the unstimulated ear to avoid cross stimulation of the contralateral ear by bone conduction. The BAEPs were recorded from conventional EEG electrodes (vertex–ear lobe, i.e., C_z to A_1 or A_2), amplified 10^5 at a band pass of 0.1 to 3.200 kHz, and averaged over a 10-msec time base. An artifact rejection device stopped triggering the averager sweeps when the EEG exceeded a preset value. A total of 2,048 clicks were presented for each averaged response. Two separate trials/averages of 2,048 responses were recorded and superimposed per ear to define reproducibility of results.

The latencies of waves I, III, and V were measured from stimulus onset to the peak of the wave (with the exception of wave V, the latency of which was chosen at the last point of upward inflection). Latencies and interpeak intervals (I–III, III–V, I–V) were considered abnormal if they were more than 2 SD above the mean of a normal population (I–III, 2.50 msec; III–V, 2.10 msec; I–V, 4.40 msec). Amplitudes were measured from the highest positive peak of the IV–V complex to the negative trough following wave V. The amplitude of the IV–V complex was considered to be reduced when it was less than the amplitude of wave I (IV–V/I ratio < 1). In all figures, positivity at the vertex electrode was in the up direction.

Clinical neurological examinations and EEG recordings were performed close to the time at which BAEPs were recorded. Posture and ocular reflexes were the main criteria used to assess the level of coma (22). Patient rectal temperature was noted at the time of BAEP recording since BAEPs are known to be affected by marked hypothermia (17). The initial study was performed within the first 3 days after injury. In many patients, follow-up studies were performed as long as 15 days after injury.

RESULTS

Comatose Head Injury Patients

Thirty patients were tested during the acute stage of coma. Most of them (19/30) had normal BAEPs with respect to latency, amplitude, and morphology.

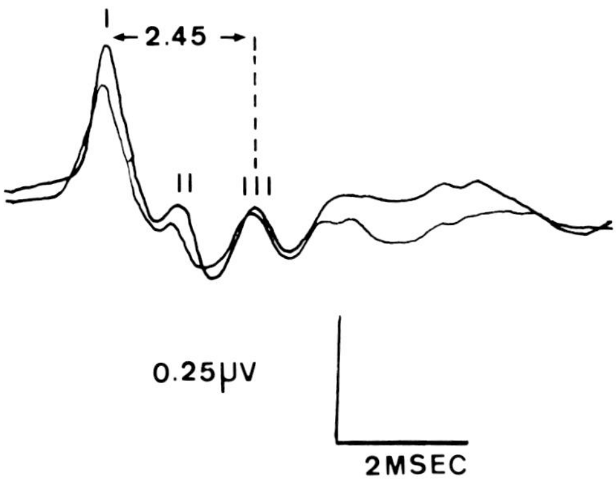

FIG. 1. Brainstem auditory evoked potentials from a comatose head injury patient recorded 4 days following the head trauma. The patient was unconscious and had marked hypertonia with decerebrate posturing. The pupils were nonreactive and dilated; the vertical oculocephalic reflex was absent. Corneal reflex was present. The BAEP showed loss of waves IV–V, suggesting a midbrain level of dysfunction.

The BAEPs were abnormal during the early acute period in 11 patients (Figs. 1 and 2). Abnormalities in BAEPs included alterations of waves IV–V, i.e., reduced amplitudes and/or prolonged III–V intervals (5 cases), alterations of waves III and IV–V (3 cases), and absence of waves III and IV–V (3 cases). Of the three comatose patients fulfilling the clinical criteria of brain death, two had bilaterally preserved waves I and II (Fig. 2) and one showed no identifiable BAEP waveform, including wave I. In this last case, transtympanic electrocochleography showed considerable reduction in amplitude of N1 but revealed preservation of cochlear microphonic that could be recorded at a normal threshold.

The BAEP revealed otologic disorders in eight patients (cophosis in four patients, conductive hearing loss in four patients).

From a clinical point of view, the loss of waves IV–V was correlated with vertical oculocephalic palsy and abnormal pupillary light responses; the loss

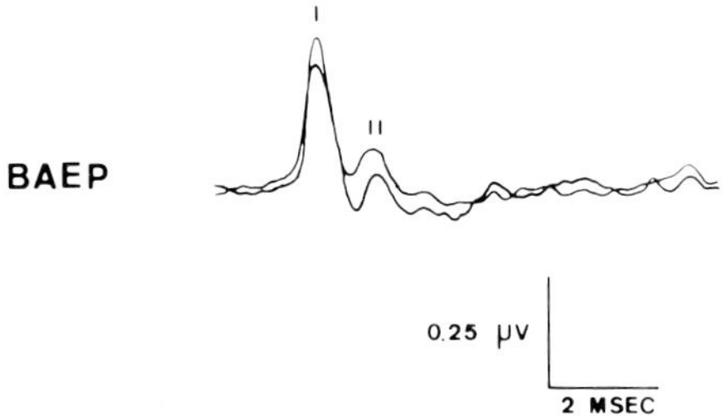

FIG. 2. Brainstem auditory evoked potentials to monaural clicks at 100 dB HL from a case of brain death showing preservation of waves I and II.

of wave III and subsequent waves was correlated with lateral oculocephalic palsy and dilated pupils. The status of the BAEP during the acute stage corresponded with patient outcome. Of the 19 patients with intact BAEPs, 14 demonstrated complete recovery within 1 month, three dropped into a persistent vegetative state, and two eventually died. In contrast, most of the patients having BAEP abnormalities died (7/11) or remained in a vegetative state (one case), whereas only three recovered completely. The loss of waves IV–V signifies a poor prognosis since all patients but one showing this type of abnormality died.

Eighteen other patients were recorded during the chronic phases of the coma. Normal BAEPs were found in 12 patients who all had normal brainstem reflexes. Completely normal BAEPs were recorded from patients rendered irreversibly comatose by diffuse bilateral cerebrocortical damage (apallic state). Six patients exhibited BAEP abnormalities including reduced amplitudes and altered morphology of waves III and IV–V (Figs. 3 and 4). These patients all had clinical signs of upper brainstem dysfunction.

Comatose Patients Following Vascular and Tumor Disorders

Of the eight comatose patients with vascular disorders, only one had normal BAEPs. That particular case was a young patient with a subarachnoidal hemorrhage following aneurysm rupture whose neurologic status gradually worsened. Four patients with intracerebral hemorrhage exhibited altered morphology of BAEPs (desynchronized pattern) and I–V interpeak latency prolongation. When coma followed intrinsic brainstem vascular damage, there were marked changes in BAEPs consisting of a loss or reduction in amplitude of waves III and IV–V. In two cases, these abnormalities were found to be markedly asymmetrical. In contrast, BAEPs were intact in a patient with coma following diffuse cortical damage from anoxia.

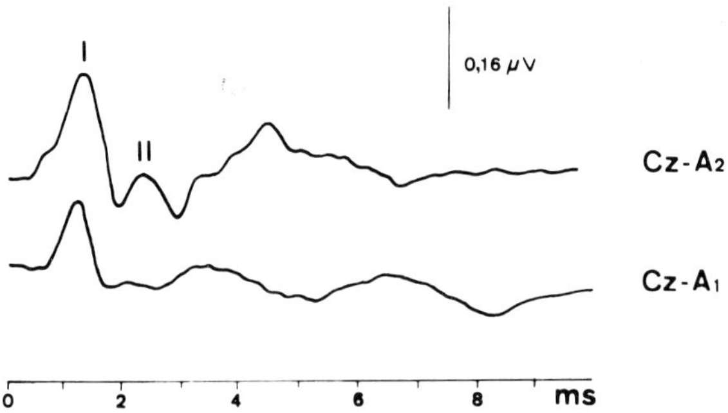

FIG. 3. Brainstem auditory evoked potentials from a young patient with amniotic embolism involving the brainstem. On neurological examination, she was found to match a "locked-in syndrome." Bilateral pinpoint pupils, ocular bobbing, and absence of corneal reflex provided evidence of lower brainstem lesion. The BAEP showed absence of waves III and IV–V on both sides.

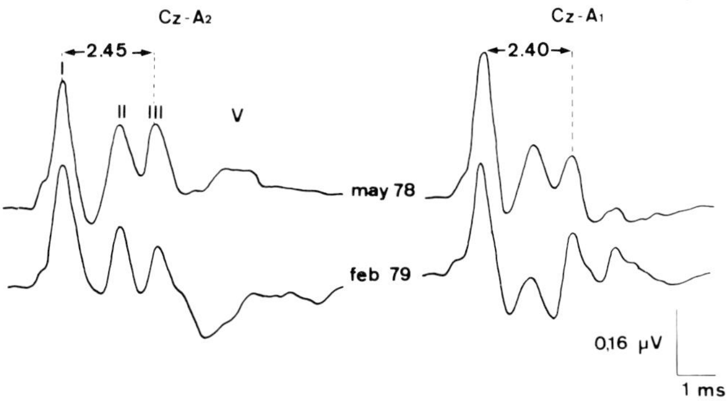

FIG. 4. Brainstem auditory evoked potentials recorded from a 19-year-old female involved in a severe head injury in May, 1976. The BAEPs were recorded in May, 1978 and February, 1979. At the time of the recordings, she was unresponsive and did not obey commands. Her pupils were sluggishly reactive; the vertical oculocephalic reflex was absent. Her BAEPs showed a strong decrease in the IV–V/I ratio, suggesting a widespread midbrain damage.

Three patients with tumor involving the brainstem showed abnormalities in either amplitude or latency of BAEPs that were correlated with the anatomical site of lesion as defined by CT scan or at surgery.

DISCUSSION

The results of the present study indicate that BAEPs can provide information as to the functional integrity of the brainstem in comatose patients. Abnormalities of both latency and amplitude of the various components provide an objective means of localizing the brainstem levels at which neurological dysfunction is occurring.

Brainstem auditory evoked potentials are useful in evaluating comas caused by severe head injury. In a previous study (22), we were able to establish a significant relationship between BAEP abnormalities and the various clinical signs usually considered evidence of known anatomical dysfunction. Three different levels of brainstem dysfunction occurring during the rostrocaudal deterioration of the CNS could be related to specific alterations of BAEP components: alteration of wave V was related to a midbrain level of dysfunction, alteration of wave III to a pontine level, and alteration of waves I and II and subsequent waves to a lower brainstem dysfunction. The present study demonstrated that a large number (63%) of comatose head injury patients had intact BAEPs. In fact, most anatomical studies have shown that primary lesions of the brainstem are rarely found in postinjury comatose patients (19,21). These findings may account for the large number of normal BAEPs in these patients.

It is reasonable to assume that the major causes of BAEP abnormalities in head trauma comatose patients may be represented by rostrocaudal deterioration following diffuse hemispheric damage or transtentorial herniation leading to upper brainstem dysfunction. Experimental studies of Nagao et al. (7,8) confirmed that altered amplitude of BAEP wave V reflected the extent of caudal displacement of the upper brainstem because of transtentorial herniation.

Measurement of the BAEP has proven useful in evaluating brain death (12). The responses were either absent or consisted of just the initial component (wave I). We have also observed, as have other authors (2,18), a third pattern in which waves I and II are preserved. This last observation indicates that a part of wave II is generated by the proximal auditory nerve. Complete absence of BAEP (including wave I) signifies a poor prognosis but requires cautious interpretation since technical and otologic problems have to be excluded. An uncommon but useful method to test auditory function may be transtympanic electrocochleography. We have already reported a case of brain death with absence of BAEP in which electrocochleography showed preservation of the cochlear microphonic (22). Stockard et al. (18) reported a similar observation with BAEPs using an acoustic coupling through a length of tubing which delayed the cochlear microphonic from the stimulus artifact.

Interpretation of BAEPs in comatose patients requires caution, since nonneurologic factors may affect the responses and produce false localizing signs. Otologic factors represent the major limitation in comatose patients with severe head injury. Temporal bone fractures may produce tympanic or ossicular injury with a conductive hearing loss. Some comatose patients in our study (15%) exhibited increased absolute latencies of the major peaks, suggesting conductive hearing loss. Fortunately, interpeak latency is not affected by conductive-type hearing loss. It is in our practice, therefore, to base our criteria of BAEP latency abnormality only on prolongation of interpeak latency. In the absence of otoscopic signs of temporal bone fractures, prolonged BAEP latencies may also represent a temporary conductive hearing deficit brought about by the inability of comatose patients to equilibrate middle ear pressure (13). Moreover, the cochlea itself may be injured by a transverse fracture of the petrous bone that results in a total loss of cochlear function. For that reason, absence of BAEP (including wave I) in a severe comatose patient must be interpreted with caution in the case of an initial recording. Thus, BAEPs are relevant for the assessment of brain death only when the patient's hearing function can be taken into consideration.

Other factors may also influence BAEPs. Hypothermia, which is often induced in comatose patients, increases I–V interpeak latency and should be considered when BAEP abnormalities are being interpreted (17).

The BAEP has been shown to have a prognostic value in posttraumatic comas (3–5). The present study confirms that BAEP's status is of value in predicting patient outcome. The loss of waves IV–V seems to have a particularly poor prognosis, since only one patient with such abnormality survived.

Abnormalities of BAEP were also found in chronically comatose patients. The major alterations concerned waves IV–V and persisted in a long-term follow-up study. Such abnormalities may result from tegmental and periacqueductal lesions commonly found in chronically comatose patients (6).

When coma follows structural damage from tumoral or vascular disorders, BAEPs may be helpful as well in evaluating the site of the lesion without any particular change due to the comatose state (14,15,16).

Brainstem auditory evoked potentials may thus provide evidence of brainstem dysfunction in comatose patients. Conversely, they can suggest the absence of brainstem lesion in toxic or metabolic comas (14) as well as in diffuse cortical processes in which the brainstem has been spared. Intactness of BAEPs in drug overdose (18) is of particular interest since high doses of barbiturates produce a flat EEG and do not allow a clinical examination. The expending use of barbiturates in acute neurologic individuals should justify a wider use of BAEPs in comatose patients.

REFERENCES

1. Becker, D. P., Vries, J. K., Sakalas, R., (1976): Early prognosis in head injury based on motor posturing, oculocephalic reflexes and intracranial pressure. In: *Head Injuries. Proceedings of the Second Chicago Symposium on Neural Trauma,* edited by R. L. McLaurin, pp. 27–30. Grune and Stratton, New York and San Francisco.
2. Goldie, W. D., Chiappa, K. H., and Young, R. R. (1979): Brainstem auditory evoked responses and short-latency somatosensory evoked responses in the evaluation of deeply comatose patients. *Neurology,* 29:581–582.
3. Greenberg, R. P., Mayer, D. J., Becker, D. P., and Miller, J. D. (1977): Evaluation of brain function in severe head trauma with multimodality evoked potentials. Part 1: Evoked brain-injury potentials, method and analysis. *J. Neurosurg.,* 47:150–162.
4. Greenberg, R. P., Becker, D. P., Miller, J. D., and Mayer, D. J. (1977): Evaluation of brain function in severe human head trauma with multimodality evoked potentials. Part 2: Localization of brain dysfunction and correlation with post-traumatic neurological conditions. *J. Neurosurg.,* 47:163–177.
5. Greenberg, R. P., Miller, J. D., and Becker, D. P. (1979): Early prognosis after severe human head injury utilizing multimodality evoked potentials. *Acta Neurochi. (Wien). [Suppl.],* 28:50–51.
6. Jellinger, K., and Seitelberger, F. (1970): Protracted post-traumatic encephalopathy. Pathology, pathogenesis and clinical implications. *J. Neurol. Sci.,* 10:51–94.
7. Nagao, S., Roccaforte, P., and Moody, R. A. (1979): Acute intracranial hypertension and auditory brainstem responses. Part 1: Changes in the auditory brainstem and somatosensory evoked responses in intracranial hypertension in cats. *J. Neurosurg.,* 51:669–676.
8. Nagao, S., Roccaforte, P., and Moody, R. A. (1979): Acute intracranial hypertension and auditory brainstem responses. Part 2: The effect of brainstem movement on the auditory brainstem responses due to transtentorial herniation. *J. Neurosurg.,* 51.846–851.
9. Perez-Dominguez, E., Frerebeau, Ph., Privat, J. M., Benezech, J., and Gros, C. (1976): The value of brainstem reflexes in coma. *J. Neurosurg. Sci.,* 20:293–298.
10. Plum, F., and Posner, J. B. (1972): *Diagnosis of Stupor and Coma.* Davis, Philadelphia.
11. Seales, D. M., Rossiter, V. S., and Weinstein, M. E. (1979): Brainstem auditory evoked responses in patients comatose as a result of blunt head trauma. *J. Trauma,* 19:347–353.
12. Starr, A. (1976): Auditory brainstem responses in brain death. *Brain,* 99:543–554.
13. Starr, A. (1977): Clinical relevance of brainstem auditory evoked potentials in brainstem disorders in man. In: *Progress in Clinical Neurophysiology, Vol. 2, Auditory Evoked Potentials in Man. Psychopharmacology Correlates of EPs,* edited by J. E. Desmedt, pp. 45–57. Karger, Basel.
14. Starr, A., and Achor, L. J. (1975): Auditory brainstem responses in neurological disease. *Arch. Neurol.,* 32:761–768.
15. Starr, A., and Hamilton, A. E. (1976): Correlation between confirmed sites of neurological lesions and abnormalities of far-field auditory brainstem responses. *Electroencephalogr. Clin. Neurophysiol.,* 41:595–608.
16. Stockard, J. J., and Rossiter, V. S. (1977): Clinical and pathologic correlates of brainstem auditory response abnormalities. *Neurology,* 27:316–325.

17. Stockard, J. J., Sharbrough, F. W., and Tinker, J. A. (1978): Effects of hypothermia on the human brainstem auditory response. *Ann. Neurol.,* 3:368–370.
18. Stockard, J. J., Stockard, J. E., and Sharbrough, F. W. (1979): Brainstem auditory evoked potentials in neurology: Methodology, interpretation, clinical application. In: *Electrophysiological Approaches to Neurological Diagnosis,* edited by M. J. Aminoff, pp. 524–567. Churchill Livingstone, New York and London.
19. Strich, S. J. (1970): Lesions in the cerebral hemispheres after blunt head injury. *J. Clin. Pathol. [Suppl.],* 4:166–171.
20. Teasdale, G., and Jennett, B. (1974): Assessment of coma and impaired consciousness: A practical scale. *Lancet,* 2:81–83.
21. Tomlinson, B. E. (1970): Brainstem lesions after head injury. *J. Clin. Pathol. [Suppl.],* 4:154–165.
22. Uziel, A., and Benezech, J. (1978): Auditory brainstem responses in comatose patients: Relationship with brainstem reflexes and levels of coma. *Electroencephalogr. Clin. Neurophysiol.,* 45:515–524.

Clinical Applications of Evoked Potentials in Neurology,
edited by J. Courjon, F. Mauguiere, and M. Revol.
Raven Press, New York © 1982.

Value of the Simultaneous Recording of Brainstem Auditory Evoked Potentials, Blink Reflex, and Short-Latency Somatosensory Evoked Potentials for the Assessement of Brainstem Function in Clinical Neurology

C. Van Nechel, P. Deltenre, S. Strul, and A. Capon

Department for Rehabilitation of Neurological Disorders, Brugmann Hospital, 1020 Brussels, Belgium

The value of BAEP, blink reflex, and short-latency SEP in the assessment of brainstem function has already been considered in some previous reports (5,8,9,11,13–15,17,18,20). The purpose of this study is to assess the value of the simultaneous recording of BAEP, blink reflex, and short-latency SEP in the diagnosis of brainstem lesions and to test the ability of the recordings to locate these lesions with precision. We therefore compared the respective diagnostic contributions of the EEG (3), ENG, and CT scan with those of evoked potentials.

MATERIAL AND METHODS

One hundred patients with no prior neurological disease but who were suffering from a single recent central nervous system disturbance were examined. Data from patients with multiple lesions in the central nervous system were not considered in this study (4).

Eighty patients, among whom 31 were comatose, suffered from a brainstem lesion. Among the noncomatose patient group, we selected 20 cases each of whom had a lesion proven to be unilateral and well located by clinical, CT scan, or anatomical data. A second group of 20 patients each with a demonstrated lesion outside the brainstem was used to assess the amount of positive data in cases without any clinical or CT scan clue for a brainstem lesion.

For the BAEP recording, we used an unfiltered click of 80 dB SPL and a negative earlobe–vertex derivation. A band-pass filter of 100 Hz to 3 kHz was connected to the input of an S.A.I.T. Save 1,024 averager (19).

For the SEP, the electrodes were located at the supraclavicular fossa and over the spinous processes of the second and seventh cervical vertebrae with a frontal reference. The positive 15 wave (P15) was studied with a central electrode using an earlobe reference (6).

TABLE 1. *Means and standard deviations (msec) of EP latencies and amplitudes*

	Mean	SD	*N*
BAEP			
I	1.59	0.143	46
II	2.65	0.174	45
III	3.72	0.172	47
IV	4.87	0.176	43
V	5.68	0.222	48
I–III	2.12	0.188	43
III–V	1.92	0.138	44
I–V	4.05	0.248	43
I–II	1.07	0.145	42
II–V	2.98	0.155	41
IV–V	0.77	0.183	38
Blink reflex			
R1	11.44	0.707	40
Short-lat. SEP			
N9	9.65	0.740	44
P15	14.35	1.098	44
N9–P15	4.70	0.625	44
Amplitude asymmetry between right and left P15 waves	26%	9.92%	44

All results were compared with those of a group of 40 normal subjects (Table 1). We considered as abnormal a BAEP with interpeak latencies greater than the mean value plus 3 SD. An amplitude asymmetry of the P 15 wave greater than 50% was considered as abnormal if the N11–N14 (6) complex was normal.

For the blink reflex, only the latency of the R1 wave or an absence of the R2 wave were considered (8,11).

RESULTS AND DISCUSSION

Conscious Patients

The respective contribution of the evoked potentials, the EEG, ENG, and CT scan recorded within the same week in the assessment of brainstem vascular or tumoral lesions is shown in Table 2. The miscellaneous group included central pontine myelinolysis, heredoataxia, and Jakob-Creutzfeld's encephalitis. The evoked potential data were obviously the most contributive to the confirmation of the clinical diagnosis, even if we consider EEG, ENG, and CT scan data together.

Table 3 summarizes these results for all of the brainstem lesions. Among the EP data, the BAEP proved to be the most contributive, although blink

TABLE 2. *Comparative value of EEG, ENG, CT scan, and EP data in conscious patients with brainstem lesions (non-MS)*

	Positive results		
	Tumors	Vascular	Miscellaneous
Cases	7	23	8
BAEP	7/7	20/23	8/8
Blink reflex	5/7	12/20	3/6
Short-lat. SEP	2/3	4/7	2/4
Total EP	7/7	20/23	8/8
EEG (+) for brainstem lesions	4/7	7/23	3/7
Normal	3/7	16/23	4/7
CT scan	5/7	6/17	1/6
EEG + ENG + CT scan	5/7	13/23	3/7

TABLE 3. *Comparative value of EEG, ENG, CT scan, and EP data in conscious patients with brainstem lesions (non-MS)*

BAEP	46/49	94%
Blink reflex	23/42	55%
Short-lat. SEP	8/14	57%
Total EP	46/49	94%
EEG (+) for brainstem lesions	19/46	41%
Normal	23/46	50%
CT scan	19/39	49%
EEG + ENG + CT scan	30/46	65%

reflex and short-latency SEP were useful to confirm the BAEP data in more than half of the cases. These two investigations were never positive in cases of lesions proving to be outside the brainstem by CT and isotopic scannings (Table 4). Nevertheless, this did not insure the absence of brainstem dysfunction. Therefore, we can not call these cases false-positive BAEP results.

Among the 20 patients with clearly one-sided lesions, we studied the correlation between BAEP data and lesion levels (Figs. 1 and 2). Each vertical line represents a new case. All I–V and IV–V interpeak latencies were found to be increased in lesions that had in common a midbrain level contralateral to the stimulation side. On the other hand, only the lower lesions caused an increased

TABLE 4. *Positive results of EP data in focal lesions outside the brainstem*

BAEP	3/18	17%
Blink reflex (wave R1)	0/18	—
Short-lat. SEP	0/10	—
Total EP	3/18	17%

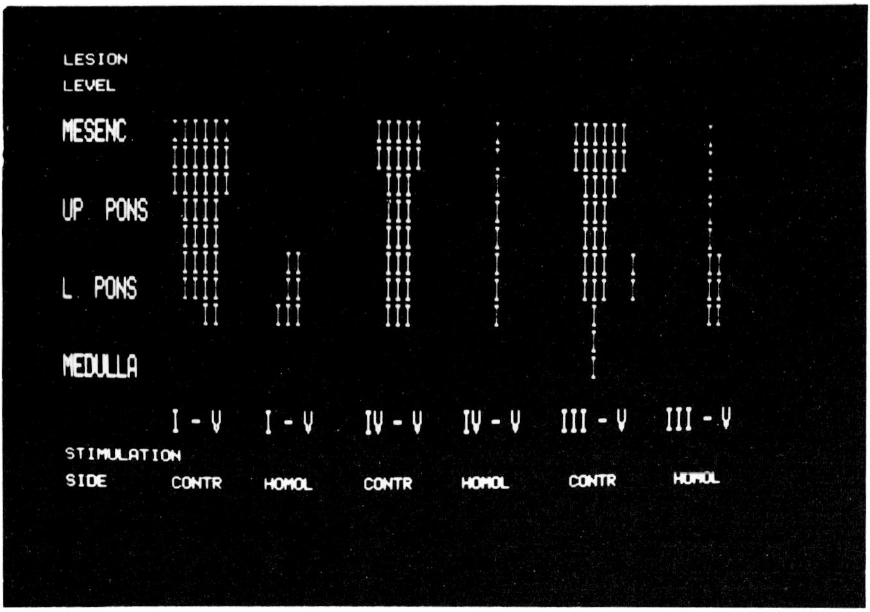

FIG. 1. Distribution of abnormal interpeak intervals in single unilateral brainstem lesions. Each *vertical line* represents the level of a lesion.

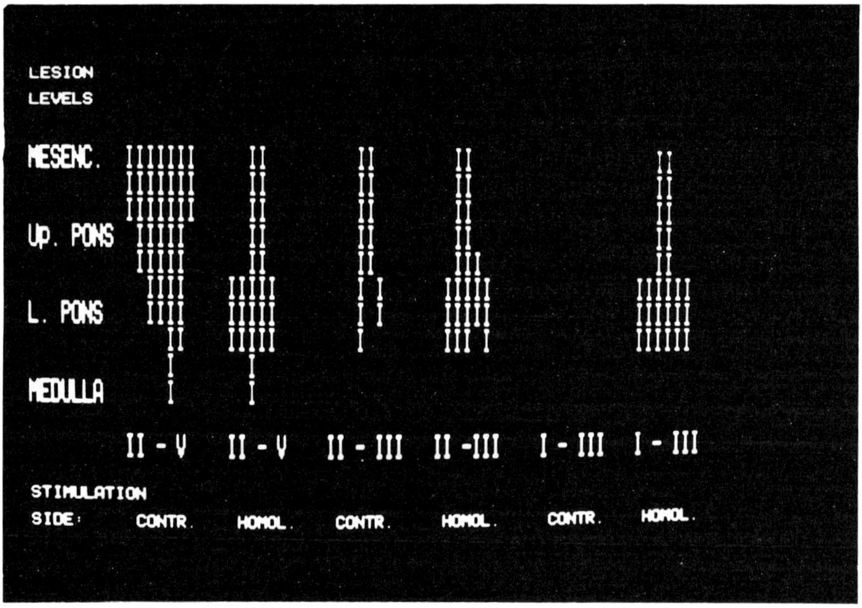

FIG. 2. Distribution of abnormal interpeak intervals in single unilateral brainstem lesions. Each *vertical line* represents the level of a lesion.

I–V interval after a homolateral stimulation. An alteration of the II–III interval also indicated a lesion at the same brainstem level but gave poor information regarding the side. Again, the II–V and especially the I–III intervals gave such information. We did not find any increased I–III interval after contralateral stimulation to a low pons lesion.

It is also noteworthy that in a few cases, alterations of the I–II interval were observed with a normal I–V interval. We view this as a clue for the existence of parallel pathways between the generators of these various waves in man.

The asymmetry between the responses obtained after left- or right-ear stimulation is an important observation that precludes the use of binaural stimulation in neurological investigations.

In this same group of 20 patients, the R1 component of the blink reflex was delayed in various pontine lesions. The bilateral disappearance of the R2 component was observed in medulla, caudal pontine, or midpontine lesions. The amplitude and latency of the P15 wave of the SEP were altered in cases of lesions located at various sites in the brainstem. This illustrates the complexity of the generators and pathways for this component (21).

Comatose Patients

We also studied the value of the BAEP and the blink reflex in a third group of 31 comatose patients (12,20). These investigations were very valuable for assessment, especially when neurological examination was made impossible by the interference of curarizing or sedative drugs used for therapeutic purposes.

The integrity of the brainstem was confirmed or revealed by the BAEP data in the six cases of toxic coma (1,2,16). For these patients, temperature was a main factor in the correct interpretation of the data (7). Such was the case of a woman who was in an areflectic coma after barbituric intoxication. The EEG and EP were simultaneously recorded, and the former indicated an absence of electrogenic cortical activity. At this time, there were many delayed latencies of the BAEP waves, and the body temperature was 34.9°C. The barbituric blood level was 3.8 mg/100 ml. Within a few hours, the temperature increased to 36.2°C, and the BAEP results became completely normal (Fig. 3). The barbituric blood level decreased from 3.8 to 3.1 mg/100 ml. The EEG remained flat for 24 hr, and the patient comatose for another 48 hr.

A differential diagnosis between brain herniation and brainstem contusion was also possible (10). In the first case, we observed a progressive deterioration of the V and preceding waves (Fig. 4).

In a case of brainstem contusions, we observed an increase of the interpeak intervals with a well-defined V wave (Fig. 5).

The last table summarizes the advantages of the use of BAEP and blink reflex recordings in comatose patients (Table 5).

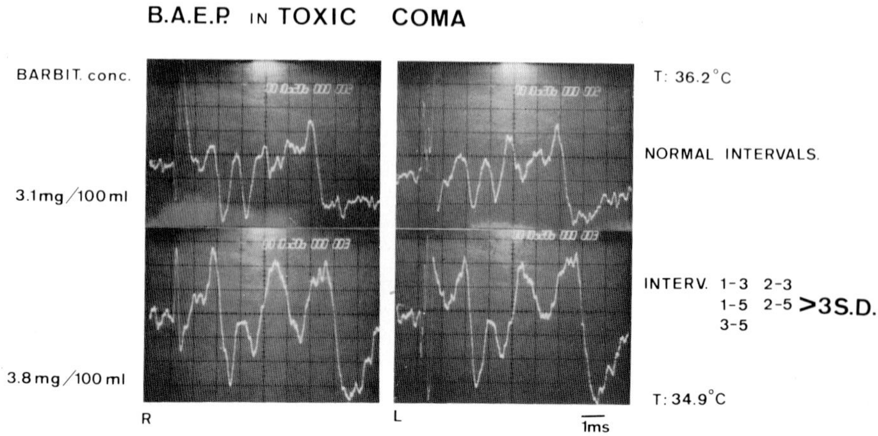

FIG. 3. Evolution of BAEP results with temperature variation in a case of toxic coma.

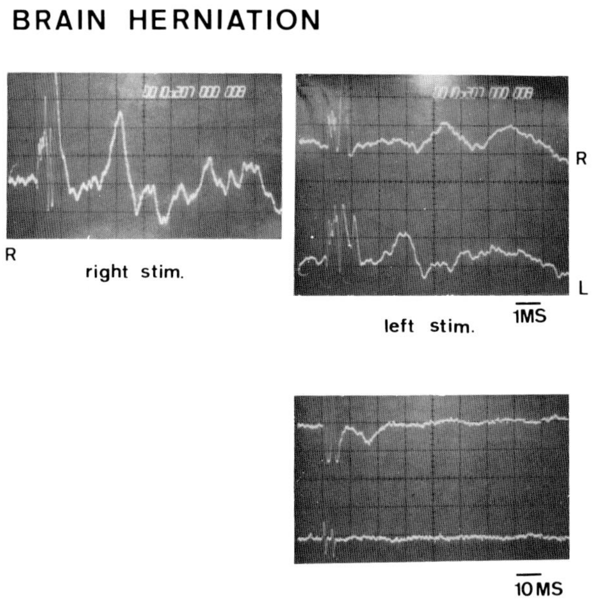

FIG. 4. BAEP and blink reflex results in a case of brain herniation. The V wave is progressively deteriorated without delayed intervals between the waves I, II, III, and IV.

CONCLUSION

The unique diagnostic contribution of brainstem EPS results from their reliability which is greater than that of EEG or CT scan, these two nevertheless being very useful for the complementary information they provide. The EP also are often the only source of information for infraclinic lesions [e.g., in

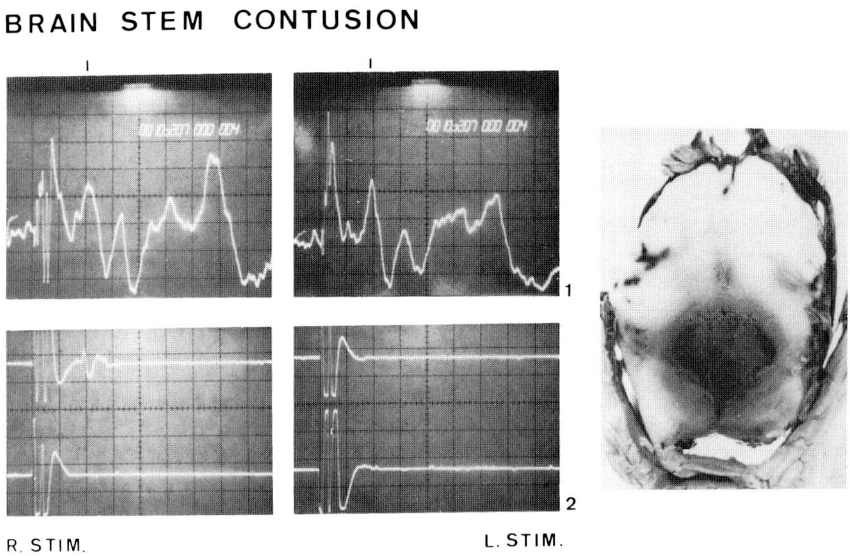

FIG. 5. BAEP and blink reflex results in a case of brainstem contusion. The interpeak intervals I–III, I–V, and II–III are increased, but the fifth wave remains well defined.

TABLE 5. *Advantages of BAEP and blink reflex recordings for comatose patients*

Easily recordable
Only two electrodes
Free of 50 Hz artifacts with stimulation frequency of $(2n + 1) \times 10$ msec
Demonstrates integrity of BAEP in most cases of toxic coma after hypothermia correction
Allows follow-up of cases with invalid clinical data because of therapeutic drugs administration
Allows differential diagnosis between brain herniation and brainstem contusion

MS patients (4)] or when the neurological examination has been made impossible by drug interference.

REFERENCES

1. Bhargava, V. K., Salamy, A., and McKean, C. M. (1978): Effects of cholinergic drugs on the brain stem auditory evoked responses (far-field) in rats. *Neuroscience,* 3:821–826.
2. Breivik, H., Safar, P., Sands, P., Fabritius, R., Lind, B., Lust, P., Mullie, A., Orr, M., Renck, H., and Snyder, J. (1978): Clinical feasability trials of barbiturate therapy after cardiac arrest. *Crit. Med.,* 6:228–244.
3. Chase, T. N., Moretti, L., and Prensky, L. (1968): Clinical and electroencephalographic manifestations of vascular lesions of the pons. *Neurology,* 18:357–368.
4. Deltenre, P., Vercruysse, A., Van Nechel, C., Ketelaer, P., Capon, A., Colin, F., and Manil, J. (1979): Early diagnosis of multiple sclerosis by combined multimodal evoked potentials. *J. Biomed. Eng.,* 1:17–21.
5. Green, J. B., and McLeod, S. (1979): Short latency somatosensory evoked potentials in patients with neurological lesions. *Arch. Neurol.,* 35:846–851.
6. Jones, S. J. (1977): Short latency potentials recorded from the neck and scalp following median nerve stimulation in man. *Electroencephalogr. Clin. Neurophysiol.,* 43:853–863.

7. Jones, T. A., Stockard, J. J., and Weidner, W. J. (1980): The effects of temperature and acute alcohol intoxication on brain stem auditory evoked potentials in the cat. *Electroencephalogr. Clin. Neurophysiol.*, 49:23–30.
8. Kimura, J., and Lyon, L. W. (1972): Orbicularis oculi reflex in the Wallenberg syndrome: Alteration of the late reflex by lesions of the spinal tract and nucleus of the trigeminal nerve. *J. Neurol. Neurosurg. Psychiatry*, 35:228–233.
9. Kjaer, M. (1980): Localizing brain stem lesions with brain stem auditory evoked potentials. *Acta Neurol. Scand.*, 61:265–275.
10. Nagao, S., Roccaforte, P., and Moody, R. A. (1979): Acute intracranial hypertension and auditory brain stem responses. *J. Neurosurg.*, 51:669–671.
11. Ongerboer de Visser, B. W., and Kuypers, H. G. J. (1978): Blink reflex in Wallenberg's syndrome. *Brain*, 101(2):285–294.
12. Sohmer, H., Gafni, M., and Chisin, R. (1978): Auditory nerve and brain stem responses. Comparison in awake and unconscious subjects. *Arch. Neurol.*, 35:228–230.
13. Starr, A., and Achor, L. J. (1975): Auditory brain stem responses in neurological disease. *Arch. Neurol.*, 32:761–768.
14. Starr, A., and Hamilton, A. E. (1976): Correlation between confirmed sites of neurological lesions and abnormalities of far-field auditory brain stem responses. *Electroencephalogr. Clin. Neurophysiol.*, 41:595–608.
15. Stockard, J. J., and Rossiter, U. S. (1977): Clinical and pathological correlates of brain stem auditory response abnormalities. *Neurology. (Minneap.)*, 27:316–325.
16. Stockard, J. J., Rossiter, V. S., Jones, T. A., and Sharbrough, F. W. (1977): Effects of centrally acting drugs on brain stem auditory responses. *Electroencephalogr. Clin. Neurophysiol.*, 43:550.
17. Stockard, J. J., Rossiter, V. S., Wiederholt, W. C., and Kobayashi, R. M. (1976): Brain stem auditory evoked responses in suspected central pontine myelinolysis. *Arch. Neurol.*, 33:726–728.
18. Stockard, J. J., and Sharbrough, F. W. (1980): Unique contributions of short latency auditory and somatosensory evoked potentials to neurologic diagnosis. In: *Progress in Clinical Neurophysiology, vol. 7,* edited by J. E. Desmedt, pp. 231–263. S. Karger, Basel.
19. Stockard, J. E., Stockard, J. J., Westmoreland, B. F., and Corfits, J. L. (1979): Brain stem auditory evoked responses. Normal variation as a function of stimulus and subject characteristics. *Arch. Neurol.*, 36:823–831.
20. Uziel, A., and Benezech, J. (1978): Auditory brain stem responses in comatose patients: Relationship with brain stem reflexes and levels of coma. *Electroencephalogr. Clin. Neurophysiol.*, 45:515–524.
21. Wiederholt, W. C. (1980): Early components of the somatosensory evoked potential in man, cat, and rat. In: *Progress in Clinical Neurophysiology, Vol. 7,* edited by J. E. Desmedt, pp. 105–117. S. Karger, Basel.

Clinical Applications of Evoked Potentials in Neurology,
edited by J. Courjon, F. Mauguiere, and M. Revol.
Raven Press, New York © 1982.

Brainstem Auditory Evoked Potentials in the Neurologic Clinic: Improved Stimulation and Analysis Methods

M. Scherg and E. W. Speulda

Max-Planck-Institute for Psychiatry, Abteilung für Klinische Neurophysiologie, D-8000 Munich 40, Federal Republic of Germany

The brainstem auditory evoked potential (BAEP) is widely considered a tool in topological and functional brainstem diagnosis (4–6). Considerable variation of the BAEP can result from stimulus and subject characteristics (7,2) as well as from peripheral influences such as audiogram shape (1). These effects are often neglected in pure neurological applications of the BAEP and might lead to false interpretations.

The purpose of this chapter is to present some examples of the dramatic influences of stimulus parameters and audiogram shape on the BAEP and to describe stimulation and analysis methods that can provide more secure BAEP parameters for the neurologic diagnosis.

METHODS

A group of 12 normal listeners (seven male, five female, age range 17–42, mean 29.2 years) was recruited from clinical staff and friends. We also recorded BAEPs from eight subjects with high-frequency hearing loss (HFHL). The three subjects presented here had occupational hearing loss (subject K.U., m., 46 years, HL O dB at 2 kHz, 70 dB at 4 kHz, 60 dB at 8 kHz, right ear), presbyacusis (subject G.R., m., 71 years, HL 5 dB at 2 kHz, 60 dB at 4 kHz, 70 dB at 8 kHz), and cochlear hearing loss caused by infection in childhood (subject B.A., m., 44 years, HL 30 dB at 4 kHz, 60 dB at 8 kHz). From over 200 clinical cases, the BAEPs of three neurologic patients were selected for demonstration (patient L.H., m., 55 years, brainstem ischemia; patient T.R., f., 24 years, multiple sclerosis; patient D.I., m., 46 years, bilateral vascular thalamic lesion).

Stimuli were generated by the DAC of a PDP 11/40 computer and delivered monaurally by TDH 39 headphones. Two stimuli were investigated (Fig. 1): a 100-μsec square wave pulse (click) and a gaussian-shaped impulse (plop) with a center frequency of 1 kHz. Stimulus level was controlled within the closed earphone volume *in situ* (70 dB HL corresponded to 95 dB peSPL). The stimuli

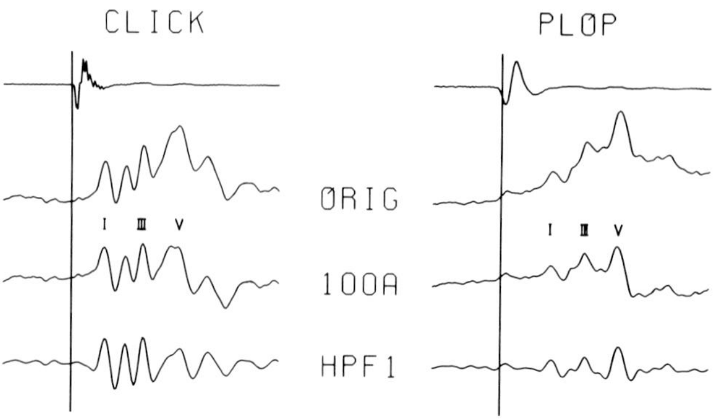

FIG. 1. Filter influences on normal BAEP (subj. HK, A-phase, 70 dB HL). *Trace 1,* acoustic stimulus waveform; *trace 2,* unfiltered BAEP (ORIG); *trace 3,* 100-Hz analog high-pass filter (100A); *trace 4,* digital high-pass filter (HPF1) used for ADA. Scale: sweep length, 16 msec (4 pre-, 12 poststimulus time); vertical distance between BAEP base lines, 500 nV.

were delivered with alternating phase at an interstimulus interval randomized between 70 and 90 msec.

Brain activity was recorded simultaneously in two channels (vertex to both earlobes) with a bandwidth of 1 Hz to 3 kHz and digitized at a rate of 10 kHz/channel. Signals were averaged into two different buffers according to stimulus phase in order to record BAEPs to rarefaction (R) and condensation (C) clicks simultaneously. Two averages (up to four in patients) of 1,000 sweeps/phase were gathered at four different stimulus levels (60, 65, 70, 75 dB HL) for both clicks (CL) and plops (PL). The alternating (A)-phase BAEP was summed up off line from the R- and C-BAEP.

Before being plotted, signals were filtered with a 100-Hz high-pass filter (6 dB/octave recursive digital filter) simulating the most widely used analog high-pass filter for comparison purposes (cf. Fig. 1). Peak latencies in the range of 1 to 10 msec were automatically determined from maxima and corrected if necessary for manual data analysis (MDA). Amplitudes were measured from the plots as peak-to-following-trough distance.

For automatic data analysis (ADA), a symmetrical digital filter was adapted with a peak frequency response at 1 kHz (HPF1 in Fig. 1) corresponding to a smoothed second derivative (17 filter coefficients: $C1 = -0.0208$, $C2 = C6 = -0.0417$, $C3 = C5 = -0.1042$, $C4 = -0.125$, $C7 = 0.1042$, $C8 = 0.2083$, $C9 = 0.25 =$ center, $C10 = C8$, etc.). The HPF1 filter had the advantage of both reducing HF noise and enhancing detection of components superimposed on others, e.g., wave V in a fused IV-V complex. Latencies and amplitudes were calculated automatically from the maxima of the filtered curves.

RESULTS

Normal subjects showed substantial variability in amplitudes and waveform of the BAEP (Fig. 2). In Table 1, normal mean values and standard deviations

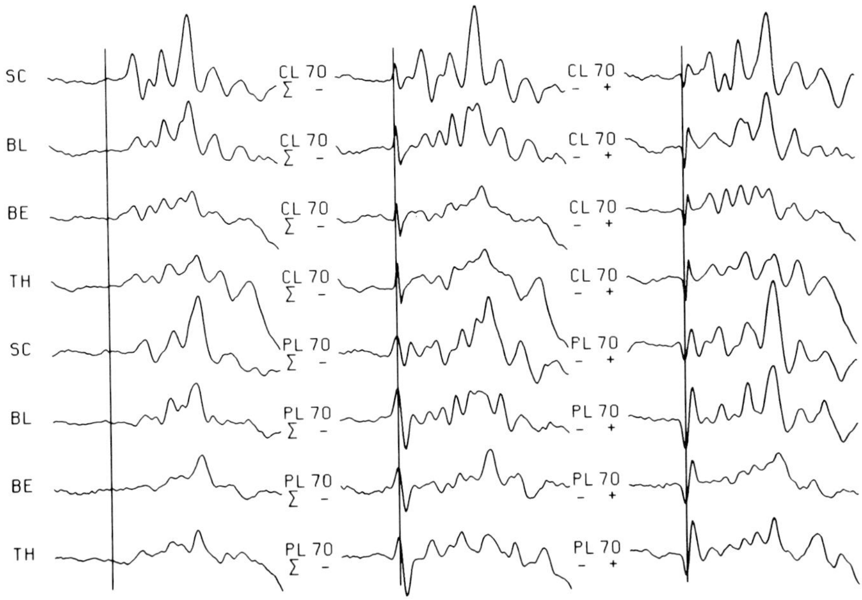

FIG. 2. Variability of BAEPs in four normal subjects (only one side shown) at 70 dB HL. Alternating (Σ, **left**), rarefaction (−, **middle**), and condensation (+, **right**) BAEPs differ considerably for both clicks (CL) and plops (PL). Scale as in Fig. 1.

(SD) of latencies (LAT) I, III, and V, interpeak latencies (IPL) I-V, I-III, III-V, and amplitude V (A5) for 70-dB HL clicks and plops are given. To underline amplitude variance, the SDs of A5 were calculated in percent.

Amplitude variation of wave V was considerable (>30%), especially in ADA because of the variations in the IV-V complex waveform. The amplitude of wave I was found to depend strongly on stimulus level in the range of 60 to 75 dB HL, whereas A5 remained fairly independent of stimulus level (Fig. 3). Interpeak latencies at 60, 65, and 75 dB HL differed no more than 0.04 msec from the 70-dB values.

A comparison of R- and C-BAEPs revealed a longer I-V IPL and a smaller A5 for rarefaction clicks. Furthermore, significant ($p < 0.05$) IPL differences for normal male and female subjects were found (male IPLs 0.12 msec greater, cf. Table 2). The lack of sufficiently stable interindividual amplitude criteria brought us to analyze intraindividually rarefaction–condensation latency differences (RCLD), interaural IPL differences (IALD), and ratios of amplitudes (IARA). These were the most sensitive parameters apart from the IPLs. In Table 2, confidence limits are given for all parameters used in clinical diagnosis.

In most cases of high-frequency hearing loss, latencies I to IV were dependent on stimulus phase, and IPL determination was handicapped by reduced wave I amplitude. The three subjects shown in Fig. 4 had prolonged I-III IPLs in some but not all stimulus conditions. In all three cases, rarefaction–condensation difference parameters were abnormal in the 85-dB CL and 80-dB PL BAEPs.

TABLE 1. *Normal values of latencies (LAT), interpeak latencies (IPL), and amplitude V (A5)*[a]

		Click stimulus			Plop stimulus		
Variable	Method	Alternating	Rarefaction	Condensation	Alternating	Rarefaction	Condensation
LAT1	ADA	1.87 ± 0.14	1.83 ± 0.15	1.92 ± 0.14	2.34 ± 0.27	2.43 ± 0.27	2.25 ± 0.34
	MDA	1.85 ± 0.15	1.82 ± 0.16	1.89 ± 0.16	2.30 ± 0.23	2.44 ± 0.26	2.27 ± 0.26
LAT3	ADA	3.99 ± 0.17	3.95 ± 0.17	4.03 ± 0.18	4.31 ± 0.35	4.41 ± 0.31	4.28 ± 0.34
	MDA	4.01 ± 0.19	3.97 ± 0.17	4.06 ± 0.21	4.39 ± 0.25	4.45 ± 0.31	4.27 ± 0.34
LAT5	ADA	5.93 ± 0.22	5.94 ± 0.23	5.93 ± 0.23	6.20 ± 0.30	6.34 ± 0.26	6.12 ± 0.30
	MDA	5.86 ± 0.22	5.87 ± 0.23	5.89 ± 0.24	6.13 ± 0.30	6.26 ± 0.27	6.06 ± 0.29
IPL15	ADA	4.06 ± 0.19	4.10 ± 0.21	4.02 ± 0.20	3.87 ± 0.18	3.92 ± 0.17	3.87 ± 0.25
	MDA	4.00 ± 0.20	4.05 ± 0.21	4.00 ± 0.22	3.83 ± 0.20	3.81 ± 0.17	3.80 ± 0.24
IPL13	ADA	2.12 ± 0.13	2.11 ± 0.12	2.11 ± 0.14	1.98 ± 0.22	1.98 ± 0.21	2.03 ± 0.24
	MDA	2.16 ± 0.15	2.14 ± 0.16	2.17 ± 0.17	2.08 ± 0.19	2.01 ± 0.15	2.00 ± 0.25
IPL35	ADA	1.94 ± 0.10	1.99 ± 0.15	1.91 ± 0.11	1.89 ± 0.15	1.94 ± 0.19	1.84 ± 0.18
	MDA	1.84 ± 0.13	1.91 ± 0.14	1.83 ± 0.17	1.73 ± 0.14	1.81 ± 0.17	1.79 ± 0.15
A5	ADA	260 ± 41%	239 ± 52%	305 ± 36%	217 ± 38%	226 ± 43%	299 ± 49%
	MDA	309 ± 31%	285 ± 36%	352 ± 29%	320 ± 36%	328 ± 44%	386 ± 37%

[a] $N = 24$ ears. All latency values in msec; amplitudes in nV.

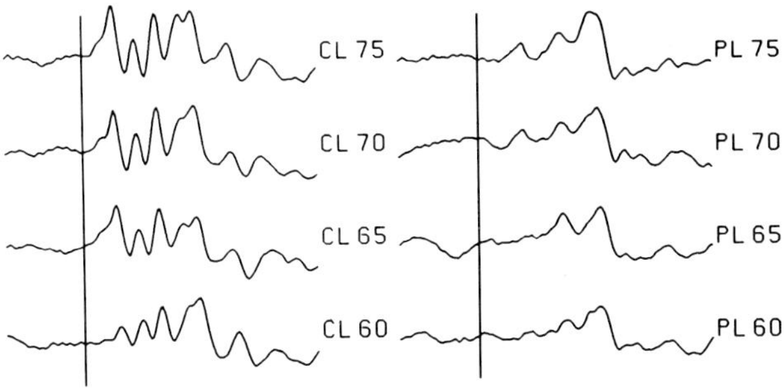

FIG. 3. Influence of stimulus level on BAEP amplitudes (subj. WA) A5 and A1 in the neurologically used intensity range of 60 to 75 dB HL. Scale as in Fig. 1.

In Fig. 5, three examples are given for the importance of the intraindividual BAEP-parameters in neurologic cases. Patient L.H. had prolonged IPLs not consistent in all stimulus conditions but showed severe differences between rarefaction and condensation BAEPs. Patient T.R., having had normal IPLs after the first attack of multiple sclerosis, showed abnormal IPL III-V (IPL35; both ears) and interaural asymmetry of wave V after the second attack. Patient D.I. exhibited an abnormal IV-V complex in the A- and R-BAEPs, whereas the C-BAEP appeared normal (right ear). In all three cases, rarefaction–condensation and interaural differences were the most significant parameters.

DISCUSSION

Because of their small variability and independence of stimulus level, IPLs turned out to be the most reliable BAEP parameters. Normal means and SDs agreed well with the values reported by most laboratories (3,7). Manual (MDA) and automatic (ADA) data analysis yielded similar results apart from slightly smaller latency variability in ADA. The IPL15 and IPL35 values were a bit longer in ADA because of the enhancement of the downslope following wave V by the ADA digital filter.

Two main effects on IPLs must not be neglected in standardizations of BAEP for neurological applications, i.e., the IPL sex differences and differences caused by stimulus phase. The cases presented here show that BAEP abnormalities may be overlooked if only single-phase BAEPs are recorded. Especially in patients with HFHL, both phases and their sum (A-BAEP) should be analyzed in order to have a reliable wave I reference for the calculation of IPLs. When stimulus levels over 70-dB HL are used, wave I detection may be obscured by the electrical stimulus artifact present in most commercially available EP equipment. Therefore, we also recommend stimulation at different levels and the use of a lower-frequency click (PL), which helped to determine wave I in two of three HFHL cases shown here.

The RC parameters were found to be abnormal both in HFHL and neurologi-

TABLE 2. *Confidence limits of BAEP parameters*

Variable[a]	Unit	Click stimulus				Plop stimulus				Comment
		Male		Female		Male		Female		
		95%	99%	95%	99%	95%	99%	95%	99%	
IPL15	msec	4.45	4.58	4.31	4.44	4.28	4.42	4.13	4.27	Add 0.04 for R-BAEP, −0.04 for C-BAEP
IPL13	msec	2.51	2.60	2.40	2.49	2.53	2.66	2.43	2.56	All phases
IPL35	msec	2.16	2.25	2.12	2.21	2.21	2.33	2.17	2.29	Add 0.04 for R-BAEP, −0.04 for C-BAEP
		Both sexes				Both sexes				
RCLD15	msec	−0.23 : 0.37	−0.32 : 0.46			−0.56 : 0.64	−0.82 : 0.74			R-IPL − C-IPL, holds also for RCLD13
RCRA5	—	0.46 : 1.68	0.37 : 2.07			0.43 : 1.79	0.33 : 2.27			R-amplitude/C-amplitude
IALD15	msec	0.28	0.36			0.36	0.47			Absolute value
IALD13	msec	0.25	0.33			0.46	0.60			Absolute value
IALD35	msec	0.28	0.36			0.46	0.60			Absolute value
IARA5	—	1.73	2.04			1.89	2.32			A(larger side)/A(opposite side)
IARA3	—	1.80	2.18			2.24	2.93			A(larger side)/A(opposite side)
RA51	—	0.67	0.49			—	—			Low limit

[a] Abbreviations: IPL, interpeak latency; RA, ratio of amplitude; IA, interaural; RC, rarefaction–condensation; LD, latency difference.

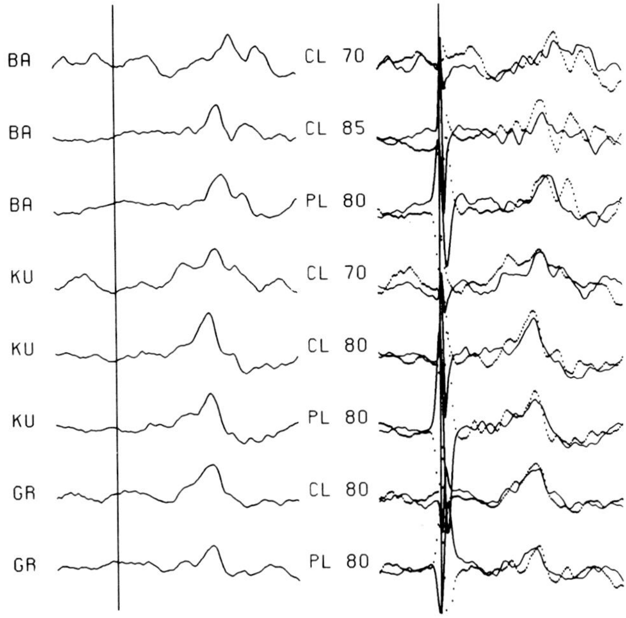

FIG. 4. Records of BAEPs of three subjects with high-frequency hearing loss. **Right side:** rarefaction *(solid lines)* and condensation *(dotted lines)* stimulation. **Left side:** alternating stimulation (sum of R- and C-BAEPs). Type of stimulus (click or plop) and level (dB HL) indicated in the middle. Scale as in Fig. 1.

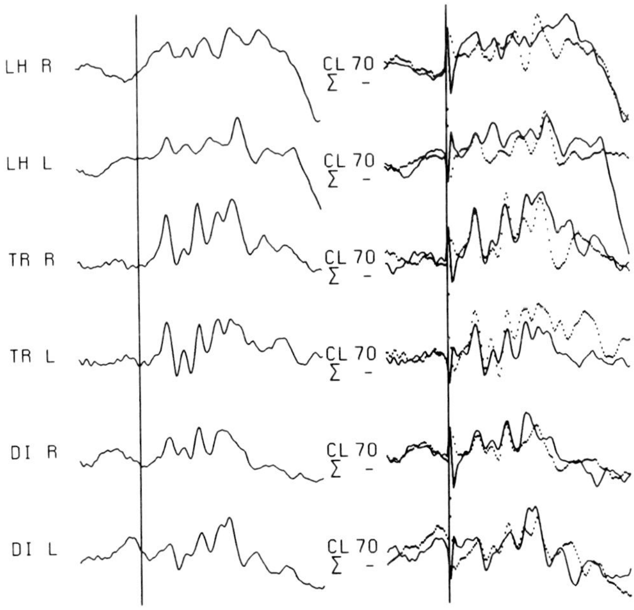

FIG. 5. Records of BAEPs of three neurologic patients. Note the differences between rarefaction (*solid lines* on the **right**) and condensation BAEPs *(dotted lines).* Alternating-phase BAEPs on the **left.** Patient code and stimulated ear (R or L) indicated on the left. Horizontal scale as in Fig. 1; vertical distance of base lines, 640 nV.

cal patients. This stresses the importance of including routine audiograms and retrocochlear tests to provide for differential diagnosis.

Finally, we suggest interaural comparison of IPLs and amplitudes instead of A5 and the ratio of A5/A1 (RA51) analysis. The RA51 may yield false negatives because of the strong dependence of A1 on stimulus level and audiological abnormalities.

The results of this study show that recording BAEPs at only one stimulus level and one phase (often undefined) can lead both to false-negative and false-positive diagnosis. In all borderline cases, stimulus phase and level should be varied, and analysis should extend beyond IPLs to rarefaction–condensation and interaural comparisons. Thus, a more reliable BAEP diagnosis can be provided for the neurologic clinic.

ACKNOWLEDGMENT

We should like to thank Mrs. C. Schmid for excellent technical assistance.

DEDICATION

This chapter is dedicated to Prof. Dr. Detlev Ploog on the occasion of his 60th anniversary.

REFERENCES

1. Coats, A. C., and Martin, J. L. (1977): Human auditory nerve action potentials and brainstem evoked responses. Effects of audiogram shape and lesion location. *Arch. Otolaryngol.,* 103:605–622.
2. McClelland, R. J., and McCrea, R. S. (1979): Intersubject variability of the auditory-evoked brain stem potentials. *Audiology,* 18:462–471.
3. Rowe, M. J. III (1978): Normal variability of the brain-stem auditory evoked response in young and old adult subjects. *Electroencephalogr. Clin. Neurophysiol.,* 44:459–470.
4. Selters, W. A., and Brackmann, D. E. (1977): Acoustic tumor detection with brain stem electric responses audiometry. *Arch. Otolaryngol.,* 103:181–187.
5. Starr, A., and Hamilton, A. (1976): Correlation between confirmed sites of neurological lesions and abnormalities of far-field auditory brainstem responses. *Electroencephalogr. Clin. Neurophysiol.,* 41:595–608.
6. Stockard, J. J., and Rossiter, V. A. (1977): Clinical and pathological correlates of brainstem auditory response abnormalities. *Neurology (Minneap.),* 27:316–325.
7. Stockard, J. E., Stockard, J. J., Westmoreland, B. F., and Corfits, J. L. (1979): Brainstem auditory-evoked responses. Normal variation as a function of stimulus and subject characteristics. *Arch. Neurol.,* 36:823–831.

Clinical Applications of Evoked Potentials in Neurology,
edited by J. Courjon, F. Mauguiere, and M. Revol.
Raven Press, New York © 1982.

Brainstem Auditory Evoked Potentials in Disorders of the Primary Sensory Ganglion

*Saty Satya-Murti and **Anthony T. Cacace

**Department of Neurology and **Division of Otolaryngology, Albany Medical College, Albany, New York 12208*

Dorsal root ganglion and primary sensory ganglion (PSG) are synonymous. The PSG is a major site of neuronal loss and degeneration in many disorders classified under the category of spinocerebellar degenerations (2). Clinical features of proprioceptive deficit and sensory nerve action potential abnormalities are explicable on this basis. In this group of disorders are included specific entities such as Friedreich's ataxia and Charcot–Marie–Tooth disease.

The spiral ganglion of the eighth nerve is also a primary sensory ganglion, although resident in a cranial nerve. We anticipated neuronal degeneration would occur in the spiral ganglion as well, since it is a cranial homolog of the PSG. Thus, we employed electrophysiological and behavioral methods to look for any auditory dysfunction that might result from such a proposed neuronal degeneration.

MATERIALS

Among the subjects examined were four patients with Friedreich's ataxia (FA), three affected and one unaffected member of a large kinship with Charcot–Marie–Tooth disease (CMT), and a single member of another family with the same diagnosis. We examined three patients with late-onset ataxia and brisk tendon reflexes whose clinical picture warranted a diagnosis of olivo–ponto–cerebellar atrophy (OPCA). In one of them (a 32-year-old female), the disease had been transmitted in an autosomal dominant fashion. A 13-year-old male, a member of a large family with hereditary spastic paraplegia (HSP) was also examined. We included the last four subjects as disease control subjects since PSG degeneration is not a major feature of their disorders.

A detailed description of the clinical pictures and peripheral nerve conduction abnormalities on the CMT and FA patients has been published (5,6).

Also available to us were patients with early-onset, slowly progressive, and longstanding sensorimotor neuropathies of a sporadic nature and an unknown etiology (PN). Classification was not possible in these instances, and they were examined without any assumptions about the location of their primary lesion. They have mild functional disabilities in their daily life but do not have any hearing difficulty. In this group, there were two males (15 and 27 years) and two females (20 and 29 years).

METHODS

Brainstem auditory evoked potentials (BAEP) were elicited using click stimuli at various intensities. Behavioral audiometric tests (BAT) were also performed whenever feasible. These included pure-tone audiograms, speech reception thresholds (SRT), tympanometry, and ipsilateral and contralateral acoustic reflexes. Two central auditory function tests were chosen for reasons of familiarity and ease of administration: the Performance Intensity Functions for Phonetically Balanced Words (PI-PB) test and Synthetic Sentence Identification Test (SSI) in the ipsilateral and contralateral competing message modes (ICM and CCM). Details about the stimulus, equipment, and testing procedures have been provided by us elsewhere (5–7). Clinical neurologic examinations had been carried out on all of our patients. Except for one of the OPCA patients, peripheral nerve conductions had been performed on all. Brainstem auditory evoked potentials were obtained using condensation clicks of 60 and 70 dB SL (sensation level). The clicks had a 2.5-kHz resonant peak and a 95 to 107 dB peSPL (peak equivalent sound pressure level). A mastoid–vertex silver cup electrode derivation (resistance less than 2,000 ohms) amplified signals at a gain of 10^5. A filter setting of 150 to 3,000 Hz was used, and the evoked potentials in response to 2,000 or more clicks were averaged twice for each intensity level. Contralateral masking noise was employed.

RESULTS

Table 1 and the illustrations provide a summary of the abnormalities found in these patients (Figs. 1–4). Normal latencies in our laboratory are (msec $\pm$ SD): waves I, III, V: 1.57 ± 0.19, 3.77 ± 0.15, 5.6 ± 0.22; interpeak latencies I–III: 2.1 ± 0.13, 1.85 ± 0.14, 4.02 ± 0.21.

DISCUSSION

As can be gathered from Table 1, patients with FA and CMT had BAEP abnormalities. Late onset ataxia patients (OPCA) and the boy with HSP had normal BAEPs. An unaffected member from the CMT family also had a normal BAEP. The degree of BAEP and BAT abnormalities correlated with peripheral nerve sensory conduction changes: those with absent sensory nerve action potentials had greater central alterations, and those with mere reduction in sensory nerve action potential amplitude had still recognizable BAEP wave forms. Fur-

TABLE 1. *Clinical data and test results*

Patient No.	Diagnosis	SNAP[a]	BAEP	BAT
1. (16-yr-old M)	CMT	↓ (5 μV)	I–III prolongation	Normal
2. (11-yr-old M)	CMT	↓ (5 μV)	I–III prolongation	Normal
3. (9-yr-old M) (cousin of above)	CMT	Absent	I–III prolongation	Normal
4. (17-yr-old M) (brother of Nos. 1, 2)	N[b]	N (22 μV)	N	N.P.[b]
5. (28-yr-old M)	FA	Absent	Unrecognizable waveforms	Mild h.f.[c] and l.f.[c] sensitivity loss and VIII N. dysfunction
6. (31-yr-old F)	FA	Absent	Unrecognizable waveforms	Mild h.f. sensitivity loss and VIII N. dysfunction
7. (28-yr-old F)	FA	Absent	Unrecognizable waveforms	Mild sensitivity loss at all f.
8. (25-yr-old M)	FA	Absent	Unrecognizable waveforms	Moderate h.f. sensitivity loss
9. (27-yr-old M)	OPCA	N.P.	N	N.P.
10. (56-yr-old M)	OPCA	N	N	N.P.
11. (34-yr-old F)	OPCA	N	N	N.P.
12. (15-yr-old M)	PN	↓ (3 μV)	I–V prolongation. Poor delineation of other waves	Mild h.f. sensitivity loss on left
13. (27-yr-old M)	PN	↓ (3 μV) (Sural N.)	I–V prolongation. Poor delineation of other waves	N
14. (29-yr-old F)	PN	Absent	N	N.P.
15. (20-yr-old F)	PN	Absent (Sural N.)	N	N.P.
16. (13-yr-old M)	HSP	N	N	N.P.
17. (51-yr-old M)	CMT	Absent	I–III prolongation	Moderate h.f. sensitivity loss

[a] SNAP: Sensory nerve action potential of median nerve (unless otherwise stated) recorded orthodromically at the wrist. Details of the abnormalities found on patients 1, 2, 6–10 are in references 5 and 6.

[b] N.P., not performed; N, normal.

[c] h.f., high frequency (4–8 kHz); l.f., low frequency (0.25–0.5 kHz).

↓, Reduced amplitude.

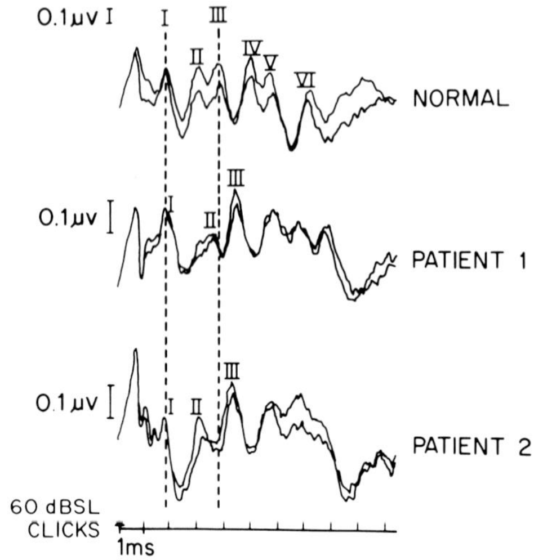

FIG. 1. I-III intervals are prolonged in the first two patients with CMT (2.64 msec and 2.57 msec) as compared with normal (2.1 ± 0.13 msec). Vertex positivity produces an upward deflection. (From Satya-Murti et al., ref. 5, with permission.)

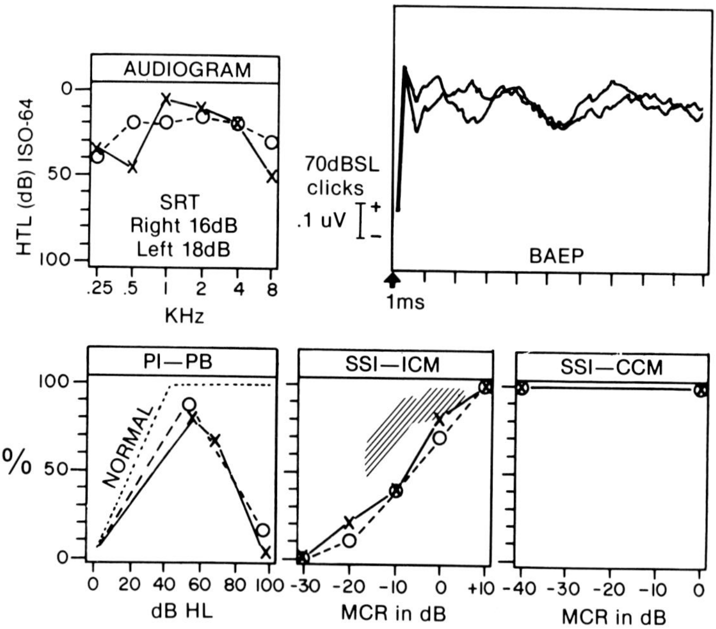

FIG. 2. Results from patient no. 4. Audiogram shows sensitivity loss at low- and high-frequency ranges. BAEP: 70 dB SL clicks presented to the left ear elicited no recognizable peaks. PI-PB: *y-axis,* correct PB word identification score in percent; *x-axis,* presentation level of PB words; *dotted lines,* normal person's score; discrimination ability is sustained as intensity in-

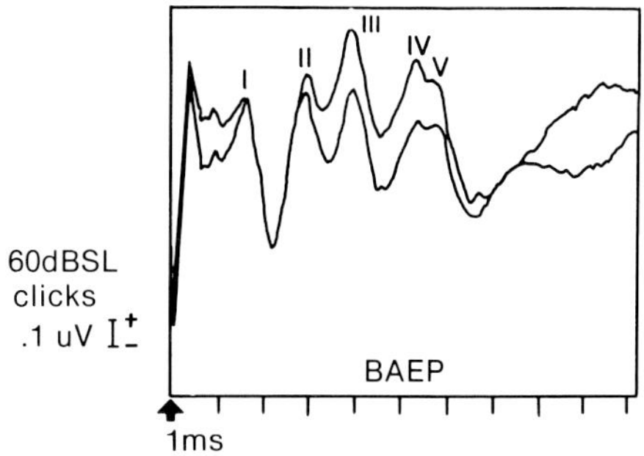

FIG. 3. Normal BAEPs are elicited from patient no. 9 who had ataxia of later onset. Clicks were applied to the right ear. Roman numerals indicate individual waves. (From Satya-Murti et al., ref. 6, with permission.)

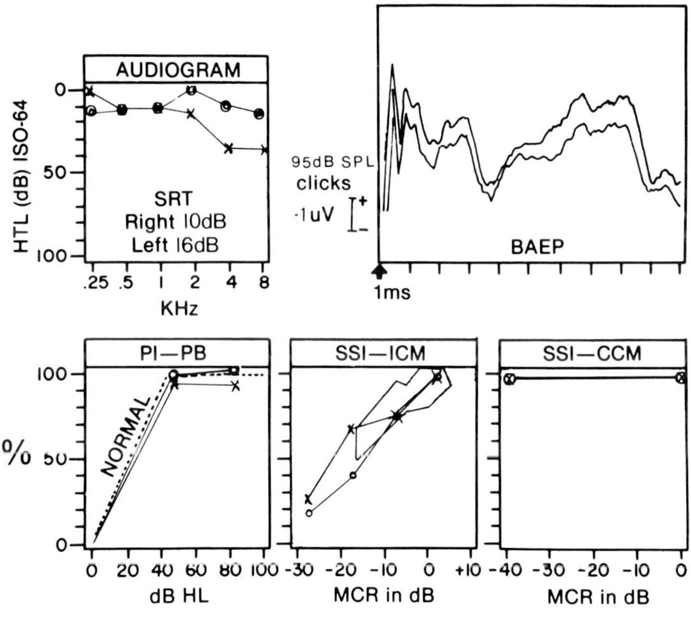

FIG. 4. Results from patient #12 who had sporadic neuropathy. The BAEP waves are poorly developed, although waves I and V are probably recognizable. Data shown for right ear stimulus. No abnormalities are evident in the BAT.

---

creases. Our patient's discrimination drops abruptly (roll-over) as intensity increases. SSI-ICM: lists of 10 synthetic sentences (message) are presented in random order to one ear. Their identification is made difficult by a story read simultaneously (competing message) to the same ear; *y-axis,* identification score in percent; *x-axis,* message-to-competition ratio (MCR); *hatched* or *boxed area,* normal performance. Note our patient's performance deficit. SSI-CCM: competing message is presented to the opposite ear; our patient's performance is normal. In all figures, O, right ear; ×, left ear. (From Satya-Murti et al., ref. 6, with permission.)

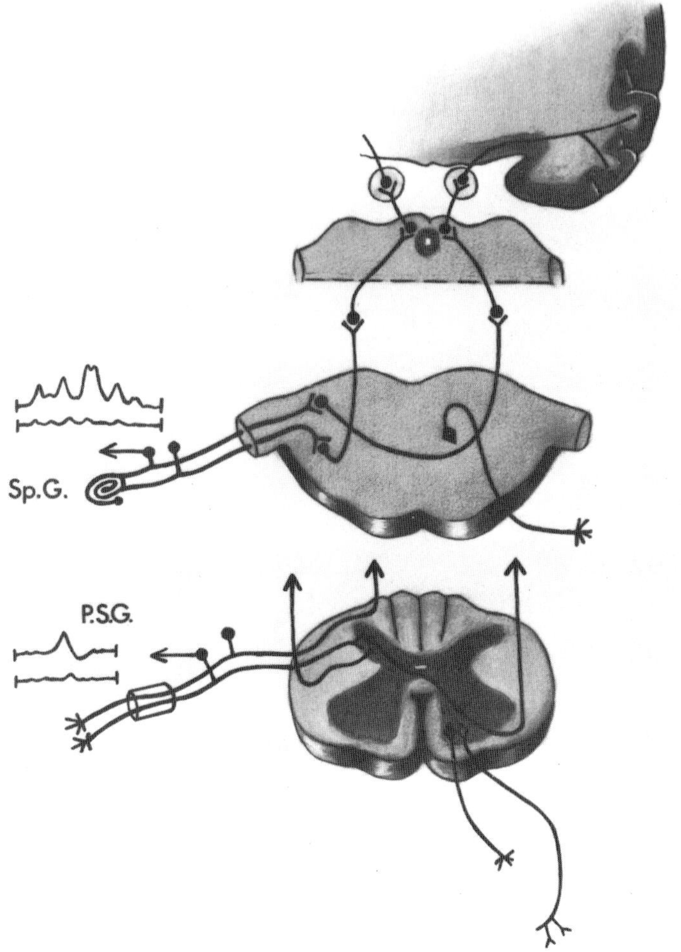

FIG. 5. Schematic diagram showing the spiral ganglion (Sp.G.) undergoing degeneration similar to that of the primary sensory ganglion (P.S.G.). Such a degeneration alters the evoked potentials much as the P.S.G. neuronal loss obliterates or diminishes the amplitude of peripheral nerve sensory evoked potentials.

ther, some degree of hearing loss, acoustic reflex abnormalities, and the roll-over phenomenon in the PI-PB test were seen only in FA patients.

Neuronal degeneration in the spiral ganglia, occurring parallel to that of primary sensory ganglion neuronal loss, could explain these abnormalities (Fig. 5). Cell loss, consequent central transneuronal degeneration (3), and asynchrony in impulse conduction can account for the distorted wave forms and prolongation of interpeak intervals. There are instances of overt deafness in these disorders (10), and even some histopathological support for spiral ganglion degeneration has been found in the literature (8).

We do not know why only two of the four PN cases reveal BAEP abnormalities. Sporadic chronic peripheral neuropathies, although bearing some resemblance to each other in their clinical manifestations, may be of diverse etiologies. Thus, asymptomatic auditory system involvement may be an inconstant feature.

None of our patients had hearing difficulties in spite of the abnormalities detected by our tests. They functioned normally in daily life, and auditory dysfunction was detected only incidentally to our study. Thus, the mechanisms responsible for production of BAEP appear to be independent of those subserving functional hearing. The two cochlear receptors, outer and inner hair cells, and their afferent systems may mediate predominantly different functions, thus accounting for the above independence (1,4,9). Studies of this nature on patients with primary sensory ganglion degeneration offer the potential for understanding some mechanisms underlying human hearing.

ACKNOWLEDGMENT

The authors are indebted to the support given by Dr. Kevin D. Barron, Dr. Jerome C. Goldstein, the Muscular Dystrophy Association, and the Robert W. Graves Memorial Fund. Sarah Crane provided secretarial assistance.

REFERENCES

1. Carlier, E., and Pujol, R. (1978): Role of inner and outer hair cells in coding sound intensity: An ontogenetic approach. *Brain Res.*, 147:174–176.
2. Dyck, P. J., and Ohta, M. (1975): Neuronal atrophy and degeneration predominantly affecting peripheral sensory neurons. In: *Peripheral Neuropathy,* edited by P. J. Dyck, P. K. Thomas, and E. H. Lambert, pp. 791–824. W. B. Saunders, Philadelphia.
3. Jean-Baptiste, M., and Morest, D. K. (1975): Transneuronal changes of synaptic endings and nuclear chromatin in the trapezoid body following cochlear ablations in cats. *J. Comp. Neurol.*, 162:111–134.
4. Kimura, R. S., Ota, C. Y., and Takahashi, T. (1979): Nerve fiber synapses on spiral ganglion cells in the human cochlea. *Ann. Otorhinolaryngol.*, 88 (Suppl. 62):1–17.
5. Satya-Murti, S., Cacace, A. T., and Hanson, P. A. (1979): Abnormal auditory evoked potentials in hereditary motor–sensory neuropathy. *Ann. Neurol.*, 5:445–448.
6. Satya-Murti, S., Cacace, A. T., and Hanson, P. A. (1980): Auditory dysfunction in Friedreich's ataxia: Result of spiral ganglion degeneration. *Neurology (Minneap.),* 30:1047–1053.
7. Satya-Murti, S., Cacace, A. T., and Swartz, S. (1979): A low-cost noise generator for masking click stimuli. *Ann. Biomed. Eng.*, 7:471–474.
8. Spoendlin, H. (1974): Optic and cochleovestibular degenerations in hereditary ataxias. II. Temporal bone pathology in two cases of Friedreich's ataxia with vestibulo–cochlear disorders. *Brain,* 97:41–48.
9. Spoendlin, H. (1978): The afferent innervation of the cochlea. In: *Evoked Electrical Activity in the Auditory Nervous System,* edited by R. F. Naunton and C. Fernandez, pp. 21–41. Academic Press, New York.
10. Tyrer, J. H. (1975): Friedreich's ataxia. In: *Handbook of Clinical Neurology, Vol. 21,* edited by P. J. Vinken and G. W. Bruyn, pp. 319–364. American Elsevier, New York.

Clinical Applications of Evoked Potentials in Neurology,
edited by J. Courjon, F. Mauguiere, and M. Revol.
Raven Press, New York © 1982.

Quantitative Survey of Uremic Brain Dysfunction by Auditory Evoked Potentials

O. Knoll, U. Harbort, K. Schulte, and F. Zimpel

Medizinische Poliklinik, University of Münster,
D-4400 Münster, Federal Republic of Germany

Uremia is a clinical syndrome occurring regularly in terminal renal failure and is regarded as a consequence of metabolic intoxication. Uremic toxins are unknown, however. Elevated urea and creatinine serum levels are unable to explain uremia. Uremic symptomatology includes anemia, bone disease, hypertension, cardiac dysfunction, gastroenteritis, pericardial and pleural effusions, fluid lung, coagulation disorders, skin changes, as well as peripheral polyneuropathy and encephalopathy. Uremic symptoms can be reversed by regular dialysis treatment (RDT), but individual dialysis requirements of different patients have proven to be very different. An essential aim of RDT is an individual adjustment of the dialysis regimen in order to guarantee sufficient treatment and to avoid unnecessarily long treatment. Since uremic toxins are unknown, laboratory measures are unsuitable for control of treatment. The observation that insufficient RDT causes persistent uremic symptoms confirms the assumption that the patient's well-being and freedom from uremic signs are until now the most reliable parameters of sufficient RDT.

Uremic encephalopathy is the most serious complication of uremia and therefore serves as an indicator of inadequate dialysis therapy. Typical complaints and signs of uremic encephalopathy—nausea, vomiting, headache, drowsiness, coma, convulsions—are either ambiguous or are very late symptoms. The actual extent of uremic brain dysfunction cannot be defined exactly by the complaints or by the neurological status. On the other hand, dialysis itself can induce an encephalopathy by rapid changes of plasma osmolarity, the so-called disequilibrium syndrome, whose symptoms are often confusingly like those of uremic encephalopathy. Therefore, too, early detection and follow-up control of brain dysfunction would be desirable for control of dialysis therapy. For the reasons given above, patients' complaints and neurological status are insufficient for such purposes.

In the search for more sensitive and more valid indicators of uremic brain dysfunction, the suitability of the EEG and of psychological tests was examined. But both tests are influenced to a considerable extent by drugs and by changes of vigilance, so that validity for follow-up studies is reduced. Quantitative neurophysiological data are required for these purposes. The suitability of EP latencies for detection of uremic encephalopathy was examined in several studies. Both VEP and SEP latencies were found prolonged in renal patients (4,5,7). Latencies of late EP components analyzed in these studies are influenced essentially by drugs, habituation phenomena, and by changes of vigilance, however, so that reproducibility is not yet sufficient (1). Latencies of early AEP components were found relatively constant and are not influenced by changes of vigilance, drugs, or habituation (3,6,8). Therefore, suitability of early AEP components for detection and follow-up control of uremic brain dysfunction was investigated in patients on RDT.

METHODS

The normal range of AEP latencies was examined in 32 healthy volunteers. Clinical investigations were done in 43 patients (19 males, 24 females) on RDT. Mean age of patients and of controls did not differ significantly.

Patients were placed in a relaxed position with eyes closed. The EEG was recorded with Ag–AgCl surface electrodes from vertex and mastoid. Artifacts were avoided by using isolation preamplifiers placed near the head of the patient. Amplifier, averager, scopes for EEG and AEP display, plotter, and stimulator were mounted in a rack and could be moved to bedside in the renal unit. The system frequency bandpass ranged from 2 to 5,000 Hz. The average of 1,024 EEG responses was calculated by a 20-bit minicomputer (NIC-527; 2,048 addresses, 40 μsec bin width, 82 msec analysis time). At least two averaged potentials, each representing 1,024 EEG responses, were plotted and compared in order to recognize the entire shape of the AEP as well as habituation phenomena. Auditory click stimuli of 0.1 msec duration were applied by earphones to both ears at 60 dB above hearing threshold at a stimulation frequency of 10/sec and, in several patients, in a random series as well.

RESULTS

Early AEP components regularly observed are shown in Fig. 1. According to their mean latencies, positive components were labeled P_2, P_7, P_{25}, P_{45}, negative components N_{15} and N_{30}. Latencies were measured from stimulus to peak. Amplitudes have not been evaluated. Latencies obtained in healthy subjects are given in Table 1. Latencies obtained at 10/sec stimulation frequency and with randomized interstimulus intervals did not differ significantly. Latencies of early AEP components were found to be exactly reproducible at different days and were obviously not influenced by drugs, changes of vigilance, or habituation phenomena (Fig 2).

The AEP latencies were found to be prolonged in most patients on RDT but were also prolonged in any patient suffering from typical uremic complaints or signs (nausea, vomiting, asterixis, drowsiness) (Fig. 3). Within the state of

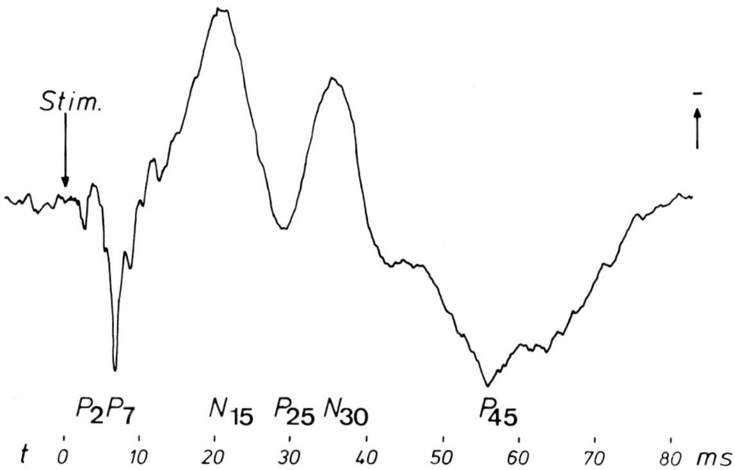

FIG. 1. Early AEP components: 2,048 responses averaged. *t,* time.

TABLE 1. *Normal range of early AEP components (mean of 32 healthy subjects)*

AEP component	Latency Mean	Latency SD
P_2	2.51	0.29
P_7	6.55	1.31
N_{15}	13.22	1.68
P_{25}	22.23	3.86
N_{30}	31.83	5.04
P_{45}	44.19	5.62

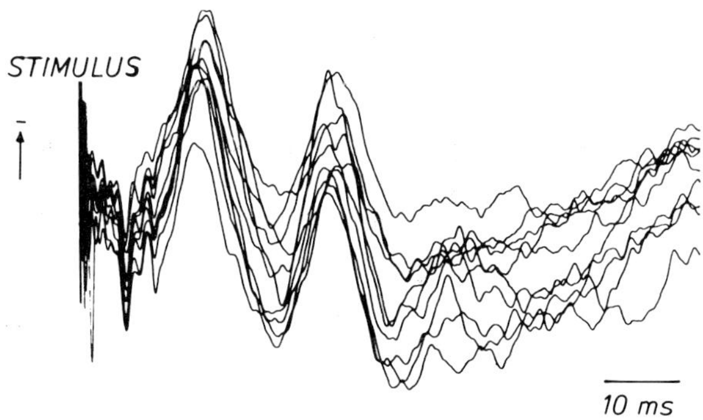

FIG. 2. Reproducibility of AEP latencies: AEP (each representing average of 1,024 responses) of the same subject on 10 different days.

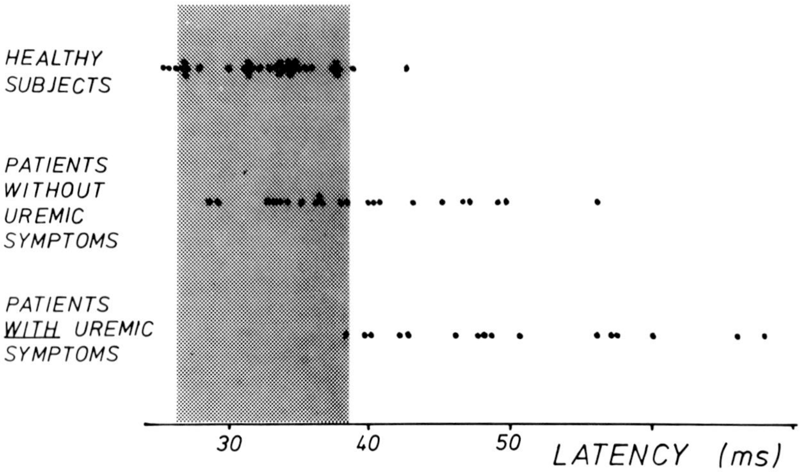

FIG. 3. Latencies of AEP component N_{30} in healthy subjects and in patients on regular hemodialysis treatment. *Hatched zone,* normal range. Uremic symptoms: nausea, vomiting, asterixis, drowsiness.

RDT initiation, the first hemodialysis caused, in some patients, an actual increase of AEP latencies, possibly because of disequilibrium, but then AEP latencies improved within a few weeks (Fig. 4).

DISCUSSION

For detection and follow-up control of uremic brain dysfunction, several neurophysiological techniques have been examined (2,4,5,7). Spectral analysis of

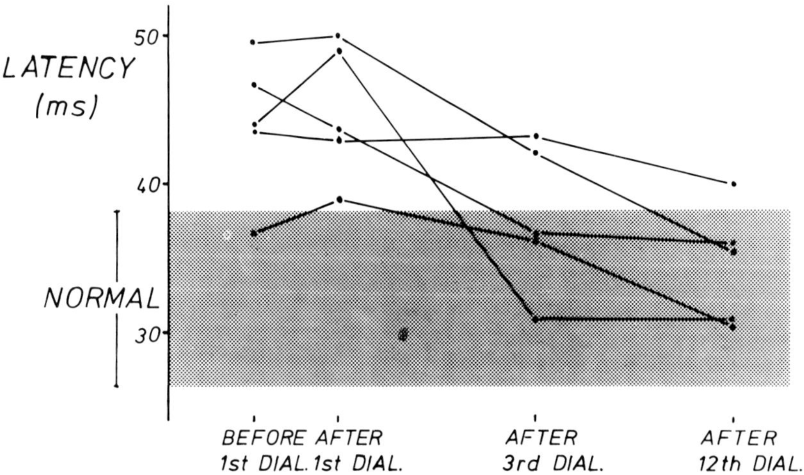

FIG. 4. Latencies of AEP component N_{30} during initiation of regular dialysis treatment.

the EEG revealed a wide range of results in healthy subjects because of interindividual variability, influences of drugs, and changes of vigilance. Latencies of late VEP and SEP components are also influenced essentially by changes of vigilance, drugs, and by habituation phenomena (1,3). Reproducibility of these measures and their suitability for monitoring purposes are therefore reduced.

An essential aim of these investigations was the examination of a more practicable neurophysiological method. Only bedside tests that can be performed by the clinical staff are suited for routine controls in severely ill patients. An AEP can be registered at bedside in the renal unit with the aid of a minicomputer. Isolation preamplifiers make EEG recordings possible even during hemodialysis treatment. Recording, on-line averaging, and plotting of AEP require about 15 min. Stimulus-to-peak latency of the distinct AEP components represents a well-defined measure of brain dysfunction. In contrast to more complicated techniques (VEP, CNV), the test is well suited for routine purposes. Patients are not traumatized by the test so that repeated controls can be done.

The sensitivity of AEP latencies in detection of uremic brain dysfunction was examined in patients on RDT suffering from no uremic complaints or signs. In most of these patients, prolonged latencies of early AEP components were found, demonstrating slight, subclinical brain dysfunction. Various VEP and SEP studies in nonrenal patients revealed that latencies of late EP components are often delayed in earlier stages of diseases because of their polysynaptic neuronal pathway. But this theoretical advantage of late EP components is compensated for by the fact that latencies of late EP components are more influenced by changes of vigilance, drugs, and habituation phenomena, so that reproducibility is often poor. Suitability for monitoring purposes is reduced, since the level of vigilance cannot be kept constant under clinical conditions.

The validity of AEP latencies was examined in patients on RDT. Auditory evoked potentials of the same subjects recorded on different days proved to be rather homogenous, although differences of drug treatment and of vigilance level must be assumed. Reproducibility of AEP latencies was obviously not reduced by bedside recording. In any patient on RDT suffering from typical uremic complaints, prolonged AEP latencies were found, demonstrating the validity of the test. Moreover, several studies revealed strong correlations between AEP latencies and changes of clinical conditions, e.g., during initiation of RDT.

First results confirm the assumption that prolonged AEP latencies are not specific patterns of uremic brain dysfunction. The CNS is reacting in a uniform way to various endogenous or exogenous influences. Permeability changes of the blood brain barrier, inhibition of cerebral enzymes, disorders of brain energy metabolism, and interference with neurotransmitters are regarded as essential pathogenetic factors of uremic encephalopathy as of other metabolic encephalopathies. Especially in renal patients, not only uremic intoxication but also severe hypertension, acidosis, dehydratation, electrolyte disturbances, and drug accumulation are able to induce encephalopathies with similar symptoms and signs. In patients suffering from severe hypertension with normal renal function, similar delays of AEP latencies were found as in patients on RDT. Auditory evoked potential latencies as well as other neurophysiological measures revealed no specific uremic patterns. But in clinical practice, early detection and sensitive monitoring of brain dysfunction are in most cases more important than detection of specific etiological factors. For such purposes, measurement of AEP latencies is a valid and sensitive test well suited for routine use.

REFERENCES

1. Aunon, J. I., and Cantor, F. K. (1977): VEP and AEP variability: Interlaboratory vs. intralaboratory and intersession vs. intrasession variability. *Electroencephalogr. Clin. Neurophysiol.*, 42:705–708.
2. Bourne, J. R., Ward, J. W., Teschan, P. E., Musso, M., Johnston, H. B., and Ginn, H. E. (1975): Quantitative assessment of the electroencephalogram in renal disease. *Electroencephalogr. Clin. Neurophysiol.*, 39:377–388.
3. Desmedt, J. E. (1977): *Progress in Clinical Neurophysiology, Vol. 2, Auditory Evoked Potentials in Man.* S. Karger, Basel.
4. Hamel, B., Bourne, J. R., Ward, J. W., and Teschan, P. E. (1978): Visually evoked cortical potentials in renal failure: Transient potentials. *Electroencephalogr. Clin. Neurophysiol.*, 44:606–616.
5. Lewis, E. G., Dustman, R. E., and Beck, E. C. (1978): Visual and somatosensory evoked potential characteristics of patients undergoing hemodialysis and kidney transplantation. *Electroencephalogr. Clin. Neurophysiol.*, 44:223–231.
6. Picton, T. W., Hillyard, S. A., Krausz, H. I., and Galambos, R. (1974): Human auditory evoked potentials. I. Evaluation of components. *Electroencephalogr. Clin. Neurophysiol.*, 36:179–190.
7. Teschan, P. E., Ginn, H. E., Bourne, J. R., Ward, J. W., Hamel, B., Nunnally, J. C., Musso, M., and Vaughn, W. K. (1979): Quantitative indices of clinical uremia. *Kidney Int.*, 15:676–697.
8. Uziel, A., and Benezech, J. (1978): Auditory brain-stem responses in comatose patients: Relationship with brain-stem reflexes and levels of coma. *Electroencephalogr. Clin. Neurophysiol.*, 45:515–529.

Clinical Applications of Evoked Potentials in Neurology,
edited by J. Courjon, F. Mauguiere, and M. Revol.
Raven Press, New York © 1982.

Brainstem Auditory Evoked Potential Abnormalities in Retarded Adults

*Nancy Squires, Jennifer Buchwald, Fasha Liley, and Joseph Strecker

Brain Research Institute and Department of Physiology, UCLA Medical Center, Mental Retardation Research Center, Los Angeles, California 90025

The possible contribution of specific sensory defects to behavioral manifestations of mental retardation has been largely ignored (7). This oversight has two bases, a theoretical and a practical one. A strong, often implicit assumption is that retardation of any etiology is primarily the result of a maturational deficit of general cognitive capacity. Thus, the retarded are called "developmentally disabled" and are characterized in terms of global measures of IQ or adaptive behavior. The difficulty in making valid discriminations between specific sensory and cognitive capacities in the retarded has also contributed to the inadequacy of research in this area. In contrast, we assume that sensory deficits may be an important contributing factor, varying in pattern and degree certainly among individuals and probably among diagnostic subgroups, and that accurate individual assessment is an essential precursor to remediation.

Electrophysiological techniques now promise to solve some of the problems in evaluating brain processes in the retarded. We chose to look first at the brainstem auditory evoked potentials because of their relative neuroanatomical specificity (4,8,15) and because of a number of reports of elevated incidence of hearing loss in the retarded (9–11). Our first target group was Down's syndrome, for which there is also limited neuroanatomical evidence for abnormalities in the brainstem (3,5,6). The BAEPs of Down's syndrome adults were compared with those of a group of retarded adults of unknown etiology and to those of a group of nonretarded adults. These data have already been published (14) and will be briefly described here along with the results of a follow-up study designed to explore some implications of the original results.

EXPERIMENT 1

Subjects

Sixteen Down's syndrome adults (mean age 29 years, mean IQ 28), 15 retarded adults of unknown etiology (mean age 29, mean IQ 36), and 15 nonretarded adults (mean age 30) participated in the experiment. All subjects were male.

**Present address:* Department of Psychology, State University of New York, Stony Brook, New York 11794.

Procedure

Brainstem auditory evoked potentials were recorded from a gold disk electrode on the scalp vertex referred to the ipsilateral mastoid (bandpass 100 Hz to 3 kHz). Monaural, 0.1-msec duration clicks were presented at three stimulus intensities (40, 55, and 70 dB above normal hearing threshold) and at three repetition rates (20, 50, and 100/sec). Each BAEP was the average of 1,500 stimulus repetitions, and two replications were performed for each condition (for other procedural details see 14).

Results and Discussion

Clear BAEPs were observed in fewer retarded subjects than in the nonretarded control subjects. At the highest stimulus intensity, clicks presented to 18% of the ears in the Down's group and to 7% of the ears in the unknown-etiology group produced no recognizable BAEPs, whereas in the nonretarded, BAEPs were evoked by clicks to both ears in all subjects.

Figure 1 shows the central transmission times (wave V latency minus wave I latency) to clicks at 70 dB, 20/sec, for each ear of all subjects in whom both waves I and V could be identified. The data of the nonretarded subjects are shown in the middle, and the dotted lines indicate ± 2 SD around the normal mean. The two retarded groups present quite different pictures with respect to transmission time: although a number of individuals in the unknown-etiology group (shown on the left) exhibit prolonged central transmission times, 33% of the ears in the Down's group had transmission times more than 2 SD below the normal mean. The rest are mostly in the lower normal range.

These transmission-time abnormalities in the Down's group were not produced by a systematic reduction in all interpeak intervals but, as shown in Fig. 2, by a selective shortening of the I-II and III-IV intervals. In the unknown-etiology group, there was, by contrast, a progressive prolongation of all peaks beyond wave I.

Figure 3 compares the effect of click repetition rate on wave V latency for the three groups. Not only was wave V latency in the Down's group shorter than normal at all rates, but it showed significantly less change with increased rate of stimulation.

In summary, this experiment demonstrated a higher than normal proportion of absent BAEPs in both groups of retarded, consistent with reports of an elevated incidence of hearing loss in the retarded. Beyond this, however, the two diagnostic categories showed distinctive patterns of BAEP abnormalities. The retarded of unknown etiology tended to have prolonged central transmission times, whereas the Down's subjects had shortened latencies of waves II and IV plus a lack of sensitivity to increased rate of stimulation. Although the pattern seen in the unknown-etiology group has also been seen in diseases such as multiple sclerosis (12,13), to our knowledge the Down's syndrome pattern does not resemble that of any other neurological disorder and therefore presents

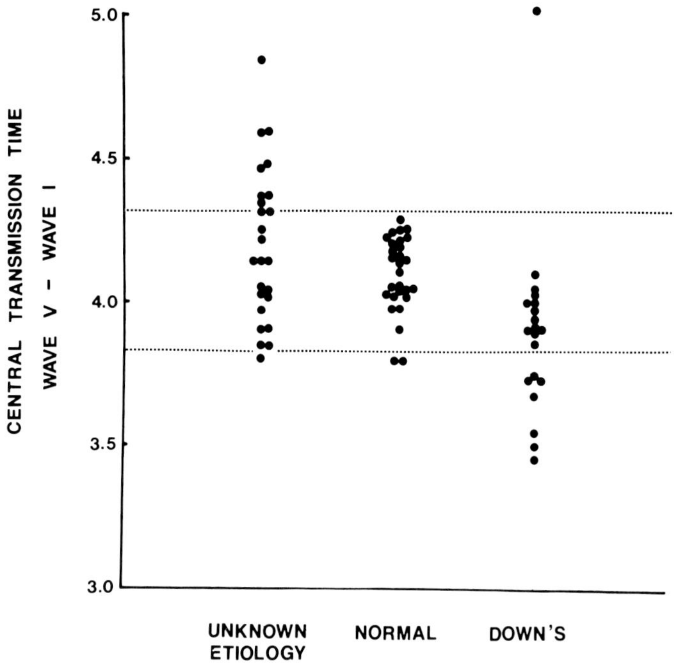

FIG. 1. Wave V minus wave I latency (central transmission time) at 70 dB, 20 clicks/sec for each experimental group. The *dotted lines* represent ±2 SD around the normal mean.

a major problem in interpretation. A second experiment was therefore designed to further examine the BAEP abnormalities in Down's syndrome.

The neuroanatomical studies on Down's syndrome retarded report two findings, a general reduction of brainstem weight (6) and an abnormally perpendicular insertion of the brainstem into the cerebrum (3,5). Because of the abnormal brainstem orientation, we considered the possibility that rather than waves II and IV being selectively shortened, we were seeing different waves in the Down's and normal subjects. Allen and Starr (1) have shown in the monkey that by varying electrode placement it is possible to observe multiple peaks in some latency regions. These extra peaks presumably reflect the activity of generators not visible to the vertex electrode when used with a mastoid reference. Therefore, in the second experiment, electrodes were placed at additional sites. We also increased the number of stimuli in each average and the number of repetition rates presented in order to determine exactly where in the sequence of BAEP peaks and at what repetition rate the Down's BAEPs diverged from normal.

EXPERIMENT 2

Subjects

The BAEPs of 20 Down's syndrome adult male subjects (mean age 25, mean IQ 23) were compared to those of 11 nonretarded male adults (mean age 21).

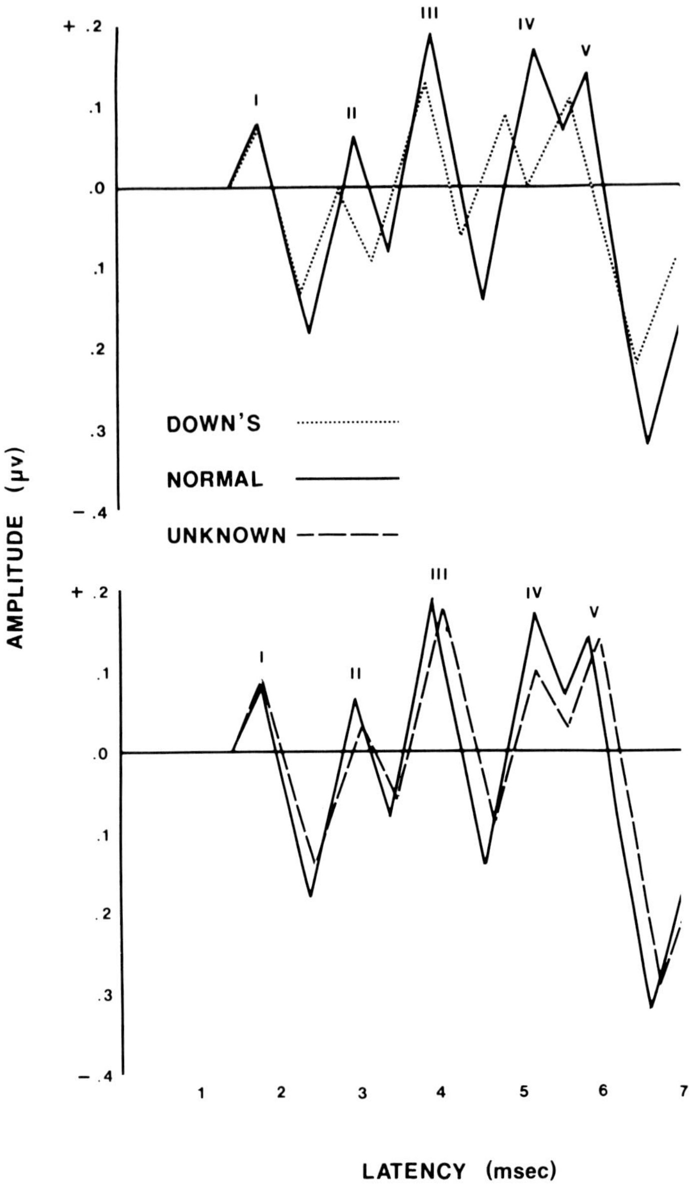

FIG. 2. Brainstem auditory evoked potentials of nonretarded *(solid lines)*, Down's syndrome *(dotted lines)*, and retarded of unknown etiology *(dashed lines)*. These schematic waveforms represent the mean amplitude and latency of each BAEP peak for 70 dB 20 clicks/sec.

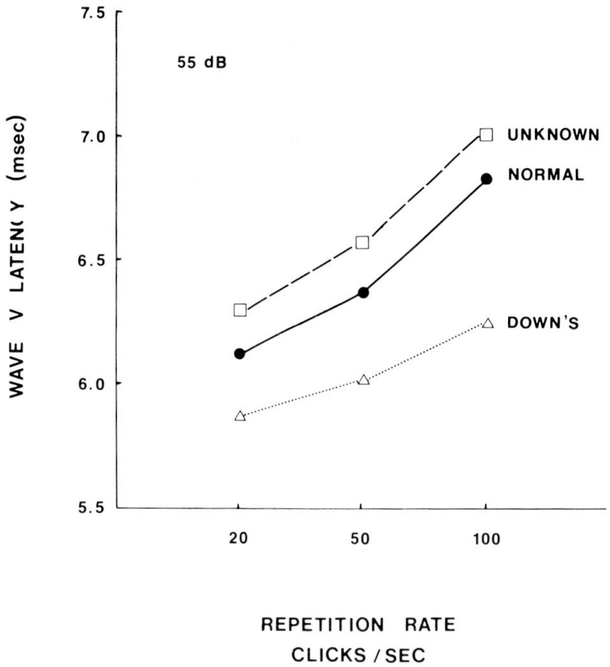

FIG. 3. Mean wave V latency as a function of click repetition rate for the three experimental groups. Only the data of subjects with wave V at all three rates are included.

The plan was to retest all of the original Down's syndrome subjects with the new protocol. In the intervening time, however, many of the higher-functioning residents had been placed in the community. We were therefore able to retest only 10 subjects from the original group, and 10 new Down's subjects were added. None of the nonretarded subjects had participated in the previous experiment.

Procedure

Clicks (65 dB HL) were presented to the right ear of each subject at rates of 10, 20, 33, 50, 75, and 100/sec. The BAEPs were recorded from C_z, right mastoid, and left mastoid, all referred to the seventh cervical vertebra (C_7).

Results and Discussion

As a result of the demographic changes in the institution, the new group of Down's syndrome subjects was of lower mean IQ than the group in the first experiment. This may account for the overall poorer quality of the BAEPs. The proportion of subjects with absent BAEPs was 40% in this experiment.

Furthermore, for three of the Down's subjects (15%), no reliable wave I was seen even at the slowest click rate, and wave V latency was greater than four standard deviations above the normal mean. In four other Down's subjects (20%), wave I was visible, but its latency was greater than four standard deviations above normal. Thus, overall, the indication of serious peripheral auditory deficit was very high (75%).[1] Yet, every one of these subjects had been described in the hospital record as having "no difficulty in hearing," based on the evaluation of the direct care staff. This probably reflects the bias towards attributing lack of auditory responsiveness in the severely and profoundly retarded to central causes.

The amount of data remaining to test the hypotheses raised by the previous study was therefore limited, particularly because the expansion of the protocol allowed for testing only in one ear of each subject. The summary waveforms of the normal subjects and the five Down's subjects without wave I prolongation are shown in the Fig. 4 for two electrodes; C_z–C_7, and ipsilateral mastoid–C_7. (The BAEPs from the contralateral mastoid are not illustrated. They resembled the vertex BAEPs in waveform and latency but were of smaller amplitude.) The BAEP waves seen at ipsilateral mastoid and vertex in the normal subjects are quite dissimilar; in very few cases do the latencies of the peaks at vertex and mastoid correspond (N. Squires, J. Buchwald, J. Strecker, and F. Liley, *unpublished data*). Thus, it does appear that the activity of different generators may be emphasized by different electrode locations. Comparing the normal and Down's syndrome subjects, however, the same latency relationships hold across electrodes. For example, there is a positive wave at the mastoid that precedes the vertex wave IV in both groups. If, in the Down's group, the vertex wave IV had aligned with the earlier mastoid wave IV, we might have concluded that different generators were reflected in the Down's and normal vertex BAEPs. The current results do not support that conclusion.

With regard to click repetition rate, insufficient data were available to determine at which BAEP peak the abnormal recovery process appears, since peaks earlier than wave V were not present in enough subjects of either group at the higher rates. The wave V latencies of seven normal and six Down's subjects who had measurable wave Vs at all rates from 10 to 75/sec are shown in Table 1. As shown in the third line, there is a progressive increase in the discrepancy between the latencies of the Down's and nonretarded as click repetition rate increased. However, it appears unlikely that the functions would converge at rates even lower than 10/sec since both functions appear to be reaching a plateau at approximately 20/sec. It thus seems safe to conclude that the latencies of the BAEPs in Down's subjects will not appear normal at any rate of stimulation.

A major remaining question raised by this research concerns the functional

[1] The large number of absent BAEPs and wave I prolongations may be attributable to the prevalence of middle ear infection in Down's infants, particularly among the most severely afflicted (2)

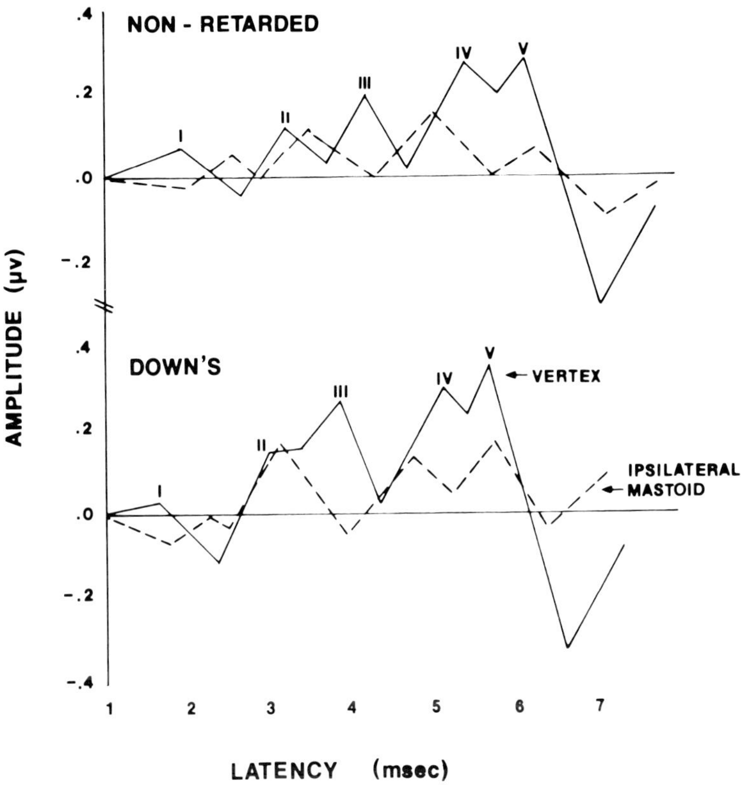

FIG. 4. Schematic BAEPs to 65 dB 10 clicks/sec for nonretarded **(top)** and Down's syndrome **(bottom)** recorded from C_z–neck *(solid lines)* and ipsilateral mastoid to neck *(dashed lines).*

implications of the unusual BAEPs seen in Down's syndrome, since an interpretation in terms of simple hearing deficit seems unwarranted. In an attempt to shed some light on this issue, the BAEP measures were correlated with other available information about the Down's subjects. Beyond the fact that the lower IQ subjects were more likely to have missing BAEPs, there was no correlation between the BAEP measures (transmission time or the slope of the recovery function) and IQ. The slope of the recovery function did relate to speech intelligibility: the more normal the recovery function, the clearer the speech ($r = 0.72$

TABLE 1. *Changes in wave V latency as a function of stimulation rate*

	10/sec	20/sec	33/sec	50/sec	75/sec
Nonretarded	6.11	6.09	6.22	6.27	6.51
Down's syndrome	5.76	5.71	5.78	5.78	5.94
Difference	0.35	0.38	0.44	0.49	0.57

for Experiment 1 and 0.76 for Experiment 2). Since speech ability did not correlate with IQ, this suggests that the BAEP recovery measure reflects an aspect of acoustic information processing in the temporal domain that is important for language acquisition, independent of overall cognitive capacity. We are currently pursuing this finding in a higher-functioning group of Down's subjects, in whom it is possible to assess the ability to discriminate a variety of acoustic features important in speech perception, with the aim of relating BAEP recovery to specific aspects of acoustic perception.

ACKNOWLEDGMENT

This work was supported by USPHS Grants HD05958 and HD04612 and USPHS Fellowship NS05725 (to N. Squires).

REFERENCES

1. Allen, A. R., and Starr, A. (1978): Auditory brain stem potentials in monkey *(M. mulatta)* and man. *Electroencephalogr. Clin. Neurophysiol.,* 45:53–63.
2. Balkany, T. J. (1979): Hearing loss in Down's syndrome. A treatable handicap more common than generally recognized. *Clin. Pediatr.,* 18:116–118.
3. Bender, C. E. (1969): *Down's Syndrome.* Grune & Stratton, New York.
4. Buchwald, J. S., and Huang, C. N. (1975): Far-field acoustic response: Origins in the cat. *Science,* 189:382–384.
5. Burger, P. C., and Vogel, F. S. (1973): The development of pathological changes of Alzheimer's disease and senile dementia in patients with Down's syndrome. *Am. J. Pathol.,* 73:457.
6. Crome, L., Cowie, V., and Stater, E. (1962): A statistical note on cerebellar and brainstem weight in mongolism. *J. Ment. Defic. Res.,* 10:69–72.
7. Gibson, D. (1978): *Down's Syndrome.* Cambridge University Press, Cambridge.
8. Jewett, D. L. (1970): Volume-conducted potentials in response to auditory stimuli as detected by averaging in the cat. *Electroencephalogr. Clin. Neurophysiol.,* 28:609–618.
9. Lloyd, L. L., and Reid, M. J. (1967): The incidence of hearing impairment in an institutionalized mentally retarded population. *Am. J. Ment. Defic.,* 71:746–763.
10. Lloyd, L. L., and Young, C. E. (1969): Pure-tone audiometry. In: *Audiometry for the Retarded,* edited by R. T. Fulton and L. L. Lloyd, pp. 1–31. Williams and Wilkins, Baltimore.
11. Matthews, J. (1971): Communication disorders in the mentally retarded. In: *Handbook of Speech Pathology and Audiology,* edited by L. E. Travis, pp. 801–818. Prentice-Hall, Englewood Cliffs, N.J.
12. Robinson, K., and Rudge, P. (1975): Auditory evoked responses in multiple sclerosis. *Lancet,* 1:1164–1166.
13. Robinson, K., and Rudge, P. (1977): The early components of the auditory evoked potential in multiple sclerosis. In: *Progress in Clinical Neurophysiology, Vol. 2,* edited by J. E. Desmedt, pp. 58–67. Karger, Basel.
14. Squires, N., Aine, C., Buchwald, J., Norman, R., and Galbraith, G. (1980): Brian stem response abnormalities in severely and profoundly retarded adults. *Electroencephalogr. Clin. Neurophysiol.,* 50:172–185.
15. Starr, A., and Achor, L. J. (1975): Auditory brainstem responses in neurological disease. *Arch. Neurol.,* 32:761–768.

Clinical Applications of Evoked Potentials in Neurology,
edited by J. Courjon, F. Mauguiere, and M. Revol.
Raven Press, New York © 1982.

The Brainstem Auditory Evoked Potential Is a Useful Diagnostic Tool in Evaluating Risk Factors for Hearing Loss in Neonatology

*P. A. Despland and **R. Galambos

**EEG-EMG and Neurophysiology Diagnostic Unit, Department of Neurology, University of Lausanne, Lausanne, Switzerland; and **Department of Neurosciences, M-008, University of California, San Diego, La Jolla, California 92093*

The brainstem auditory evoked potential (BAEP) is proving to be increasingly useful in the diagnosis of adult and infant disorders (3,6,10,12–14). It thus provides precise neurophysiological data to aid both otological and neurological diagnosis. The actual incidence of significant hearing loss in the intensive care nursery has been estimated at around 1:20 to 1:14 (4,11). In this chapter, we report BAEP measurements made on 100 babies in an intensive care unit. Our primary aim was to identify every baby with a hearing loss and to specify its magnitude and type. Thereafter, we examined the clinical histories of the entire group in an attempt to uncover otonoxious risk factors and arrange them in order of importance.

METHOD

The babies were all tested in isolettes or open basinettes by the same person. Disk electrodes were attached to the vertex and both mastoids by standard techniques, as explained elsewhere (5,10). Stimuli were clicks delivered monaurally through an earphone (TDH-39) taped over the ear. Testing on most babies was about 30 min post-feeding and while they were in natural sleep.

A relatively simple two-step procedure will in most cases separate the newborn infant with neurological disorder from one with audiological disease. Step 1 involves stimulation with 60- or 70-dB clicks at a rate of 37 Hz in an effort to develop the BAEP. If no response appears, the baby obviously suffers a severe peripheral hearing loss which calls for stimulation at still higher intensities in search of his threshold. If, as is usually the case, a response appears, the latencies of its waves I and V are measured and compared with those expected for a normal infant of the same age. Table 1 summarizes the changes in the latencies of waves I and V with age and stimulus intensity. Finally, the time interval required for conduction through the brainstem to the inferior colliculus

TABLE 1. *Brainstem auditory evoked potential latencies and standard deviations obtained from premature infants presumed to be normal audiologically and neurologically*

Gestational age at test (weeks)	Wave V latency (msec), stimulus rate 37 Hz/sec ($N = 135$ ears)		Latencies to 60 dB, 10 Hz/sec stimulus ($N = 74$ ears)		
	60 dB	30 dB	Wave I	Wave V	I-V interval
30–31	9.43 ± 0.60	11.08 ± 0.81	3.50 ± 0.53	9.10 ± 0.32	5.60 ± 0.55
32–33	9.22 ± 0.80	10.88 ± 0.87	2.78 ± 0.22	8.36 ± 0.54	5.62 ± 0.30
34–35	8.57 ± 0.38	10.10 ± 0.69	2.56 ± 0.25	8.00 ± 0.28	5.44 ± 0.29
36–37	8.09 ± 0.34	9.27 ± 0.39	2.53 ± 0.19	7.80 ± 0.45	5.27 ± 0.38
38–39	7.97 ± 0.38	9.12 ± 0.50	2.30 ± 0.19	7.42 ± 0.19	5.09 ± 0.16
40–41	7.62 ± 0.36	8.65 ± 0.40	2.28 ± 0.27	7.35 ± 0.46	5.07 ± 0.41
42–43	7.56 ± 0.15	8.55 ± 0.14	2.28 ± 0.20	7.17 ± 0.10	4.89 ± 0.20

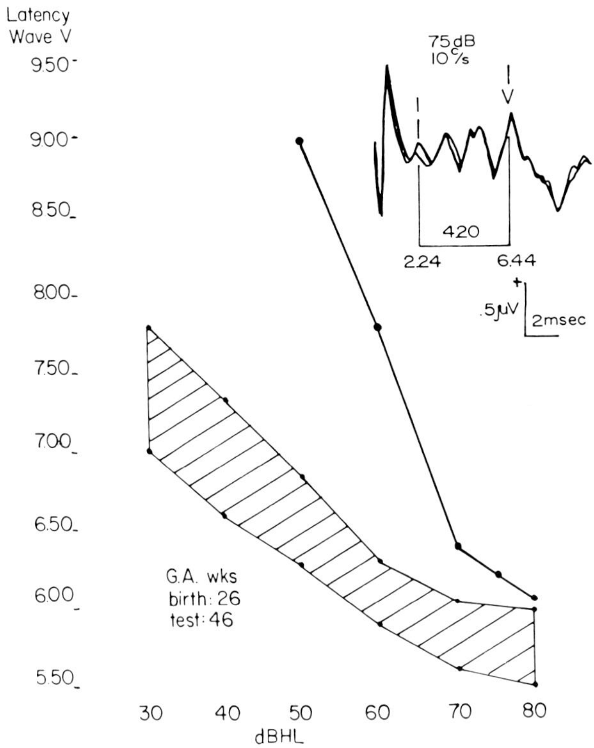

FIG. 1. Example of a sensorineural hearing loss.

level is measured at 10 Hz. The measurements of waves I and V make possible several diagnostic statements. If wave V is normal, the I-V interval will also be normal, and so neurological disorder is unlikely. If wave V is prolonged, but the I-V interval is normal, a hearing loss is indicated. And if the I-V interval is prolonged with wave I normal, a neurological disorder is probable. Neurological and audiological disorders are both suggested if wave I and the I-V interval are prolonged.

Step 2 aims to produce the definitive audiological diagnosis. Threshold sensitivity is estimated by establishing the weakest stimulus that produces wave V, and the type of hearing loss (conductive or sensorineural) can often be identified from a graph showing the manner in which wave V latency shortens as intensity increases (Fig. 1).

RESULTS

Detection of Hearing Loss

In the 100 babies tested at 26 to 42 weeks estimated gestational age, 86 fulfilled the criteria for normal hearing. The 14 infants who failed to meet the

BAEP criteria for normal hearing consisted of 11 prematures and three newborns. The intensity series of these babies demonstrated the following abnormal data: three infants produced no BAEP to clicks at a level of 90 dB; nine infants with elevated auditory threshold (40 dB or more) had a normal neurological status; and two infants had BAEP responses permitting a diagnosis of both audiological and neurological disorder.

The type of deviation of the intensity curves from the normal graph characterized conductive or sensorineural hearing loss. The losses found included 12 of the sensorineural type and two involving the conductive apparatus.

Identifying Risk Factors for a Hearing Loss

An effort to identify the clinical factors predisposing for these hearing losses began with a search through the charts of the affected babies for probable or likely causes. Our search detected nine categories of apparently relevant information as plotted in Table 2. These include weight and gestational age at birth, Apgar scores at 1 and 5 min, acidosis, ototoxic drugs, various signs of central nervous disorder, the number of days on assisted ventilation, and cardiac or face malformations. A risk factor is identified when the number of babies with abnormal BAEPs exceeds or approximates the number of normals. All of the factors included in this list, except for the factor acidosis, are either known or suspected risk factors for hearing loss.

By acidosis, we mean a blood pH level of 7.25 or below within an hour or two of birth and/or 2 or more days during treatment in which blood pH fell below 7.25.

DISCUSSION

According to this study, the BAEP method can reliably identify hearing-impaired infants in neonatology. The method uncovered a total of 14 in the population of 100 tested. Two died within a few days of birth, and eight were discharged home. The incidence of peripheral hearing loss in such population (8 to 12%) seems reasonable. Somewhere between 1:10 and 1:20 of the babies from an intensive care nursery may leave for home with a significant peripheral hearing loss. In our series, about half of the babies retested showed that the losses appear to be permanent, but this conclusion needs confirmation.

Most of the nine risk factors identified in this study have already been recognized. Our sample did not contain certain other well-known factors (e.g., baby whose parents were deaf, rubella infection by mother, hyperbilirubinemia). Thus, our list is not exhaustive; it gives only factors detected from the histories of this particular sample of 100 babies. An examination of Table 2 which lists the risk factors found in the clinical records of the babies with abnormal BAEPs suggests the following considerations:

1. Infants with cleft palate are obviously at high risk, a fact already stated in the literature (1,8).

TABLE 2. *Clinical factors predisposing for hearing loss*

	Tested by BAEP				
			Abnormal		
Clinical data	Total	Normal	Audio-logical[a]	Neuro-logical	Risk factor?
Gestational age at birth (weeks)					
26–30	23	15	6	2	Yes
31–34	27	25	1(2)		
35–38	30	26	0(2)		
39–42	20	18	2		
Weight at birth (g)					
<1,000	9	2	6	1	Yes
1,000–1,500	16	13	1(2)	1	
1,600–2,500	44	43	0(1)		
2,600–4,000	31	28	1(3)	1	
Apgar scores at 1 and 5 min					
5/6	22	11	9(10)	1	Yes
6/7	78	75	0(2)	1	
Postnatal blood pH					
>7.26	90	86	0(3)	1	
<7.25	10	0	9	1	Yes
Neurological status					
Brain hem.	8	3	3	2	Yes
Deep coma	10	4	6		Yes
Normal	82	79	2(3)		
Seizures					
1–5 days	9	6	1	2	Perhaps
Status epil.	2	0	2		Perhaps
None	89	80	6(9)		
Respiratory distress syndrome: days on ventilation					
<1	27	25	0(2)		
1–10	63	59	2(3)	1	
>11	10	2	7	1	Yes
Congenital malformation					
Cardiac	9	3	5	1	Yes
Face	7	4	3		Yes
Trisomy-18	1	0	1		Perhaps
None	83	79	3	1	

[a] Number in parenthesis adds infants with craniofacial malformation.

2. The factors most frequently represented in Table 2 are low Apgar scores (11 cases) and acidosis (10 cases).
3. Since low Apgar scores appear most frequently, hypoxia may be the most important of the perinatal factors predisposing for hearing loss.

However, in our sample, we detected 22 babies with unusually low Apgar scores at birth. Of these, only half showed audiological disorders. The measurements of blood pH suggest that hypoxia at birth alone was not the main cause of hearing loss. Instead, babies showed impaired auditory function when the hypoxia-related acidosis persisted for a prolonged period at birth and/or when several periods of severe acidosis appeared postnatally during treatment.

Our analysis indicates that acidosis is a more important predictor of hearing loss than any other physiological variable. It has already been pointed out that in the presence of severe hypoxia, the prevention or correction of an acidosis can have important beneficial consequences. In his monograph, Dawes summarizes recent animal studies in this field (2). Hrbek et al. demonstrated that the degree of brain dysfunction at a given level of hypoxia depended on how much the pH of the circulating blood had dropped (9).

Our hypothesis that prolonged acidosis at and after birth is closely related to irreversible hearing loss is being advanced for the first time, so far as we are aware, and, of course, more data will be required to confirm it (7). If, as the analysis suggests, the events associated with the acidosis, not the hypoxia, were mainly responsible for the peripheral hearing loss measured by BAEPs, any neonate in whom acidosis is a problem during the postnatal period should be considered at risk for hearing loss. This group obviously includes babies with cardiac anomalies and those requiring long periods of assisted ventilation.

SUMMARY

Fourteen of 100 babies in an intensive care nursery showed abnormal BAEPs. An analysis of the clinical records identified nine risk factors. Neonatal asphyxia appeared to be associated with hearing loss only when repeated episodes of acidosis accompanied it.

We conclude that the BAEPs can identify hard-of-hearing babies and estimate the type and amount of peripheral hearing loss. Prolonged perfusion of the cochlea with blood low in pH level may be the most common cause of hearing disorder in our group of nine identified risk factors.

REFERENCES

1. Bess, F. H., Schwarth, D. M., and Redfield, N. P. (1976): Audiometric, impedance, and otoscopic findings in children with cleft palates. *Arch. Otolaryngol.*, 102:665–669.
2. Dawes, G. S. (1969): *Foetal and Neonatal Physiology: A Comparative Study of the Changes at Birth.* Year Book Medical Publishers, Chicago.
3. Despland, P. A., and Galambos, R. (1979): Les propriétés neurophysiologiques des ondes précoces auditives du tronc cérébral et leur utilité en clinique. *Schweiz. Med. Wochenschr.*, 109:781–787.
4. Despland, P. A., and Galambos, R. (1980): The auditory brainstem response is a useful diagnostic tool in the intensive care nursery. *Pediatr. Res.*, 14:154–158.
5. Despland, P. A., and Galambos, R. (1980): Use of the auditory brainstem responses by prematures and newborn infants. *Neuropaediatrie*, 11:99–107.
6. Galambos, R., and Despland, P. A. (1980): The auditory brainstem response evaluates risk factors for hearing loss in the newborn. *Pediatr. Res.*, 14:159–163.
7. Galambos, R., and Hecox, K. (1978): Clinical applications of the auditory brainstem response. *Otolaryngol. Clin. North Am.*, 11:709–722.
8. Graham, M. D. (1963): A longitudinal study of ear disease and hearing loss in patients with cleft lips and palate. *Trans. Am. Acad. Ophtalmol. Otolaryngol.*, 67:213–222.
9. Hrbeck, A., Karlsson, K., Kjellmer, I., Olsson, T., and Riha, M. (1974): Cerebral reactions during intra uterine asphyxia in the sheep. II. Evoked electroencephalogram responses. *Pediatr. Res.*, 8:58–63.

10. Schulman-Galambos, C., and Galambos, R. (1975): Brainstem auditory evoked responses in premature infants. *J. Speech Hear. Res.*, 18:456–465.
11. Schulman-Galambos, C., and Galambos, R. (1979): Brainstem evoked response audiometry in newborn hearing screening. *Arch. Otolaryngol.*, 105:86–90.
12. Starr, A., Amlie, R. N., Martin, W. H., and Sanders, S. (1977): Development of auditory function in newborn infants revealed by auditory brainstem potentials. *Pediatrics,* 60:831–839.
13. Starr, A., and Hamilton, A. (1976): Correlation between confirmed sites of neurological lesions and abnormalities of far-field auditory brainstem response. *Electroencephalogr. Clin. Neurophysiol.*, 41:595–608.
14. Stockard, J. J., Stockard, J. E., and Sharbrough, F. W. (1977): Detection and localization of occult lesions with brainstem auditory responses. *Mayo Clin. Proc.*, 52:761–767.

Clinical Applications of Evoked Potentials in Neurology,
edited by J. Courjon, F. Mauguiere, and M. Revol.
Raven Press, New York © 1982.

Brainstem Evoked Responses in Prematures

*A. Morgon, **B. Salle, **H. Mycek, and **J. M. Chanal

**Centre d'Audiophonologie de Lyon and **Service de Néonatologie de Lyon, Hôpital Edouard Herriot, Lyon, France*

A study of human auditory system maturation was carried out in the Premature Unit of Professor Salle at the Edouard Herriot Hospital, Lyon. Brainstem evoked responses to auditory stimuli were recorded as previously described (1).

SUBJECTS

Thirty-nine cases were analyzed in the present study. They were divided into three groups according to gestational age at birth: group A (16 cases) had gestational age of 32 to 35 weeks; group B (15 cases), 36 to 37 weeks; and group C (eight cases), 38 to 39 weeks.

The groups were further subdivided on the basis of the interval between birth and testing, i.e., less than 2 weeks or greater than 30 days.

LATENCY MEASUREMENTS

The study included analyses of wave patterns, amplitudes, and latencies; the present chapter deals only with our findings with regard to latencies.

Means and standard deviations of latencies were calculated for each stimulus used, for each stimulus intensity, and for each group of subjects. Latency variations of peaks J_I, J_{III}, and J_V were studied first as a function of stimulus within each group and then according to group for each stimulus.

Within Groups

It was clearly found that, in all cases, the latency values increase when the intensity of a stimulus decreases (Fig. 1).

Another phenomenon was clearly apparent: the latency of waves evoked by 2 kHz stimuli was greater than those evoked by 4 kHz stimuli or by nonfiltered click (NFC) stimuli. Moreover, this effect was most pronounced with group A (low gestational age) subjects and was less pronounced with groups B and C. In addition, the phenomenon was more clearly apparent near threshold stimulus strength and less so at higher stimulus intensity (Figs. 2 and 3). For 4

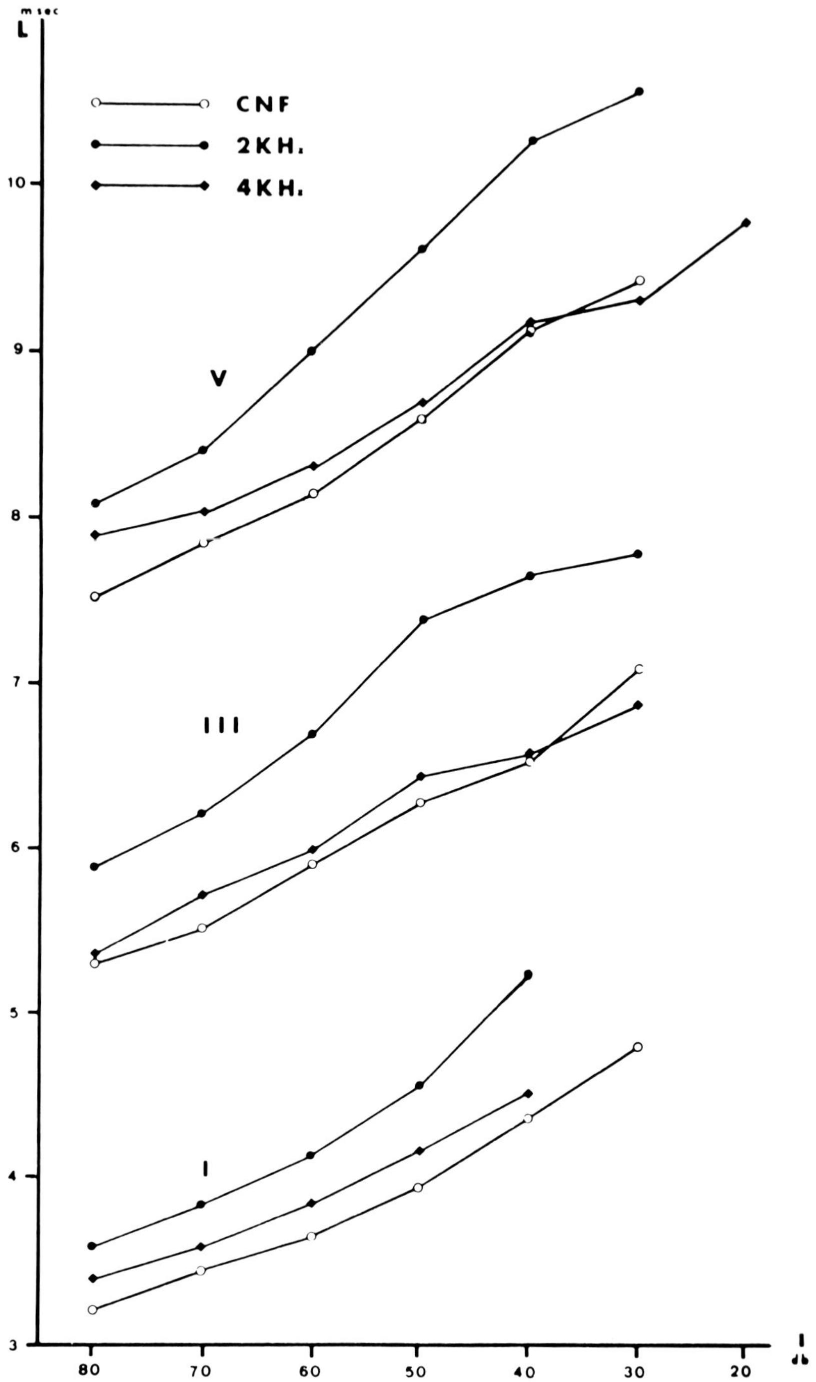

FIG. 1. Latencies of subjects in group A. Note that the latencies of responses to 2 kHz stimuli exceed those of responses to other stimuli; this is most pronounced for J_{III} and J_{V}. The responses to a nonfiltered click (CNF) and to a 4 kHz tone are nearly superimposed.

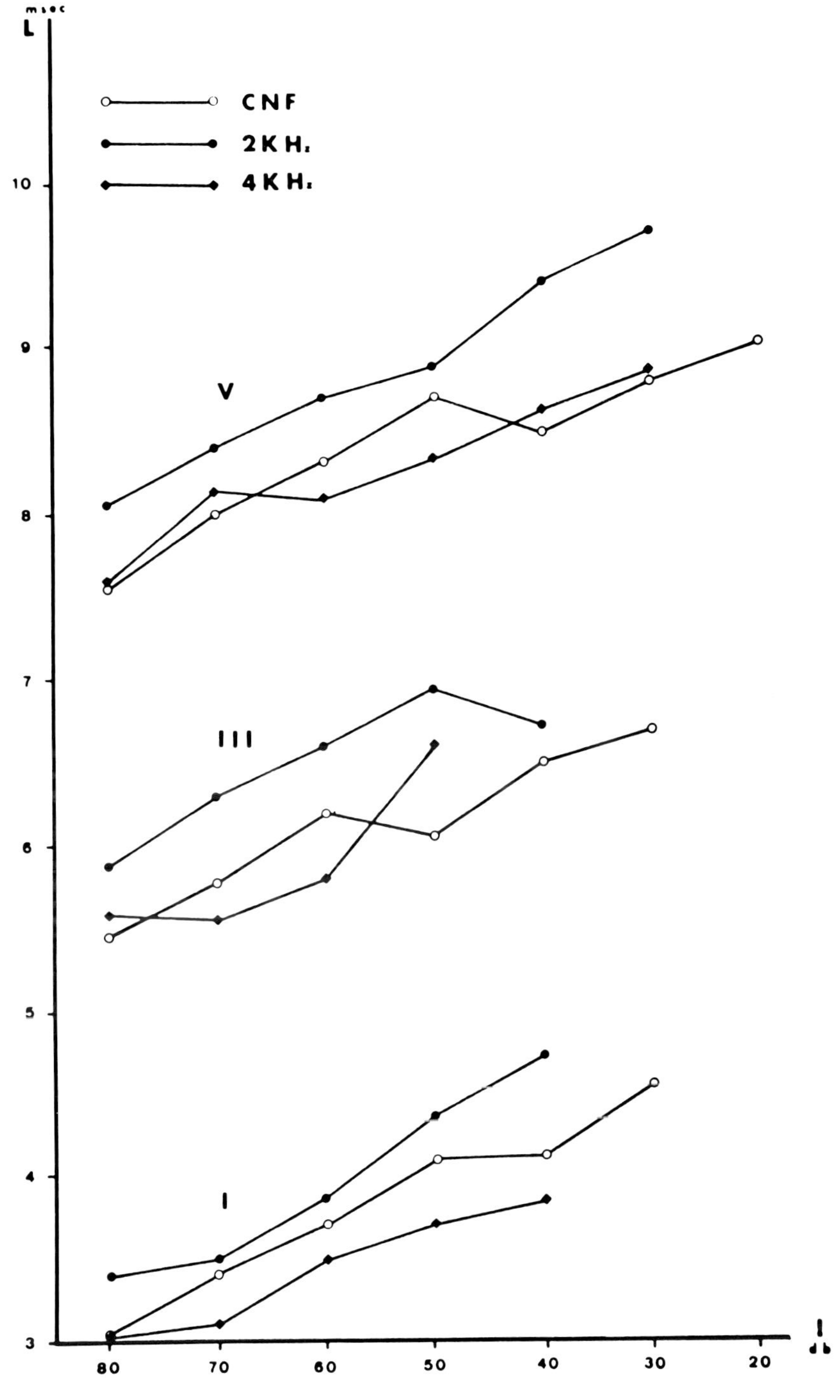

FIG. 2. Latencies of subjects in group B. Note that the phenomenon observed with group A (Fig. 1) is greatly diminished.

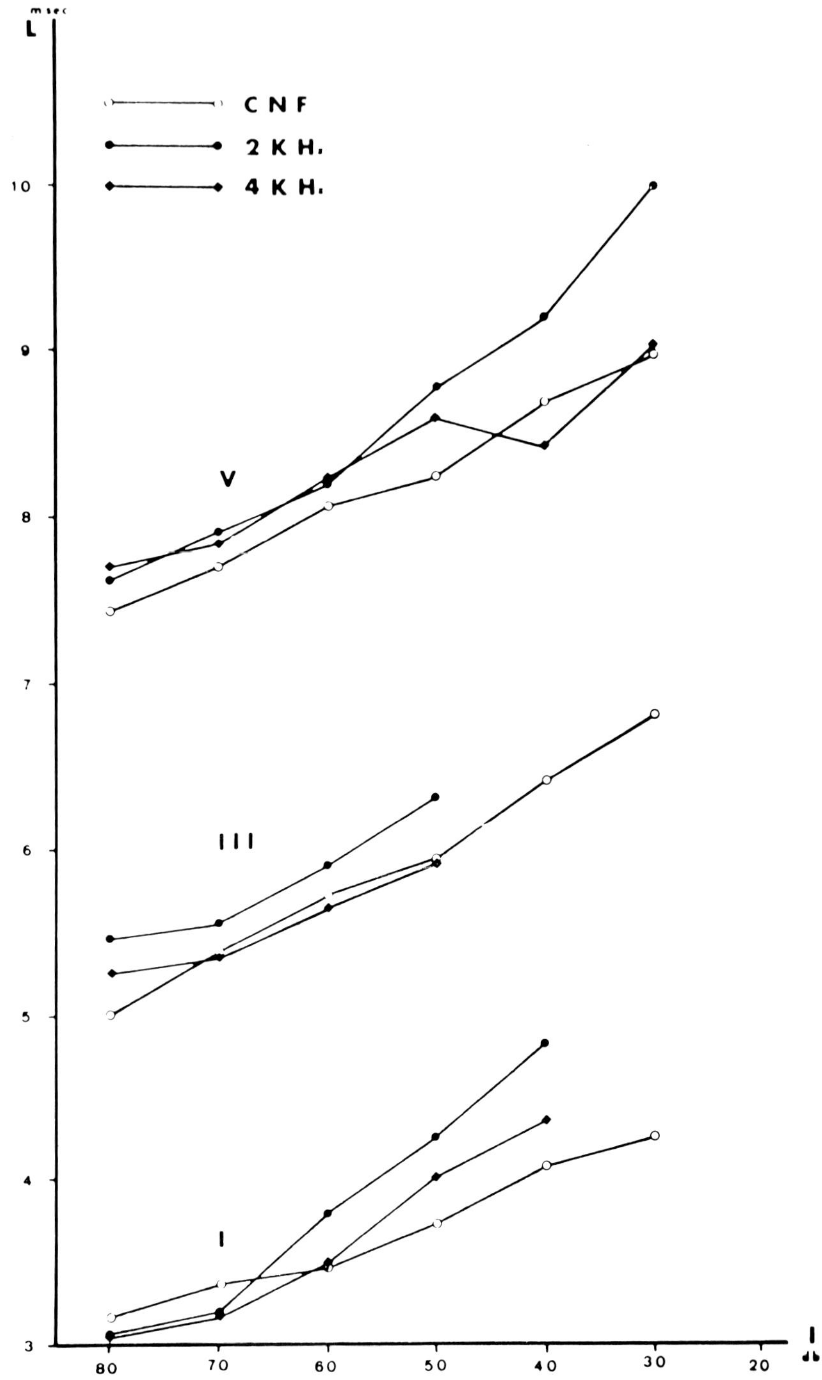

FIG. 3. Latencies of subjects in group C. Note that the difference between the latencies of responses to 2 kHz stimuli and of those produced by other stimuli (Figs. 1 and 2) have all but disappeared except at low stimulus intensities.

kHz or NFC stimuli, the gradation of latency with intensity was not apparent for groups B and C but was present, although not clearly pronounced, for group A (Fig. 4).

For Each Frequency

For 2 kHz stimuli only, there was a clear variation of each of the three measured latencies (J_I, J_{III}, J_V) among the three groups of subjects, from the youngest to the oldest prematures. This observation was not so pronounced for the NFC and 4 kHz stimuli for which the graphs approximately coincide. However, if a distinction is made between high and low intensities, one can observe that near the threshold, the latencies of group A are markedly greater than those of the other groups of subjects. This is most apparent for the latency of wave J_V.

Influence of Weight

As already mentioned, each of the three groups was subdivided into those tested early (weighing less than 1,500 g) and those tested later (weighing over 1,500 g). We considered the possibility that weight differences might be significant to the extent that weight differences reflect changes in lipid metabolism that might have an impact on myelinogenesis. A comparison was made between subgroups of each group for the latency of the J_V wave. In our population, there was no effect of subject weight.

Interwave Intervals

Analysis was made first of the V–I latency difference and then of its two measurable components, the III–I and V–III differences. Only the data on the V–I interval are presented here.

The V–I Interval

Examination of the figures might produce the impression that no measurable information can be obtained from these data. This may reflect the fact that we made it a point to keep the same time scales for these diagrams as for the others. It must be remembered that changes in the interpeak intervals are minimal and that they must, therefore, be magnified.

With this in mind, the recordings may be considered from two viewpoints: the V-I interval as a function of age, and the interval as a function of stimulus.

Although the value of this interval is independent of intensity and frequency in groups B and C, in group A, the interval progressively increases, irrespective of frequency, when the intensity decreases. Here again, the 2 kHz frequency gives a greater interval and faster extension near the threshold. With regard

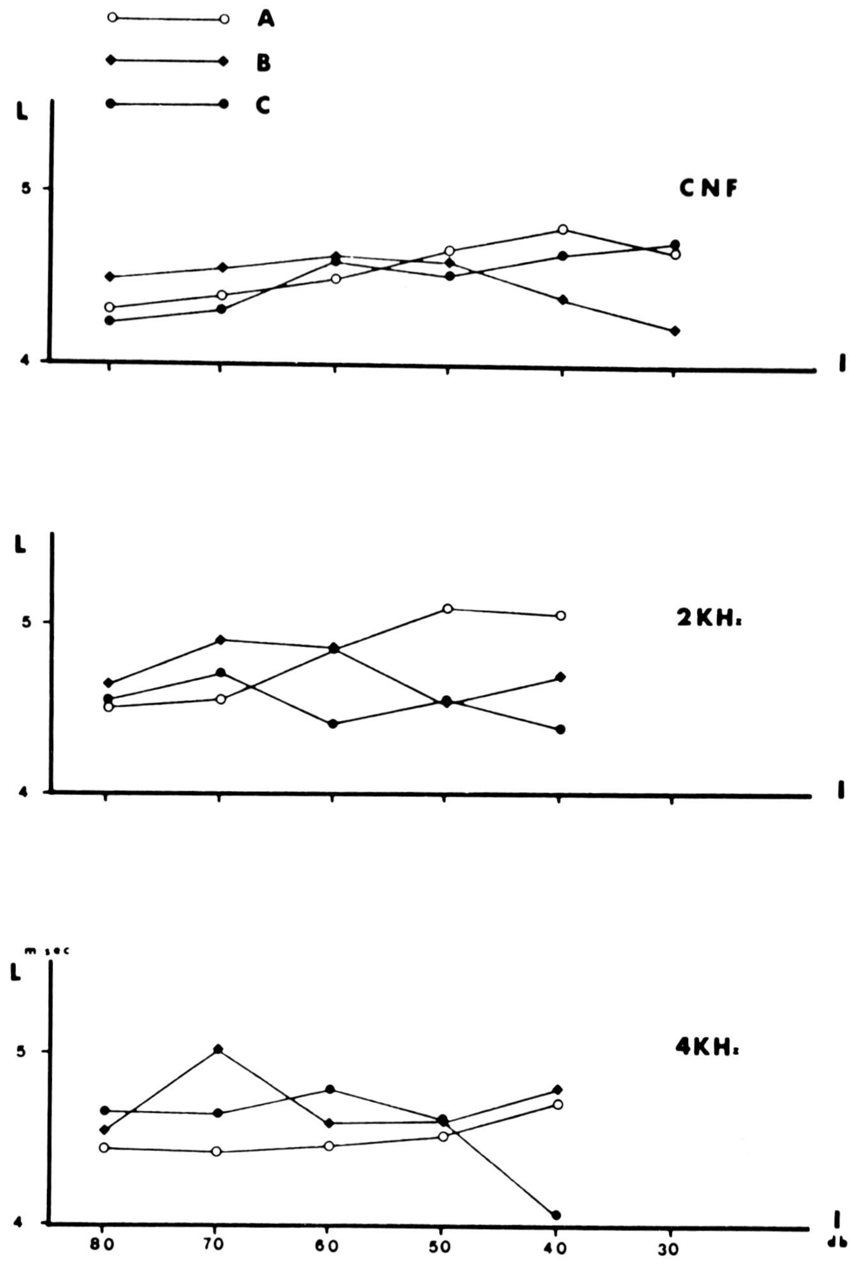
A
B
C
L
5
4
CNF
I
L
5
4
2KHz
I
m sec
L
5
4
4KHz
I
80
70
60
50
40
30
db

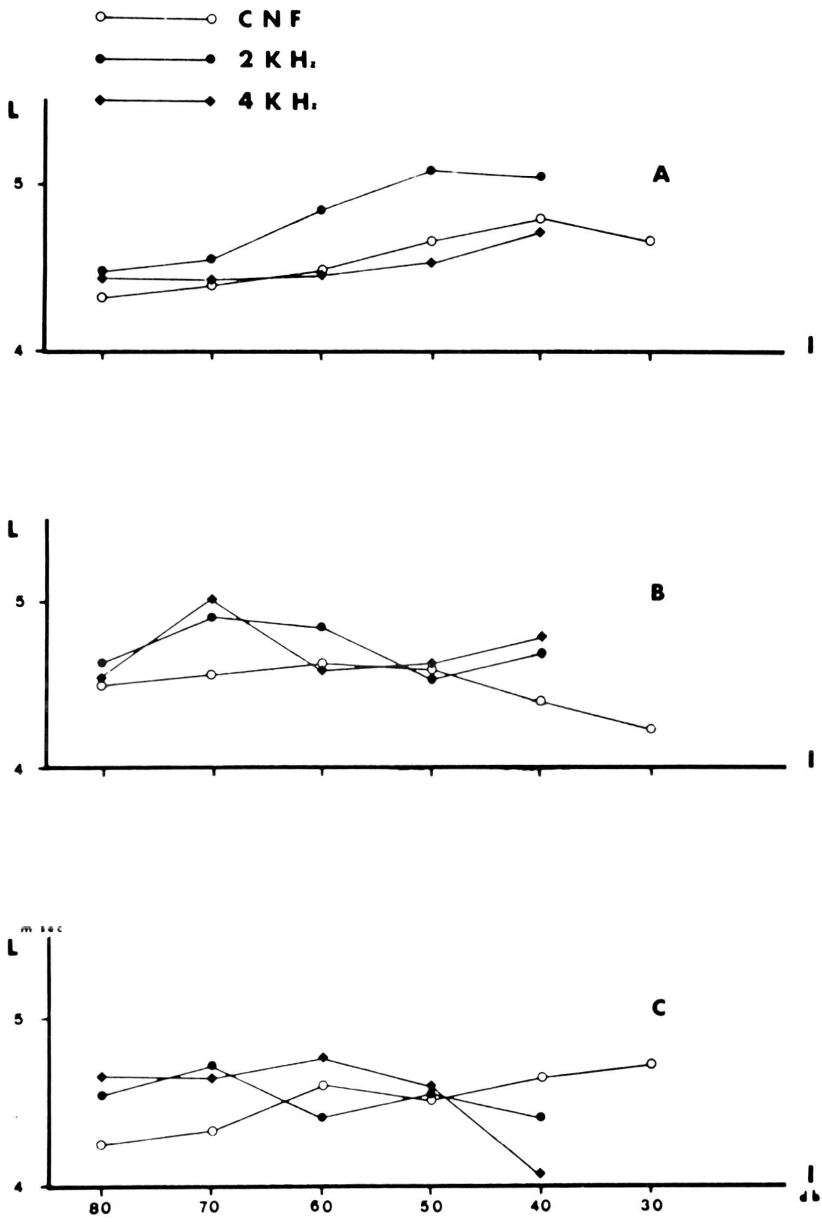

FIG. 4. Interpeak intervals between peaks J_I and J_V. The response of group A is clearly different from those of other groups in that the latency of the response to the 2 kHz stimulus clearly exceeds that of responses to other stimuli used and also shows a clear dependence on stimulus intensity.

to V-I intervals according to frequency, these data are confirmed, and we find that only the interpeak intervals of group A rise at low intensities; it is difficult to reach any conclusion with the other groups.

Influence of the Age at Testing

As already described, we formed subgroups based on the conceptional age–gestational age difference: subgroup 1 for those under 2 weeks; subgroup 2 for those over 30 days. We then compared the different latencies of J_V for these A_1–A_2, B_1–B_2, and C_1–C_2 groups. The latencies of subgroups 2 are higher than those of subgroups 1.

DISCUSSION

The study of auditory evoked potential latency made possible an approach to the maturation of the hearing system.

The auditory system seems to evolve rapidly until the 35th week, and it appears that the 2 kHz frequency is the most appropriate to demonstrate this temporal maturation as it best brings out the differences among the groups of subjects.

The 2 kHz frequency also produces longer latencies than do 4 kHz or NFC stimuli. It is, therefore, possible to conclude that the structures that conduct 2 kHz tones are less mature than those conducting low frequencies and 4 kHz tones.

REFERENCES

1. (1980): A study of brain stem evoked responses in prematures. *Acta Otorhinolaryngol. Belg.*, 89:370–375.

Clinical Applications of Evoked Potentials in Neurology,
edited by J. Courjon, F. Mauguiere, and M. Revol.
Raven Press, New York © 1982.

Right Hemianacousia Without Language Deficit

F. Michel, F. Peronnet, and F. Mauguière

Unité 94, INSERM, 69500 Bron, France

When a lesion involves the supratemporal plane and damages the konio- and the parakoniocortex (1), areas that receive direct afferents from the medial geniculate body, or when a lesion cuts the auditory geniculocortical pathways, patients exhibit two striking features among other clinical deficits: an extinction of the messages in the contralateral ear during a dichotic test; and a reduction if not a complete disappearance of the late components of the auditory evoked potentials (AEP) in the mastoid and temporal leads facing the damaged hemisphere.

We propose to call these abnormalities "hemianacousia" (6,10) in analogy to similar sensory deficits, hemianopia and hemianesthesia.

Neurologists will certainly agree that a fair number of left hemianacousias could pass unnoticed if the right temporal lesion is relatively small and restricted to the supratemporal plane (see ref. 4). Usually attention is attracted to a right temporal lesion by an accompanying deficit (hemiplegia, hemianesthesia, or hemianopia) that is the result of a subcortical white matter involvement.

The situation is different for left hemisphere lesions since, as is well known, language disturbances are a prominent feature of the clinical picture when the left temporo–parietal area is damaged. In this chapter, we shall not present cases of apparently isolated left hemianacousia by a right temporal lesion because it is not a surprising entity. We shall refer to patients who, as a result of a left hemisphere lesion, present a right hemianacousia without language disturbances or with only negligible ones.

The great majority of aphasic patients in our experience show a clear and often nearly complete extinction of the right ear messages in a dichotic test if one uses pairs of words or short sentences (and not only digits). Among them, a good proportion do not show abnormalities of their AEP over the mastoid and temporal leads. This is not surprising, since the lesions that induce aphasic disturbances and right ear extinction in the dichotic test may obviously be located outside the supratemporal plane, for example, in the third frontal gyrus, the second temporal gyrus, or the parietal area.

But a fair number of patients exhibit both a deficit at the subjective dichotic test and abnormalities of their left AEP. It is only in this case that we use the term hemianacousia. Until recently, we were tempted to think that a clear anomaly of the left AEP was only seen in the context of obvious and often severe language disturbances. And evidently, patients who have the most severe aphasic symptoms are likely to have the largest lesions and, consequently, lesions damaging the auditory cortex or its afferents.

But some observations that we tended at first to neglect oblige us to reconsider this point of view. We indeed have seen a few apparently unquestionable cases in which there are both a recovery of language disturbances and a persisting anomaly of the left AEP.

The interested reader may find in former articles the technical data concerning the recording of the AEP (5,10). We shall discuss five patients with left hemisphere lesions and one patient with bilateral lesions.

CLINICAL DATA

Case 1: Mr. S.

Transient aphasia: phonemic paraphasias; excellent comprehension; no disturbances of reading and writing; normal visual field; no sensorimotor deficit. Almost perfect recovery, but complete right ear extinction to the dichotic test. Clear asymmetry of the AEP (Fig. 1A).

Case 2: Mr. I.

Right hemiplegia and hypoesthesia predominant at the superior limb because of a thrombosis of a sylvian artery branch. Sudden motor and sensory deficit predominantly at the right superior limb, global aphasia, normal visual field. Complete recovery of the aphasic disturbances except some articulatory distortions and few phonemic paraphasias. But complete right ear extinction, and AEP clearly asymmetric (Fig. 1B).

Case 3: Mme K.

Emboli in a rolandic and a parietal branch of the sylvian artery; hypoesthesia of the right arm and paraphasic speech but normal comprehension. After a few months, persistence of the sensory deficit (with hyperpathy) but normal language.

Almost complete extinction of the right ear to the dichotic test. The left AEPs are hardly visible over the mastoid and temporal left leads (Fig. 1C).

Case 4: Mr. P.

Transient expressive aphasia. Right ear extinction to the dichotic test. Clear asymmetry between the left and the right AEPs, especially over the mastoid and temporal leads (Fig. 1D).

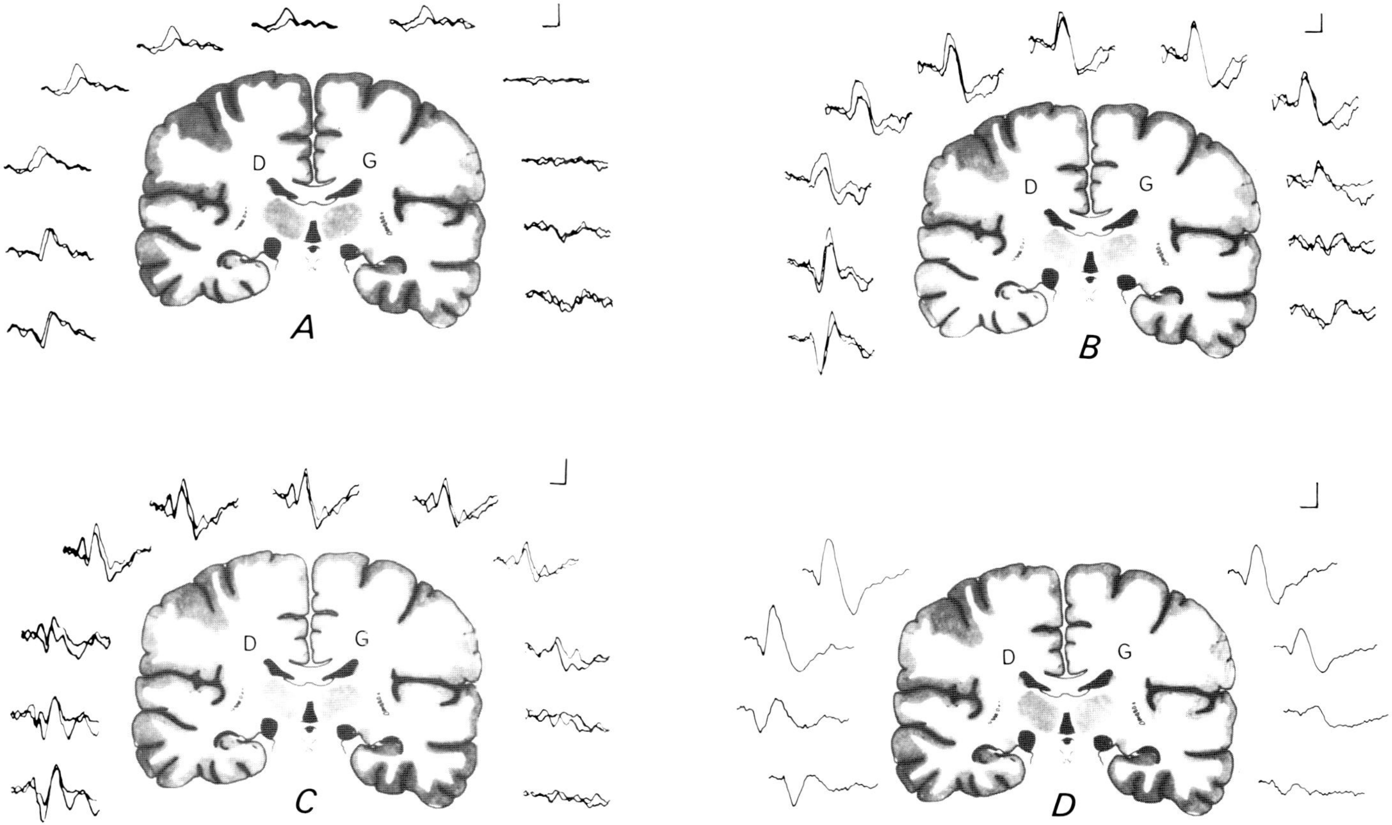

FIG. 1. Auditory evoked potentials of the first four cases (see text). One observes a clear asymmetry between right and left AEP in the mastoid, temporal, and low parietal leads. Calibration: 100 msec, 5 mV.

Case 5: Mr. T.

In a left-handed subject, thrombosis of a parietal branch of the left sylvian artery; amusia without language disturbances (7). Complete right ear extinction to the dichotic test. The left AEPs are obviously abnormal (Fig. 2).

Case 6

The complete history of this patient has already been published (8). Left temporal and right parieto–temporal lesions leading to a cortical deafness without any linguistic defect. At two separate sessions, complete absence of AEP over a coronal chain of electrodes (after 500 stimulations), although VEPs were immediately extracted on the same leads in only 25 summations.

COMMENTS

Our data show, to our surprise, that an abolition or at least a reduction of N1 and P2 components of the left AEP does not imply that the patient exhibits severe or even mild persistent aphasic disturbances.

Clinically, our patients (those with a left unilateral lesion) at first show language disturbances that resemble conduction aphasia. We particularly insist on the lack of comprehension deficits in these cases. The lesion responsible for conduction aphasia is classically located in the arcuate fasciculus, often under the supramarginal gyrus. In three of our cases, the arteriograms or the CT scan precisely favor such a localization of the lesions. Obviously, a supramar-

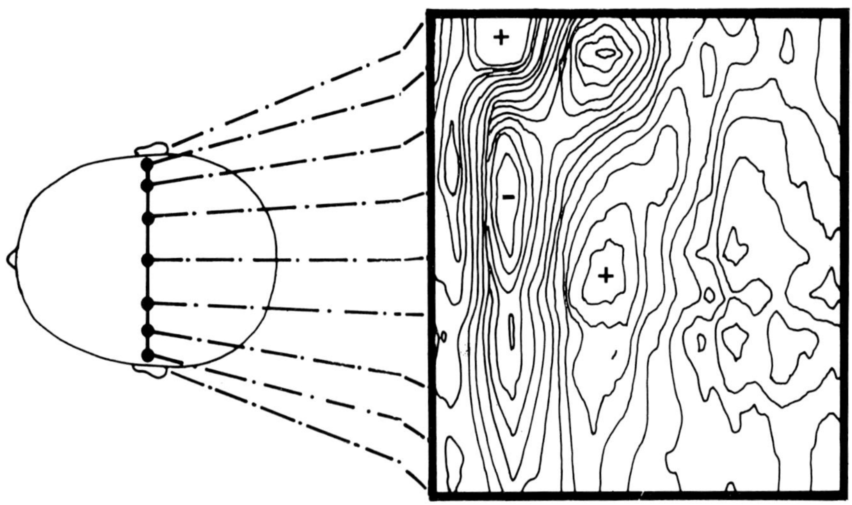

FIG. 2. Case 5 in text: the spatial-temporal map (9) shows a clear right–left asymmetry (11 sites of recording).

ginal gyrus lesion should not destroy the acoustic supratemporal area except in its most posteromedial part. We assume that the lesions in the present cases must spread forward into the supratemporal plane. A white matter lesion cutting the acoustic radiations would indeed be the ideal lesion to account for a sensory deficit without an integrative one. It is also possible that the lesions spare a very small part of the acoustic area and that this remnant of acoustic cortex is able to ensure speech sound processing without being able to generate an AEP. But, in the absence of postmortem examination, we can only hypothesize.

These data are in accordance with the classical idea that a left temporal lesion will lead to verbal deafness only if, at the same time, the left acoustic radiations and the right callosal afferents are involved (3). In a case of left supratemporal lesions, it takes a few weeks or months for the patient to learn the use of this callosal contingent and then recover.

These data also seem to show that the left acoustic cortical area apparently has no special skill compared to the right for decoding speech material and that the right temporal area is able to supply the damaged left one. This is less of a surprise if one remembers that a good part of the left occipital lobe (and certainly the calcarine area) has no special skill for decoding written material. In other words, the functional asymmetry between left and right hemispheres does not lie at the level of the konio- and parakoniocortex, and this fits rather well with the anatomical data (2) showing a morphological and cytoarchitectonic asymmetry only for the area Tpt, i.e., in the integration area caudal to the konio- and parakoniocortex.

REFERENCES

1. Galaburda, A., and Sanides, F. (1980): Cytoarchitectonic organization of the human auditory cortex. *J. Comp. Neurol.,* 190:597–610.
2. Galaburda, A., Sanides, F., and Geschwind, N. (1978): Human brain. Cyto-architectonic left–right asymmetries in the temporal speech region. *Arch. Neurol.,* 35:812–817.
3. Geschwind, N. (1965): Disconnection syndromes in animals and man. *Brain,* 88:237–294,585–644.
4. Lhermitte, F., Chain, F., Escourolle, R., Ducarne, B., Pillon, B., and Chedru, F. (1971): Etude des troubles perceptifs auditifs dans les lésions temporales bilatérales. *Rev. Neurol.,* 124:329–351.
5. Maraval, G., Pernier, J., Peronnet, F., Echallier, J. F., Gerin, P., and Mauguière, F. (1980): EVØQ: Système configurable de stimulation automatique et d'enregistrement des potentiels évoqués moyens sur mini-ordinateur. *Int. J. Biomed. Comput.,* 11:225–239.
6. Michel, F., Peronnet, F., Labourel, D., and Martin, M. M. (1973): Confrontation entre les données du test d'écoute dichotique et les données de l'enregistrement des potentiels évoqués acoustiques dans divers cas d'aphasie. *Rev. Neurol.,* 129:295–296.
7. Michel, F., Peronnet, F., and Schott, B. (1976): A propos d'un cas de surdité de l'hémisphère gauche (hémianacousie droite). *Rev. Electroencephalogr. Neurophysiol. Clin.,* 6(2):175–178.
8. Michel, F., Peronnet, F., and Schott, B. (1980): A case of cortical deafness: Clinical and electrophysiological data. *Brain Lang.,* 10:367–377.
9. Pernier, J., Bruckert, R., Maraval, G., Perrin, F., and Echallier, J. F. (1977): Technique de tracé de courbes isovales sur ordinateur. *Int. J. Biomed. Comput.,* 8:95–108.
10. Peronnet, F., and Michel, F. (1977): The asymmetry of the auditory evoked potentials in normal man and in patients with brain lesions. In: *Auditory Evoked Potentials in Man. Progress in Clinical Neurophysiology,* edited by J. E. Desmedt, pp. 130–141. Karger, Basel.

Clinical Applications of Evoked Potentials in Neurology,
edited by J. Courjon, F. Mauguiere, and M. Revol.
Raven Press, New York © 1982.

Ideomotor Apraxia and P300: A Preliminary Study

*R. Ragot, **C. Derouesne, *B. Renault, and *N. Lesevre

**Laboratoire d'Electrophysiologie et de Neurophysiologie Appliquée and **Clinique des Maladies du Système Nerveux, Hôpital de la Salpêtrière, 75651 Paris Cédex 13, France*

As far as we know, there has not yet been a study of event-related potentials recorded from patients with ideomotor apraxia (IMA). The main reason for this might be that, on a conceptual level, there is still relatively little interaction between neuropsychology and electrophysiology. On the other hand, for practical reasons, the testing procedures ordinarily used to investigate the IMA syndrome do not apply easily to electrophysiological recordings. Moreover, it could be difficult for patients to fulfill the types of tasks designed for normal subjects, since patients with a clear syndrome of IMA with no paralysis, aphasia, or any associated sign are very rare.

The IMA is a syndrome that is relatively well defined by the clinical examination procedure. However, whether there is only one or several physiopathological mechanisms involved and at which level in sensorimotor processing the disturbances take place remain unsettled.

Recent electrophysiological studies of human brain activity have established that the late positive component of the evoked potential—the "P300" (approximately 300 msec latency)—is related to cognitive information processing. Indeed, the P300 is visible only when some kind of mental processing, especially stimulus identification followed by response choice, is required (3). Moreover, this wave usually exhibits a high correlation factor with the reaction time (RT). The purpose of this investigation is, therefore, to see whether P300 characteristics are modified in the IMA syndrome and if modifications with respect to the RT could shed some light on the neurophysiological mechanisms involved.

METHODS

Two patients showing a clear IMA syndrome were studied. Both of them were admitted to the Hôpital de la Salpêtrière (Clinique des Maladies du Système Nerveux) for a circumscribed ischemic infarct in the area of the middle cerebral artery (Fig. 1). Both were right-handed and were free from major sensorimotor impairment and from severe aphasia. A group of seven healthy subjects from a previous study (5) has provided data for comparison in task 2 (see below).

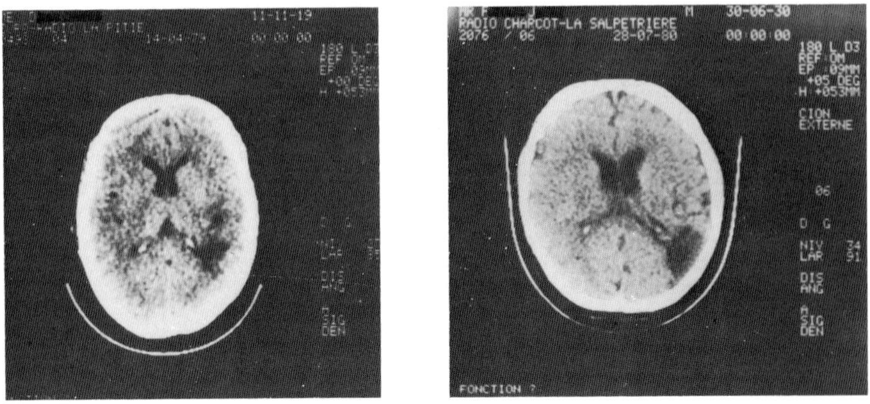

FIG. 1. CT scans of patient Y.D. **(left)** and J.F. **(right),** both showing left parieto-occipital lesions caused by middle cerebral artery thromboses. Sections are 53 mm above the orbitomeatal plane.

The subjects of this control group (CG) were four men and three women, aged between 20 and 36, all right-handed.

Two experimental situations were used:

1. Subjects who fixated on a visual stimulator, had to press one of two buttons, either with the right or with the left index finger, according to the color of the stimulus.
2. The same situation as described above, except that the stimuli appeared either on the right or on the left of a fixation point. If the response (R), still dictated by the color, had to be given on the same side as the stimulus (S) (case 2a), the S–R pairs are said to be matched, since there is a spatial correspondence between the S and the R; if the R was to be given on the side opposite to the S (case 2b), there is a spatial mismatch between the S and the R (5).

These tasks (1, 2a, and 2b) were designed to represent a gradual order of complexity.

Seven collodion-affixed Beckman electrodes were placed on a transverse line extending from the right to the left external auditory meatus with the midline electrode situated on the vertex. The potentials were recorded with respect to a linked earlobe reference. Horizontal and vertical ocular movements were also recorded in order to check that no eye movements were made during the off-axis stimulus presentation.

The time constant of the amplifiers was 1.5 sec, with an upper bandpass limit of 130 Hz. The data were A/D converted on line and later processed on a BGE M40 computer. Data processing consisted of 50 Hz notch filtering, eliminating artifactual S/R pairs and wrong responses, averaging with the stimulus as a trigger, and plotting the results and the corresponding spatial-temporal maps that display simultaneously the amplitude, timing, and topography of electrical events (7).

RESULTS

While they were being tested, both patients exhibited, as did the CG, large P300 components, whatever the task, stimulus, and response location (Fig. 2). But the results from the patients compared to those of the CG differed as far as the P300 and RT were concerned (see Table 1 and Fig. 3).

P300 Component

During task 2, which was also performed by the CG, the topography and amplitude characteristics of the P300 elicited by both patients were not markedly different from those of the CG. Only the latency showed a tendency to be slightly longer (mean P300 latency: 410 msec for Y.D.; 430 msec for J.F.; 349 msec for the CG). For both subjects as well as for the CG, however, a slight but gradual increase in the P300 latency according to the task difficulty was noticed (Fig. 3).

Reaction Time

As opposed to the relatively constant P300 latency described above, the RT of both patients was largely increased with respect to that of the CG (mean values in task 2: 861 msec for Y.D.; 653 msec for J.F.; 443 msec for the CG).

Moreover, the RT also tended to increase with the difficulty of the task, as did the P300 latency. For both patients, this RT increase was much more important than that of the P300 latency, in particular for patient Y.D. It must be also noted that the RT for both patients was longer when responding with their right hand, whatever the task (965 msec versus 759 msec for Y.D.; 710 msec versus 592 msec for J.F.).

DISCUSSION

The following comments can be made concerning the validity of the results.

As mentioned earlier, it was not obvious that the patients could fulfill the tasks designed for normal subjects. In fact, the tasks were accomplished by both patients, providing that they began with the simpler task (task 1), which had not been used for the normal group.

Subject Y.D. (Fig. 2) exhibited noisy responses together with an unstable electrooculogram. In spite of this, the P300 component was clearly observed, because the disturbances were not time-locked with the stimulus, contrary to blinking which very often is and which has been eliminated from the average.

Concerning the results themselves, the most striking effect that differentiates

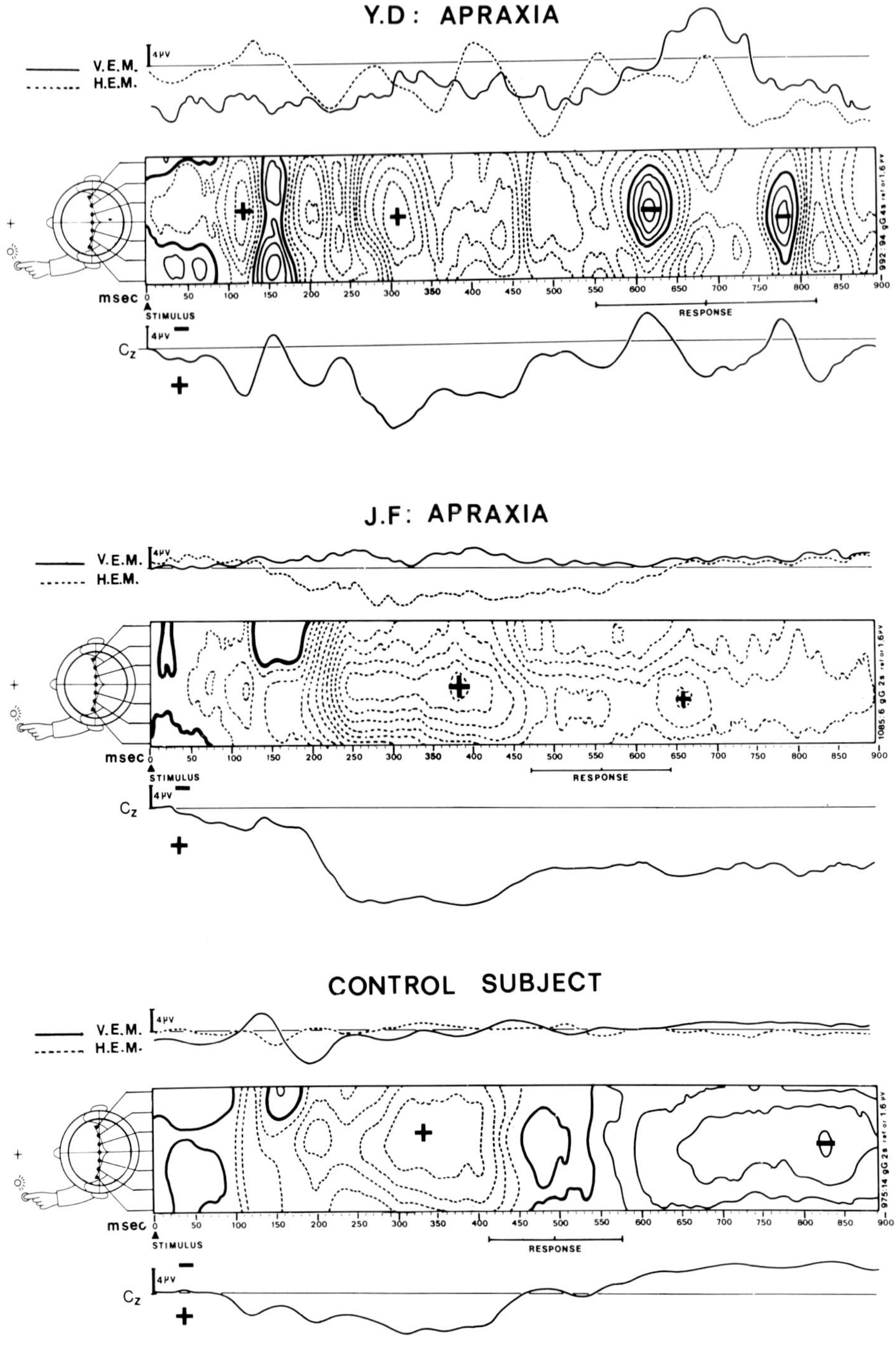

FIG. 2. Examples of averaged spatial-temporal maps showing the P300 component accompanying a left index finger button press after a visual stimulus appearing on the left. Transverse montage, linked earlobes reference; 1.6 μV between *thin isopotential lines; thicker lines* indicate potential zero. Vertical and horizontal electrooculograms above; conventional representation of C_z derivation under each map.

TABLE 1. *Mean value and SD (σ) of RTs and P300 latencies for the two subjects and controls*

	Patient Y.D.			Patient J.F.			7 Controls	
Task	1	2a	2b	1	2a	2b	2a	2b
RT								
mean RT	583	784	939	506	657	645	429	457
σRT[a]	123	138	153	78	137	29	29	26
P300 latency								
mean P300	335	382	439	387	432	430	339	358
σP300[a]							40	32

[a] Standard deviations for the RTs represent interindividual differences (intraindividual differences range from 32 to 97 msec). Standard deviations for the RTs of the patients are intraindividual (calculated from approx. 140 responses). These cannot be given for the P300 latencies, since the data in this case are obtained from only two average spatial-temporal maps (one for a right and one for a left index flexion).

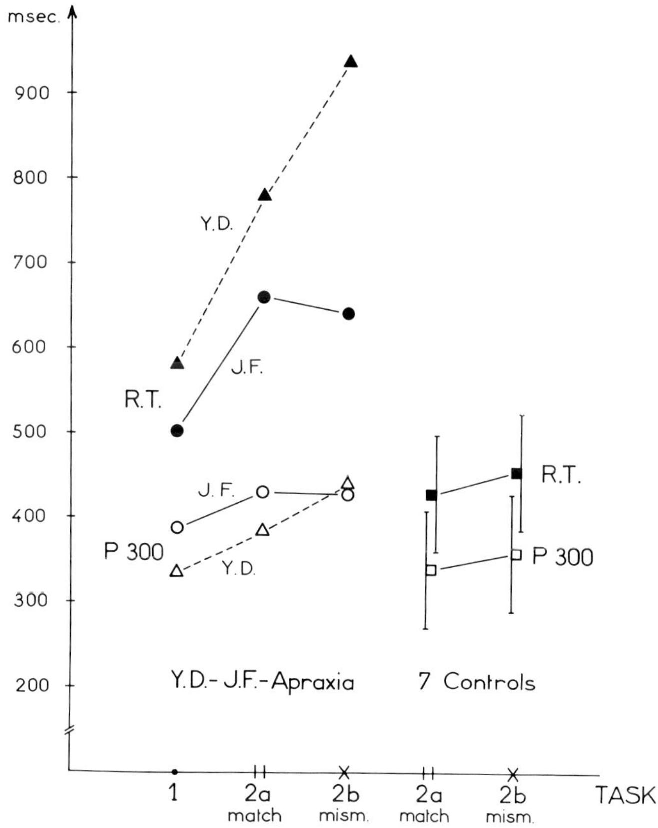

FIG. 3. Averaged data for the two patients **(left)** and for the controls **(right).** P300 and RT are delayed with the difficulty of the task. The P300 latency of the patients is not markedly greater than that of the controls, but their RT is largely increased. Confidence intervals for the controls are indicated by *vertical segments.*

the two patients from the CG is the important lengthening of the RT as opposed to the P300 latency which is not markedly increased.

In fact, the slight lengthening of the P300 latency of both patients (Fig. 3) can be explained, since the patients are older than the controls. Indeed, this difference stays between the limits related to age (8). The generation of P300 is classically known to be linked to the processes associated with stimulus evaluation when there is a decision involved. Moreover, it is generally agreed that the P300 reflects the time taken to evaluate the stimulus sufficiently to perform the task but is independent of the execution of the task itself. Indeed, whenever the motor execution is delayed, the latency of the P300 does not change (4). It has also been shown with normal subjects that when the complexity of the motor execution stage of the task increases, the RT increases too, whereas the latency of the P300 remains the same (6). According to this current interpretation of the P300, it can then be ascertained that the perturbation associated with IMA is not related to the stimulus evaluation stage during which the matching between the stimulus and the required task is accomplished. Thus, the present data seem to rule out afferent theories of IMA and be in favor of IMA being linked rather to the motor execution stage.

The very important lengthening of RTs could reflect several factors. First of all, it has been mentioned that the motor response of both patients was delayed when they were using the right hand. This is probably because of sequelae of right sensorimotor defects and could contribute to the lengthening of RTs as shown in Fig. 3 in which equal numbers of right- and left-hand responses were averaged. Nevertheless, the left-hand RTs are still abnormally increased compared to those of the controls. The effect of age must also be taken into account, since both patients are older than the controls, and it is well known that RTs increase with age. However, the differences observed between both patients and the controls are much too important to be explained by this factor alone (2). It must be recalled that the effect of all brain lesions on reaction times interacts with that of age in such a way that all acquired brain lesions lead to a more pronounced retardation in RT in older patients (1). Therefore, this important RT increase which characterizes our two patients can surely be interpreted as a defect in the motor programming and execution stage of information processing; however, it cannot be concluded so far that the dissociation that permits an abnormally long RT to occur with a normal P300 latency is specific to IMA. This question could be answered by studying patients with other brain lesions and other neuropsychological defects under the same conditions.

SUMMARY

Event-related cerebral potentials and reaction time were studied in two patients with left parietal lesions inducing ideomotor apraxia and in seven control subjects. Results showed no marked increase of P300 latency in the patients with respect to the control group, whereas the RT was largely lengthened. This suggests that the decision-making processes are left intact in IMA and that only the motor execution stage is impaired.

ACKNOWLEDGMENTS

The authors wish to thank Mrs. L. Farrugia, M. T. Martin, and Mr. R. Grob for their technical assistance.

REFERENCES

1. Benton, A. L. (1977): Interactive effects of age and brain disease on reaction time. *Arch. Neurol.,* 34:369–370.
2. Dee, H. L., and Van Allen, M. W. (1973): Speed of decision-making processes in patients with unilateral cerebral disease. *Arch. Neurol.,* 28:163–166.
3. Desmedt, J. E. (1979): *Cognitive Components in Cerebral Event-Related Components and Selective Attention.* Karger, Basel.
4. Kutas, M., McCarthy, G., and Donchin, E. (1977): Augmenting mental chronometry: The P$\overline{300}$ as a measure of stimulus evaluation time. *Science,* 197:792–795.
5. Ragot, R., and Rémond, A. (1979): Event-related scalp potentials during a bimanual choice R.T. task: Topography and interhemispheric relations. In: *Human Evoked Potentials: Applications and Problems,* edited by D. Lehmann and E. Callaway, pp. 303–316. Plenum Press, New York and London.
6. Ragot, R., Renault, B., and Rémond, A. (1981): The P$\overline{300}$, indexing the spatial match–mismatch between stimulus and hand position, but irrelevant to motor spatial programming. In: *EEG Correlates of Information Processing (in press.)* North-Holland, Amsterdam.
7. Rémond, A. (1961): Integrated and topographical analysis of the EEG. *Electroencephalogr. Clin. Neurophysiol.* [*Suppl.*] 20:64–67.
8. Squires, N. K., Goodin, O., and Starr, A. (1979): Event-related potentials in development, aging and dementia. In: *Human Evoked Potentials: Applications and Problems,* edited by D. Lehman and E. Callaway, pp. 383–396. Plenum Press, New York and London.

Clinical Applications of Evoked Potentials in Neurology,
edited by J. Courjon, F. Mauguiere, and M. Revol.
Raven Press, New York © 1982.

Anosognosia with Hemiplegia: Auditory Evoked Potential Studies

*F. Mauguière, **S. Brechard, †J. Pernier, *J. Courjon, and **B. Schott

**EEG Department and **Department of Medical Neurology, Hôpital Neurologique, Lyon, France; and †C.E.M.I., Lyon, France*

Since the first detailed descriptions by Anton (1,2) and Babinski (3–5), it is widely admitted that anosognosia associated with left-sided hemiplegia in right-handed patients cannot be merely the consequence of a somatosensory deafferentation of the minor hemisphere. However, one may hypothesize that sensory deprivation does facilitate the occurrence of this neglect phenomenon, because clinical observations clearly suggest that most of these patients have a left-sided hypesthesia which may be associated with a left visual field defect (see 10 for a review). Moreover, Green and Hamilton (7) demonstrated that the contralateral somatosensory evoked potentials (SEPs) are absent following left median nerve stimulation in these patients. The purpose of this chapter is to examine the topographical organization of the auditory evoked potentials (AEPs) in patients suffering from left-sided hemiplegia associated or not with anosognosia. Auditory evoked potential recording and a dichotic listening test (DLT) were used in order to investigate separately the auditory function of each hemisphere, since clinical examination alone is inappropriate for this kind of study.

PATIENTS AND METHODS

Patients

Ten right-handed patients (seven females, three males; mean age ± SD, 59 ± 14 years) were selected for this study. All of them had a left-sided hemiplegia of vascular origin with a gross left hemianesthesia. In all cases, the N20, P25, P40, and N70 potentials usually evoked in the right parietal region by stimulation of the left median nerve were absent (see F. Mauguiere, A. M. Brunon, J. F. Echallier, and J. Courjon, *this volume* for a description of the SEP recording procedure).

Group I comprised five patients (three females, two males; mean age ± SD, 57 ± 20 years) who had been transiently anosognosic for their hemiplegia; the verbal and behavioral anosognosia was associated with a left-sided asomatognosia in four cases.

In Group II were the five other patients (four females, one male; mean age ± SD, 62.4 ± 11 years) who always remained clearly aware of their motor deficit.

None of the patients had dementia or trouble with consciousness. A left lateral homonymous hemianopsia was observed in six patients; four of them belonged to group I. A left-sided visual extinction was noted in one patient of group II.

Evoked Potential Recording Procedure

Somatosensory and auditory EP recording sessions were carried out 2 weeks to 3 months after the onset of the disease. All the patients of group I had recovered a full consciousness of their hemiplegia when the EP study was performed. In both groups, the left hemiplegia and hemianesthesia were still present in all cases.

The procedure described by Peronnet et al. (15) was used for the recording of AEPs. The patients were lying in a dimly lit sound-treated room. Auditory stimuli were 1,000 Hz 80 db SL tones of 150 msec duration (rise and fall times, 10 msec) delivered at a rate of 1/sec randomly to the right or left ear through the same earphone. Eight disk electrodes were regularly spaced from the right to the left mastoids, the two upper ones being situated 1 cm apart from C_Z on each side; the reference electrode was placed on the tip of the nose and the ground on the forehead. The EEG was amplified by eight 7P5 Grass amplifiers with a filter band-pass of 1 to 35 Hz. The averaging was conducted on line by means of a LABO 16 computer (11): 500 to 1,000 sweeps were averaged for each ear with an analysis time of 360 msec (512 samples).

CT Scans

CT scans were available for eight patients, three in group I and five in group II. The size and sites of lesions were evaluated using the atlas of De Armond et al. (6).

Dichotic Listening Test

A DLT with pairs of figures, words, and short sentences was performed in eight subjects (three in group I, five in group II).

RESULTS

AEP Study

In both groups of patients, the topographical organization of AEPs on the vertex and left hemisphere were identical, for both ears, to those described by

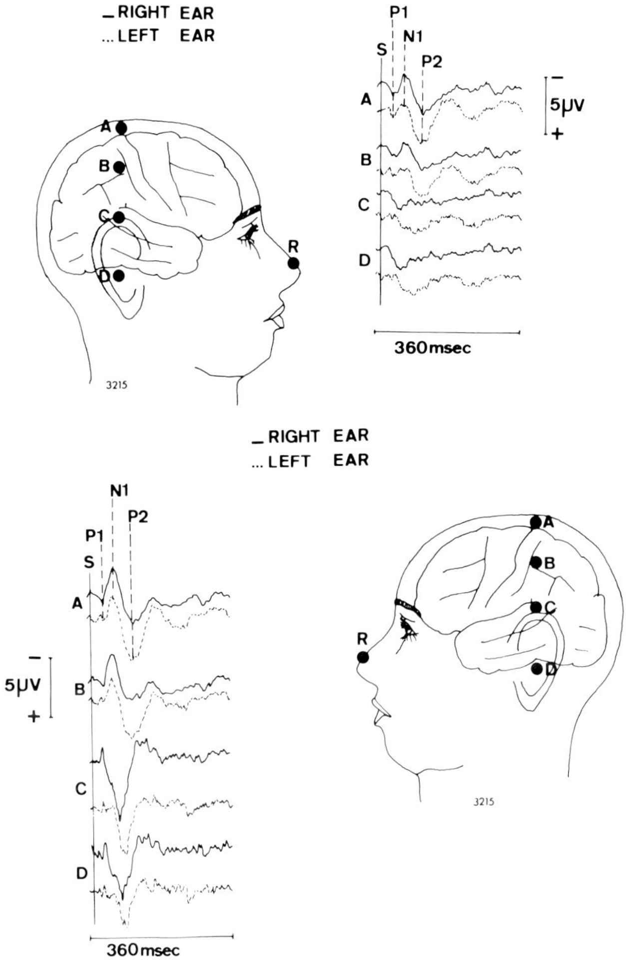

FIG. 1. Auditory evoked potentials in a patient with anosognosia and left-sided hemiplegia. In the right temporal region, auditory evoked responses are lowered in amplitude. (The CT scan of this patient is in C in Fig. 3.)

Peronnet et al. (15) using the same recording technique in the same laboratory. The vertex response was a P_1, N_1, P_2 complex according to Picton's nomenclature (16), and an aspect of polarity reversal was present over the left temporal region (Figs. 1 and 2).

The two groups of patients were clearly different as to their right temporal AEPs. In patients in group I (with anosognosia), no aspect of phase reversal was observed at the level of the right sylvian fissure (T_4 electrode), and no potential was recorded by right temporal and mastoid electrodes (Fig. 1). In patients in group II (without anosognosia), the topographical organization of the AEP's was symmetrical over the right and left hemispheres (Fig. 2). No difference was found in either group between left ear and right ear stimulations.

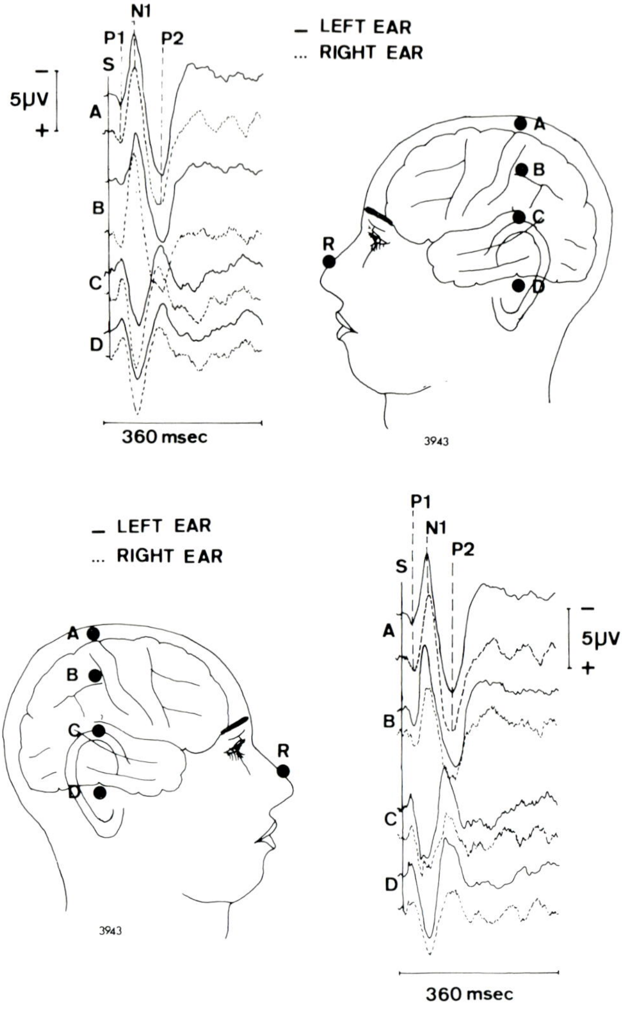

FIG. 2. Auditory evoked potentials in a patient without anosognosia (case B in Fig. 4). Note the symmetrical responses in the temporal regions.

CT Scans

In the eight patients with CT scans, the sites of the lesions also differed between the two groups. Of the three patients in group I, two had large cortical and subcortical ischemic lesions of the right temporal lobe involving the auditory cortex of the minor hemisphere (Fig. 3A,B).

The remaining patient of this group (Fig. 3C) had undamaged temporal cortex on the right side, but the auditory fibers running from the medial geniculate

A
B
C

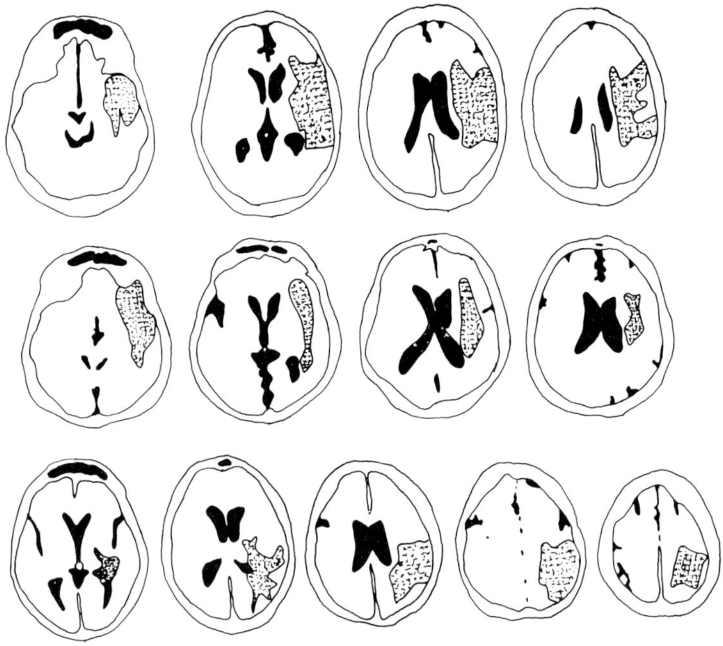

FIG. 3. CT scan data in patients in group I (with anosognosia). Only the slices that demonstrated abnormalities *(hatched areas)* are represented for each patient.

body to the right auditory cortex were probably interrupted at the level of the temporal isthmus.

In five patients in group II (Fig. 4), neither the right auditory cortex nor the auditory geniculo–cortical fibers were obviously damaged.

In agreement with clinical and SEP data, the somesthetic thalamo–cortical pathways and/or the parietal cortex were damaged on the right side in all patients.

Dichotic Listening Test

In all tested patients, an extinction phenomenon was observed for left ear stimulation.

DISCUSSION

Our data suggest that in right-handed patients with left hemiplegia and absent cortical SEPs over the minor hemisphere, the occurrence of anosognosia may be correlated with absent cortical AEPs over the right temporal lobe. Much controversy still exists as to the number and the location of the generators of the AEPs recorded on the scalp during the 40 to 200 msec following the stimula-

A

B

C

D

E

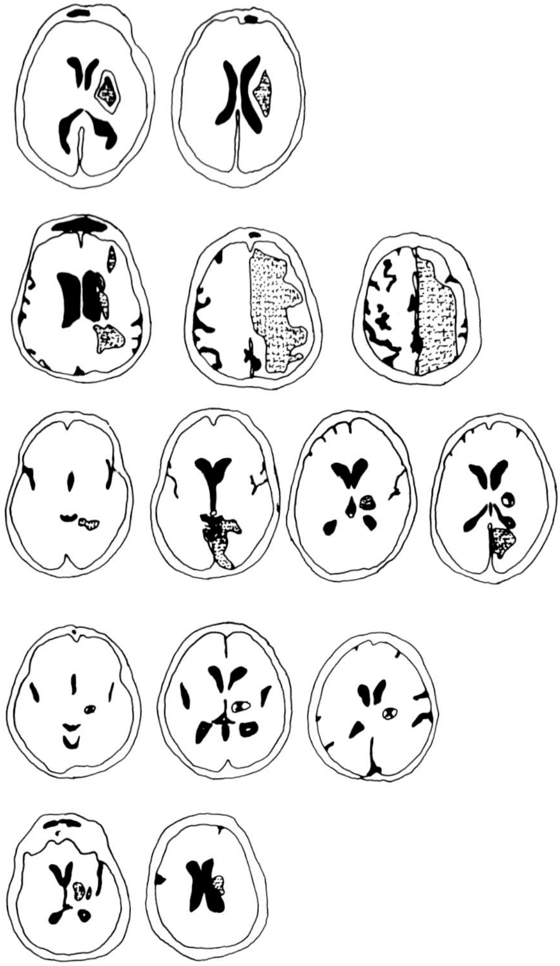

FIG. 4. CT scan data in patients of group II (without anosognosia). Same representation as for Fig. 3.

tion (for a review see refs. 8 and 9). Recently, Knight et al. (9) reported normal N_1 amplitudes in one case of bilateral destruction of primary auditory cortex and observed a bilateral lowering of amplitude of the N_1 potential in patients with unilateral temporal–parietal lesions. In our patients, we did not study the amplitudes of the N_1 potential recorded with each lead statistically since, with our recording technique, the reduction of AEP amplitudes and the absence of phase reversal at the mastoid electrode were obvious over the damaged hemisphere in patients in group I. Previously published electroclinical studies using the same recording technique in patients with unilateral hemispheric lesions are in agreement with our findings and lend substance to the idea that a clear-cut asymmetry between the AEPs recorded in the temporal regions is associated with damaged or deafferented auditory cortex on the side where AEPs are absent or lowered in amplitude (12–14).

A second step in the interpretation would be to conclude that the right hemisphere did not process normally auditory inputs in patients in group I (with anosognosia). The results of AEPs, DLT, and CT scans converge to support the view that such a defect was present in anosognosic patients, but psychophysical evidence of normal auditory function of the right hemisphere is lacking in patients in group II, since an extinction of the left ear was observed in all of these cases. However, DLT may certainly reveal an impairment of auditory input processing by the minor hemisphere in patients without anatomical damage to the primary or associative auditory cortex (12). In such cases, the left ear extinction phenomenon may be caused by an interhemispheric disconnection or equivalent to a lateralized sensory neglect, both interpretations that may be valid in our patients in group II.

The last point to be discussed is the existence of a pathophysiological link among AEP abnormalities, defect of auditory input processing by the right hemisphere, and anosognosia itself. Since the lesion sites largely differed between our two groups of patients, one may suppose that other structures than those involved in the processing of sensory inputs by the minor hemisphere were selectively damaged in patients with anosognosia and spared in the other group. Moreover, in the five patients in group I, DLT, SEP, and AEP abnormalities persisted when the anosognosia had completely cleared, and four of them were still hemianopic on the left side. This strongly suggests that plurimodal deafferentation of the minor hemisphere is not sufficient, per se, to produce anosognosia in left hemiplegic patients. However, such a deafferentation could facilitate the occurrence of anosognosia in the acute stage of the disease, since when the minor hemisphere is deprived of visual and somesthetic imputs with spared auditory afferences, anosognosia does not occur.

To conclude, it must be emphasized that evoked potential studies may help to elucidate the pathophysiology of asomatognosia even though they are not appropriate to investigate the mechanisms underlying the recovery of a full consciousness of hemiplegia.

REFERENCES

1. Anton, G. (1898): Ueber Herderkrankungen des Gehirns, die von Patienten selbst nicht wahrgenommen werden. *Wien Med. Wochenschr.*, 48:1282–1283.
2. Anton, G. (1899): Ueber die Selbstwahrnehmung der Herderkrankungen des Gehirns den Kranken bei Rindenblindheit und Rindentaubheit. *Arch. Psychiatr. Nervenkr.*, 32:86–127.
3. Babinski, J. (1914): Contributions à l'étude des troubles mentaux dans l'hémiplégie cérébrale (anosognosie). *Rev. Neurol.*, 27:845–847.
4. Babinski, J. (1918): Anosognosie. *Rev. Neurol.*, 31:365–367.
5. Babinski, J. (1923): Sur l'anosognosie. *Rev. Neurol.*, 36:731–732.

6. De Armond, J. J., Fusco, M. M., and Devwey, M. M. (1976): *A Photographic Atlas: Structure of the Human Brain, Second Edition.* Oxford University Press, New York.
7. Green, J. B., and Hamilton, W. J. (1976): Anosognosia for hemiplegia: Somatosensory evoked potential studies. *Neurology,* 26:1141–1144.
8. Hillyard, S. A., and Picton, T. W. (1979): Event-related brain potentials and selective information process in in man. In: *Progress in Clinical Neurophysiology, Vol. 6, Cognitive Components in Cerebral Event-Related Potentials and Selective Attention,* edited by J. E. Desmedt, pp. 1–52. Karger, Basel.
9. Knight, R. T., Hillyard, S. A., Woods, D. L., and Neville, H. T. (1980): The effects of frontal and temporal–parietal lesions on the auditory evoked potential in man. *Electroencephalogr. Clin. Neurophysiol.,* 50:112–124.
10. Lhermitte, F., and Cambier, J. (1960): Les perturbations somatognosiques en pathologie nerveuse. In: *Congrès de Psychiatrie et de Neurologie de Langue Française, LVIIIème Session, Lille,* pp. 465–544. Masson, Paris.
11. Maraval, G., Pernier, J., Peronnet, F., Echallier, J. F., Gerin, P., and Mauguière, F. (1980): EVØQ: système configurable de stimulation automatique et d'enregistrement des potentiels évoqués moyens sur mini-ordinateur. *Int. J. Biomed. Comput.,* 11:225–239.
12. Michel, F., and Peronnet, F. (1974): Extinction gauche au test dichotique, lésion hémisphérique ou lésion commissurale? (Apport de l'étude des potentiels évoqués acoustiques). In: *Les Syndromes de Disconnexion Calleuse Çhez l'Homme,* edited by F. Michel and B. Schott, pp. 85–117. Colloque International de Lyon, SPCM, Lyon.
13. Michel, F., Peronnet, F., Labourel, D., and Martin, M. (1973): Confrontation entre les données du test d'écoute dichotique et les données de l'enregistrement des potentiels évoqués acoustiques dans divers cas d'aphasie. *Rev. Neurol.,* 129:295–296.
14. Peronnet, F., and Michel, F. (1977): The asymmetry of the auditory evoked potentials in normal man and in patients with brain lesions. In: *Progress in Clinical Neurophysiology, Vol. 2, Auditory Evoked Potentials in Man, Psychopharmacology Correlates of E.P.s,* edited by J. E. Desmedt, pp. 130–141. Karger, Basel.
15. Peronnet, F., Michel, F., Echallier, J. F., and Girod, J. (1974): Coronal topography of human auditory evoked responses. *Electroencephalogr. Clin. Neurophysiol.,* 37:225–230.
16. Picton, T. W., Hillyard, S. A., Krausz, H. I., and Galambos, R. (1974): Human auditory evoked potentials. Evaluation of components. *Electroencephalogr. Clin. Neurophysiol.,* 36:179–190.

Clinical Applications of Evoked Potentials in Neurology,
edited by J. Courjon, F. Mauguiere, and M. Revol.
Raven Press, New York © 1982.

Long-Latency Event-Related Potentials in Normal Aging and Dementia

*Karl Syndulko, *Edward C. Hansch, *Stanley N. Cohen, *James W. Pearce, *Zev Goldberg, *Barbara Montan, *Wallace W. Tourtellotte, and **Alfred R. Potvin

**Neurology and Research Services, VA Wadsworth Medical Center, Los Angeles, California 90073 and Department of Neurology, University of California at Los Angeles School of Medicine, Los Angeles, California 90024; and **Department of Bioengineering, University of Texas, Arlington, Texas 76019*

Recent reports have suggested that P300, a long-latency endogenous component of the auditory event-related potential (ERP) to low-probability target stimuli, shows progressive increases in latency in healthy adults with advancing age (2). Healthy, elderly subjects showed significantly prolonged P300 latencies as compared to young subjects (1,7). The P300 component was thought to reflect age-related changes in orienting (7) or other aspects of cognitive function (1,2). A potential clinical application for P300 was reported for the diagnosis and evaluation of dementia (3,8) and other neurocognitive disorders (6).

The present study was designed as a partial replication of the work of Goodin et al. (3) in assessing the utility of P300 in the diagnosis of dementia of the Alzheimer type. To this end, we also report control data on normal aging effects over the adult range for P300 and other components of the auditory ERP.

METHODS

The patient group ($N = 12$, mean age = 66.9 years, range 50 to 84 years) was selected on the basis of a clinical neurological diagnosis of moderate progressive dementia of unknown etiology (presumed Alzheimer type) and Folstein mini-mental-state (MMS) scores less than 27 (mean = 20.9; SD = 4.2). Only patients able to clearly differentiate the tone pip frequencies were included. Normal controls ($N = 45$, mean age = 49 years, range 18 to 85 years) were recruited from hospital and community sources and were selected on the basis of a brief medical screening questionnaire and evaluation and Folstein MMS scores of 30. Criteria for inclusion of controls included an absence of a history of signs or symptoms of major neurological or medical disorders.

For the auditory ERP, recordings were made at F_z, C_z, and P_z and referenced to linked mastoid electrodes. Electrodes above and below the right eye were used to record electrooculograms (EOG) in order to monitor blinks and other electrooculographic artifacts. The amplifier bandpass was 0.04 to 60 Hz (3 dB points).

The stimulus paradigm was a target detection or "odd-ball" paradigm. Tone pips (1,000 Hz or 2,000 Hz, 50 msec duration, 5 msec rise–fall time, and 95 dB SPL) were presented binaurally from a tape recorder at the rate of 1 per 1.5 sec. A run consisted of a sequence of 400 tone pips in which 85% were 1,000 Hz (common or nontarget tone) and 15% were 2,000 Hz (rare or target tone), with the two stimulus types randomly intermixed. The subjects' task was to maintain a running mental count of the number of rare tone pip occurrences which was reported at the end of each run sequence. Three identical runs were presented.

The ERP waveforms were averaged for 1,000 msec with a 1 msec dwell initiated by a trigger pulse 95 msec prior to tone pip onset. Separate averages of 20 to 40 trials each were obtained for ERP to the rare (runs 1 and 2) and common (run 3) tone pips. Trials in which electrical artifacts, including eye movements, exceeded the analog-to-digital converter input voltage range were automatically excluded from the averages.

Latencies of the N100, P200, and P300 ERP components to the rare stimulus only were derived by intersecting visually "best-fit" slope lines on either side of the component peaks and by using the points of intersection as component latency. Amplitudes were measured both peak to peak (for N100–P200) and base to peak (for all components). Base line was defined as the average waveform voltage over the 95-msec epoch prior to tone pip onset.

RESULTS

Normal Controls

Figure 1 shows grand mean waveforms to the rare stimulus for the five oldest (mean age = 80.6 years) and five youngest (mean age = 21.4 years) normal controls. The ERP waveform configurations are essentially the same, except that older subjects show prolonged P200 and P300 latencies and reduced amplitudes for P300.

Separate linear regressions of age versus components N100, P200, and P300 for the three electrode sites (F_z, C_z, and P_z) were performed for both latency and amplitude measures. Significant age-related latency increases were obtained for P200 at all three electrode sites. Pearson product–moment correlation coefficients *(r)* were 0.54, 0.50, and 0.51 for the F_2, C_z, and P_z sites, respectively; $p < 0.01$ at all sites. No significant linear regression effects were found for N100 latency. Figure 2 shows the normal latency data and regression results for P200 and N100. Aging effects were also noted for N100 and P200 amplitude, although the correlation coefficients were smaller and the standard errors of estimate about the regression line were relatively larger. Significant negative correlations

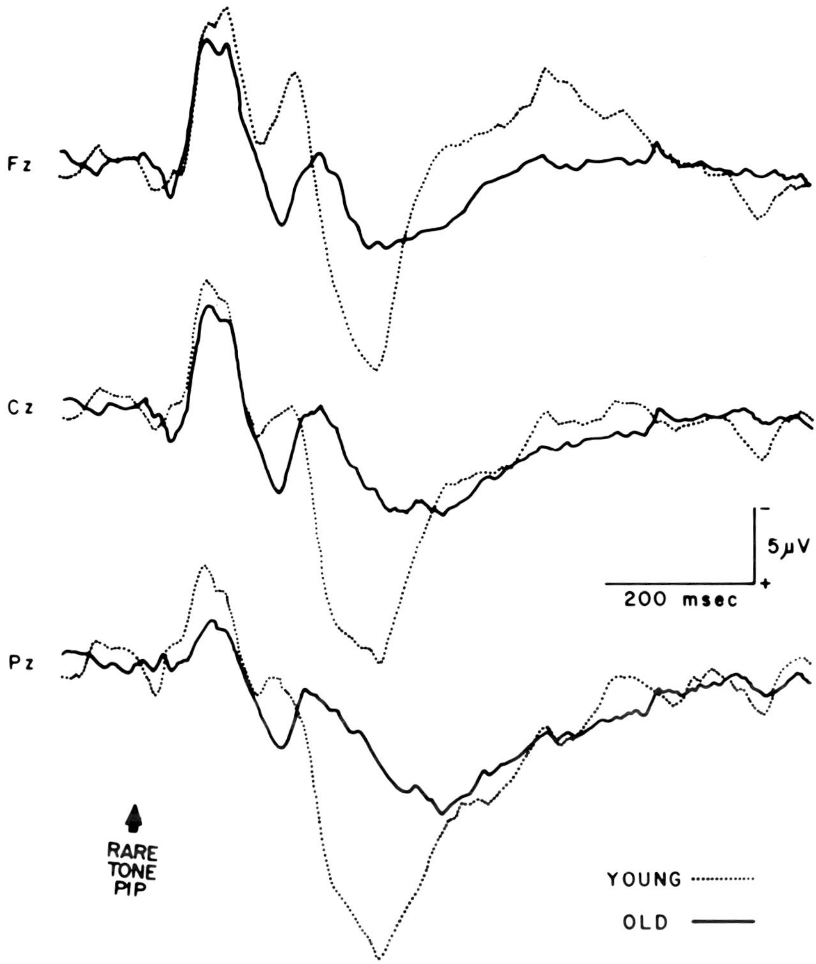

FIG. 1. Grand mean ERP waveforms for the five oldest and five youngest normal controls in response to the rare tone pip.

with age were found for N100 amplitude only at P_z ($r = 0.45$, $p < 0.01$). The P200 amplitude showed significant positive correlations with age (i.e., P200 amplitude increased with increasing age) at F_z and C_z ($r = 0.50$ and 0.41, respectively; $p < 0.01$).

The strongest correlations with age were found for P300. Latency of P300 increased with increasing age at all three sites ($r = 0.50$, 0.63, and 0.68 for F_z, C_z, and P_z sites, respectively, $p < 0.01$ at all sites). The slopes of the regression equations for P300 provided an index of the magnitude of latency shift with age and equaled 0.7, 1.0, and 1.1 msec per year for F_z, C_z, and P_z, respectively. Figure 3 shows P300 latency recorded at P_z plotted as a function of age for

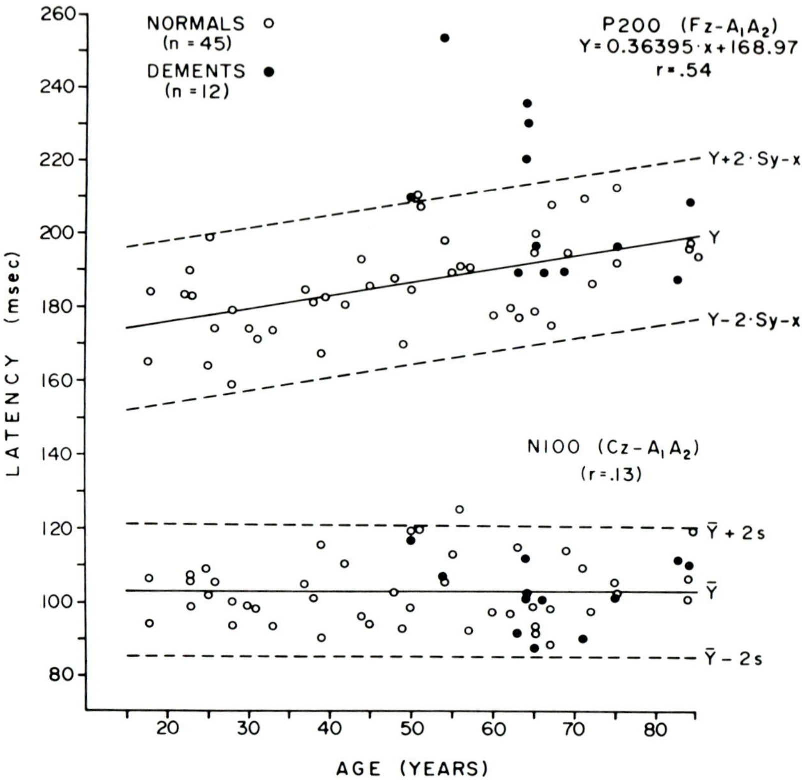

FIG. 2. N100 and P200 latencies measured on ERP waveforms to the rare tone pip for 45 normal controls and 12 dementia patients. The linear regression line for both components is displayed along with limits for plus and minus 2 standard errors of the estimate *($S_{y \cdot x}$)* for the regression lines. Also indicated are the respective regression equations in the form $Y = AX + B$ and the Pearson product–moment correlation coefficients *(r)* for age versus latency.

the normal group regression line and two standard errors of the estimate (1 $S_{y \cdot x}$ = 22.4 msec) around the regression line are shown. Two normals had P300 latencies greater than two standard errors from the regression line. This is within the number expected by chance (2.25 expected for each 45 subjects).

Patients

Figure 4 shows grand mean waveforms for the dementia patients and a subgroup of age-matched normal controls. The most striking difference in waveforms between the groups is for the P300 component. The latency data for the 12 dementia patients are plotted in Fig. 2 for component N100 at C_z and P200 at F_z, the respective electrode sites of maximum age effects in normals. None of the patients showed abnormal latencies (i.e., greater than two standard errors

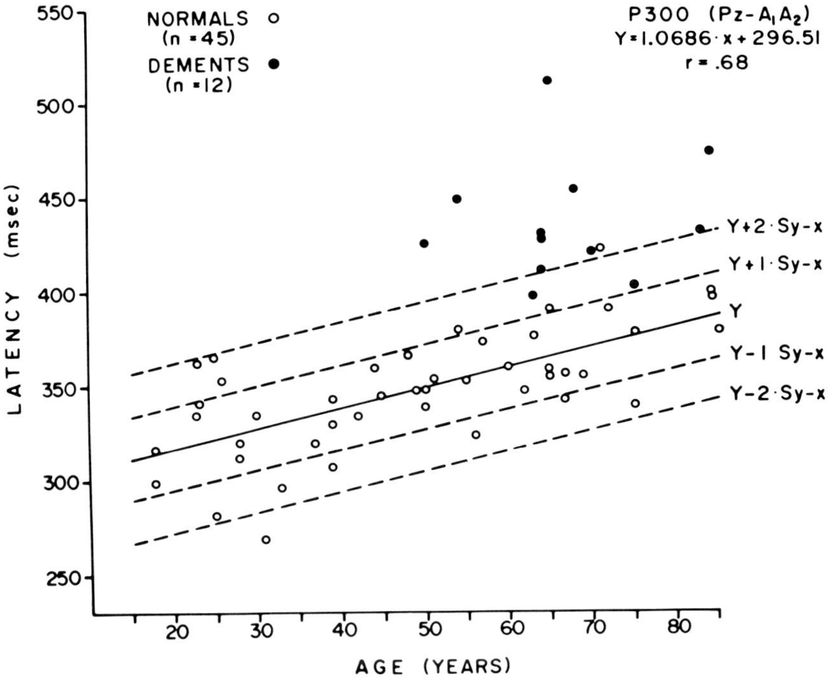

FIG. 3. P300 latencies measured from the rare tone pip ERP waveforms for 45 normals and 12 dementia patients. The linear regression line for P300 latency is displayed along with limits for plus and minus 2 standard errors of the estimate *($S_{y \cdot x}$)* for the regression line. Also indicated is the regression equation in the form $Y = AX + B$ and the Pearson product–moment correlation coefficient *(r)* for age versus latency.

above the regression line at their age) for N100. Five of the patients (42 %) showed abnormal P200 latencies at P_z. The remaining patients all fell within one standard error for P200.

Maximum differentiation between patients and controls was found for P300 latency. The latency data at P_z for patients is also plotted in Fig. 3. At P_z and C_z electrode sites, 10 of the 12 patients (83%) showed abnormal P300 latencies, whereas nine of 12 showed abnormal latencies at F_z. For P300 at P_z, the mean deviation from the controls' regression line was 3.05 standard error units. A comparison of abnormal responses for P300 and P200 latencies showed that all five patients with abnormal P200 were also abnormal on P300.

DISCUSSION

The ERP data for normal aging controls confirm, in most respects, the findings reported by others. Both P200 and P300 latency showed significant positive correlations with age in agreement with Goodin et al. (2). The correlation coeffi-

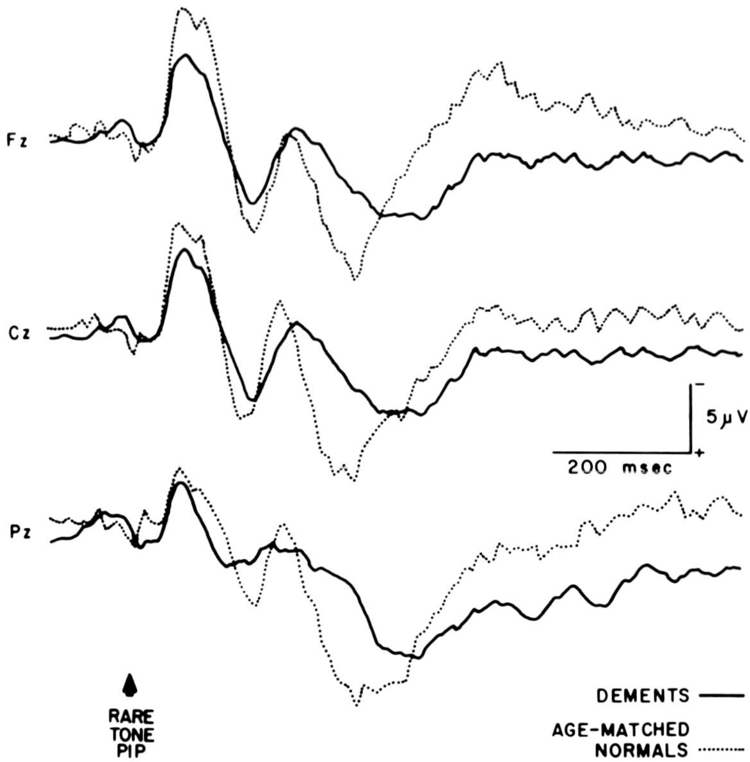

FIG. 4. Grand mean ERP waveforms for the 12 dementia patients and for a subgroup of 12 normal controls age-matched to the patients.

cients and the maximal slopes of the regression lines were somewhat less than reported by Goodin et al. (2). This was especially the case for P300 (1.1 msec/year versus 1.8 msec/year). Differences in composition of the normal control group, especially in regard to the mental status of older subjects, could conceivably account for these variations. We found no significant change in N100 latency with age, again in agreement with other results (2,4,5). Similarly, results for P300 amplitude were nearly identical to those of Goodin et al. (2), with both studies finding a significant decrease with age. We found significant decreases in N100 amplitude and significant increases in P200 amplitude with age. No significant N100–P200 amplitude effect was found; Goodin et al. (2) reported a decrease in N100–P200 amplitude with aging.

Our N100 and P200 results for the dementia patients are also in substantial agreement with those of Goodin et al. (3). Using P300 latency abnormality as a criterion, 83% of the dementia patients were correctly classified in the present study. None of the patients showed abnormal N100 latency, whereas five patients showed abnormal P200 latency. However, the patients with P200 abnormalities also showed abnormal P300. Thus, P200 did not add useful diagnostic information. The patients in the present study were diagnosed as suffering dementia of the Alzheimer type and were of moderate severity. The results support the potential diagnostic utility of P300 in dementia. Goodin et al. (3) have indicated that P300 latency is abnormal in dementia patients regardless of etiology, implying that it is not a useful tool in the differential diagnosis of dementia. However, recent data suggest that P300 may have a role in differentiating the etiology of cognitive impairment in questions of functional versus primary dementing disorders (8). The eventual utility for P300 in such major diagnostic problems as differentiating mild cognitive deficits in the elderly as resulting primarily from depression or other reversible causes versus the initial stages of a progressive dementing disease awaits future study. The general sensitivity of P300 to mild cognitive deficits in early dementia also has yet to be assessed.

ACKNOWLEDGMENTS

We thank Mark Ivey for technical assistance, Karen Cohen for editorial assistance, and Diane Guntrip and Diane Varnas for clerical assistance. The research was supported by the Neurology Research Service.

REFERENCES

1. Ford, J. M., and Pfefferbaum, A. (1980): The utility of brain potentials in determining age-related changes in central nervous system and cognitive functioning. In: *Aging in the 1980s,* edited by L. W. Poon, pp. 115–124. American Psychological Association, Washington.
2. Goodin, D., Squires, K., Henderson, B., and Starr, A. (1978): Age-related variations in evoked potentials to auditory stimuli in normal human subjects. *Electroencephalogr. Clin. Neurophysiol.,* 44:447–458.
3. Goodin, D., Squires, K., and Starr, A. (1978): Long latency event related components of the auditory evoked potential in dementia. *Brain,* 101:635–648.
4. Pfefferbaum, A., Ford, J. M., Roth, W. T., Hopkins, W. F. III, and Kopell, B. S. (1979): Event-related potential changes in healthy aged females. *Electroencephalogr. Clin. Neurophysiol.,* 46:81–86.
5. Pfefferbaum, A., Ford, J. M., Roth, W. T., and Kopell, B. S. (1980): Age-related changes in auditory event-related potentials. *Electroencephalogr. Clin. Neurophysiol.,* 49:266–276.
6. Pfefferbaum, A., Horvath, T. B., Roth, W. T., and Kopell, B. A. (1979): Event-related potential changes in chronic alcoholics. *Electroencephalogr. Clin. Neurophysiol.,* 47:637–647.
7. Smith, D. B. D., Thompson, L. W., and Michalewski, H. J. (1980): Averaged evoked potential research in adult aging—status and prospects. In: *Aging in the 1980s,* edited by L. W. Poon, pp. 135–151. American Psychological Association, Washington.
8. Squires, K. C., Chippendale, T.J., Wrege, K. S., Goodin, D. S., and Starr, A. (1980): Electrophysiological assessment of mental function in aging and dementia. In: *Aging in the 1980s,* edited by L. W. Poon, pp. 125–134. American Psychological Association, Washington.

Clinical Applications of Evoked Potentials in Neurology,
edited by J. Courjon, F. Mauguiere, and M. Revol.
Raven Press, New York © 1982.

Evoked Potentials in the Assessment of Brain Function in Senile Dementia

*S. Laurian, *J.-M. Gaillard, and **J. Wertheimer

**Clinique Psychiatrique Universitaire de Lausanne, CH-1008 Prilly, Switzerland; and*
***Hôpital Psycho-Gériatrique de Prilly, CH-1008 Prilly, Switzerland*

A number of investigations have been devoted to the study of EPs in aging; only a few of them, however, concern the modifications of EPs in senile dementia. Straumanis et al. (13), in subjects with severe arteriosclerotic cognitive disorders, and Visser et al. (15), in patients suffering from a degenerative senile dementia, found increased latencies of some late components of VEPs. Similar observations were made by Hendrickson et al. (5) for AEPs and Levy et al. (9) for SEPs (especially for the N50 wave). These last authors also reported that the peak 5 (negative, mean latency = 89 msec) was often absent or very flat in senile demented patients. Goodin et al. (4) found a significant correlation between the cognitive disorders in dementia and the increased latency and diminished amplitude of P300. A more functional approach was used by Gerson et al. (3); by studying the interhemispheric covariance of the AEPs, they showed that the two hemispheres of the brain are significantly less well coordinated in senile patients than in normal aged subjects.

In our studies, we investigated many facets of brain evoked electrical activity: (a) the topographical aspect of responses to visual stimuli; (b) the differences among the reactivity to stimuli pertaining to various sensory modalities; and (c) the fast habituation to auditory stimuli. We present here the results of two studies on the modifications of EPs in senile dementia.

A preliminary study (7) was performed in 12 patients with a diagnosis of senile dementia and in 12 young controls. The VEPs to flashes were recorded at C_z and O_z. Significant topographical differences between patients and controls were observed; in several patients, the VEPs at the vertex were of very low amplitude or missing, whereas the VEPs at the occipital lead were quite similar to the VEPs recorded in controls. The most altered vertex responses were observed in patients suffering from Alzheimer's disease or a senile dementia evolving towards an Alzheimer condition.

FIRST STUDY

The aims of this investigation were: (a) to verify the observations made in the preliminary study; (b) to examine the correlations between the modifications of EPs and the clinical diagnosis; (c) to investigate the responses to another sensory modality (auditory); and (d) to have a control group matched for age.

Method

Subjects were 10 patients suffering from a simple senile dementia (SD), seven patients presenting an Alzheimer's disease or a senile dementia evolving towards an Alzheimer condition (AD), and five nondemented controls. Mean age was 83.4 years for SD (range 71–94), 73.5 years for AD (range 67–84) and 73.3 years for controls (range 68–77). The brain electrical activity was recorded using monopolar leads with occipital (O_z) and vertex (C_z) active electrodes and a reference on the linked ear lobes. After a proper amplification of the signals with a Grass 78 EEG polygraph, data were stored on magnetic tape (PCM System) and processed off line with a Nicolet Med-80 System. For each subject, 128 visually evoked responses to flashes delivered at 0.5 cps, intensity 4, by a Grass PS2 Photostimulator were averaged, as well as 128 auditory evoked responses to tone pips of 1,000 Hz, 75 dB SL delivered at 0.5 cps by a loudspeaker placed behind the subject's head.

The individual averaged responses were superimposed and plotted separately by group, sensory modality, and scalp electrode site; the grand mean EPs averaged across the subjects were also obtained by group, sensory modality, and scalp electrode site.

Results

The superimposed individual averages to flashes showed a considerable interindividual variability of the waveforms in the occipital region (Fig. 1). However, the configuration of the grand means was quite similar for the three groups. At the vertex, by contrast, the responses in the AD group differed strikingly from those recorded in the SD and controls. In these last two groups, the VEPs presented the usual configuration with a N_1–P_2 component always identifiable, whereas in the AD group, the N_1–P_2 component was almost not discernible or completely missing, being replaced on the grand mean curve by a positive wave of low amplitude. The interindividual variability was greater in SD than in controls.

The profile of AEPs was quite different (Fig. 2). At the occipital lead, the response was not discernible, whereas at the vertex, the waveforms had a similar configuration in the three groups. A response was present in all subjects, including the AD patients. The N_1 and P_2 latencies were longer in both patient groups than in controls.

SECOND STUDY

The aim of this investigation was to evaluate brain function in senile dementia by studying the fast habituation to auditory stimuli.

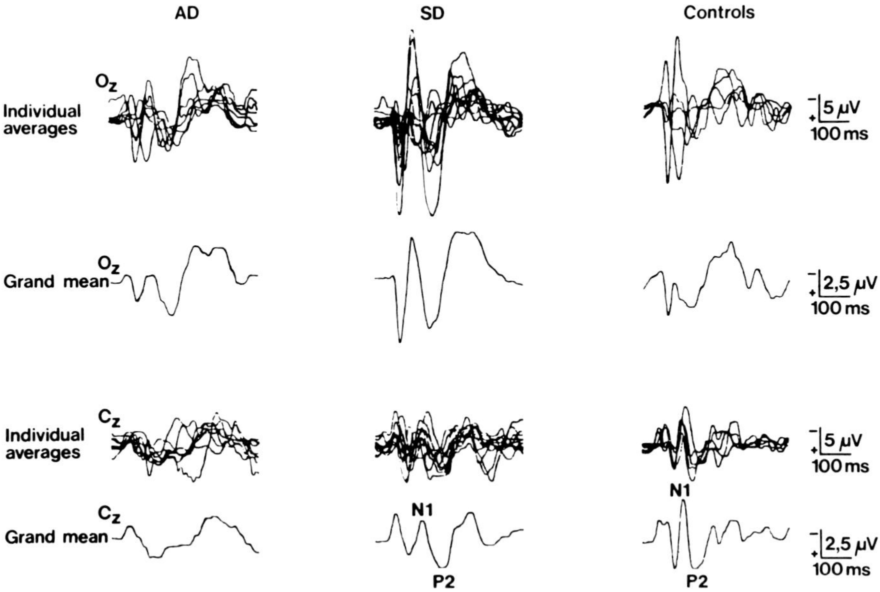

FIG. 1. Visual EPs in AD patients ($N = 7$), SD patients ($N = 10$), and control subjects matched for age ($N = 5$). Individual averages of 128 responses are superimposed by group and scalp electrode site; below the individual traces are represented the grand mean waveforms.

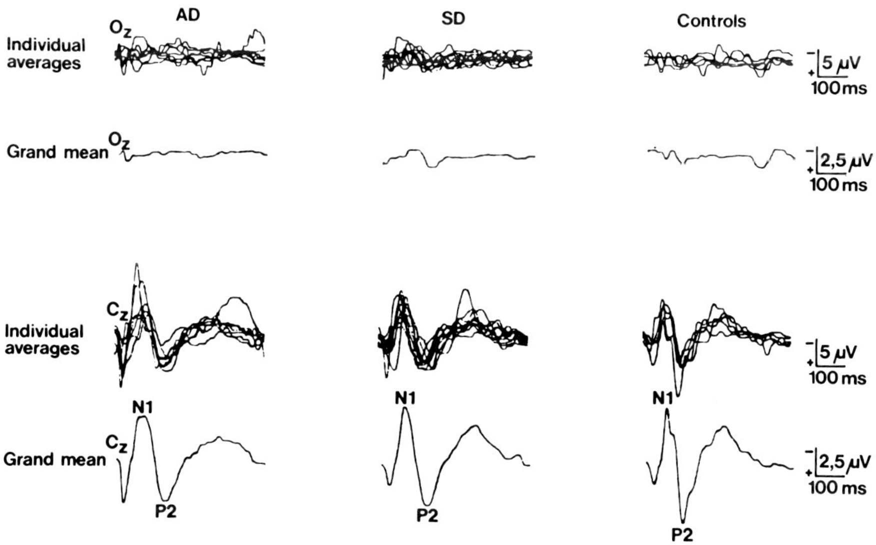

FIG. 2. Auditory EPs in AD patients ($N = 7$), SD patients ($N = 10$), and control subjects matched for age ($N = 5$). Individual averages of 128 responses are superimposed by group and scalp electrode site; below the individual traces are represented the grand mean waveforms.

Habituation can be defined as a decline in the size of response with repetitive stimulation; it may be considered as an apprenticeship to prevent needless stereotyped responses to repeating stimuli.

The fast habituation is a reduction in EP amplitude that occurs when less than 10 sec elapse between presentations of stimuli and is generalized to most components from 100 to 300 msec (1). It can be demonstrated by presenting trains of two or more stimuli separated by 2 sec, with intertrain intervals of 10 sec or more. Generally, the amplitude of the stimulus occuring second or later in the train represents about 50% of the amplitude of the first one (12). This form of habituation was not studied in psychogeriatric patients.

Method

Subjects were 18 young adults (mean age 24.2 years, range 21–40) and 15 senile patients (mean age 78.7 years, range 64–89). Of these patients, 12 suffered from a simple senile dementia, and three presented a senile dementia evolving towards an Alzheimer condition. Ten patients and eight controls (first series) received 12 trains of 5 tone pips (1,000 Hz, 20 msec duration) presented by a loudspeaker situated behind the subject's head. In an attempt to enhance the signal-to-noise ratio, a second series of five patients and 10 controls received 32 trains of clicks presented by earphones. The intertrain interval was 10 sec, and the interstimulus interval was 2 sec; the stimulus intensity was 70 dB SL. The brain electrical activity was recorded at the vertex with a reference on the linked earlobes and stored on FM analog magnetic tape using a 3968A HP recorder. The EEG amplification with a low-frequency cutoff at 1 Hz and a high-frequency cutoff at 70 Hz was provided by a Grass Model 8–18 EEG. The stored data were submitted to a second filtering (active filters with an attenuation of 40 dB between 30 and 38 Hz) and processed using a Nicolet Med-80 System.

Data Processing

The EPs were averaged by ordinal position; so we obtained for each subject five averages: the average of responses to the first stimulus in the train, the average of responses to the second stimulus, and so on. The N_1–P_2 wave of the vertex auditory response is the only component that could be identified in all subjects and declined systematically over a session of repetitive stimulation. Latencies and peak-to-peak amplitudes of this component were measured on the computer oscilloscope by a cursor program that displayed the coordinate values of any wanted point of the response in milliseconds and microvolts. Another measure of the amplitude was performed by integrating, in absolute values, the samples between the following limits: $N_1 - 20$ msec and $P_2 + 20$ msec for each AEP obtained by ordinal averaging. These integrated values were used to calculate the habituation curve by plotting the relative amplitude of responses 2, 3, 4, and 5 as percentages of the amplitude of the first one.

Results

The individual responses averaged across trains by ordinal position showed a drop in amplitude greater than 20% in all controls but one. The mean decrement of the amplitude of the second response with respect to the first one was about 47%. The same value was obtained when we compared the average amplitude of responses 2 to 5 to the amplitude of the first one (Fig. 3). This indicates that the main drop in amplitude occurs between the first two responses, with no modifications, on the average, after the second response. In contrast, only three patients presented a decrement in amplitude from stimulus 1 to stimulus 2 greater than 20%; the mean group values indeed show an increment of this amplitude. The differences between the two groups are statistically significant (Mann–Whitney *U* test).

DISCUSSION

The scalp distribution of VEPs in the group of patients suffering from an Alzheimer's disease or a senile dementia evolving towards an Alzheimer condition shows an interesting peculiarity. Whereas the responses obtained from the occipital scalp are generally preserved and comparable to those recorded in SD and controls, the N_1–P_2 component of the vertex response is very flat or missing; it is replaced on the grand mean VEP by a low-amplitude positive wave. In contrast, the vertex AEPs are present in all AD patients with a normal configuration.

It is generally admitted that the human vertex potential is a nonspecific response, able to be evoked by any stimulus (clicks, tones, flashes, electric shocks) but, nevertheless, with a certain degree of modality specificity (11). Our results emphasize rather a modality specificity of the vertex response, which may be evoked by auditory stimuli but not by visual stimuli in AD patients. The func-

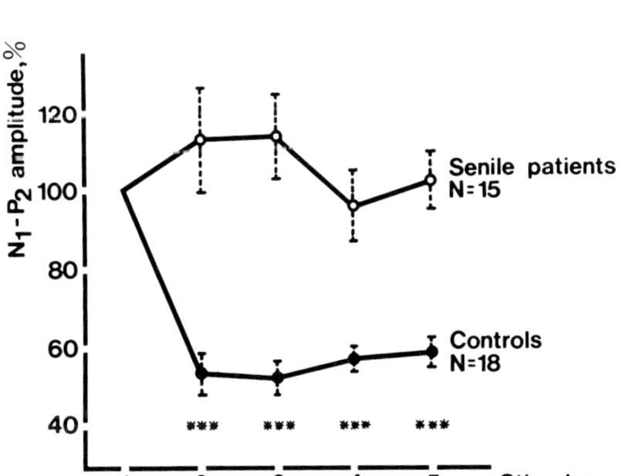

FIG. 3. Fast habituation of AEPs. N_1–P_2 amplitudes of responses 2, 3, 4, and 5 are expressed as percentages of the amplitude of the first one. Each point represents the group mean amplitude ± SEM. *** $p < 0.001$ (Mann–Whitney *U* test).

tional significance of the vertex visual EP is an open question. It does not exhibit the same degree of stimulus control as the corresponding component recorded over the occipital lobe; the interstimulus interval has different effects on the occipital and vertex responses. The data reported here confirm the assumption that the vertex and occipital VEP probably have their origins at different cortical generators and that they represent different neurophysiological phenomena (6,8,14). We can infer that the structures responsible for the genesis of the vertex VEP are impaired in AD and that the lack of an important alteration of the vertex VEP may constitute an objective sign of a severe mental impairment.

Concerning the fast habituation, it is clearly impaired in most of our senile patients. At this time, we don't know which is the effect of normal aging on the fast habituation; further studies are necessary. This type of habituation is a central phenomenon, probably independent of peripheral adjustments, and may include a recovery cycle component (1). Consequently, it is highly improbable that the increment in the acoustic threshold in aging could play a role in the lack of habituation observed in our patients. Roth and Kopell (12) showed that the rate of habituation is not dependent on the intensity of stimuli; in addition, all of our patients were able to perceive them.

Two psychological variables, the level of arousal and the direction of attention, which are impaired in aging, are known to influence the parameters of EPs. It seems that these variables have only a limited effect on the habituation of the vertex EP (10). Nevertheless, attention influences the amplitude of the response to the first stimulus in the train, being larger in an attentive state than in inattentive state (2).

Another parameter that can affect the size of the response to the first stimulus is the intertrain interval. The extremely slow recovery of the AEP at the vertex is known, an interval of about 10 sec being necessary for its complete recovery. We can wonder whether this interval was sufficient for the complete recovery of the auditory vertex response in our patients. To answer this question, we tested five senile patients using two intertrain (ITIs) intervals: 10 sec and 20 sec. Three of these patients presented an amplitude of the first stimulus greater with an ITI of 20 sec than with an ITI of 10 sec, but the two others showed the opposite.

We suppose that no single mechanism can account for the loss of fast habituation in all senile patients. We can infer that at least two factors may interfere with the function of habituation: impaired attention and the lengthening of the recovery cycle of the vertex AEP.

CONCLUSIONS

Using the EP technique, we investigated many facets of the evoked brain electrical activity to stimuli pertaining to various sensory modalities in senile dementia. Some of the differences found between the senile patients and the control groups may be related to normal aging, but others, such as the loss of the vertex response to flashes, are very probably linked with a deep brain organic and/or functional disorder. The almost constant lack of habituation noticed in our patients may be associated with the decreased learning abilities observed in senile dementia, if we consider habituation to be an elemental form of learning.

The EPs appear to constitute a valuable clue for the study of the brain dysfunction in senile dementia.

REFERENCES

1. Callaway, E. III (1973): Habituation of averaged evoked potentials in man. In: *Habituation, Vol. II,* edited by H. V. S. Peeke and M. J. Herz, pp. 153–174. Academic Press, New York.
2. Fruhstorfer, H., Sovieri, P., and Järviletho, T. (1970): Short-term habituation of the auditory evoked response in man. *Electroencephalogr. Clin. Neurophysiol.,* 28:153–161.
3. Gerson, I. M., John, E. R., Bartlett, F., and Koenig, V. (1976): Average evoked response (AER) in the electroencephalographic diagnosis of the normally aging brain: A practical application. *Clin. Electroencephalogr.,* 7:77–91.
4. Goodin, D. S., Squires, K. C., Henderson, B. H., and Starr, A. (1978): Age-related variations in evoked potentials to auditory stimuli in normal human subject. *Electroencephalogr. Clin. Neurophysiol.,* 44:447–458.
5. Hendrickson, C., Levy, R., and Post, F. (1979): Averaged evoked responses in relation to cognitive affective state of elderly psychiatric patient. *Br. J. Psychiatry,* 134:494–501.
6. Kress, G. (1976): Effect of visual stimulation on the evoked response recorded at the vertex. *Brain Res. Bull.,* 1:337–339.
7. Laurian, S., Reigner, J., Heimann, H., Gruber, G., Wertheimer, J., and Lobrinus, A. (1973): Visual evoked responses in elderly psychiatric patient. *Electroencephalogr. Clin. Neurophysiol.,* 34:760.
8. Lethonen, J. B. (1973): Functional differentiation between late components of visual evoked potentials recorded at occiput and vertex: Effect of stimulus interval and contour. *Electroencephalogr. Clin. Neurophysiol.,* 35:75–82.
9. Levy, R., Isaacs, A., and Behrman, J. (1971): Neurophysiological correlates of senile dementia. II. The somatosensory evoked response. *Psychol. Med.,* 1:159–165.
10. Öhman, A., and Lader, M. (1977): Short-term changes of the human auditory evoked potentials during repetitive stimulation. In: *Progress in Clinical Neurophysiology, Vol. 2, Auditory Evoked Potentials in Man. Psychopharmacology Correlates of EPs,* edited by J. E. Desmedt, pp. 93–118. Karger, Basel.
11. Picton, T. W., Hillyard, S. A., and Galambos, R. (1976): Habituation and attention in the auditory system. In: *Handbook of Sensory Physiology,* edited by W. D. Keidel and W. D. Neff, pp. 343–389. Springer, New York.
12. Roth, W. T., and Kopell, B. S. (1969): The auditory evoked response to repeated stimuli during a vigilance task. *Psychophysiology,* 6:301–309.
13. Straumanis, J. J., Shagass, C., and Schwartz, M. (1965): Visually evoked cerebral response changes associated with chronic brain syndromes and aging. *J. Gerontol.,* 20:498–506.
14. Vaughan, H. G. (1969): The relationship of brain activity to scalp recordings of event-related potentials. In: *Average Evoked Potentials. Methods, Results and Evaluation,* edited by E. Donchin and D. B. Lindsley, pp. 45–94. National Aeronautics and Space Administration, Washington.
15. Visser, S. L., Stam, F. C., van Tilburg, W., Op Den Velde, W., Bloom, J. L., and de Rijke, W. (1976): Visual evoked response in senile and presenile dementia. *Electroencephalogr. Clin. Neurophysiol.,* 40:385–392.

Clinical Applications of Evoked Potentials in Neurology,
edited by J. Courjon, F. Mauguiere, and M. Revol.
Raven Press, New York © 1982.

Recent Progress in the Understanding of Subcortical Somatosensory Evoked Potentials

J. E. Desmedt and G. Cheron

Brain Research Unit, University of Brussels, B-1000 Brussels, Belgium

The somatosensory evoked potentials (SEP) recorded with scalp electrodes can provide invaluable data about clinical disorders involving either the peripheral nerve or the central nervous system (6,9,14,19). The diagnostic uses of SEP emphasize the early components that can be more reliably elicited by electrical stimulation of the median nerve at the wrist or of fingers of the hand. The method is based on the accurate estimation of the time of arrival of the corticopetal volley at the primary cortical projection on the contralateral postcentral gyrus. Therefore, it is worth considering the evidence that validates the use of the onset time of the negative N_{22} component of the SEP for estimating the cortical SEP latency (7,10).

Components of the SEP are designated by the polarity (N for negative or P for positive) and peak latency, following recent recommendations (12). Methods used have been discussed in detail (6). Current studies following the lead of Cracco (3,4) concur in the distinction in the scalp-recorded SEP between (a) far-field components that are generated subcortically and are volume-conducted towards the entire scalp and (b) cortical components that are generated by more or less extensive cortical regions. In view of the widespread scalp distribution (see Fig. 9 of ref. 7), the far-field components are small or even absent when the reference electrode (leading to grid 2 of the amplifier) is also placed on the scalp; they are more apparent when a reference on the earlobe is used (Fig. 1C,D) and considerably larger with a noncephalic reference (Fig. 1A,B).

On this basis, it should be possible to distinguish the earliest cortical components by superimposing a recording from the primary contralateral postcentral focus on a recording from another scalp region that does not lie over the primary projection. In Fig. 1, the paired traces recorded in the same run were superimposed as closely as possible for the larger far-field P_{17} component rather than for the prestimulus record level. Notice that the P_{17} far-field to finger stimulation thus displayed corresponds to the P_{14} far-field of the SEP elicited by median nerve stimulation at the wrist (there being about 3 msec conduction time between finger and wrist).

In agreement with previous findings (11), the ipsilateral SEP has little, if

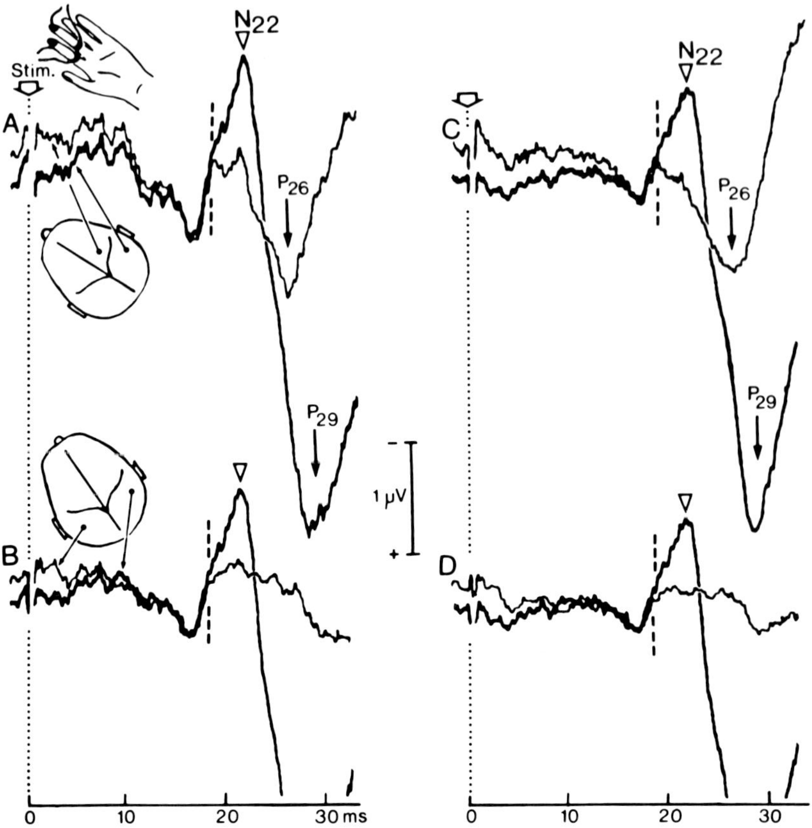

FIG. 1. Identification of the onset latency of the cortical SEP in a male subject of 22 years. Negativity of the active electrode records upwards in this and all other figures. Same calibration for all traces. The *thicker trace* in each of the four superimpositions is the averaged SEP recorded from the postcentral scalp on the side opposite to the fingers stimulated. In **A** and **B**, a noncephalic reference on the right hand is used. In **C** and **D**, the reference is the earlobe on the same side. The *thinner trace* is recorded from the precentral scalp on the side contralateral to the finger stimulation in **A** and **C** (see the *figurines*), and from the postcentral scalp on the side ipsilateral to the finger stimulation in **B** and **D**. The peak of the parietal N_{22} is indicated by a *hollow triangle*. The time of divergence of the traces is indicated by a *vertical interrupted line,* and this is taken to correspond to the onset of the cortical negative response in the projection areas of the contralateral parietal cortex. The peaks of the precentral P26 and of the postcentral P29 are indicated. (From Desmedt and Cheron, ref. 7, with permission.)

any, significant negativity during the time slot of the contralateral N_{22}, and there is also little positivity thereafter during the large contralateral positive P_{29} component, both with noncephalic reference (Fig. 1B) or with earlobe reference (Fig. 1D). This profile of the ipsilateral response may be related to the lack of callosal connections from the primary somatosensory cortex for the projection areas of the distal parts of the limb, as documented anatomically in the monkey (15,20). The divergence of the traces in these superimpositions corresponds roughly to the initial upgoing limb of the contralateral N_{22} which takes off virtually when the preceding P_{17} far-field is reaching baseline.

Because thalamocortical radiation potentials are elicited from the thalamus contralateral to the hand stimulated one could argue that the ipsilateral SEP might provide no adequate reference for delineating the contribution of the radiation volley to the scalp recording. An answer to this question is provided by the superimposition of the precentral SEP on to the postcentral response, because both traces are then recorded from scalp areas only 5 cm apart which lie over the contralateral hemisphere. The positive far-field and P_{17} are virtually identical at these two scalp locations, as indeed is to be expected for a volume-conducted subcortical activity. However, the onset of the subsequent N_{22} also diverges from the precentral trace (Fig. 1A,C) which presents little early negativity before the characteristic precentral positive P_{26} component that has recently been identified by Papakostopoulos and Crow (21) and by Desmedt and Cheron (7). One must conclude that the marked divergence of the negative postcentral N_{22} reveals that it is to be taken as the true onset of the cortical response in the primary projection area (7,8).

The time slot between the peripheral stimulus and the arrival of the afferent volley at the cerebral cortex (onset of N_{22}) is made up of conduction times along several neurons, but one can start by considering the two parts that correspond to (a) the conduction along the peripheral nerve up to the spinal cord and (b) the transit time from spinal entry to cortex. The spinal entry time has been evaluated first by recording sensory nerve action potentials along the peripheral nerve trunk (5,10), and then by direct recording of the spinal SEP with an electrode placed on the lower neck (2,17).

One current problem with the interpretation of neck SEP traces appears to be related to the use of different references, namely, a scalp reference electrode whereby the scalp positive far-fields are mixed with the genuine spinal potentials. For a clear appreciation of the different components seen at the neck or scalp, it is necessary to simultaneously record with different montages using both cephalic and noncephalic references (7). Furthermore, an essential control can be provided by the comparison of conduction of sensory nerve potentials along the nerve up to Erb's point with the neck and scalp records as in Fig. 2.

In such experiments, one should stimulate fingers rather than a mixed nerve in order to exclude the interference from the potentials of the group I muscle afferents and of the antidromically stimulated motor axons. The sensory nerve potentials (needle recording; averaging with bin width of 20 μsec) have a triphasic profile, and the first negative-going phase indicates the arrival of the volley under the active recording electrode (7,13). Latency data between wrist and Erb's point over the brachial plexus consistently fit a linear regression with a calculated mean conduction velocity (CV) of 72 m/sec (Fig. 2, A–E). The mean CV over the median nerve for afferents from fingers is 71.1 $\pm$ 4.0 m/sec in 25 young adults (8).

Extrapolation of the regression line to the lower neck recording site fits remark-

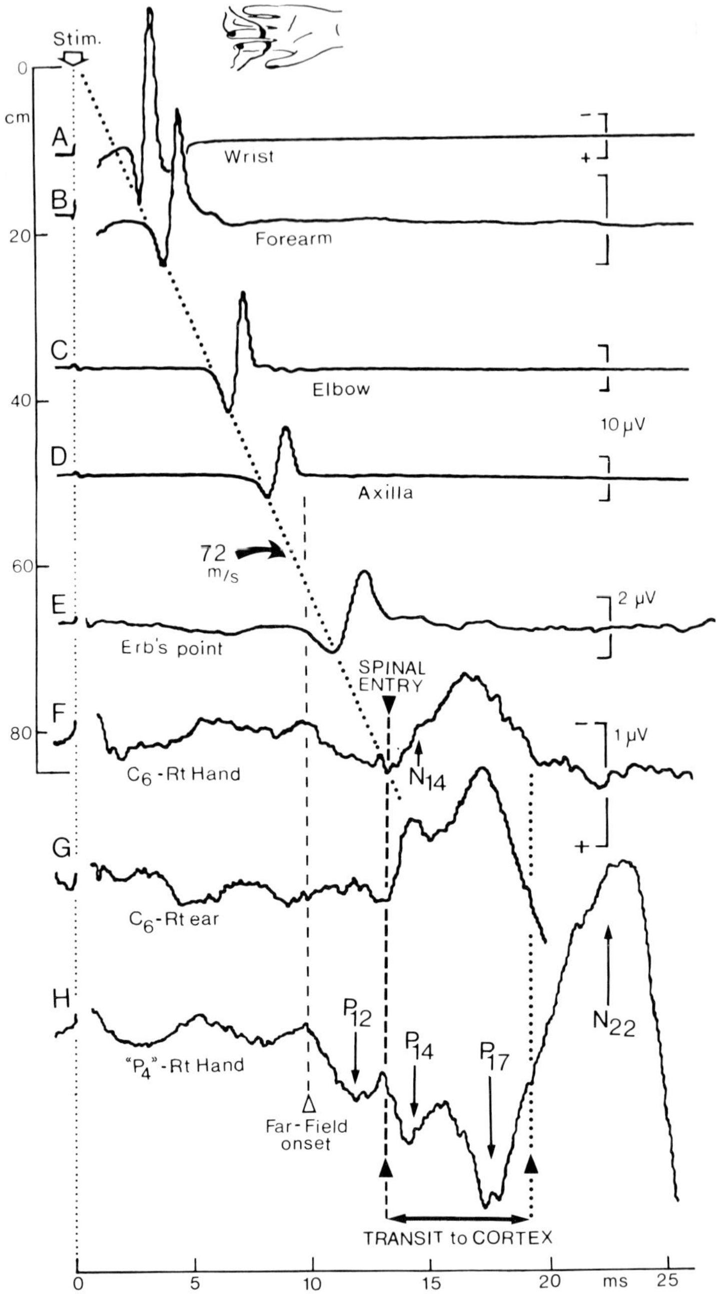

FIG. 2. Sensory nerve potentials recorded from the median nerve at wrist, forearm, elbow, axilla, and Erb's point **(A-E)** with different amplifications. Stimulation at three times subjective threshold of fingers I-II-III of the left hand. The vertical separation of the averaged traces is proportional to the conduction distances between the recording sites. The calculated linear regression gives a CV of 72 m/sec. Extrapolation of CV to the lower neck recording site fits the onset of the negative spinal component N14 **(F,G),** and the onset of the second positive scalp far-field P14 **(H).** The onset of the cortical N22 recorded from the contralateral parietal scalp with a noncephalic reference **(H)** indicates a spino-cortical transit time of 6.0 msec. The onset of the first scalp far-field P12 *(white arrowhead and vertical interrputed line)* is earlier than the Erb's point potential but later than the nerve potential at the axilla. (From Desmedt and Cheron, ref. 7, with permission.)

ably well, in different subjects, the onset of the spinal negative component N_{14} (displayed with an earlobe reference in Fig. 2G, and with a noncephalic reference in F). It also fits the concomitant onset of the scalp-recorded second far-field FF_2 or P_{14} (Fig. 2H). Notice that these N_{14} at neck and P_{14} at scalp are homologous to the N_{11} and P_{11}, respectively, recorded when stimulating the median nerve at the wrist. These data enable one to define with no ambiguity the true spinal entry time of the afferent volley (7).

The first far-field FF_1 is positive-going (noncephalic reference) all along the neck and at the scalp, in contrast to the second potential that is negative at the neck (N_{14}), but positive at the scalp (P_{14}). The first far-field starts at about 10 msec for finger stimulation (Fig. 2F,H). This first far-field onset precedes the arrival of the peripheral volley at Erb's point (Fig. 2E), but it is later than the onset of the nerve potential at the axilla (Fig. 2D). These data confirm that the first positive far-field FF_1 is a volume-conducted potential generated by peripheral nerve activity just proximal to the axilla (4).

The next point is to consider the spinal potentials recorded along the neck. When using a noncephalic reference, we found a clear difference of onset latencies for the first negative component recorded over the neck between the levels of C_6 (Fig. 3B) and C_2 (Fig. 3E), respectively. The negative component is delayed at C_2 by a mean of 0.95 ± 0.15 msec (7). This result confirms a suggestion by Cracco (2), but it is at variance with the claim by Matthews et al. (17) and Jones (16) that the neck SEP negativity would present a stable latency along the neck as if it were related to a fixed generator. Briefly put, this controversy appears to be resolved by the identification of the location of the reference electrode as the critical variable. Thus, the latency shift is clearly recorded when using a noncephalic reference. By contrast, when a scalp reference is used, the large scalp positive far-fields are injected into grid 2 of the amplifier whereby the nerve far-field P_9 is obliterated and even transformed into a negative N_9 (Fig. 3C,D). Moreover, a negative N_{14} component (that does not belong to the spinal cord but is generated above the foramen magnum) is spuriously added on top of the neck SEP by the third positive scalp far-field P_{14} injected into grid 2 of the amplifier. Finally, the addition of the second positive far-field P_{11} by the scalp reference obliterates the latency shift from lower to upper neck (Fig. 3C,D). Thus, the neck-to-scalp montage may be practically useful in diagnostic applications, but it can be misleading in any detailed discussion of the neural generators of SEP components (7).

Since the latency shift along the neck may reasonably be interpreted as reflecting the ascending conduction along the dorsal columns, these data have been used in conjunction with anatomical observation on dissected bodies to estimate a maximum CV of 58 m/sec in the dorsal columns and an arrival time at the cuneate nucleus at 1.2 msec after spinal entry time. Consideration of timing and synaptic delays suggest that the ascending volley only arrives at the thalamus 3.2 msec after spinal entry. As a corollary, the third far-field P_{14} must be generated above the foramen magnum but below the thalamus, and hence, in the

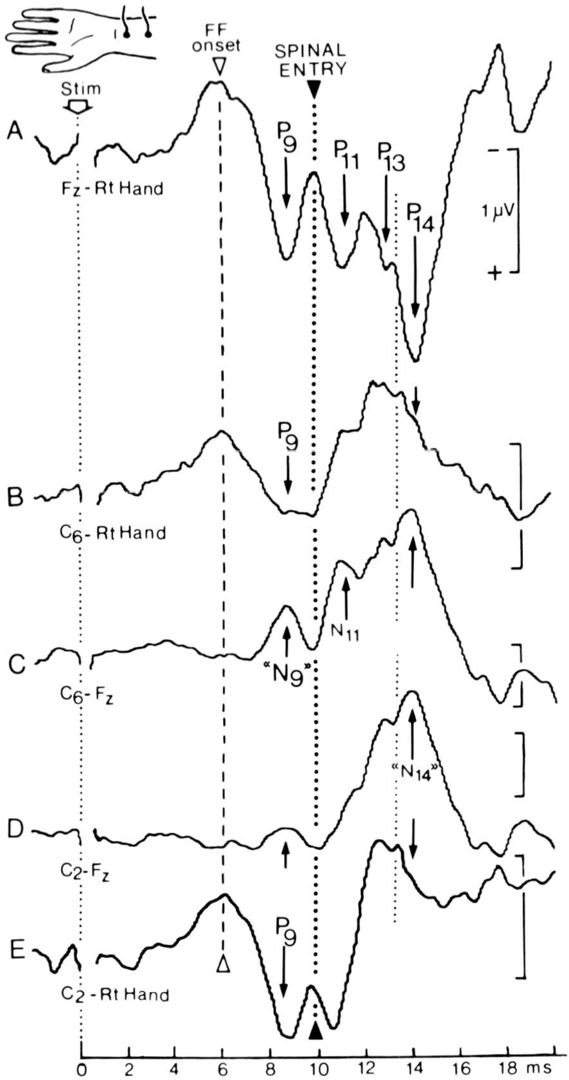

FIG. 3. Analysis of SEP components recorded from the lower or upper neck and the effect of the location of the reference electrode. The SEPs are elicited by electrical stimulation of the left median nerve at the wrist at the time indicated by the first *vertical dotted line.* **A:** Scalp far-fields recorded by a midfrontal electrode F_z with a noncephalic reference on the right hand. **B:** Neck SEP recorded from lower neck, at spinal level C_6, with a noncephalic reference. **C:** Recording from the same neck electrode but with the reference at the F_z scalp location. This eliminates the first far-field P_9 and introduces a negative N_9 and a negative N_{14}. Notice that the amplification has been reduced to half. **D:** Recording from upper neck at C_2 with a scalp F_z reference. This shows no significant latency shift with respect to the preceding trace. **E:** Recording from the same neck electrode but with a noncephalic reference. The onset of the spinal negative component is clearly delayed by about 1 msec with respect to the spinal entry time indicated by the trace in **B** *(vertical row of thick dots and black arrow-head).* (From Desmedt and Cheron, ref. 7, with permission.)

medial lemniscus (see ref. 7 for a detailed discussion). There are several supporting data. Clinical evidence indicates that P_{14} recorded from scalp is present in patients with a thalamic lesion, so that its generator must be located below the thalamus (18). Furthermore, the third far-field P_{14} is significantly larger in voltage at the contralateral earlobe than at the ipsilateral earlobe (noncephalic reference), as indeed should be the case if P_{14} is indeed related to a lemniscal generator located above the decussation of the somatosensory pathway (7).

ACKNOWLEDGMENT

This research has been supported by grants from the Fonds de la Recherche Scientifique Médicale, Belgium.

REFERENCES

1. Albe-Fessard, D., Arfel, G., Guiot, G., Derome, P., Herran, J., Korn, H., Hertzog, E., Vourch, G., and Aleonard, P. (1963): Activitiés électriques caractéristiques de quelques structures cérébrales chez l'homme. *Ann. Chir.*, 17:1185–1214.
2. Cracco, R. Q. (1973): Spinal evoked response: Peripheral nerve stimulation in man. *Electroencephalogr. Clin. Neurophysiol.*, 35:379–386.
3. Cracco, R. Q. (1980): Scalp-recorded potentials evoked by median nerve stimulation: Subcortical potentials, traveling waves and somato–motor potentials. In: *Progress in Clinical Neurophysiology, Vol. 7, Clinical Uses of Cerebral, Brainstem and Spinal Somatosensory Evoked Potentials*, edited by J. E. Desmedt, pp. 1–14. Karger, Basel.
4. Cracco, R. Q., and Cracco, J. B. (1976): Somatosensory evoked potentials in man: Far-field potentials. *Electroencephalogr. Clin. Neurophysiol.*, 41:460–466.
5. Desmedt, J. E. (1971): Somatosensory cerebral evoked potentials in man. In: *Handbook of Electroencephalography and Clinical Neurophysiology, Vol. 9*, edited by A. Remond, pp. 55–82. Elsevier, Amsterdam.
6. Desmedt, J. E. (1977): Some observations on the methodology of cerebral evoked potentials in man. In: *Progress in Clinical Neurophysiology, Vol. 1, Attention, Voluntary Contraction and Event-Related Cerebral Potentials*, edited by J. E. Desmedt, pp. 12–29. Karger, Basel.
7. Desmedt, J. E., and Cheron, G. (1980): Central somatosensory conduction in man: Neural generators and interpeak latencies of the far-field components recorded from neck and right or left scalp and earlobes. *Electroencephalogr. Clin. Neurophysiol.*, 50:382–403.
8. Desmedt, J. E., and Cheron, G. (1980): Somatosensory evoked potentials to finger stimulation in healthy octogenarians and in young adults: Wave forms, scalp topography and transit times of parietal and frontal components. *Electroencephalogr. Clin. Neurophysiol.*, 50:404–425.
9. Desmedt, J. E., and Noël, P. (1973): Average cerebral evoked potentials in the evaluation of lesions of the sensory nerves and of the central somatosensory pathway. In: *New Developments in Electromyography and Clinical Neurophysiology, Vol. 2*, edited by J. E. Desmedt, pp. 352–371. Karger, Basel.
10. Desmedt, J. E., Noël, P., Debecker, J., and Namèche, J. (1973): Maturation of afferent conduction velocity as studied by sensory nerve potentials and by cerebral evoked potentials. In: *New Developments in Electromyography and Clinical Neurophysiology, Vol. 2*, edited by J. E. Desmedt, pp. 52–63. Karger, Basel.
11. Desmedt, J. E., and Robertson, D. (1977): Differential enhancement of early and late components of the cerebral somatosensory evoked potentials during fast sequential cognitive task in man. *J. Physiol. (Lond.)*, 271:761–782.
12. Donchin, E., Callaway, E., Cooper, R., Desmedt, J. E., Goff, W. R., Hillyard, S. A., and Sutton, S. (1977): Publication criteria for studies of evoked potentials: Report of a committee. In: *Progress in Clinical Neurophysiology, Vol. 1, Attention, Voluntary Contraction and Event-Related Cerebral Potentials*, edited by J. E. Desmedt, pp. 1–11. Karger, Basel.
13. Gilliatt, R. W., and Sears, T. A. (1958): Sensory nerve action potentials in patients with peripheral nerve lesions. *J. Neurol. Neurosurg. Psychiatry*, 21:109–118.

14. Hume, A. M., and Cant, B. R. (1978): Conduction time in central somatosensory pathways in man. *Electroencephalogr. Clin. Neurophysiol.,* 45:361–375.
15. Jones, E. G., and Powell, T. P. S. (1969): Connexions of the somatic sensory cortex of the rhesus monkey. Contralateral cortical connexions. *Brain,* 92:717–730.
16. Jones, S. J. (1977): Short latency potentials recorded from the neck and scalp following median nerve stimulation in man. *Electroencephalogr. Clin. Neurophysiol.,* 43:853–863.
17. Matthews, W. B., Beauchamp, M., and Small, D. G. (1974): Cervical somatosensory evoked responses in man. *Nature,* 52:230–232.
18. Mauguière, F., and Courjon, J. (1981): The origin of short-latency somatosensory evoked potentials in man: A clinical contribution. *Ann. Neurol.,* 9:607–611.
19. Noël, P., and Desmedt, J. E. (1980): Cerebral and far-field somatosensory evoked potentials in neurological disorders involving the cervical spinal cord, brainstem, thalamus and cortex. In: *Progress in Clinical Neurophysiology, Vol. 7, Clinical Uses of Cerebral, Brainstem and Spinal Somatosensory Evoked Potentials,* edited by J. E. Desmedt, pp. 205–230. Karger, Basel.
20. Pandya, D. N., and Vignolo, L. A. (1969): Interhemispheric projections of the parietal lobe in the rhesus monkey. *Brain Res.,* 15:49–65.
21. Papakostopoulos, D., and Crow, H. J. (1980): Direct recording of the somatosensory evoked potentials from the cerebral cortex of man and the difference between precentral and postcentral potentials. In: *Progress in Clinical Neurophysiology, Vol. 7, Clinical Uses of Cerebral, Brainstem, and Spinal Somatosensory Evoked Potentials,* edited by J. E. Desmedt, pp. 15–26. Karger, Basel.

Clinical Applications of Evoked Potentials in Neurology,
edited by J. Courjon, F. Mauguiere, and M. Revol.
Raven Press, New York © 1982.

Short-Latency Somatosensory Evoked Potentials in Man, Monkey, Cat, and Rat: Comparative Latency Analysis

T. Allison, C. C. Wood, G. McCarthy, A. L. Hume, and W. R. Goff

Neuropsychology Laboratory, Veterans Administration Medical Center, West Haven, Connecticut 06516 and Department of Neurology, Yale University School of Medicine, New Haven, Connecticut 06510

Short-latency SEPs generated in afferent pathways and the somatosensory cortex are useful in the evaluation of neurological disorders (9,12,13). The specificity of inferences about the location of a lesion depends on how well each component of the surface-recorded SEP can be ascribed to neuronal activity in a particular structure or level of the neuraxis. In human recordings, several techniques have been used to infer neural origins including analysis of latency and topography, recovery functions, and pathophysiological correlates (5,9, 10,12,13,15–17,20). Progress has been made, but disagreement remains.

In this chapter we show that, when recorded from similar electrode derivations, short-latency SEPs in the four species studied are very similar in appearance. We then show that comparison of latencies across species provides another way of assessing the correspondence of components. Some results have been presented elsewhere (2).

METHODS

Recordings have been made in 93 normal humans (age 10–84 years), five monkeys (three *Macaca* spp. and two *Ateles* spp.), nine cats, and six rats. Stimulating and recording conditions in all species were similar to those described previously (5,13). Stimuli were 0.5 msec duration, 5/sec constant-current shocks to the median nerve at the wrist at an intensity producing a detectable twitch of the first digit. Electrodes on the body surface were placed comparably in all species, except that in humans, F_z was used as a reference for neck and shoulder recordings, whereas in animals, "Fp_z" (a screw electrode in frontal bone) was used. After preamplification (−3 dB at 0.03 and 3 kHz), SEPs were digitized (80 μsec/pt), summed by a Fabri-Tek Model 1074 four-channel averager, and transferred to a LINC computer. The humans were in a relaxed waking state. The animals were initially anesthetized with 30 to 45 mg/kg sodium pentobarbital and maintained under light anesthesia by supplemental doses as required; their body temperature was maintained at 37 ± 1°C.

RESULTS AND DISCUSSION

Representative human recordings are illustrated in Fig. 1A. The top trace shows the median nerve volley (N10) recorded from the ipsilateral shoulder. The middle trace shows the N12–N13–N14 complex recorded from an electrode over the seventh cervical spinous process (C_7) and described previously (4,9, 13,15,17,20). The lower trace, from contralateral scalp, begins with a scalp-positive amalgam of potentials corresponding in latency with the N13–N14 components as recorded in the C_7 derivation and terminating in a small peak or inflection labeled P15. P15 is followed by a scalp-negative potential typically interrupted by two inflections labeled P16 and P18 and terminating in N20.

Somatosensory evoked potentials similarly recorded from monkey, cat, and rat are shown in Fig. 1B–D. For each derivation, the morphology of the waveforms is similar in all species, with the one exception that the initial activity of somatosensory cortex recorded in man and monkey as a negativity (4,8) is recorded in cat and rat as a positivity (14,19). A schematic summary of typical human waveforms in the three channels of Fig. 1 and in a C_2 cervical derivation is shown in Fig. 2A. With the exception of the P16–N20 sequence of potentials, Fig. 2A also typifies activity recorded in the other species. These cross-species similarities of waveform and topography have led us to hypothesize that the sequence of components in each species reflects similar neuronal events. For this reason, and to avoid using four sets of polarity/latency nomenclatures, animal components are labeled according to their presumptive human counterparts.

To investigate the neural origins of this sequence of activity, we made simultaneous surface and depth recordings in animals and determined the effects of lethal dosages of sodium pentobarbital (for details, see 6). Figure 2B is a schematic summary of the postulated origin of each component. To assess correspondences between SEPs in animals and humans, we compared across species the effects of different rates of stimulation. As would be expected from previous studies (7,19), in both humans and animals, the earlier components are less affected by this manipulation than are later components, but the effects are not specific enough to demonstrate direct correspondences.

Another way of assessing correspondence of components is by comparison of their latency. Since the somatosensory system of mammals is highly similar in structure and function, it may be assumed that the sequence of neuronal activity in afferent pathways and somatosensory cortex is also similar. However, absolute latencies obviously cannot be compared directly because of differing lengths of the conduction pathways. Table 1 gives peak latencies of all components and shows systematic decreases with decreasing body size. Such differences

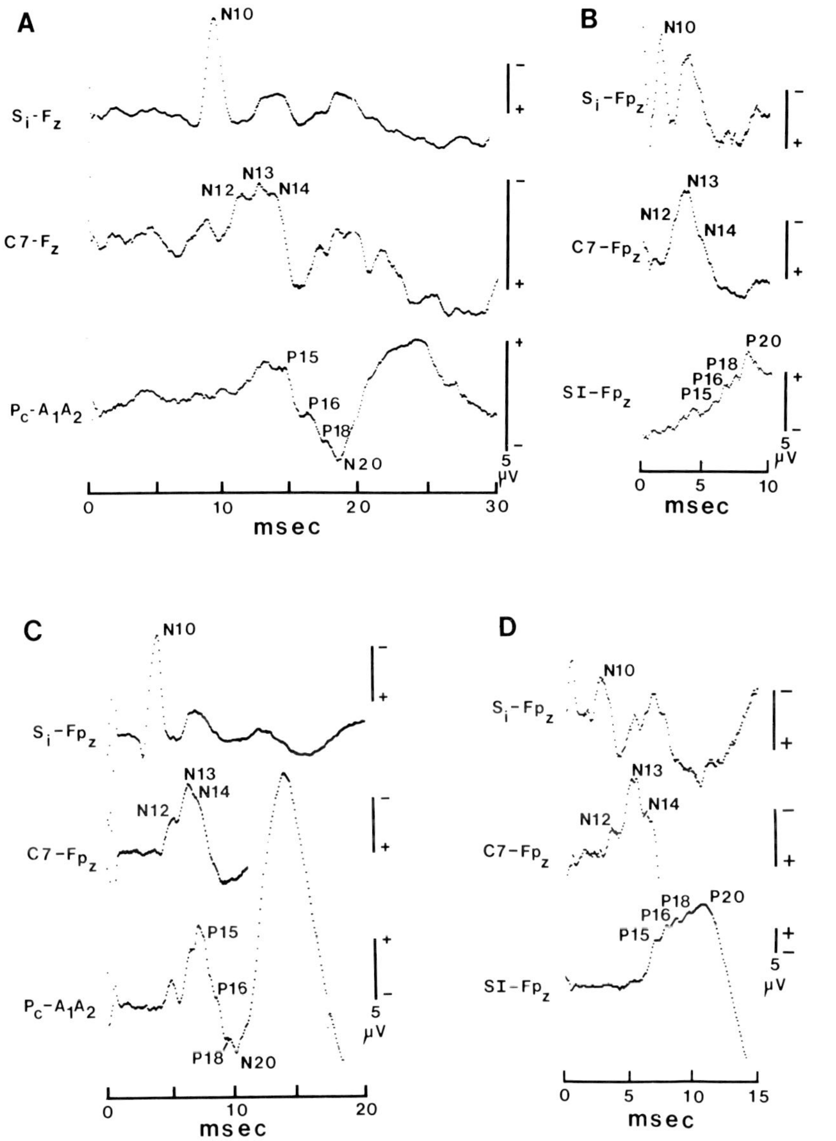

FIG. 1. Short-latency SEPs to median nerve stimulation in human **(A)**, rat **(B)**, monkey **(C)**, and cat **(D)**. Simultaneous recordings from ipsilateral shoulder (S_i, located midway along the clavicle), neck (C_7), and contralateral parietal area (P_C) or somatosensory cortex (SI) referred to linked-ear (A_1A_2) or midfrontal (F_z or Fp_z) electrodes. In this and following figures, polarity at electrode location specified first is noted on the voltage calibration.

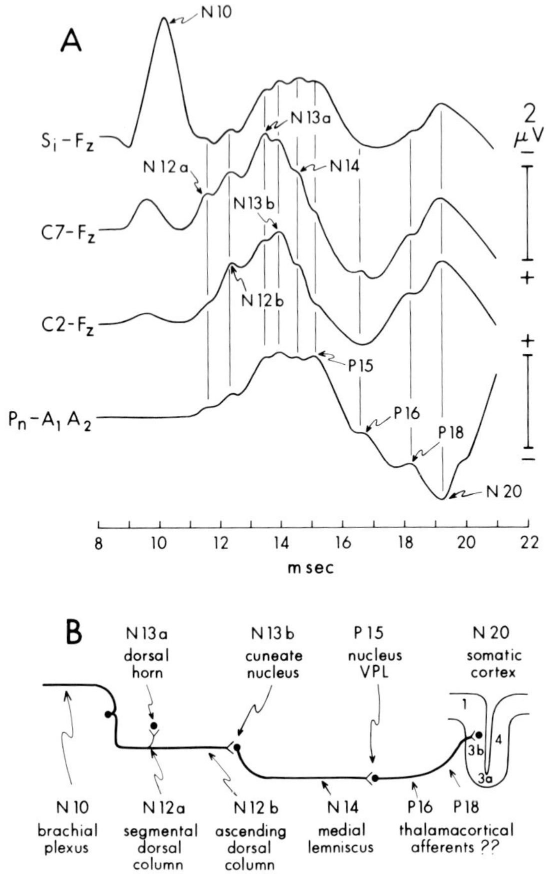

FIG. 2. A: Schematic waveform of the human SEP as recorded in a four-channel array for clinical purposes. In most humans and animals, two fractions of N12 and N13 can be distinguished; typical topographic differences in these components are illustrated. Voltage calibrations are approximate. **B:** Schematic illustration of the structures thought to be the primary generators of each component, based on animal recordings. Some components appear to derive mainly from cell bodies **(top),** whereas others appear to derive mainly from fiber tracts **(bottom).**

are also observed in recordings of humans of varying arm length and body height (e.g., 13,16,17) and account for about two-thirds of the across-subject latency variance in humans.

The effect of body size on latency can be taken into account if we assume that monkey, cat, and rat somatosensory systems are progressively linearly compressed versions of the human somatosensory system and if at least one component of undoubted correspondence is available to serve as a benchmark. (For a similar analysis of BAEPs see ref. 1.) In the recordings of Fig. 1, two such components are available, N10 and N20/P20. In man, N10 reflects the median

TABLE 1. *Peak latency of SEP components in man, monkey, cat, and rat*

	N10	N12a	N12b	N13a	N13b	N14	P15	P16	P18	N20/ P20
Human ($N = 93$)	10.1[a]	11.6	12.2	13.5	13.8	14.4	15.1	16.6	18.3	19.2
SD	0.9[b]	1.1	1.1	1.1	1.2	1.1	1.1	1.1	1.1	1.2
Monkey ($N = 5$)	5.3	5.9	6.4	7.5	8.0	8.7	9.3	10.4	11.3	12.0
SD	1.2	1.2	1.2	1.5	1.5	1.6	1.7	1.8	1.9	2.0
Cat ($N = 9$)	2.8	3.6	4.2	5.4	5.8	6.6	7.7	9.0	10.2	11.3
SD	0.3	0.4	0.4	0.4	0.4	0.5	0.6	0.5	0.7	0.7
Rat ($N = 6$)	1.5	1.7	2.5	3.0	3.4	4.0	4.9	5.7	6.6	7.5
SD	0.2	0.1	0.4	0.3	0.4	0.5	0.5	0.5	0.5	0.5

[a] Mean.
[b] Standard deviation.

nerve afferent volley at the level of the brachial plexus (9,10,13,15,20). In animals, the latency of N10 is consistent with such an origin, and in terminal recordings, we consistently find that N10 is present after all activity recorded from neck or scalp is abolished. In animals in which most of somatosensory cortex lies on the cortical surface, the classical "primary" evoked potential consists of an initial surface positivity followed by a negativity. In cat and rat, this positivity is labeled P20 in Fig. 1. In man and monkey, this activity is recorded as a postivity anterior to the central sulcus but as a negativity posterior to the sulcus, as in Fig. 1, because of the different orientation of somatosensory cortex in primates (4,8). Thus, N20/P20 reflects initial activity in the somatosensory cortex and provides a second benchmark.

Figure 3, top trace, is a schematic human SEP based on the latencies given in Table 1. For the other species, the peak latencies of N10 and N20/P20 are set equal to the human values, and intermediate peaks are plotted proportionally over the range between N10 and N20/P20, based on the data of Table 1. In other words, the animal SEPs are "stretched" linearly such that N10 and N20/P20 are aligned in time. If the time between N10 and N20/P20 is taken as 100%, the difference between an animal component and its presumed human counterpart can be expressed as a percentage of the total. Averaged over all components, the mean discrepancy between human and animal components is small: 3.6, 4.0, and 6.4% for monkey, cat, and rat, respectively. For components N14 and later, the discrepancy averaged across animals is quite small (2%), and no trend is apparent; some components occur earlier, and others later than expected. However, components earlier than N14 show systematic deviation from expected values; mean discrepancies across species are 8, 6, 7, and 4% for N12a, N12b, N13a, and N13b, respectively and increase with decreasing body size. This suggests either that these components do not reflect similar

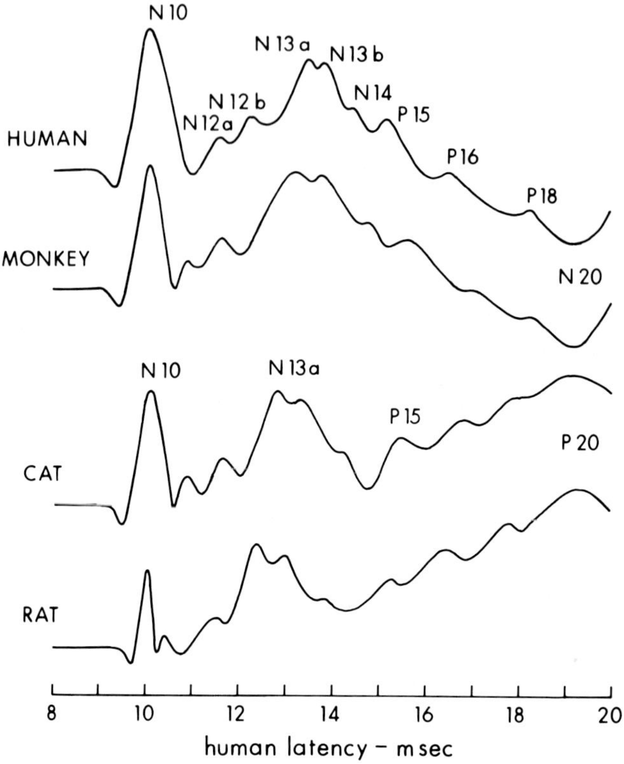

FIG. 3. Relative latencies of human and animal early SEP components, where the latencies of N10, and N20/P20 are set equal on the *x axis* (human latency in msec), and latencies of other components in animals are plotted proportionally; see text for details. For illustrative purposes, activity recorded in multiple channels (Figs. 1 and 2) is collapsed into a single waveform.

neural events in the four species or that increasing and nonlinear departures from the assumptions of the method occur with decreasing body size. Several possibilities may be considered.

1. The somatosensory afferent pathway changes in some manner with decreasing body size. To explore this question, we compared latencies for relatively tall and short humans and monkeys (Fig. 4). For the N12a-N13b sequence, the relative latencies of short humans are as discrepant with those of tall humans as are those of the monkeys. Since there is no reason to assume systematic errors of component identification in short as compared with tall humans, Fig. 4 suggests some systematic change in relative length of portions of the afferent pathway as it becomes progressively shorter. To assess this question, we measured the length of the following interelectrode distances in tall and short humans: S_i-C_7, C_7-C_2, and C_2–somatic cortex (approximated by a linear measurement from C_2 to vertex). When expressed as a percentage of the total, these distances

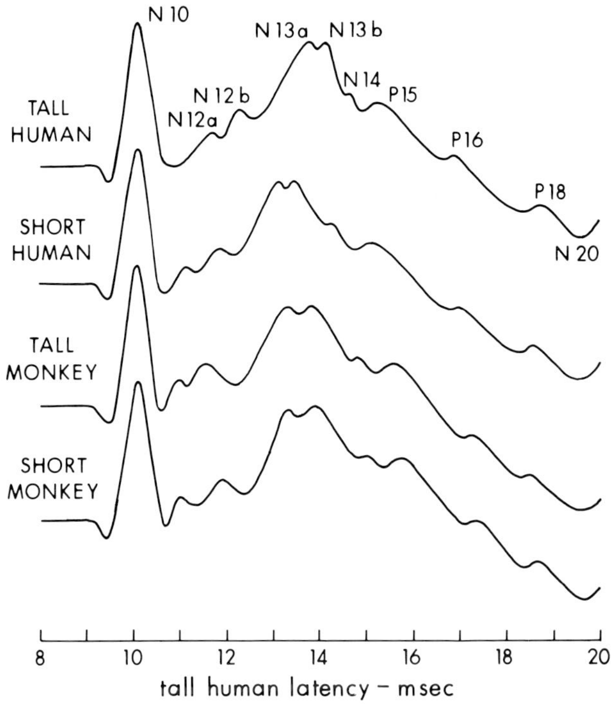

FIG. 4. Relative latencies derived as in Fig. 3. Tall humans: three 25- to 30-year-old males, mean height 1.80 m; short humans: three 10-year-old boys, mean height 1.30 m; tall monkeys: two adult spider monkeys (*Ateles* spp.); short monkeys: three adult *Macaca* spp.

are 38, 22, and 40%, and 30, 23, and 47% in tall and short humans, respectively; that is, the S_1-C_7 segment of the pathway is relatively shorter in small humans than in tall ones. This is not surprising, since the brain has achieved about 95% of its maximum volume by the age of 10, whereas body height has reached only about 80% of its maximum value (11). Much of the discrepancy in relative latency between small and large humans may be attributed to this change in relative pathway length. For example, N12a and N13a are thought to be generated approximately at the C_7 level (Fig. 2B) and should thus occur about 8% earlier in relative time in small humans; the empirical values from Fig. 4 are 6% and 7%, respectively. Unfortunately, length measurements were not obtained from most of the animals, and it is unclear to what extent differences in their relative pathway lengths contribute to the observed discrepancies.

2. There are (at least) three synapses in the dorsal column–medial lemniscal–somatic cortex pathway. It is reasonable to assume that the synaptic delay of about 0.8 msec in VPL (18) is representative of the delays at all synapses of the pathway and in the different species. In humans, the total conduction time from brachial plexus to somatic cortex (N10-N20) is about 9.1 msec, of which

a relatively small portion (2.4/9.1, or 26%) reflects synaptic delay. This percentage necessarily increases with decreasing body size and, for example, is 2.4/6.0, or 40%, in the rat. This has the direct effect of increasing the relative latency of N20/P20 in small species and hence has the indirect effect of decreasing the relative latency of earlier components, especially those reflecting activity prior to the first synapse. However, it is not clear how to obtain quantitative estimates of this effect.

3. The animals were anesthetized, whereas the humans were not. Anesthesia might be expected to increase peak latencies, particularly of later components. Furthermore, since the effects of anesthesia are primarily synaptic rather than axonal, such an effect would be relatively greater for smaller animals for the reasons discussed above. Again, this would have the indirect effect of decreasing the relative latency of earlier components. Our data cannot address this problem directly, since we have not recorded from animals in the unanesthetized and anesthetized state. In the monkey, Arezzo et al. (7) noted slight but cumulative increments in latency in light compared with deep anesthesia across components but did not compare latencies in the waking and anesthetized states. Comparison of the latencies of P20 [(Table 1) 11.3 msec] with those obtained under roughly comparable conditions in unanesthetized cats [(3); 10.1 msec] indicates that anesthetic effects can account for some of the discrepancy in relative latencies of the N12 and N13 components.

In summary, on the basis of this preliminary study, the following observations seem justified. (a) The general agreement in relative latency across species is good, suggesting that similarly labeled components reflect similar neural events. (b) Systematic deviations from expected relative latencies are apparent in those components thought to be generated in the cervical cord and lower brainstem (N12a-N13b), and at least some of the discrepancy results from differences in body size since the same trend is apparent in short as compared with tall humans. (c) Other factors, particularly delays introduced by synaptic transmission and enhanced by barbiturate anesthesia in the animal studies, probably contribute as well to discrepancies in relative latency. These complicating factors cannot be assessed quantitatively at this time but suggest that similar recordings in unanesthetized animals will be useful.

REFERENCES

1. Allen, A. R., and Starr, A. (1978): Auditory brain stem potentials in monkey *(M. mulatta)* and man. *Electroencephalogr. Clin. Neurophysiol.*, 45:53–63.
2. Allison, T. (1979): Short latency SEPs in man: Generator sources and clinical application. In: *Symposium on Clinical Applications of Somatosensory Evoked Potentials.* American EEG Society Meeting, Atlanta, September, 1979.
3. Allison, T., Goff, W. R., and Sterman, M. B. (1966): Cerebral somatosensory responses evoked during sleep in the cat. *Electroencephalogr. Clin. Neurophysiol.*, 21:461–468.
4. Allison, T., Goff, W. R., Williamson, P. D., and Van Gilder, J. C. (1980): On the neural origin of early components of the human somatosensory evoked potential. In: *Clinical Uses of Cerebral, Brainstem and Spinal Somatosensory Evoked Potentials,* edited by J. E. Desmedt, pp. 51–68. Karger, Basel.

5. Allison, T., Goff, W. R., and Wood, C. C. (1979): Auditory, somatosensory and visual evoked potentials in the diagnosis of neuropathology: Recording considerations and normative data. In: *Human Evoked Potentials,* edited by D. Lehmann, and E. Callaway, pp. 1–16. Plenum Press, New York.
6. Allison, T., and Hume, A. L. (1981): A comparative analysis of short-latency somatosensory evoked potentials in man, monkey, cat and rat. *Exp. Neurol.,* 72:592–611.
7. Arezzo, J., Legatt, A. D., and Vaughan, H. G., Jr. (1979): Topography and intracranial sources of somatosensory evoked potentials in the monkey. I. Early components. *Electroencephalogr. Clin. Neurophysiol.,* 46:155–172.
8. Arezzo, J. C., Vaughan, H. G., Jr., and Legatt, A. D. (1981): Topography and intracranial sources of somatosensory evoked potentials in the monkey. II. Cortical components. *Electroencephalogr. Clin. Neurophysiol.,* 51:1–18.
9. Chiappa, K. H., Choi, S. K., and Young, R. R. (1980): Short-latency somatosensory evoked potentials following median nerve stimulation in patients with neurological lesions. In: *Clinical Uses of Cerebral, Brainstem and Spinal Somatosensory Evoked Potentials,* edited by J. E. Desmedt, pp. 264–281. Karger, Basel.
10. Cracco, R. Q., and Cracco, J. B. (1976): Somatosensory evoked potential in man: Far field potentials. *Electroencephalogr. Clin. Neurophysiol.,* 41:460–466.
11. Dekaban, A. S., and Sadowsky, D. (1978): Changes in brain weights during the span of human life: Relation of brain weights to body heights and body weights. *Ann. Neurol.,* 4:345–356.
12. Desmedt, J. E. (1980): *Clinical Uses of Cerebral, Brainstem and Spinal Somatosensory Evoked Potentials.* Karger, Basel.
13. Hume, A. L., and Cant, B. R. (1978): Conduction time in central somatosensory pathways in man. *Electroencephalogr. Clin. Neurophysiol.,* 45:361–375.
14. Iragui-Madoz, V. J., and Wiederholt, W. C. (1977): Far-field somatosensory evoked potentials in the cat: Correlation with depth recording. *Ann. Neurol.,* 1:569–574.
15. Jones, S. J. (1977): Short latency potentials recorded from the neck and scalp following median nerve stimulation in man. *Electroencephalogr. Clin. Neurophysiol.,* 43:853–863.
16. Kritchevsky, M., and Wiederholt, W. C. (1978): Short-latency somatosensory evoked potentials. *Arch. Neurol.,* 35:706–711.
17. Matthews, W. B., Beauchamp, M., and Small, D. G. (1974): Cervical somatosensory evoked responses in man. *Nature,* 252:230–232.
18. Tsumoto, T. (1974): Characteristics of the thalamic ventrobasal relay neurons as a function of conduction velocities of medial lemniscal fibers. *Exp. Brain Res.,* 21:211–224.
19. Wiederholt, W. C., and Iragui-Madoz, V. J. (1977): Far-field somatosensory potentials in the rat. *Electroencephalogr. Clin. Neurophysiol.,* 42:456–465.
20. Yamada, T., Kimura, J., and Nitz, D. M. (1980): Short latency somatosensory evoked potentials following median nerve stimulation in man. *Electroencephalogr. Clin. Neurophysiol.,* 48:367–376.

Clinical Applications of Evoked Potentials in Neurology,
edited by J. Courjon, F. Mauguiere, and M. Revol.
Raven Press, New York © 1982.

Subcortical and Cortical Somatosensory Evoked Potentials: Characteristic Waveform Changes Associated with Disorders of the Peripheral and Central Nervous System

S. J. Jones and A. M. Halliday

Medical Research Council, National Hospital, London WC1, England

Although it is now convincingly demonstrated that somatosensory evoked potentials (SEPs) may be affected by a variety of disorders involving the peripheral nerves (2), dorsal columns (4), brainstem (7), and cerebral hemispheres (3), the nature of the abnormalities described in the literature has generally been fairly nonspecific as to the type and locus of the underlying pathology. It seems that a general attenuation of cortical SEP amplitude may be encountered with a lesion at any level of the sensory pathway from the far periphery to the cerebral cortex, and likewise, a prolongation of latency is frequently reported whether the lesion is at peripheral, spinal, or subcortical (but not cortical) level. Attempts have occasionally been made to recognize more subtle alterations of the cortical waveform (namely, the attenuation or enhancement of individual components) and to relate these to specific lesions at cortical and subcortical level, but the recent development of techniques for recording potentials generated in the periphery and the spinal cord as well as in subcortical and cortical cerebral structures has opened the way towards recognition of many patterns of abnormality that may be characteristic of, if not absolutely unique to, a particular condition involving the peripheral or central nervous system.

The recordings illustrated were obtained using a standard eight-channel montage (not all channels are shown in Figs. 1, 2, and 5) with an extended high-frequency bandpass (−3 dB at 5 kHz) and an averager sampling rate of 8 points per millisecond. Stimuli were delivered at 2 Hz to the median nerve at the wrist (sometimes the median or ulnar nerve at the elbow) with intensity sufficient to induce a slight motor twitch. Evoked potentials occurring in the first 35 msec after the stimulus (an epoch of up to 128 msec was employed when the responses were severely delayed) were averaged in groups of 400 and subsequently combined off-line to obtain a grand average consisting of up to 1,600 sweeps. Conditions most extensively studied in our laboratory include brachial plexus injuries, Charcot–Marie–Tooth disease, Friedreich's ataxia, multiple sclerosis, and various myoclonic syndromes.

BRACHIAL PLEXUS TRACTION LESIONS

Somatosensory evoked potential components recorded from the upper cervical region and the scalp overlying the somatosensory cortical hand area contralateral to the stimulated arm (Fig. 1) (the reference was situated over the midfrontal scalp) were attenuated, delayed, or absent, depending on the severity of the lesion and the number of roots involved. The supraclavicular N9 component, however, might be attenuated to a greater or lesser degree than the cervical N13 and was occasionally entirely normal. An attenuation of N9 greater than or equal to that of N13 should be indicative of a lesion on the distal side of the dorsal root ganglia (although this does not preclude the possibility of a double lesion with involvement on the proximal side also), whereas the converse situation with N9 relatively unattenuated is likely to be caused by a proximal root avulsion with functional continuity preserved in the peripheral sensory axons.

Surgical exploration of 16 cases has confirmed the value of preoperative electro-

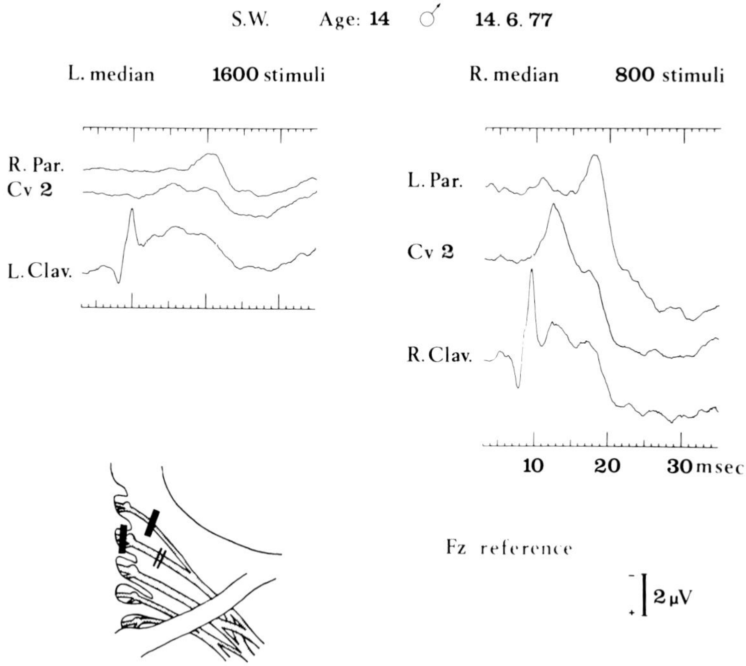

FIG. 1. Somatosensory evoked potentials recorded from the clavicle, second cervical vertebra, and parietal scalp in a patient with a traction lesion of the left brachial plexus. Subsequent surgical exploration revealed an avulsion of the C6 root (ruptured proximal to the dorsal root ganglion) consistent with a marked attenuation of the cervical response (N13) but with relative preservation of the clavicular potential (N9). A more distal rupture of the C5 root, with some damage to C6 distal to the dorsal root ganglion, may have been responsible for the slight attenuation of N9.

physiological recordings, the conclusions from which were found to be substantially accurate in 13 cases (6). The responses to median nerve stimulation were found to reflect the integrity of the C6 and C7 roots, whereas the ulnar nerve was used to investigate C8 and T1. The location of a root lesion proximal or distal to the dorsal root ganglia is of great significance with regard to the likely extent of spontaneous recovery or the outcome of surgical grafting.

CHARCOT–MARIE–TOOTH DISEASE (HEREDITARY SENSORY–MOTOR NEUROPATHY)

Cortical SEPs are generally of low amplitude but are present (with normal latency or delayed by as much as 25 msec) even when SNAPs and subcortical SEPs are absent. Conduction velocity (CV) in surviving sensory fibers can be measured by the change in cortical SEP latency when the stimulus is delivered to the elbow instead of the wrist. Out of 13 cases so far studied, sensory CV in the forearm was normal in two (60–70 m/sec) but slowed in the remainder, ranging from 50 to 10 m/sec. The degree of peripheral slowing was generally thought to be sufficient to account for the total delay of the cortical SEP, and the likely absence of involvement of central sensory pathways in the majority of cases was confirmed by the finding of a normal separation between cervical (when present) and cortical SEP components. In three cases, however, there was evidence of a slight increase in the separation between N13 and the initial cortical negativity (N20), and in two of these, extrapolation of the increase in wrist–elbow conduction time to the estimated point of entry into the spinal cord did not quite account for the total delay of N20.

FRIEDREICH'S ATAXIA

The characteristic SEP pattern in this disease (Fig. 2) (5) is an attenuated peripheral nerve component without evidence of slowed conduction in the surviving fibers, a less attenuated but possibly slightly broadened cervical response, and a markedly delayed cortical waveform with a prolonged (or multiple, see ref. 8) initial negativity. A normal shift in the latency of N20 when the stimulating electrode is removed from the wrist to the elbow confirms that, in spite of the peripheral neuropathy (predominantly axonal), it is likely to be degeneration of the central sensory pathway that is responsible for the prolongation of cortical SEP latency. This SEP pattern is clearly distinguishable from that encountered in Charcot–Marie–Tooth disease or multiple sclerosis (see below).

MULTIPLE SCLEROSIS

In view of the large number of possible manifestations of this disease, it is not surprising that several patterns of SEP abnormality are encountered (see Figs. 3 and 4). These have in common, however, preservation of the peripheral

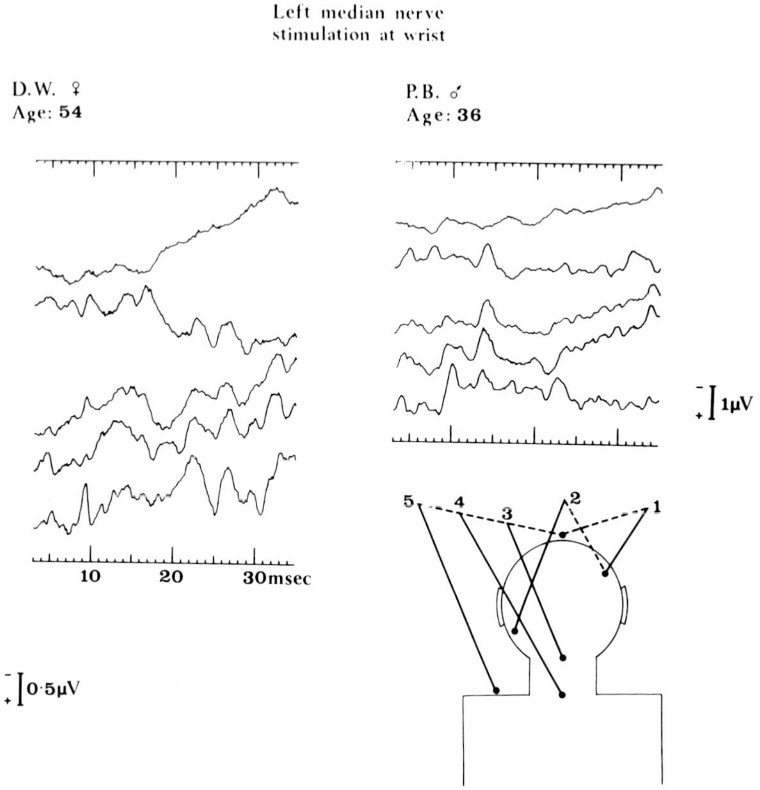

FIG. 2. Clavicular, cervical, mastoid, and scalp SEP recordings in two cases of Friedreich's ataxia. N9 (Ch. 5) is of very low amplitude but normal latency; N13 (Ch. 3 and 4) is somewhat broadened on the **left;** N14 (Ch. 2) is slightly delayed on the left and absent on the **right;** and N20 (Ch. 1, peak just visible at 32 and 34 msec) is severely delayed with a prolonged onset-to-peak duration.

nerve component. Subsequent potentials are usually attenuated, often with fragmentation of the cervical response and prolongation of cortical SEP latency, although the cervical N11 potential may also be preserved (Fig. 3, left). In less severely affected cases, there may be attenuation of N13 with the following brainstem (N14) and cortical components preserved (Fig. 3, right) or a converse pattern with N14 and N20 delayed while N13 is relatively preserved (Fig. 4). The observation that N14 and N20 are often delayed to a very similar degree suggests that both may depend on the transmission of input via the dorsal columns (4), but the relative independence of N13 suggests an origin outside the main dorsal column/medial lemniscal pathway, possibly in the spinal gray matter. Many groups have explored the possibility of using SEPs in the diagnosis of MS and have noted that abnormalities may be present even following stimulation of an asymptomatic limb. The characteristic waveform changes are distin-

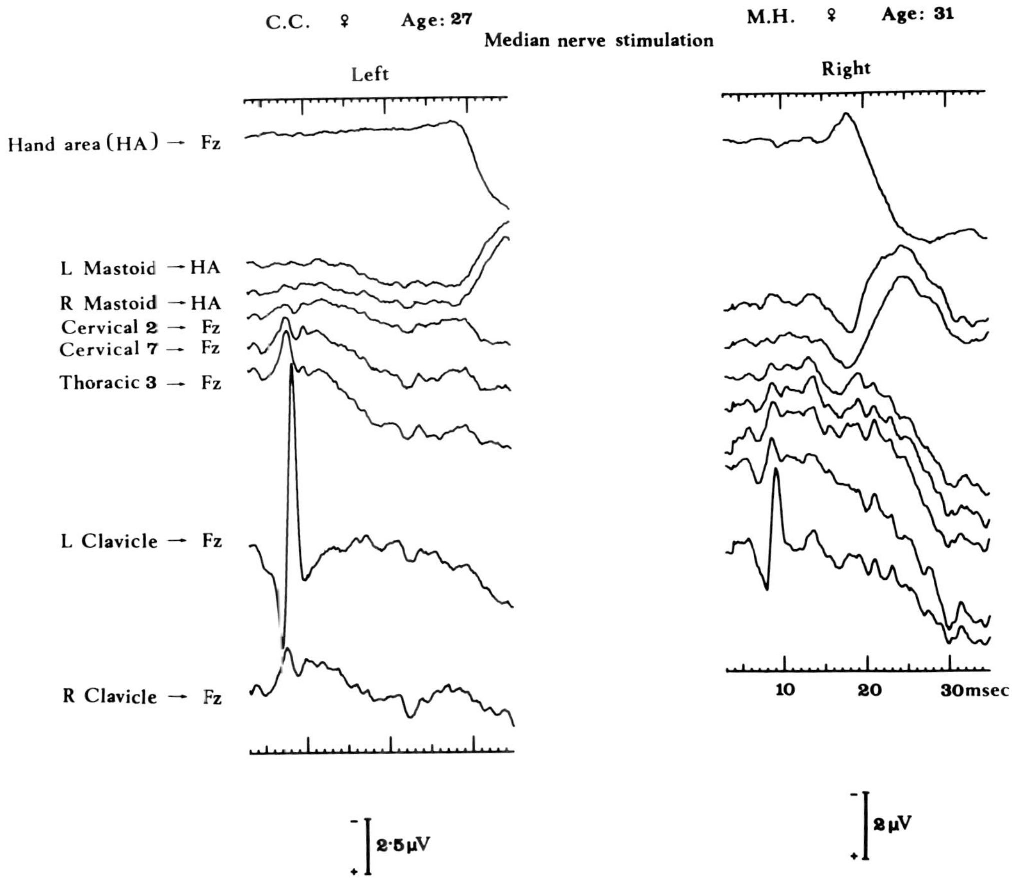

FIG. 3. Somatosensory evoked potential recordings in two cases of multiple sclerosis, demonstrating characteristic SEP abnormalities. On the **left,** N13 and N14 are doubtfully visible above a low level of background noise, and N20 is markedly delayed. On the **right,** N14 and N20 are well preserved (N14 seen in all subcortical channels), but N13 (normally sharp with an amplitude of at least 1.2 μV in Ch. 4) is apparently absent.

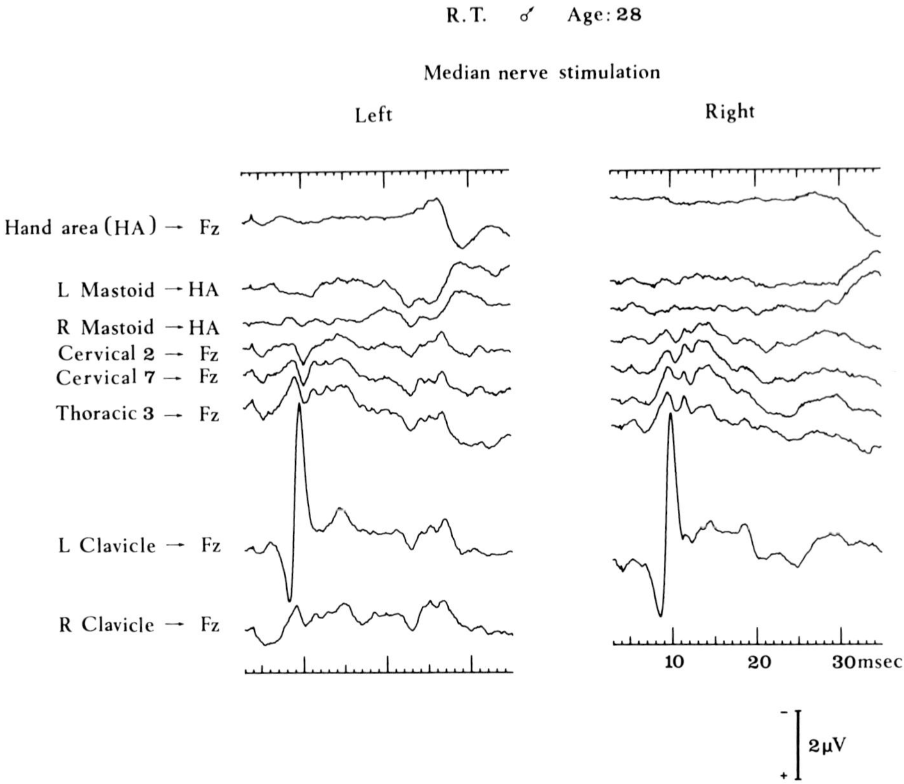

FIG. 4. Left and right median nerve responses in a patient with multiple sclerosis. All potentials up to N13 are present with normal latency, although the latter (Ch. 4–6) is of very low amplitude. N14 (Ch. 2 and 3) is delayed on the left (20 msec) and absent on the right, and N20 is bilaterally delayed.

guishable from those encountered in neuropathic conditions and, although perhaps not uniquely associated with MS, may further enhance the diagnostic power of the SEP technique.

PROGRESSIVE MYOCLONIC EPILEPSY

The well-known exaggeration of cortical SEP amplitude first described by Dawson (1) may be useful in distinguishing between progressive and benign myoclonic conditions. Although large-amplitude SEPs have been recorded in association with lesions of the spinal cord, brainstem, and other structures, the most extreme enhancement (with amplitudes of up to 10 times normal) is characteristic of progressive myoclonic epilepsy when there is jerking present in the appropriate limb. Subcortical potentials are not similarly enhanced, but other abnormalities (including absence of N20; see Fig. 5) have been observed.

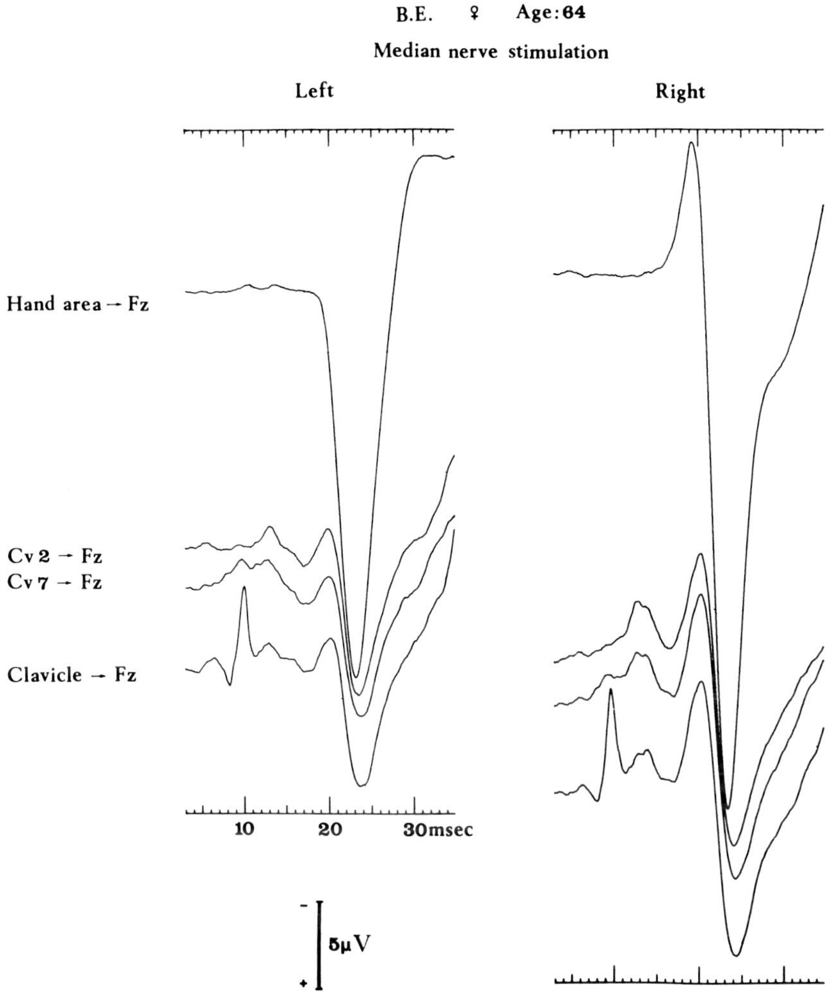

FIG. 5. Clavicular, cervical, and scalp SEPs in a case of progressive myoclonic epilepsy. The enhanced cortical potentials are not matched by enhancement of subcortical components, and N14 and N20 appear to be absent on the left in spite of normal sensation.

With further refinement of recording techniques and acquisition of suitable clinical material, many further characteristic patterns of abnormality may be recognized, extending the usefulness of SEPs in the investigation and diagnosis of neurological disease. Cervical spondylosis and syringomyelia, for example, appear particularly appropriate for study by established techniques. Ulnar nerve responses have been studied less extensively but may be of interest in the context of, for example, thoracic outlet syndromes. Finally, the techniques of lower limb, dermatomal, and facial nerve stimulation should be capable of further development and exploitation.

REFERENCES

1. Dawson, G. D. (1947): Investigations on a patient subject to myoclonic seizures after sensory stimulation. *J. Neurol. Neurosurg. Psychiatry,* 10:141–162.
2. Desmedt, J. E., and Noël, P. (1973): Average cerebral evoked potentials in the evaluation of lesions of the sensory nerves and the central somatosensory pathway. In: *New Developments in Electromyography and Clinical Neurophysiology, Vol. 2,* edited by J. E. Desmedt, pp. 352–371. Karger, Basel.
3. Giblin, D. R. (1964): Somatosensory evoked potentials in healthy subjects and in patients with lesions of the nervous system. *Ann. N.Y. Acad. Sci.,* 112:93–142.
4. Halliday, A. M., and Wakefield, G. S. (1963): Cerebral evoked potentials in patients with dissociated sensory loss. *J. Neurol. Neurosurg. Psychiatry,* 26:211–219.
5. Jones, S. J., Baraitser, M., and Halliday, A. M. (1980): Peripheral and central somatosensory nerve conduction defects in Friedreich's ataxia. *J. Neurol. Neurosurg. Psychiatry,* 43:495–503.
6. Jones, S. J., Wynn Parry, C. B., and Landi, A. (1981): Diagnosis of brachial plexus traction lesions by sensory nerve action potentials and somatosensory evoked potentials. *Injury,* 12:376–382.
7. Noël, P., and Desmedt, J. E. (1975): Somatosensory cerebral evoked potentials after vascular lesions of the brainstem and diencephalon. *Brain,* 98:113–128.
8. Noël, P., and Desmedt, J. E. (1980): Cerebral and far-field somatosensory evoked potentials in neurological disorders involving the cervical spinal cord, brainstem, thalamus and cortex. In: *Progress in Clinical Neurophysiology, Vol. 7, Clinical Uses of Cerebral, Brainstem and Spinal Somatosensory Evoked Potentials,* edited by J. E. Desmedt, pp. 205–230. Karger, Basel.

Clinical Applications of Evoked Potentials in Neurology,
edited by J. Courjon, F. Mauguiere, and M. Revol.
Raven Press, New York © 1982.

Early Somatosensory Evoked Potentials in Thalamo-Cortical Lesions of the Lemniscal Pathways in Humans

*F. Mauguière, *A. M. Brunon, **J. F. Echallier, and *J. Courjon

**EEG Department, Hôpital Neurologique, 69394 Lyon Cédex, France; and **C.E.M.I., 69394 Lyon Cédex 3, France*

Most authors agree that electrical stimulation of the median nerve at the wrist elicits scalp-recorded potentials that are successively positive, negative, and positive. According to the classification of the Brussels committee they are currently referred to in literature as P14 (or P15), N18 (or N20), P24 (or P25), and P40 (6,7,12,16–18,20). However, much controversy still exists as to the exact origins of these early SEP components in humans (see ref. 1 for a review), and the clinical interpretation of SEP may be uncertain. The aim of this chapter is to study the abnormal patterns of SEP in patients with thalamic or parietal lesions in order to correlate them with clinical, radiological, and CT scan data. Such a clinical approach has been shown to increase the diagnostic value of SEP recordings in clinical practice (2,5,15,24–26) and may contribute (in parallel with experimental data in animals and with cortical or subcortical recordings in man) to the localization of the SEP generators in humans.

SUBJECTS AND METHODS

Subjects

Normal Subjects

Normative data were obtained from 18 members of the medical staff aged 32 ± 11 (SD) years and without previous history of neurological disease.

Patients

Either of two criteria was used for the selection of our 27 patients.

1. A clinical history of somatosensory loss caused by a well-localized unilateral cortical or subcortical lesion investigated by computerized tomography (18 cases) or radionuclide scanning (one case). The lesions were of vascular origin in 15

patients; the four remaining cases were patients with cortical atrophy resulting from head trauma (two cases) or following neurosurgery for an intracerebral hematoma (one case) or a meningioma (one case).

2. A well-limited vascular thalamic lesion with or without somatosensory loss (eight cases).

Among the 19 patients selected with the first criterion (nine males, 10 females, mean age 56 ± 13 years), two categories could be differentiated. Thirteen patients had large ischemic (nine cases), hemorrhagic (three cases), or atrophic (one case) lesions involving either the subcortical structures only (eight cases), or both the white fibers and the cortex of the parietal lobe (five cases). Lesions were left-sided in 10 cases and right-sided in three cases. As shown on Fig. 1A, the afferent fibers to the parietal lobe could be considered to be interrupted in all of these cases. The six remaining patients, aged 47 ± 16 (SD) years, had superficial cortical lesions (three right-sided, three left-sided) that were well-limited parietal ischemic (three cases) or atrophic (three cases) lesions. Computerized tomography data of five patients are presented in Fig. 1B. One patient of this group was investigated only with radionuclide scanning, which showed a superficial posterior parietal infarction (Fig 2). In two cases, the lesions seemed to be restricted to the postcentral gyrus.

The group with thalamic lesions is composed of eight patients, five females and three males aged 48 ± 15 (SD) years. The lesions were bilateral ischemic lacunar hypodensities in two cases, right-sided hemorrhage in two cases, ischemic hypodensities in three cases (right-sided in two cases, left-sided in one case). The remaining patient had been operated on for a posttraumatic epilepsy: CT scan showed a large hypodense area involving most of the right thalamic mass and adjacent parietal subcortical structures. As shown in Fig. 1C, lesions were scattered along the whole rostro–caudal extent of the thalamus; the ventroposterolateral nucleus (VPL) was obviously damaged in four cases.

Methods

Clinical Examination

Clinical examination was performed in all patients by the same investigator (FM) on the day of the SEP recording session. Sensations of temperature, pain, vibration, and joint position were tested in all subjects. In patients with minimal sensory loss, two-point discriminative sense was studied on both sides at the tip of the second finger and on the dorsum of the hand and forearms; stereognosis was tested for both hands with familiar objects using both verbal and visuo–tactile recognitions; graphesthesia was studied on the dorsum of hands and of forearms and on hand palms; tactile extinction phenomena for bilateral stimulation were systematically looked for.

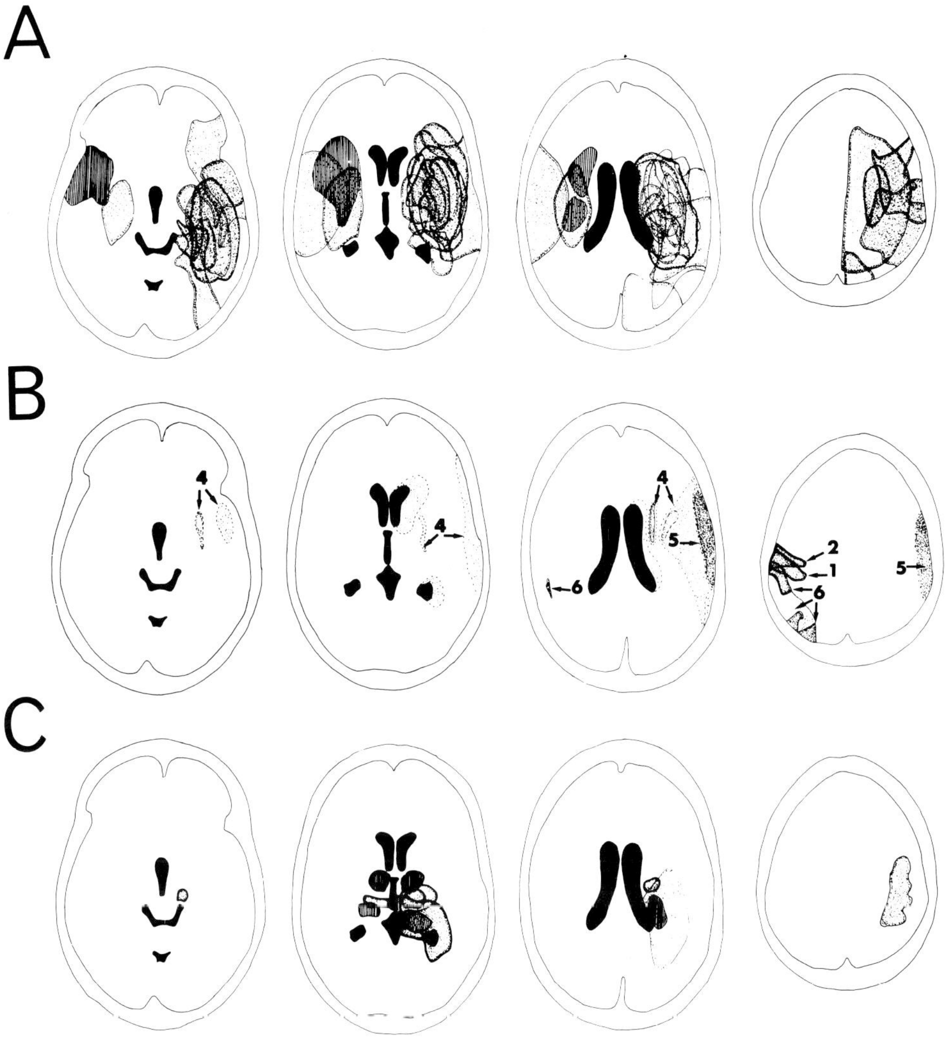

FIG. 1. Localization of lesions according to CT scans. The lesions that were not associated with a clinical sensory loss are represented as hatched areas. **A:** Large subcortical and cortical lesions. **B:** Cortical lesions: the numbers indicate the sites of the CT scan abnormalities for each patient and refer to the case numbers listed in Table 2 and in Figs. 5–7. **C:** Thalamic lesions.

SEP Recording Procedure

In most patients, SEPs were repeatedly recorded; all the data reported and discussed in this chapter were obtained 3 months or more after the acute stage for both vascular and traumatic lesions.

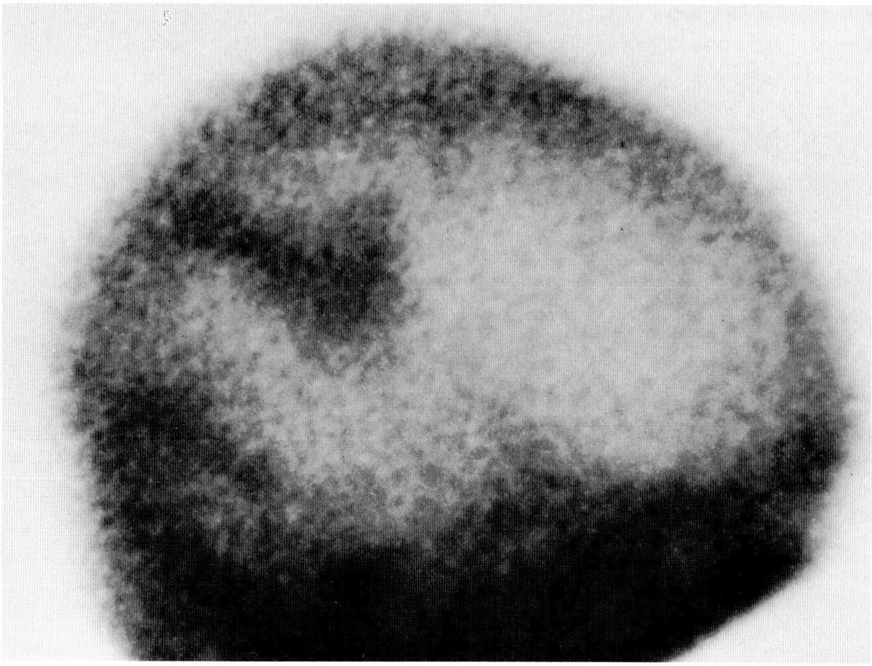

FIG. 2. Radionuclide scan showing a right-sided parietal infarct in the only patient without a CT scan.

Standard recording

The SEP recording was carried out in a dimly lit shielded room with the subject lying on a bed. The median nerve was electrically stimulated with a square-wave pulse of 0.2 msec duration delivered at a rate of 2/sec through a pair of surface electrodes placed 3 cm apart, just proximal to the wrist. The stimulus intensity was adjusted to the motor threshold for contraction of the opponens pollicis. Both median nerves were stimulated succesively; in patients, the unaffected side was stimulated first. The signal was amplified by Grass 7P5 amplifiers (filter bandpass 1 to 3,000 Hz, 6 dB down); 1,000 sweeps were averaged by a Solar Labo 16 computer as described elsewhere (21) with 1,024 samples per channel for an analysis time of 60 msec. The stimulation was triggered by the computer. In all subjects, a five-channel montage of cup electrodes was used to record the activity: at Erb's point; C_7 and C_2 spinal processes using a F_Z reference; and at two sites on the scalp situated, respectively, 2 cm behind C_Z on the midline and 2 cm behind C_Z, 7 cm contralaterally to the stimulated side. The scalp electrodes were referred to the interconnected earlobes. Two ground electrodes were used, one midfrontal, the other on the forearm on the side of the stimulation.

Additional studies

In patients with purely cortical lesions *(vide infra)* and in some others, additional recordings were performed to study the topography of the responses. Two different montages were used in these cases: a coronal montage with six to eight electrodes situated in a frontal plane 2 cm behind C_Z, referred to the interconnected earlobes and disposed contra- and ipsilaterally to the stimulated side; and a longitudinal montage of six electrodes (three on each side) situated in the parietal regions (as described above), in C_4 and C_3 and in F_4 and F_3 referred to the ipsilateral earlobe.

An analysis time of 140 msec was used for these complementary studies. In four cases of cortical lesions, the study of the early parietal responses was completed by a recording using a shorter analysis time of 48 msec with the same sampling rate of 1,024.

SEP nomenclature

The peak latencies were automatically calculated using the cursors of the data processor. The polarity latency nomenclature recommended by the Donchin committee (9) was used for the classification of the different peaks.

RESULTS

Normative Data

Normative data are summarized in Table 1. As shown in Fig. 3, the following potentials were constantly observed in normals: a negative N11 potential at Erb's point; a negative N14 cervical potential; a positive scalp-recorded P15 potential; followed by negative N20 and positive P25 peaks. The P15 peak was found to be widely distributed on the scalp, whereas N20 and P25 peaks were recorded only in the parietal region contralateral to the stimulated side. The mean amplitudes indicated in Table 1 were calculated from the baseline for N14 and P15; for N11, N20, and P25, the peak-to-peak amplitudes between the apexes of the peak itself and of the immediately preceeding potential were chosen because of the difficulty in determining the exact level of the base line.

TABLE 1. *Normative data*

	Erb's point N11	C_2 N14	Scalp largely distributed P15	Contralateral parietal region N20	P25	P40
Peak latency mean ± SD (msec)	10.8 ± 0.8	14.4 ± 0.9	15.4 ± 1.3	20 ± 1.2	24.5 ± 2.4	40.2 ± 5.5
Amplitude mean ± SD (μV)	6.9 ± 3.6	3.6 ± 1.1	1.4 ± 0.6	2.9 ± 1.2	4.4 ± 2.9	4.7 ± 2

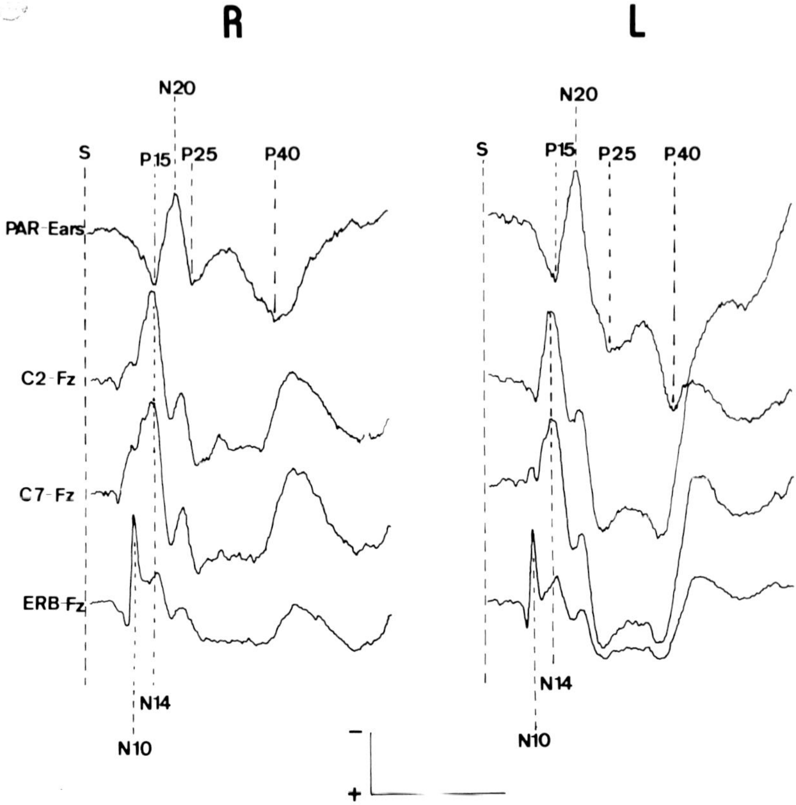

FIG. 3. Normal SEPs (see text for details). **R:** Right median nerve stimulation. **L:** Left median nerve stimulation. PAR, contralateral parietal lead. Calibration: 5 μV, 25 msec.

A parietal P40 potential was observed in 16 subjects with much interindividual variability of amplitudes and peak latencies. For this potential, the amplitude was estimated from base line because of the varying size of an N30 potential which may be interposed between P25 and P40 and which is maximal over the prerolandic area.

Other subcomponents such as an N11 peak and a positive notch on the descending phase of P15 were observed in some subjects. These potentials are known to be recorded more easily with a noncephalic reference electrode (2,8); in our recording conditions, they were found to be very inconsistent and therefore were not studied in patients. With an analysis time of 140 msec, an N70 potential was constant over the parietal region of the intact hemisphere in patients. This component was not studied in our normals; for this reason, the abnormalities observed in patients will not be discussed in detail in this chapter.

SEP in Patients

Our patients may be classified into three groups according to the aspects of their SEP. Group I (five cases) consisted of patients with normal SEP whichever side was stimulated (type I SEP). Group II (16 cases) consisted of patients with normal N11, N14, and P15 potentials and absent N20, P25, and P40 peaks following stimulation of the abnormal side (type II SEP, Fig. 4). Group III (six cases) included those patients with asymmetrical N20, P25, and P40 potentials between normal and abnormal sides and normal N11, N14, and P15 potentials (type III SEP, Figs. 5–7).

Patients of Group I

Normal SEPs were observed in patients without any clinically obvious somatosensory loss and in patients with only a "tactile extinction" phenomenon on the affected side when symmetrical stimulations were applied on both sides of the body. The former group was made of three patients, two with transient hypokinetic mutism resulting from bilateral anterior thalamic infarcts (Fig. 1C) and one with a left thalamo–capsular hypodensity (Fig. 1C). Clinical examination of somatosensory function showed only a reduced reactivity to pain in the two cases with anterior thalamic lesions; right-sided paresthesias were the only somatosensory symptom in the third case.

The latter group was composed of two patients, one with a right posterior thalamic hemorrhage (Fig. 1C) and the other with a large ischemic lesion involving the white matter, which, on CT scans, could reasonably be supposed to interrupt most of the afferent fibers to the left parietal lobe (Fig. 1A). In this latter patient, an additional study with a 140-msec analysis time was performed, and the N70 potential was found to be absent following right median nerve stimulation. Synchronous stimulation of both median nerves in the first of these patients evoked normal and symmetrical parietal responses on both hemispheres.

Patients of Group II

All patients with type II SEP were hemiplegic, with complete sensory loss for light tactile stimuli, vibrations, joint position, and passive movements. Of the patients with lesions confined to the minor hemisphere, six had a left asomatognosia with complete anosognosia. The causal lesions were large cortico–subcortical lesions in most cases (12 patients), but thalamic or capsulo–thalamic lesions with damage to VPL were observed in four cases (Fig. 1C).

Patients of Group III

Type III SEPs were correlated with minimal somatosensory loss of the cortical type; clinical data concerning these six patients are detailed in Table 2. None of them was hemiplegic; all had normal tactile exploration.

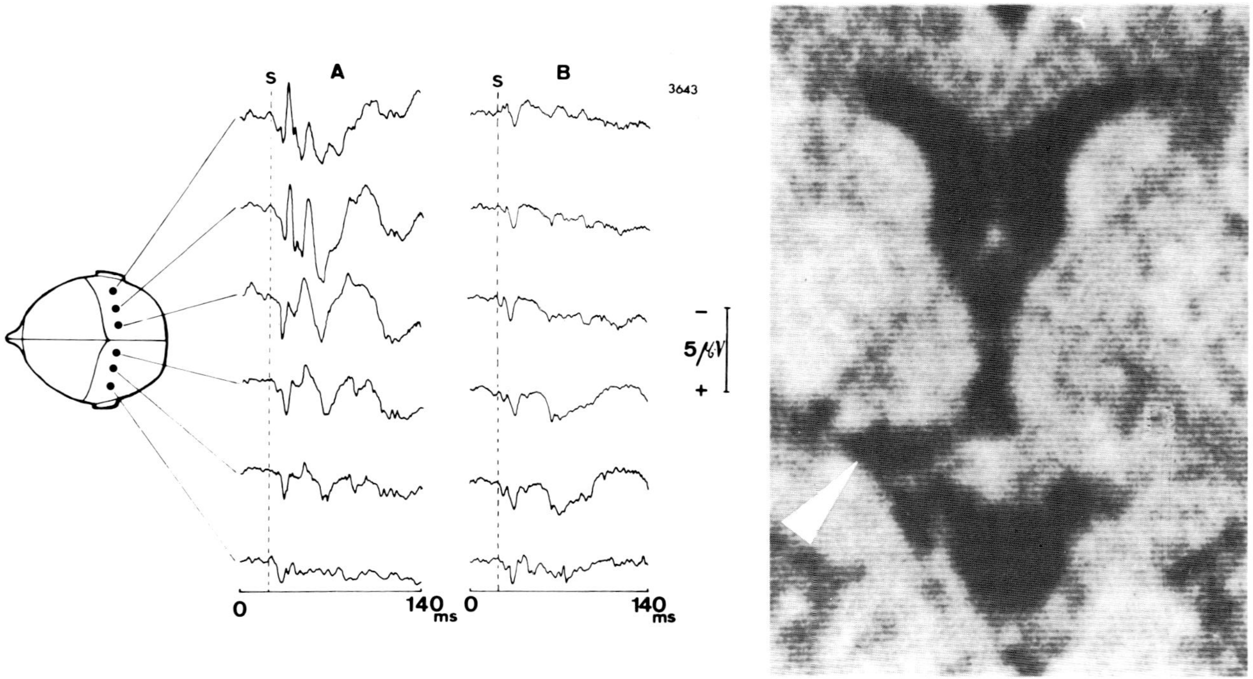

FIG. 4. Abnormal SEPs in one case of left-sided posterior thalamic infarct *(white arrowhead)* showing normal contralateral responses following left median nerve stimulation **(A)** and absent N20, P25, and P40 peak over the left parietal region following right median nerve stimulation. **(B)** Note in **B** that the first positive component P15 is present.

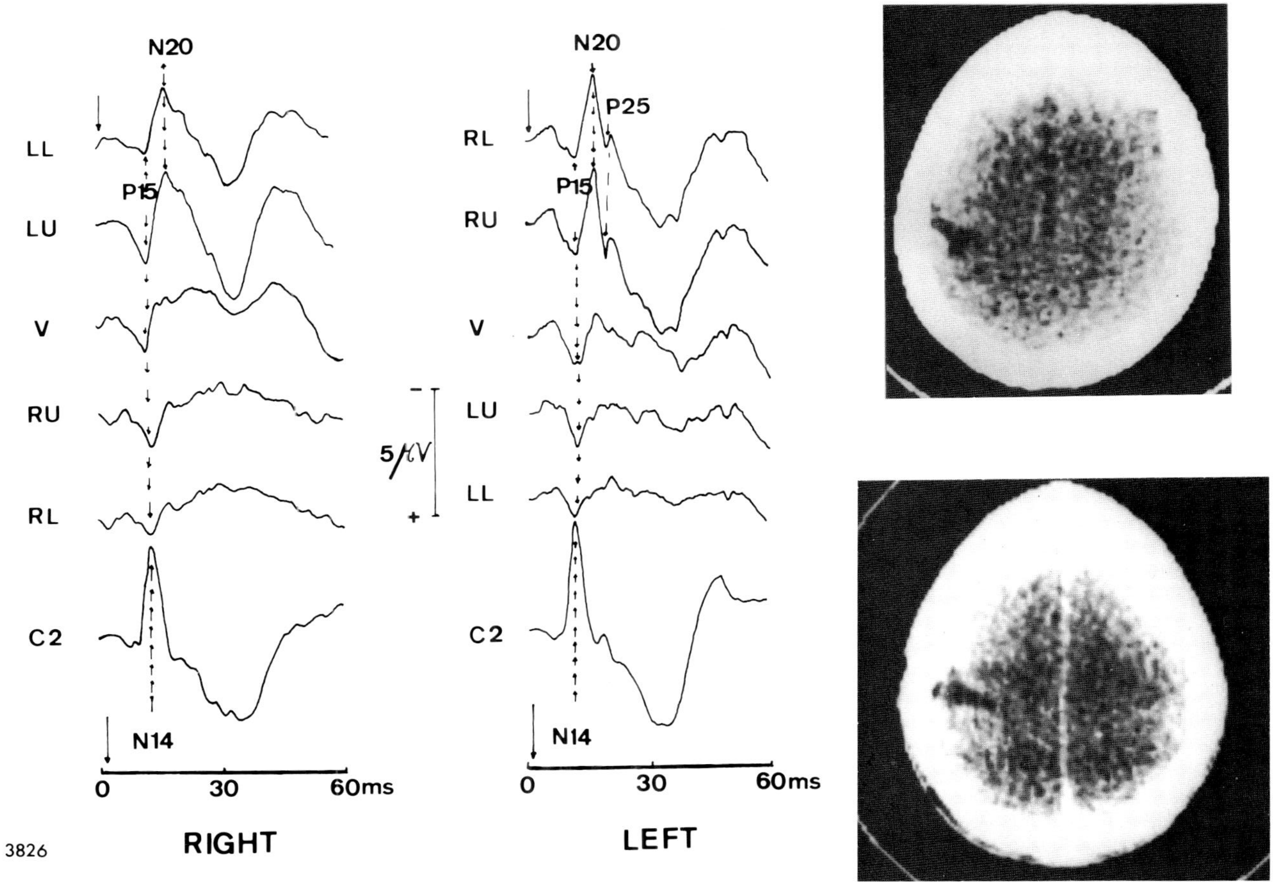

FIG. 5. Abnormal SEPs following right **(right)** and left **(left)** median nerve stimulation in one patient with a small-sized cortical infarct in the left parietal lobe on CT scans (case 1). Note the absence of the P25 component and the abnormal aspect of the N20 potential in the left parietal region. Derivations C2, second cervical spinal process–F_Z; RL, right lower parietal lead; RU, right upper parietal lead; V, vertex lead; LU, left upper parietal lead; LL, left lower parietal lead. All parietal electrodes are referred to the interconnected earlobes. The CT scan of this patient is the **upper** one; the **lower** CT scan concerns patient 2 (see Fig. 1B).

TABLE 2. *Somatosensory impairment in patients of group III*

Case	Age (years)	Pain, temperature	Touch	Vibration sense	Position sense	Graphesthesia	Stereognosis	Tactile extinction
1	36	N	N	N	↘	↘	↘ O	NO
2	31	N	↘	N	N	↘	↘ O	YES
3	75	N	N	N	N	↘	↘ O	YES
4	43	N	↘	N	↘	↘	↘	NO
5	41	N	↘	N	N	↘	↘ O	YES
6	57	N	↘	↘	↘	↘ O	↘ O	NO

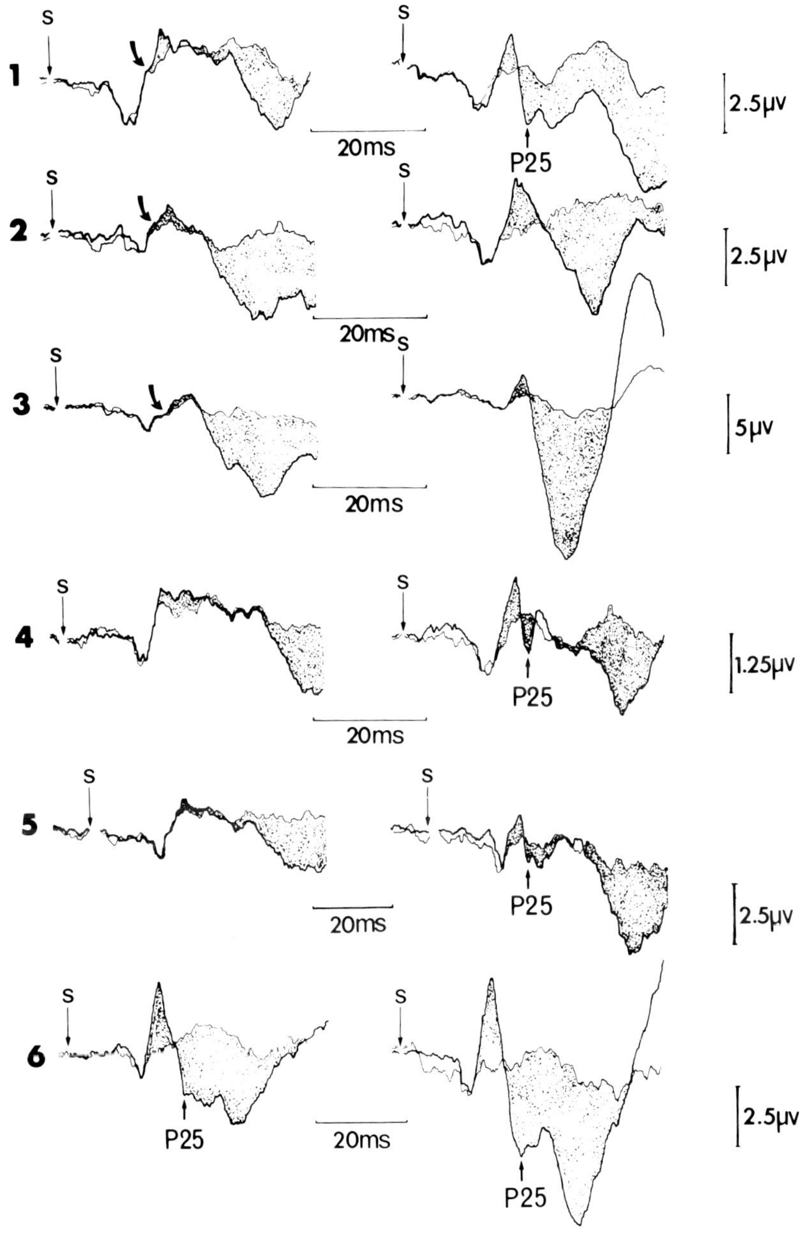

FIG. 6. Superimposed contralateral and ipsilateral parietal responses to the stimulation of the median nerve on the normal side **(right column)** and on the side of the somatosensory loss **(left column)** in six patients with unilateral small-sized lesions of the parietal lobe. Note that in all cases but one, the amplitude of the N20 is lowered. The case numbers are the same as in Table 2 and in Fig. 1B.

Type III SEP may be characterized by one or more of the following abnormalities: delayed N20 (three cases); N20 of reduced amplitude (five cases); absent P25 (four cases); and P40 with reduced amplitude (six cases).

Moreover, in agreement with earlier studies (28,29), a lowering of the amplitude of the N70 potential was found in these six patients.

As demonstrated in Figs. 5 and 6, the traces must be carefully studied for a correct analysis of these changes (the case numbers refer to the same patients for Figs. 1B, 5, and 6 and for Table II). In Fig. 5, the SEPs observed in a case of small-sized left parietal infarct caused by a thrombosis of the left internal carotid artery (case 1) are represented; on the left parietal traces following the stimulation of the right median nerve, the N20 potential could be considered to be within normal limits, whereas the P25 was obviously absent.

However, if one superimposes the ipsi- and contralateral parietal responses to evaluate the amplitude of the N20, as proposed by Desmedt and Cheron (8), it becomes clear (trace 1 of Fig. 6) that the N20 peak for right-sided stimulation is delayed with a little hump on its ascending phase and largely reduced in amplitude. A similar study was performed for the six patients of this group, and the results are represented on Fig. 6.

Moreover, as shown in Fig. 7, the recording of central responses may also be useful in these patients not only to appreciate the amplitude of N20 wave but also to analyze the shape of the N20–P25 complex. It has been demonstrated by multichannel topographical studies that N20 is recorded with maximal amplitude from lateral and posterior parietal electrodes and is not recorded more anteriorly than the level of the central fissure (10). The recording of central responses and the study of the coronal parietal responses were found to be necessary to make sure of the correct placement of the parietal leads in this group of patients with slightly asymmetrical N20 potentials. The electrode placement is probably of less importance for P25 and P40 peaks, since these potentials are of a larger amplitude than N20 and are distributed over a wider zone, posterior to the C_3 and C_4 electrodes (10). However, as shown in Fig. 6, the P25 potential was absent over the normal hemisphere in two patients; in these cases, the absence of the P25 wave on the affected side was, therefore, not significant.

Correlations with other complementary investigations were quite easy in four patients (cases 1, 2, 3, and 6) with well-limited cortical parietal lesions (see Figs. 1B and 5 for cases 1, 2, 6 and Fig. 2 for case 3). In the two remaining cases, such clear-cut correlations were impossible because the CT scans showed large unilateral cortical heterogeneous zones of retractive atrophy with an enlarged lateral ventricle.

In one patient only (case 6), the N20 wave was found to be within normal limits over the damaged hemisphere. In this case, the lesion was mainly confined to the posterior parietal region (Fig. 1B); this patient was the only one in this group who developed an optic ataxia in the right visual field.

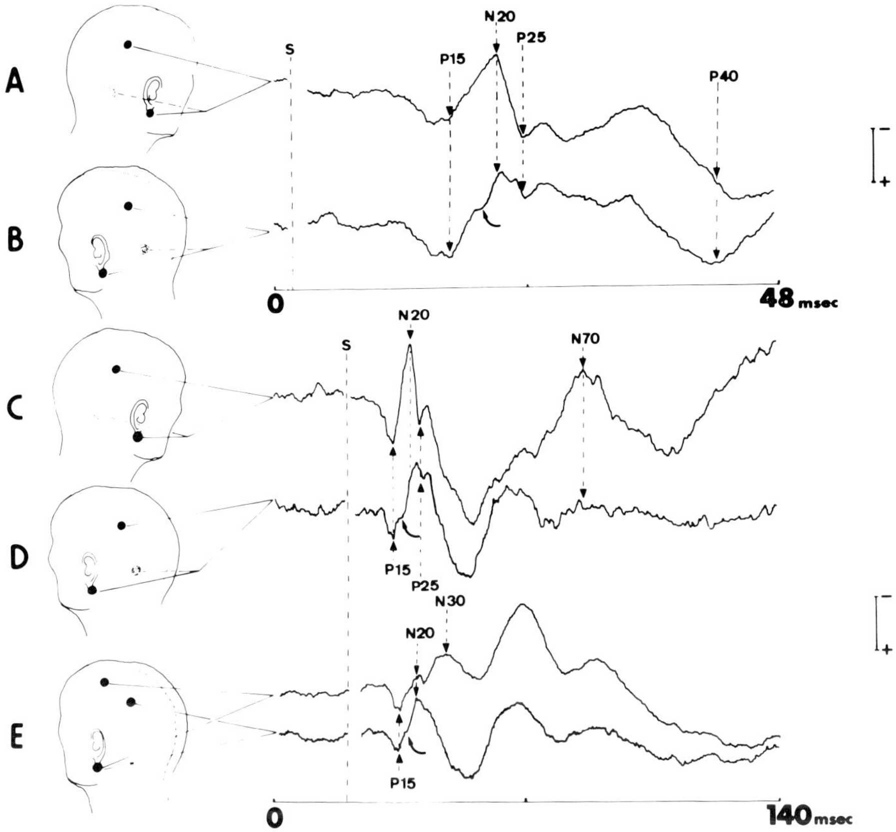

FIG. 7. Complementary EP studies in one case of right astereognosis caused by a left parietal infarct (case 1 of group III). **A:** Normal right parietal response following left median nerve stimulation. **B:** Abnormal left parietal response following right median nerve stimulation with a retarded and lowered N20 and absent P25. **C:** Right parietal response following left median nerve stimulation showing the normal N70 potential. **D:** Left parietal response with absent N70 component following right median nerve stimulation. **E:** Central *(upper trace)* and parietal *(lower trace)* responses on the left side following right median nerve stimulation. Note in the central region the presence of an N30 potential and the almost complete disappearance of the N20 component. Calibrations: for **A** and **B** 3 μV; for **C** through **E,** 1.5 μV.

DISCUSSION

Since the study of Halliday and Wakefield (15), it is widely accepted that the scalp-recorded N20 peak is mediated by the lemniscal pathway and is normal in lesions of the spinothalamic tract. Correlations have already been attempted between the degree of sensory loss and the scalp-recorded SEP occuring during the 100 msec following stimulation of the median nerve in patients with lesions of the parietal lobe (see 19, 28 for reviews). These studies demonstrated a reduced amplitude of contralateral SEPs corresponding roughly to the P40 and N70 components of this chapter in patients with moderate somatosensory deficits (see, for instance, cases B, F, and J of ref. 28). Using simultaneous stimulation of both median nerves, Yamada et al. (29) showed that the N70 potential recorded contralaterally to the clinically affected side was modified in patients with parietal lesions and normal pain, temperature, vibration, and joint position sense. This was observed even in patients with normal and symmetrical SEP following unilateral stimulation; no description of stereognosis is available in this study. Such a lowering of the amplitude of N70 was present in our six patients with cortical lesions (group III), but our study indicates that more precise correlations may be envisaged between the earlier scalp-recorded SEPs (P15, N20, P25, P40) and the degree of the clinical somatosensory loss and the site of the lesion. These correlations will be discussed in parallel with data pertaining to the localization of the sources of the scalp-recorded SEP.

Correlations with Clinical Data

The SEPs were found to be normal in patients without permanent somatosensory loss. It may be surprising that "tactile extinction" phenomenon was associated with normal SEP in two patients; however, one may suppose that this phenomenon is mostly a result of an unbalanced activity between the two hemispheres when they process competitive sensory information and is not the direct consequence of a mere unilateral deafferentation of the parietal cortex. In one of these patients, the contralateral SEPs were identical following unilateral or synchronous bilateral stimulation of the median nerves; this suggests that, in this peculiar case, the extinction phenomenon was caused by "hemiinattention" (see 11 for a recent review of the concept) and not by a temporary "switch off" of somatosensory information processing by the damaged hemisphere when both sides were simultaneously stimulated. A similar discrepancy is known to occur for audition between extinction of one ear in a dichotic listening test and normal auditory evoked potentials in both temporal regions (23).

In patients of group II, a gross sensory loss was associated with the absence of all scalp-recorded potentials, P15 excepted. This result is in agreement with recent studies of early SEPs in similar patients (2,22,24).

We do not know of any previous description of N20 and P25 abnormalities in patients with astereognosis associated with minimal somatosensory loss. The "N1" potential, which corresponds to our N20, was absent in one of the cases recently reported by Anziska and Cracco (2); this patient (case 30) had a right cortical infarct on CT scan with impaired sensation for position and vibration, but the degree of the somatosensory deficit was not detailed. Green and McLeod (13) observed an abnormal positive peak in the central region in one patient with right parietal infarct and mild sensory loss on the left side of the body; this potential might correspond to our P25, although its latency was shorter in normals [20.5 $\pm$ 1.2 (SD) msec].

Our finding is in agreement with previous well-detailed clinical studies, suggesting that the integration of somatosensory impulse patterns into spatial information about objects may take place in the hand area of the primary sensory cortex (SI) when the hand is used for stereognostic discrimination (27). The lowering of the N20 potential and the absence of the P25 component could be considered to be the electrophysiological correlates of the functional disorder of SI neurons in these patients. In one patient only (case 6 of group III), both EP and CT scan data favored the hypothesis of an intact SI area coexisting with a gross astereognosis.

Correlations with the Site of the Lesions

Neck-recorded early potentials and P15 scalp-recorded potentials (earlobe reference) were normal in all of our patients with thalamo–cortical lesions; this result suggests that all these components have a subthalamic origin and confirms previous clinical studies (14,22,24). Desmedt and Cheron (8), using a noncephalic reference electrode, demonstrated in normals that the early positive far-field scalp-recorded potential following median nerve stimulation is a complex polyphasic event made, in this study, of four successive potentials, the last of which (P14) is supposed to have its origin in the medial lemniscus and corresponds closely to our P15 potential recorded with earlobe reference. With a reference electrode on the dorsum of the hand, Anziska and Cracco (2) confirmed that this far-field early positivity (which is named P3 in their study) is normal in thalamo–cortical lesions.

In our patients, the N20, P25, and P40 were absent in thalamic and subcortical lesions but, although present, were also clearly abnormal in five patients out of six with cortical parietal lesions. Two conclusions may be drawn from this finding: the first is that lesions of the soma or of the axons of the thalamo-cortical neurons of the lemniscal pathway are associated with the same SEP pattern (i.e., absent N20 and following potentials); the second is that the N20 and P25 potentials could have origins in or near the primary sensory cortex of area SI.

The P25 (or equivalent events with slightly different latencies) is considered by most authors to be generated in the somatosensory cortex (1,4,5,18), but the origin of the N20 is still unclear. Detailed studies in normals strongly suggest that N20, which is recorded only in the parietal region contralateral to the stimulated side, results from the synchronous postsynaptic potentials generated by the cortical neurons of area SI in response to the afferent thalamo–cortical volley (see 1,7,8 for recent reviews). However data obtained in patients have been presented as evidence against the above hypothesis by Chiappa et al. (4,5) who reported normal N20 waves in patients with severe centrum semiovale leucoencephalopathy or neocortical death from anoxia and suggested a thalamic origin for N20. These results are in contradiction with ours, since we found the N20 potential to be absent in lesions of thalamo–cortical white fibers at the centrum semiovale level (one case excepted; see below) and abnormal in well-limited cortical lesions. Such a discrepancy might perhaps reflect methodological differences. In the study by Chiappa (3), the criteria for the selection of patients were very different from ours; moreover, a single C_4–F_Z channel was used to record the activity in the centro–parietal region. With this montage, the P15 component is almost completely canceled, and the N20 potential is not recorded with its maximal amplitude.

It seems important in this kind of study to choose patients in whom clinical data concerning somatosensory impairment may be obtained. This necessity is well illustrated in one of our patients with a left ischemic lesion (Fig. 1A); on the CT scan performed 3 months after the ischemic attack, most of the thalamo-cortical fibers could be reasonably considered as interrupred by the lesion. Nevertheless, at the same period, the only somatosensory deficit was a tactile extinction phenomenon on the right side, and N20 was normal following right median nerve stimulation. The same kind of discrepancy between CT scan and electro-clinical data was observed in two patients with astereognosis and abnormal but present N20 and P25 (suggesting well-limited cortical lesions) in whom large cortical and subcortical atrophic lesions were observed on CT scans (cases 4 and 5, see Fig. 1B). Multichannel scalp recordings were useful to make sure of the electrode placement and to correctly interpret the N20 potential. The amplitude of the N20 wave is difficult to evaluate by peak-to-peak or base line-to-peak measurements; the superimposition of ipsi- and contralateral responses was found to be more valuable since the slight differences of amplitude between ipsi- and contralateral P15 (or P14) observed with noncephalic reference (8) may be negligible with an earlobe reference (this point merits checking). Because of these methodological difficulties, attempts to localize the SEP generators by mere correlations between scalp recordings and CT data may be hazardous in some cases.

CONCLUSIONS

From our results, it may be concluded that SEP patterns are different in thalamic and cortical parietal lesions of the somesthetic pathways. The modifications of the N20 potential in patients with cortical lesions may result either from a desynchronized thalamo-cortical afferent volley or from a disorganized postsynaptic response of the cortical neurons of area SI. The latter hypothesis would be in better agreement with current concepts concerning the pathophysiology of astereognosis and is supported by scalp and pial recordings in man (1,7,8). A higher degree of correlation between the activity of cortical SI neurons and N20–P25 waves was suggested by Allison et al. (1) who concluded from direct pial recordings of the postcentral gyrus in man that N20 could be generated in the posterior bank of the central sulcus (Brodman's area 3) and P25 in the surface of the postcentral gyrus (Brodman's area 1). Should the hypothesis of a cortical origin of N20 be valid, a question would remain in regard to the absence of scalp-recorded events related with the postsynaptic response of the VPL neurons, since the positive P15 far-field component seems to be generated in the subthalamic white fibers of the medial lemniscus and is probably not the scalp-recorded correlate of the large positive potential constantly recorded with intrathalamic electrodes in man following stimulation of the median nerve (see 3 for a review). Even in patients with "small cortical lesions," it seems obvious that both the cortical neurons and the presynaptic ends of thalamo-cortical fibers are damaged; therefore, electroclinical correlations in these patients cannot be pertinent for a precise localization of the generator of the N20 potential.

ACKNOWLEDGMENTS

The authors are grateful to Ms M. Piccolo and B. Demarcq for their invaluable contribution to the preparation of the manuscript.

REFERENCES

1. Allison, T., Goff, W. R., Williamson, P. D., and Vangilder, J. C. (1980): On the neural origin of early components of the human somatosensory evoked Potential. In: *Progress in Clinical Neurophysiology, Vol. 7, Clinical Uses of Cerebral Brainstem and Spinal Somatosensory Evoked Potentials,* edited by J. E. Desmedt, pp. 51–68. Karger, Basel.
2. Anziska, B., and Cracco, R. Q. (1980): Short latency somatosensory evoked potentials: Studies in patients with focal neurological disease. *Electroencephalogr. Clin. Neurophysiol.,* 49:227–239.
3. Celesia, G. G., (1979): Somatosensory evoked potentials recorded directly from human thalamus and SMI cortical area. *Arch. Neurol.,* 36:399–405.
4. Chiappa, K. H., Choi, S. K., and Young, R. R. (1980): Short latency somato-sensory evoked potentials following median nerve stimulation in patients with neurological lesions. In: *Progress in Clinical Neurophysiology, Vol. 7, Clinical Uses of Cerebral Brainstem and Spinal Somatosensory Evoked Potentials,* edited by J. E. Desmedt, pp. 264–281. Karger, Basel.
5. Chiappa, K. H., Young, R. R., and Goldie, W. D. (1979): Origin of the components of human short latency somatosensory evoked responses. *Neurology (Minneap).,* 29:598.
6. Cracco, R. Q. (1972): The initial positive potential of the human scalp-recorded somatosensory evoked response. *Electroencephalogr. Clin. Neurophysiol.,* 32:623–629.
7. Desmedt, J. E., and Brunko, E. (1980): Functional organization of far-field and cortical components of somatosensory evoked potentials in normal adults. In: *Progress in Clinical Neuropathology, Vol. 7, Clinical Uses of Cerebral Brainsten and Spinal Somatosensory Evoked Potentials,* edited by J. E. Desmedt, pp. 27–50. Karger, Basel.
8. Desmedt, J. E., and Cheron, G. (1980): Central somatosensory conduction in man: Neural generators and interpeak latencies of the far-field components recorded from neck and right or left scalp and earlobes. *Electroencephalogr. Clin. Neurophysiol.,* 50:382–403.
9. Donchin, E., Callaway, E., Cooper, R., Desmedt, J. E., Goff, W. R., Hillyard, S. A., and Sutton, J. (1977): Publication criteria for studies of evoked potentials: Report of committee. In: *Progress in Clinical Neurophysiology, Vol. 1, Attention, Voluntary Contraction and Event-Related Cerebral Potentials,* edited by J. E. Desmedt, pp. 1–11. Karger, Basel.
10. Duff, T. A. (1980): Multichannel topographic analysis of human somatosensory evoked potentials. In: *Progress in Clinical Neurophysiology, Vol. 7, Clinical Uses of Cerebral Brainstem and Spinal Somatosensory Evoked Potentials,* edited by J. E. Desmedt, pp. 69–86. Karger, Basel.
11. Friedland, R. P., and Weinstein, E. A. (1977): Hemi-inattention and hemisphere specialization: Introduction and historical review. In: *Advances in Neurology, Vol. 18, Hemi-inattention and Hemisphere Specialization,* edited by E. A. Weinstein and R. P., Friedland, pp. 1–31. Raven Press, New York.
12. Goff, G. D., Matsumiya, Y., Allison, T., and Goff, W. R. (1977): The scalp topography of

human somatosensory and auditory evoked potentials. *Electroencephalogr. Clin. Neurophysiol.*, 42:57–76.
13. Green, J. B., and McLeod, S. (1979): Short latency somatosensory evoked potentials in patients with neurological lesions. *Arch. Neurol.*, 36:846–851.
14. Greenberg, R. P., Bercker, D. P., Miller, J. D., and Mayer, D. J. (1977): Evaluation of brain function in severe human head trauma with multimodality evoked potentials. Part 2: Localization of brain dysfunction and correlation with posttraumatic neurological conditions. *J. Neurosurg.*, 47:163–177.
15. Halliday, A. M., and Wakefield, G. W. (1963): Cerebral evoked potentials in patients with dissociated sensory loss. *J. Neurol. Neurosurg. Psychiatry*, 26:211–219.
16. Hume, A. L., and Cant, B. R. (1978): Conduction time in central somatosensory pathways in Man. *Electroencephalogr. Clin. Neurophysiol.*, 45:361–375.
17. Jones, S. J. (1977): Short latency potentials recorded from the neck and the scalp following median nerve stimulation in man. *Electroencephalogr. Clin. Neurophysiol.*, 43:853–863.
18. Kritchevsky, M., and Widerholt, W. C. (1978): Short latency somatosensory evoked potentials. *Arch. Neurol.*, 35:706–712.
19. Laget, P., Mamo, H., and Houdart, R. (1967): De l'intérêt des potentiels évoqués somesthésiques dans l'étude des lésion du lobe pariétal de l'homme. *Neurochirurgie*, 13:841–853.
20. Lesser, R. P., Koehle, R., and Lueders, H. (1979): Effect of stimulus intensity on short latency somatosensory evoked potentials. *Electroencephalogr. Clin. Neurophysiol.*, 47:377–382.
21. Maraval, G., Pernier, J., Peronnet, F., Echallier, J. F., Gerin, P., and Mauguiere, F. (1980): EVØQ: Systeme configurable de stimulation automatique et d'enregistrement des potentiels évoqués moyens sur mini-ordinateur. *Int. J. Biomed. Comput.*, 11:225–239.
22. Mauguiere, F., and Courjon, J. (1981): The origin of short-latency somato-sensory evoked potentials in man: A clinical contribution. *Ann. Neurol.*, 9:607–611.
23. Michel, F., and Peronnet, F. (1974): Extinction gauche au test dichotique: Lesion hemisphérique ou lésion commissurale. In: *Les Syndromes de Disconnexion Calleuse Chez l'Homme, Vol. 1*, edited by F. Michel and B. Schott, pp. 85–117. S.P.C.M., Lyon.
24. Nakanishi, T., Shimada, Y., Sakuta, M., and Toyokura, Y. (1978): The initial positive component of the scalp-recorded somato-sensory evoked potential in normal subjects and in patients with neurological disorders. *Electroencephalogr. Clin. Neurophysiol.*, 45:26–34.
25. Noël, P., and Desmedt, J. E. (1975): Somatosensory cerebral evoked potentials after vascular lesions of the brainstem and diencephalon. *Brain*, 98:113–128.
26. Noël, P., and Desmedt, J. E. (1980): Cerebral and far-field somatosensory evoked potentials in neurological disorders involving the cervical spinal cord, brainstem, thalamus and cortex. In: *Progress in Clinical Neurophysiology, Vol. 7, Clinical Uses of Cerebral Brainstem and Spinal Somatosensory Evoked Potentials*, edited by J. E. Desmedt, pp. 205–230. Karger, Basel.
27. Roland, P. E., (1976): Astereognosis: Tactile discrimination after localized hemispheric lesions in man. *Arch. Neurol.*, 33:543–550.
28. Williamson, P. D., Goff, W. R., and Allison, T. (1970): Somatosensory evoked response in patients with unilateral cerebral lesions. *Electroencephalogr. Clin. Neurophysiol.*, 28:566–575.
29. Yamada, T., Kimura, J., Young, S., and Powers, M. (1978): Somatosensory-evoked potentials elicited by bilateral stimulation of the median nerve and its clinical application. *Neurology (Minneap.)* 28:218–223.

Clinical Applications of Evoked Potentials in Neurology,
edited by J. Courjon, F. Mauguiere, and M. Revol.
Raven Press, New York © 1982.

Diagnostic Significance of Cortical Somatosensory Evoked Potentials Following Trigeminal Nerve Stimulation

*U. W. Buettner, **F. Petruch, *K. Scheglmann, and *M. Stöhr

**Department of Neurology, University of Tübingen, D-7400 Tübingen, Federal Republic of Germany; and **Psychiatric Hospital, Department of Neurology, D-800 Ansbach, Federal Republic of Germany*

Larsson and Previc (5) investigated the trigeminal system with the somatosensory evoked potential (SEP) method, applying mechanical stimuli. Stöhr and Petruch (7), using electrical stimulation, described an easy and routinely applicable method for the investigation of the "trigeminal SEP" which gives reproducible results in normals and patients. In the meantime, Bennet and Jannetta (1) and Drechsler (2) reported similar methods using a somewhat different stimulation.

This chapter describes the standardization of stimulus parameters in our laboratory and discusses the clinical relevance of the trigeminal SEP in different groups of patients.

METHODS

More than 200 subjects were investigated including healthy volunteers, patients without involvement of the central nervous system, and patients with established or suspected diagnosis of multiple sclerosis (definite MS–46 patients), trigeminal neuralgia (20 patients), brainstem ischemia (Wallenberg's syndrome—seven patients) or tumors in the cerebello–pontine angle (11 patients). For stimulation, bipolar surface electrodes (Medelec EL 21 M) and the Disa stimulator (15 C 25) were used. Generally, the branches V_2 and V_3 of the trigeminal nerve were stimulated simultaneously at both lips, the electrode covering upper and lower lip at the corner of the mouth. In some patients, the second and third divisions were separately stimulated at upper and lower lip, respectively. Stimulus duration was 0.1 msec. Stimulus strength ranged between 2 and 10 mA depending on the sensory threshold of the subject and was usually set to three times sensory threshold at onset of stimulation. It was below the threshold of pain in all cases. The frequency of stimulation was varied in volunteers from 1 to 20 Hz, whereas routinely, a 2- or 3-Hz pulse sequence was applied. Whenever possible, direct motor action of the orbicularis oris muscle was avoided. The

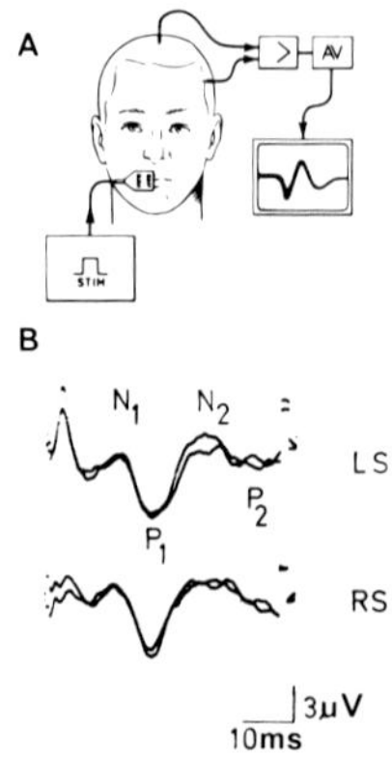

FIG. 1.A: Schematic experimental procedure described in the text. (From Stöhr, ref. 6, with permission.) **B:** An example of a normal trigeminal SEP with reproducible recordings on the left side (LS) and right side (RS). Nomenclature of the waves is indicated.

active recording electrode (Disa 25 C 04; platinum needle electrode) was placed subcutaneously at C_5 or C_6 (10–20 system) above the face region of the primary sensory cortex. A midfrontal reference electrode (F_Z) was used. The bandpass of the amplifier (Disa 15 C 01) was set at 10 Hz to 2 kHz (sometimes 1 kHz). There were 64 to 512 (in a few instances, 1,024) stimulus responses averaged (Disa Digital Averager 15 G 07). The resolution of the 50-msec analyzing period was 1,024 data points. To ascertain reliability, all recordings were repeated at least once. In this investigation, only the latency of the first positive wave (P_1) was considered. The schematic recording procedure and a normal trigeminal SEP are shown in Fig. 1.

RESULTS

Results in Normals

Measurements in healthy volunteers were performed to investigate the influence of frequency, site, and strength of stimulation on the trigeminal SEP.

The general wave form (Fig. 1B) consists of two negative and two positive peaks within an analysis time of 50 msec. The mean latency of P19 of a normal trigeminal SEP according to Stöhr and Petruch (7) is 18.5 msec. This value includes the results of interpolation whenever P19 was W-shaped. A pathologically delayed P19 is assumed to occur with a latency >22.3 msec (mean + 2.5 SD), and a pathological side difference >1.9 msec (mean + 2.5 SD). It can be shown that frequency changes of stimulation between 1 and 20 Hz do not affect the latency of P19 (Fig. 2) and that the amplitude (N13/P19, peak to peak) remains near maximum until 5 Hz. High-frequency stimulation did not cause discomfort to the subject whenever the low-frequency stimulus was not painful.

In these and earlier investigations, the lips were chosen as the site of stimulation because they are easily accessible and because they are more densely endowed with cutaneous receptors than the adjacent skin.

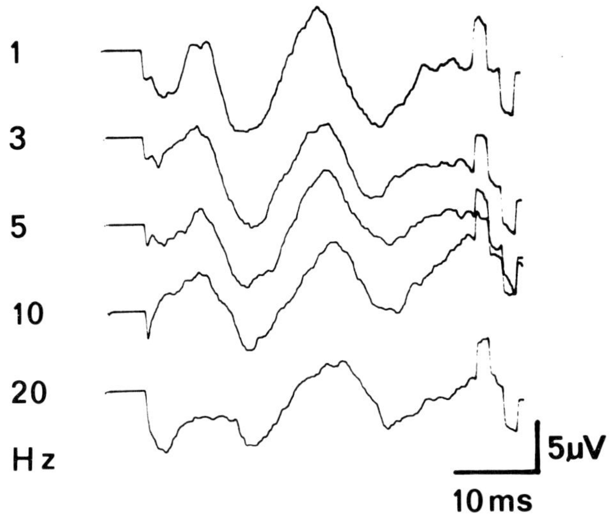

FIG. 2. Influence of stimulus frequency on the SEP. Note that P19 latency is not affected. For suppression of stimulus artifact, 5 msec of the traces is blocked.

Separate stimulation of the upper and lower lip on each side results in considerable differences of the wave form of the SEP. N19 is much sharper and more pronounced, P19 latencies are, on average, about 1 msec shorter in recordings following V_3 stimulation than with V_2 stimulation. This fact could explain the W shape of P19 in some recordings. The differential stimulation of V_2 and V_3 was, therefore, applied in normal volunteers and in patients with trigeminal neuralgia confined to single branches. The same procedure was applied in some cases without reproducible recordings from simultaneous stimulation of V_2 and V_3 in order to possibly detect a mutual masking of the V_2 and V_3 components of the trigeminal SEP.

Several points affect the choice of an appropriate stimulus strength. The sensory threshold for electrical stimulation ranged in our experimental design from 1.0 mA up to 5 mA in normal subjects and changed its value considerably during stimulation in most subjects. Stimulation strength is limited by the sensation of pain, since pain prevents relaxation. Another factor is the direct local motor response of orbicularis oris muscle which in part distorts the P19 peak to higher latency values. The last factor limiting the stimulus strength is the stimulus artifact itself.

Most of the experiments could be done with stimuli below motor threshold at about 4 to 8 mA which is on average three times the threshold intensity. The dependence of the trigeminal SEP on stimulus strength is shown in Fig. 3. Based on these experiments, we now determine the sensory threshold in all cases before each trial and choose double- or triple-threshold stimulus strength.

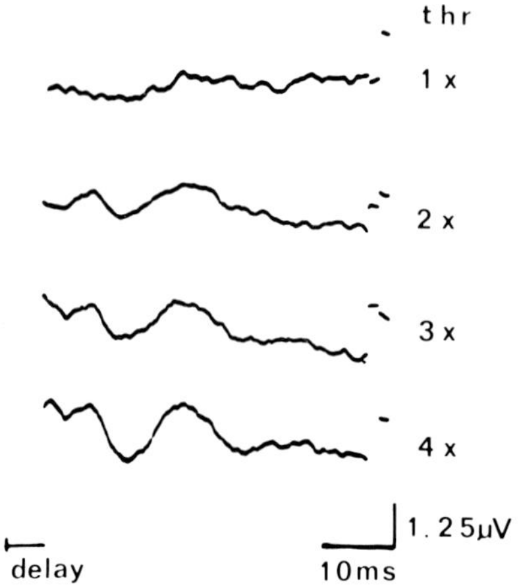

FIG. 3. Increase of stimulus strength above threshold (thr.). The higher the stimulus current is, the larger is the amplitude of the P19 wave.

Results in Patients

Patients with trigeminal neuralgia involving the second and third branches (10 subjects), the second branch alone (five subjects), the third branch alone (four subjects), and the first and second division (one subject) were investigated (Table 1). Seventeen patients were exclusively treated by medication; three subjects had undergone a fractionated root section or thermocoagulation of the gasserian ganglion. The mean latency of P19 (only patients with idiopathic neuralgia and exclusively conservative treatment) was 21.1 msec (SD, 1.9 msec) on the involved side, 19.8 msec (SD 1.3 msec) on the normal side. The average difference of 1.3 msec between the two sides is statistically significant (*t*-test; $\alpha = 0.005$; Table 1). Seven of 17 patients with only conservative treatment showed a pathological side difference. An example of a patient with symptomatic neuralgia of the third branch is shown in Fig. 4. The latency of the SEP following stimulation of the mandibular branch is prolonged (bottom trace). Since the patient had undergone surgery of the mandible, it must be assumed that demyelinization in the course of the nerve has occurred.

From the whole group of patients with definite multiple sclerosis, 28 (61%) exhibited pathologically prolonged P19 latencies (Fig. 5), a pathological side difference, or a lack of the P19 wave (Table 2). Eighteen of the patients with

TABLE 1. *Latency of P19 in trigeminal neuralgia*

	Mean (msec)	SD (msec)
Normal side	19.8	1.3
Involved side	21.1	1.9
Difference between sides	1.3[a]	

[a] Significance of side difference, $\alpha = 0.005$ (*t*-test).

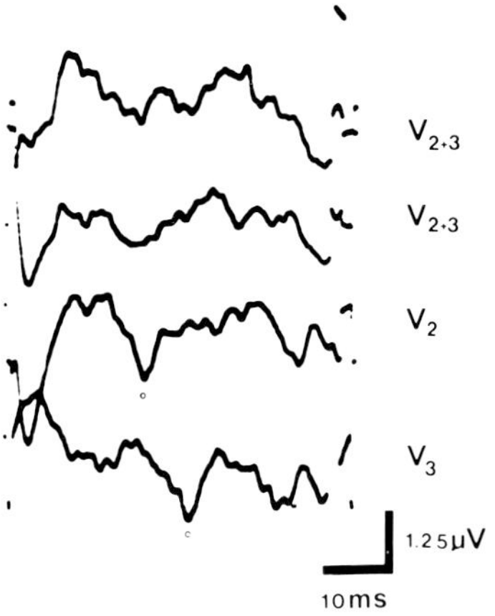

FIG. 4. An SEP of a patient with symptomatic trigeminal neuralgia (V_3). The branches were stimulated simultaneously *(traces 1 and 2)* and separately *(traces 3 and 4)*. It can be shown that P19 is considerably delayed in V_3 compared to V_2.

a pathological trigeminal SEP did not reveal symptoms or signs of sensory disturbances in the area of the trigeminal nerve.

Ischemic lesions with the syndrome of the lateral medulla oblongata (Wallenberg's syndrome) almost regularly (six of seven cases) showed disturbances of the trigeminal SEP. In three cases, the SEP was absent; in the other three cases, there was a prolonged latency or reduction of amplitude of P19.

Compression of the trigeminal nerve by tumors in the cerebello–pontine angle or brainstem led to a pathological latency or side difference in a total of six out of 11 patients investigated.

DISCUSSION

The trigeminal SEP supplements other noninvasive diagnostic procedures such as the brainstem evoked acoustic response, the orbicularis occuli reflex (V_1),

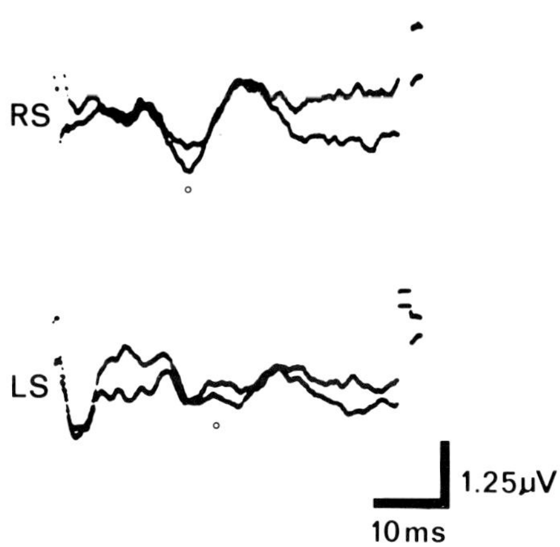

FIG. 5. Recording in a patient known to suffer from multiple sclerosis. Latency of P19 (W-shaped) is delayed on the left side (LS).

TABLE 2. *Trigeminal SEP findings in multiple sclerosis (definite)*

	No sensory impairment	Sensory impairment
Normal Trigeminal SEP	16	2
Pathological side difference only	3	1
Prolonged latency of P19	6	4
Prolonged latency of P19 and pathological side difference	8	3
Lack of Trigeminal SEP on one side	1	2

ENG, and computer-assisted tomography. The method of stimulating the two branches separately or simultaneously at both lips and recording over the contralateral somatosensory face region can routinely be applied without considerable discomfort to the patient and allows for separate investigation of both the second and third branches. The applied frequency of stimulation is not very critical, although 5 Hz should be the upper limit in order to get sufficiently high amplitudes of the response. The determination of thresholds in a large number of subjects reveals adaptation, and the current for threshold stimulation must be increased in successive measurements. When the stimulus is set to twice or three times the threshold, it can be safely assumed that stimulation is effective, is not painful, and does not cause larger artifacts contaminating the reliability of the response.

When separate and simultaneous stimulation of V_2 and V_3 are compared, a shorter P19 latency for V_3 is found in most subjects; this seems to be the cause of the occasional W-shaped P19. In patients suffering from trigeminal neuralgia, separate stimulation is favorable, since prolonged latencies in one branch only can be masked by simultaneous stimulation. However, even with combined stimulation of the upper and lower lips, there is a pathological delay of the P19 latency in 40% of these patients (8). This leads to the assumption that demyelinization of one or more trigeminal roots may occur by compression through abnormal vessels or occult tumors (3,4,).

The most frequent indication for recording evoked potentials is suspected multiple sclerosis. As can other evoked potential methods, the trigeminal SEP may reveal demyelinization at times when no symptom or sign directs attention to the trigeminal pathway. About 60% of patients with definite MS exhibit pathologically delayed trigeminal SEPs, 60% of them without sensory disturbances in the face.

Ischemic lesions of the brainstem, especially the lateral medulla oblongata, lead to pathologically delayed or abnormally shaped SEPs in a high proportion of cases, probably indicating an involvement of the main sensory nucleus. The trigeminal SEP can therefore help to determine the extent of the lesion.

There is now enough evidence to suggest that examination of the trigeminal SEP should belong to the set of established evoked potential techniques supporting the attempt to determine the patient's disease before invasive diagnostic procedures are applied.

REFERENCES

1. Bennet, M. H., and Jannetta, P. J. (1980): Trigeminal evoked potentials in humans. *Electroencephalogr. Clin. Neurophysiol.,* 48:517–526.
2. Drechsler, F. (1980): Short and long latency cortical potentials following trigeminal nerve stimulation in man. In: *Evoked Potentials,* edited by C. Barber, pp. 415–422. MTP Press, Lancaster.
3. Jannetta, P. J. (1977): Observations on the etiology of trigeminal neuralgia, hemifacial spasm, acoustic nerve dysfunction and glossopharyngeal neuralgia. Definite microsurgical treatment and results in 117 patients. *Neurochirurgia,* 20:145–154.
4. Jannetta, P. J., and Rand, R. W. (1967): Arterial compression of the trigeminal nerve at the pons in patients with trigeminal neuralgia. *J. Neurosurg.,* 26(Suppl.):159–162.
5. Larsson, L. E., and Previc, T. S. (1970): Somato-sensory responses to mechanical stimulation as recorded in the human EEG. *Electroencephalogr. Clin. Neurophysiol.,* 28:162–172.
6. Stöhr, M. (1980): *Iatrogene Nervenläsionen.* Georg Thieme, Stuttgart, New York.
7. Stöhr, M., and Petruch, F. (1979): Somatosensory evoked potentials following stimulation of the trigeminal nerve in man. *J. Neurol.,* 220:95–98.
8. Stöhr, M., Petruch, F., and Scheglmann, K. (1981): Somatosensory evoked potentials following trigeminal nerve stimulation in trigeminal neuralgia. *Ann. Neurol.,* 9:63–66.

Clinical Applications of Evoked Potentials in Neurology,
edited by J. Courjon, F. Mauguiere, and M. Revol.
Raven Press, New York © 1982.

Diagnostic Value of Segmental Somatosensory Evoked Potentials in Cases with Chronic Progressive Para- or Tetraspastic Syndromes

J. Jörg, W. Düllberg, and S. Koeppen

Neurologische Universitätsklinik Essen, D-4300 Essen 1, West Germany

In the majority of transsectional lesions, diagnosis can clearly be established by history taking, clinical findings, CSF examination, and occasionally myelography; thus, additional neurophysiological investigations are not needed. Each neurologist knows, however, less easily classifiable chronic progressive para- or tetraspastic syndromes with or without sensory disturbance. In these cases particularly, spinal multiple sclerosis (MS) or cervical myelopathy (CM) has to be taken into consideration (9). Concerning the differential diagnosis of spinal MS or CM, the application of segmental SEP recording is useful for objective registration and localization of a spinal lesion if VEPs are normal and cervical myelography reveals no definite abnormal findings.

MATERIAL AND METHODS

Bilateral stimulation of up to 17 dermatomes (C4–L5) is performed by surface electrodes giving rectangular stimuli of 2 Hz frequency and three to four times the voltage of the sensory threshold (Fig. 1a). The person under examination should be relaxed in a prone position in a room of moderate temperature and is asked to stay awake. A sequence of 256 responses per segment is averaged with an analysis time of 100 msec. The recording electrodes (thin steel needles) are arranged according to the international 10–20 system modified by Shagass and Schwartz (17) as follows: C3/P3 against F3 and C4/P4 against F4, respectively, are used for arm and trunk recordings, CZ/PZ against FZ for leg recordings. The band-pass amplifier ranges from 2 Hz to 2 kHz. Segmental stimulation is repeated three to four times if necessary. Results obtained from 28 control subjects aged 15 to 76 years serve as normal reference values. Assessment of the findings in patients is made by taking the mean and standard deviation of each age group as well as the normal skin temperature and the length of the extremities into account.

Dermatomes are selected for examination according to the clinical findings. Nomenclature and criteria of SEP assessment are described in a previous study (10,11).

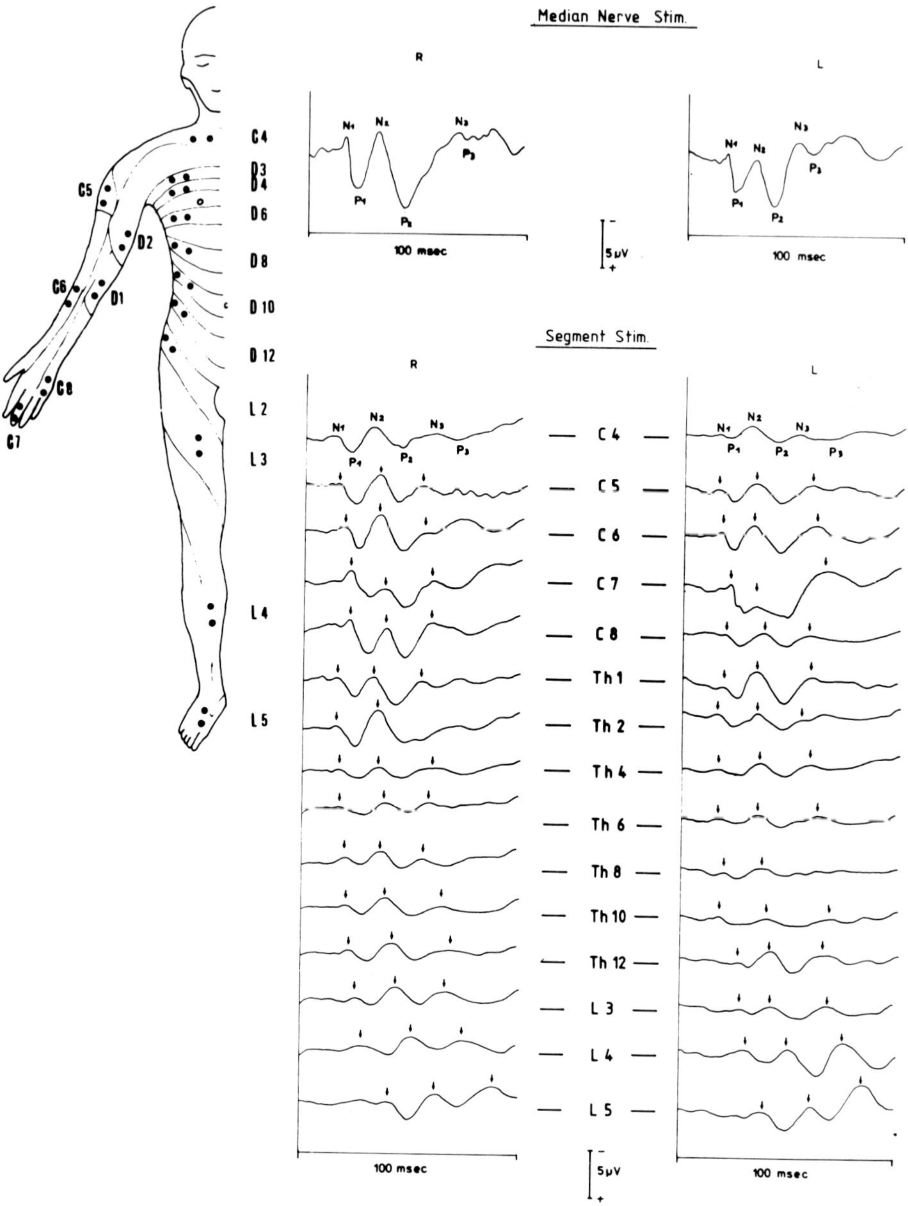

FIG. 1. Left: Arrangement of stimulation electrodes in the 17 dermatomes C4 to L5. **Right:** Average medianus and segmental SEPs of a 23-year-old control subject (PH).

Our examination comprised 43 patients with chronic progressive para- or tetraspasticity who showed exclusively or predominantly motor deficits; there were 15 cases with probable spinal MS and 28 cases with spondylogenic cervical myelopathy.

In 28 cases the diagnosis of spondylogenic CM was established; most of these patients underwent laminectomy or methacrylate fusioning and occasionally excision of disk protrusions. In 10 of the 28 patients, the pre- and postoperative SEP examination was repeated up to three times.

In 15 cases a probable diagnosis of spinal MS was made because there was no evidence either of an intraspinal tumor or of vascular or cervical myelopathy; moreover, the VEPs had always been normal. A CSF examination showed increased IgG levels in only five of the 15 cases, cells being in normal range. Myelography carried out in most cases showed normal findings corresponding to the patient's age. A 2-year follow-up study of three of the 15 spinal patients confirmed the diagnosis, because in these cases VEP alteration occurred as a sign of a multilocular disease process.

RESULTS

In normal subjects three negative and three positive peaks are usually demonstrable within the first 100 msec after stimulation of the segments C4 through L5. The peaks N1 through N3 and P1 through P3 (Fig. 1b) are defined by latencies and amplitudes. Means and standard deviations of one of the three age groups are listed in Table 1. For amplitude values as well as comparative values obtained by median nerve stimulation, previous reports should be transferred to (10,11). According to the results of median nerve stimulations, there is no significant difference between right and left segmental SEP recordings from the segments C8 and L5. With the present recording technique, early so-called P 15 peaks, as reported by numerous authors, particularly from the active electrode mastoid-C/P on median nerve stimulation, arc not obtainable. Based on an equal peripheral distance, the spinal CV in adults aged 38 to 50 years is 75 m/sec within the distance T4 to T10.

In the majority of CM patients (19 of 28) a typical transsectional pattern was seen, with amplitude diminution or conduction block being demonstrable mainly in the lower cervical or upper thoracic segments (Figs. 2a and b and 3a—d). Conduction block or amplitude reduction was the most common abnormality, although 10 of these patients had no definite sensory disturbance clinically. Compared to the results in spinal MS, a significant latency delay, particularly of the first peak, was less common and less distinct.

The majority of the nine patients without a transectional pattern showed some abnormal or missing segmental cervical SEPs. Occasionally, SEPs could be recorded again from lower lumbar segments (especially L4 and L5). This was considered an indicator of a ventrally located spinal cord compression, since neurophysiological evaluation revealed no involvement of the most dorsally located posterior columns.

TABLE 1. *The mean and standard deviations of the segmental SEP peaks (msec) (C4 to L5) in 10 normal control subjects, ages 38 to 50 years*

	N1	P1	N2	P2	N3	P3
C 4	13.3 ±1.8	20.9 ±1.1	31.5 ±2.6	44.4 ±3.2	65.7 ±4.3	79.4 ±4.4
C 5	17.2 ±2.7	25.4 ±3.0	36.4 ±2.4	50.2 ±5.9	68.3 ±9.1	85.9 ±5.6
C 6	19.7 ±1.5	27.3 ±2.5	38.9 ±2.3	51.9 ±3.0	71.7 ±4.7	88.5 ±4.6
C 7	22.7 ±3.4	30.3 ±4.3	41.8 ±7.0	50.6 ±6.7	70.3 ±7.7	86.5 ±7.4
C 8	23.4 ±2.1	31.6 ±2.4	41.9 ±1.9	55.6 ±3.3	73.3 ±5.5	86.6 ±6.5
Th1	18.9 ±1.3	25.8 ±2.6	36.0 ±2.5	51.4 ±7.0	72.8 ±6.8	87.0 ±4.3
Th2	18.1 ±1.4	26.4 ±2.4	37.0 ±2.8	54.2 ±5.9	69.8 ±7.5	83.5 ±4.4
Th3	18.5 ±1.1	25.7 ±1.8	37.5 ±2.2	54.9 ±5.4	72.5 ±6.4	86.6 ±5.1
Th4	18.4 ±2.2	26.4 ±1.8	38.1 ±1.8	51.1 ±6.6	68.5 ±6.6	83.8 ±5.8
Th6	19.8 ±1.6	27.2 ±1.9	38.3 ±3.8	49.5 ±5.5	66.3 ±5.5	83.4 ±3.9
Th8	21.0 ±2.3	28.6 ±4.5	41.6 ±4.0	52.6 ±4.6	70.4 ±7.2	82.6 ±6.9
Th10	21.7 ±1.6	30.0 ±4.0	43.6 ±5.7	53.4 ±7.3	68.5 ±3.6	82.8 ±3.0
Th12	22.2 ±1.3	30.0 ±1.1	40.3 ±2.2	56.3 ±4.0	72.1 ±5.5	86.4 ±5.0
L 2	24.0 ±1.2	31.1 ±2.7	40.9 ±1.7	55.4 ±4.6	70.7 ±5.4	85.6 ±6.5
L 3	26.1 ±1.5	32.9 ±2.1	45.0 ±5.1	57.9 ±5.5	73.9 ±4.6	87.9 ±5.0
L 4	31.4 ±3.6	39.5 ±5.6	49.7 ±5.4	62.1 ±8.6	78.7 ±5.9	89.8 ±5.6
L 5	34.9 ±8.5	42.2 ±9.0	53.7 ±9.5	65.8 ±9.8	78.2 ±11.1	88.5 ±8.3

FIG. 2 (a and b). This 68-year-old woman (EP) had developed a feeling of heaviness in her arms within the past 15 years and a stiff gait during the past 5 years. Neurological examination revealed a mainly left-sided tetraspasticity with moderate paresis of small muscles of her hand. Sensory testing showed only impairment of vibration sensation in hands and feet. Radiography showed Klippel-Feil syndrome at C2 to C3 and spondylosis, particularly at C4 to C5 with signs of a narrow spinal channel. Cervical myelography confirmed these findings. After laminectomy at the C3 to C6 levels, marked improvement of tetraspasticity, gait disturbance, and delicate hand movements was seen. Segmental SEP evaluation shows absent potentials below C7, distinct latency delay at C7, and normal SEPs at C5 and C6 on the right. Postoperatively, repeatedly evocable responses from C8, T10, and possibly L3 were demonstrable. A further SEP assessment 1½ years after laminectomy shows no responses from T10 and L3 and evident response from L5 and C8, corresponding to further improvement for the tetraspasticity.

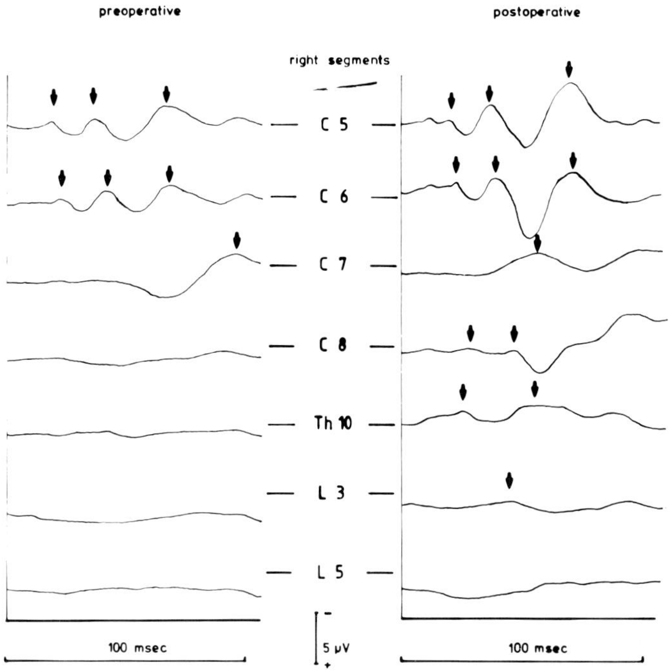
preoperative
postoperative
right segments
C 5
C 6
C 7
C 8
Th 10
L 3
L 5
100 msec
5 µV
100 msec

a

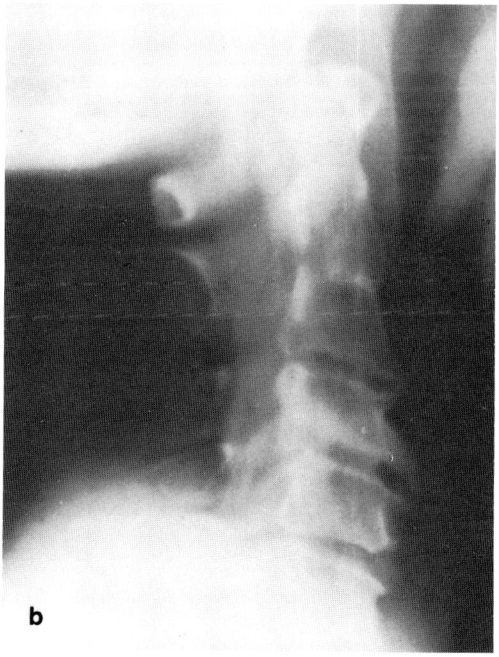

b

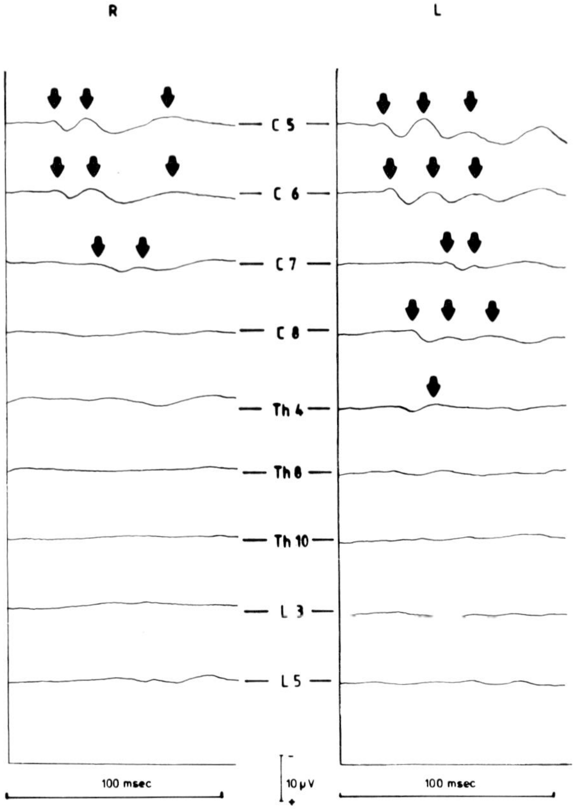

a

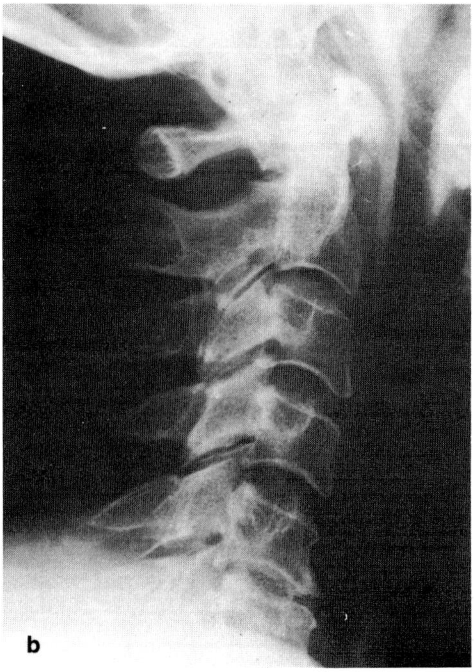
b

Spinal MS could be excluded because there was no disseminated SEP alteration and latency delays were less marked than in MS. Postoperative clinical and neurophysiological examination of 10 patients showed deterioration in two cases, no change in three cases, and slight or good improvement of SEPs and clinical findings in five cases. Results obtained from the latter group are displayed in Figs. 2a and b and 3a–d.

In the majority of the 15 patients with probable spinal MS, segmental SEP recording showed a characteristic disseminated SEP alteration with some absence of peaks and SEPs with delayed latencies. The most common abnormality was not conduction block but amplitude reduction associated with marked latency delay; this was significantly increased in comparison to the contralateral recording (Figs. 4a and b). The onset of some potentials could not easily be recognized because of their small amplitude or distorted waveform. The SEPs detected subclinical lesions by showing abnormality in a proportion of MS patients who had no corresponding abnormal clinical signs. Only three of the 15 patients showed a transectional pattern without disseminated SEP alteration. Therefore, these cases could not be differentiated from CM or other spinal monolocular disease process simply by SEP recording.

DISCUSSION

In normal subjects of all age groups, latencies and amplitudes of the segmental SEPs obtained from C4 through L5 are well defined and correlate with reports on SEP recording on cutaneous or nerve stimulation (1,4). The calculable spinal CV corresponds to values reported by Cracco et al., those values ranging from 62 to 80 m/sec inside the lumbar–cervical distance (3).

When the patient's age and size and the peripheral sensory nerve CV are taken into account, and the bilateral comparative evaluation is stressed, application of segmental SEP recording is of special value in the diagnosis of spinal cord diseases (5). However, normal peripheral nerve function as well as normal cerebral and brainstem function are essential for SEP application as a spinal diagnostic procedure (6).

Whereas segmental SEP recording showing absence or change of potentials at certain levels only confirms diagnosis in the case of clinically defined pictures

FIG. 3a and 3b. This 53-year-old man (RM) had a tickling in his hands and a stiff gait that had been progressive for 1 year. Neurological examination revealed bilateral tetraspasticity, mild hemihypesthesia below T7 on the right, and a slight cerebral organic psychosyndrome. A CSF examination revealed a slight barrier disturbance (889 mg/liter). Neurophysiological evaluation showed absent potentials below C8 on the right, and below C8 on the left. Normal responses were obtained only at C5 and C6 bilaterally and at C8 on the left. Findings in the native X-ray film, showing marked cervical spondylochondrosis with protrusion and subluxation at the C5 and C6 level, as well as generalized marked spondylochondrosis, were confirmed by cervical myelography presenting a functional stop at c C5 to C6 with the head in reclined position.

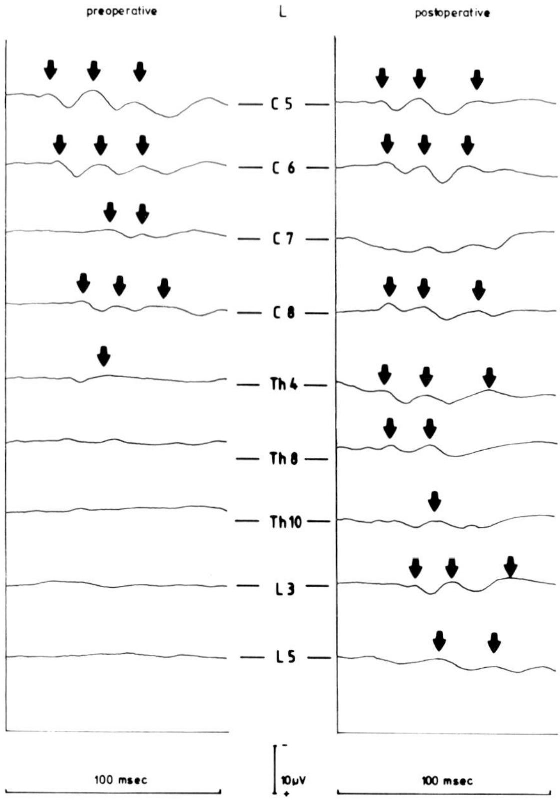
preoperative
L
postoperative
C 5
C 6
C 7
C 8
Th 4
Th 8
Th 10
L 3
L 5
100 msec
10µV
100 msec

c

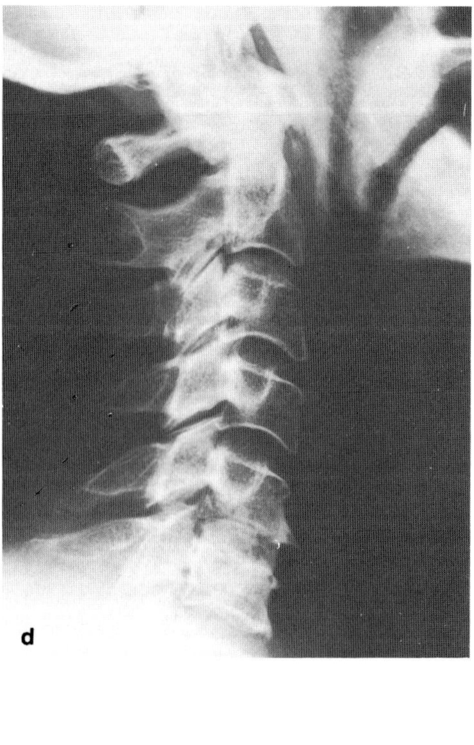

d

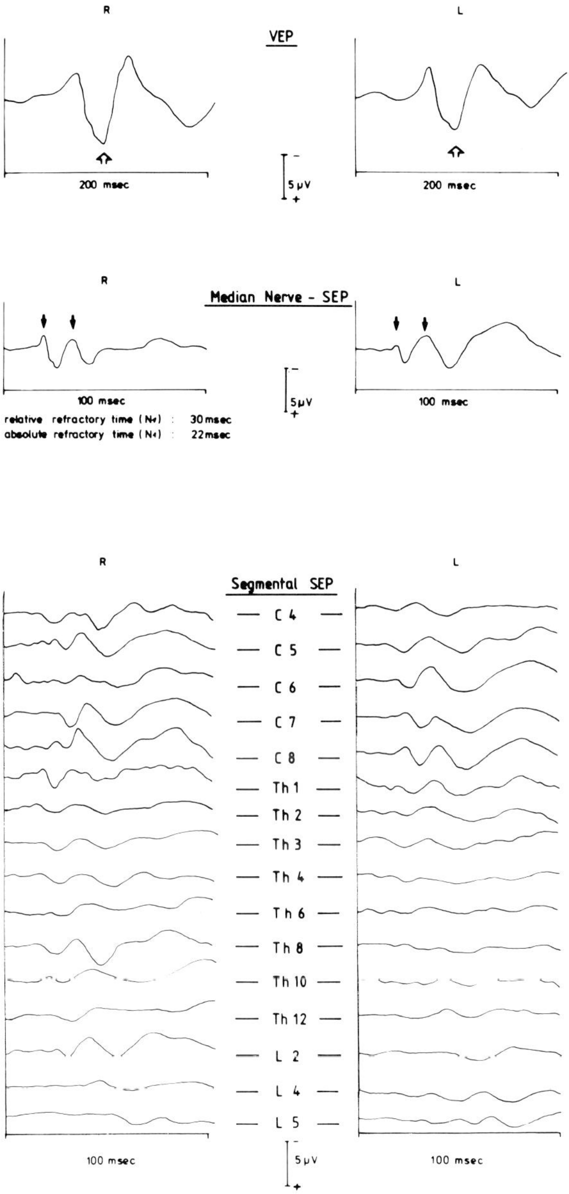

a

FIG. 4a. Spinal MS in a 40-year-old woman (JS). Neurophysiological techniques in confirming the diagnosis (MS). Chronic, progressive tetraspacticity, especially of the legs, with normal clinical sensory testing. (See Fig. 4b. for explanation.)

FIGS. 3c and 3d. Same patient (RM) as discussed in Figs. 3a and 3b. Operative therapy consisted of methacrylate fusion of C5 to C6, as can be seen on this second X-ray film. Postoperatively, a painful stiffness of the right shoulder predominated initially; 1 year after surgery, no spasticity of the lower extremities was present. Sensory testing revealed only a slight glove-shaped hypesthesia of the right hand. Neurophysiological examination performed 1 year after surgery demonstrated SEPs obtained from thoracic and lumbar segments; these had been absent preoperatively.

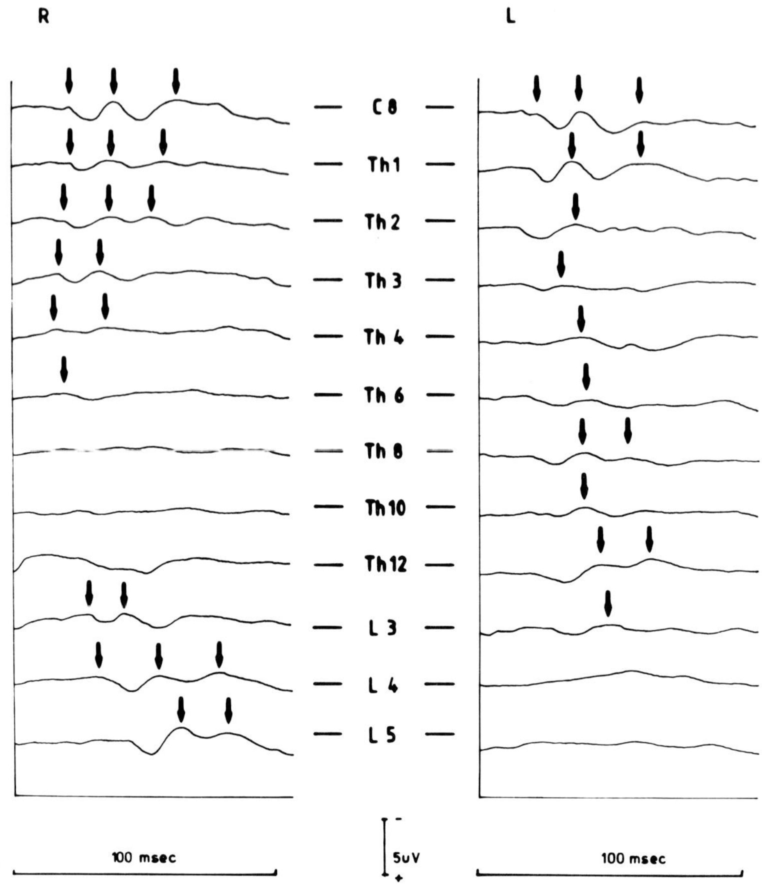

b

FIG. 4b. Multiple sclerosis in a 30-year-old woman (Chr. K). In both patients with spinal MS (Figs. 4a and 4b), segmental SEP evaluation does not show a transectional pattern. The clinical examination of both patients (JS and Chr. K) with disseminated SEP alterations revealed no sensory disorder.

such as spinal cord tumors, it is diagnostically useful in unclear para- or tetraspasticities with normal VEP and CSF findings. This applies particularly to the results in CM with the frequently presented transectional pattern in lower cervical or upper thoracic segments even without clinical sensory disturbance. Comparable results were obtained by Schramm in 18 CM patients (15) and he is correct in emphasizing that normal segmental SEPs nearly exclude CM (10). This conclusion is also important for the reason that CM is not necessarily associated with marked cervical osteochondrosis apart from the fact that in almost all patients beyond the age of 40 osteochondrosis is demonstrable radiographically, and myelography as well as electromyography often only provide additional information.

The most relevant differential diagnosis of the CM is from spinal MS. In the latter, Schramm et al. (16) found, consistent with our results, no transectional pattern but, typically, a disseminated SEP alteration beside normal SEPs. The predominant latency delay of N1 and P1, repeatedly mentioned in the literature (8) as an indicator of demyelination, is seen independently of any sensory impairment that is either still present or already restored. It is still questionable whether recording of spinal responses to median and tibial nerve stimulation can be useful for the differential diagnosis of spinal MS and CM. In adults, the amplitudes are often smaller than 0.2 μV (3), and in our opinion, absence of a potential in a tracing recorded from the cervical spine after median nerve stimulation does not necessarily support CM just as latency delay does not necessarily support MS (18).

The interhemispheric difference in latency of the early negative component N1 after median nerve stimulation is considered by numerous authors to be a sign of CNS demyelination (12,13); however, it is not MS specific (2,7). Therefore, Noël and Desmedt (14) evaluated SEPs after finger and sural nerve stimulation in the differential diagnosis of cervical compression or spinal MS. In the latter, they found marked latency delay of SEPs obtained by finger stimulation, whereas in CM, increased SEP latency was more evident after sural nerve stimulation. We also found a similar SEP constellation in some other spinal space-occupying disease processes.

An undoubted disadvantage of segmental SEP examination is the time consumption of this diagnostic procedure. With regard to diagnostically difficult cases, it should be kept in mind that a more detailed neurophysiological study of segmental SEPs reveals more abnormal findings than does a recording restricted to two or three peripheral nerve stimulations. In clinical application, it has to be noted that no specific but only a typical SEP pattern exists for specific spinal diseases.

REFERENCES

1. Chippa, K. H., Choi, S. K., and Young R. R. (1980): Short-latency somatosensory evoked potentials following median nerve stimulation in patients with neurological lesions. In: *Clinical Use of Cerebral, Brainstem and Spinal SEPs,* edited by J. E. Desmedt, pp. 264–281. Karger, Basel.
2. Clifford-Jones, R. E., Clarke, G. P., and Mayles, P. (1979): Crossed acoustic response combined with visual and somatosensory evoked responses in the diagnosis of multiple sclerosis. *J. Neurol. Neurosurg. Psychiatry,* 42:749–752.
3. Cracco, R. Q., Cracco, J. B., Sarnowski, R., and Vogel, H. B. (1980): Spinal evoked potentials. In: *Clinical Use of Cerebral, Brainstem and Spinal SEPs,* edited by J. E. Desmedt, pp. 87–104. Karger, Basel.
4. Desmedt, J. E., and Brunko, E. (1980): Functional organization of far-field and cortical components of SEPs in normal adults. In: *Clinical Use of Cerebral, Brainstem and Spinal SEPs,* edited by J. E. Desmedt, pp. 27–50. Karger, Basel.
5. Desmedt, J. E., and Cheron, G. (1980): Somatosensory pathway and evoked potentials in normal

human aging. In: *Clinical Use of Cerebral, Brainstem and Spinal SEPs,* edited by J. E. Desmedt, pp. 162–169. Karger, Basel.
6. Dorfmann, L. J., Bosley, T., and Cummins, K. L. (1978): Electrophysiological localisation of central somatosensory lesions in patients with multiple sclerosis. *Electroencephalogr. Clin. Neurophysiol.,* 44:742–753.
7. Duff, T. A. (1980): Multichannel topographic analysis of human somatosensory evoked potentials. In: *Clinical Use of Cerebral, Brainstem and Spinal SEPs,* edited by J. E. Desmedt, 69–86. Karger, Basel.
8. Eisen, A., Stewart, J., Nudemann, K., and Cosgrove, J. B. R. (1979): Short-latency somatosensory responses in multiple sclerosis. *Neurology,* 29:827–834.
9. Jörg, J. (1974): Die cervicale Myelopathie als differentialdiagnostische Erwägung bei Gehstörungen im mittleren und höheren Lebensalter. *Nervenarzt,* 45:341–353.
10. Jörg, J. (1977): *Die elektrosensible Diagnostik in der Neurologie.* Springer-Verlag, Berlin.
11. Jörg, J., Gerhard, H., and Lehmann, H. J. (1980): Somatosensorische Reizantwortpotentiale bei Normalpersonen nach Einzel- und Doppelstimulation des N. medianus. *Z. EEG-EMG,* 11:211–217.
12. Jörg, J., Mehdorn, H. M., and Podemski, R. (1980): Cerebral refractory period of somatosensory system. EEG and clinical findings before and after vascular surgery in cerebrovascular diseases. *Excerpta Med.,* 526:181–190.
13. Lehmann, D., Gabathuler, U., and Baumgartner, G. (1979): Right/left differences of median nerve evoked scalp potentials in multiple sclerosis. *J. Neurol.* 221:15–24.
14. Noël, P., and Desmedt, J. E. (1980): Cerebral and far-field somatosensory evoked potentials in neurological disorders involving the cervical spinal cord, brainstem, thalamus and cortex. In: *Clinical Use of Cerebral, Brainstem and Spinal SEPs,* edited by J. E. Desmedt, pp. 205–230. Karger, Basel.
15. Schramm, J. (1980): Clinical experience with the objective localization of the lesion in cervical myelopathy. *Adv. Neurosurg.,* 8:26–32.
16. Schramm, J., Dettle, G. J., and Pichert, T. (1980): Clinical application of segmental somatosensory evoked potentials (SEP)—experience in patients with non-space-occupying lesions. In: *Proceedings of the Nottingham International Evoked Potentials Symposium, Lancaster.* pp. 455–464. MTP Press, Lancaster.
17. Shagass, Ch., and Schwartz, M. (1964): Recovery functions of somatosensory peripheral nerve and cerebral evoked responses in man. *Electroencephalogr. Clin. Neurophysiol.,* 17:126–135.
18. Small, D. G., Beauchamp, M., Matthews, W. B. (1980): Subcortical somatosensory evoked potentials in normal man and in patients with central nervous system lesions. In: *Clinical Use of Cerebral, Brainstem and Spinal SEPs,* edited by J. E. Desmedt, pp. 190–204. Karger, Basel.

Clinical Applications of Evoked Potentials in Neurology,
edited by J. Courjon, F. Mauguiere, and M. Revol.
Raven Press, New York © 1982.

Somatosensory Evoked Potentials Before and After Percutaneous Thermocoagulation of the Gasserian Ganglion for Trigeminal Neuralgia

G. Salar, I. Iob, and S. Mingrino

Department of Neurosurgery, University of Padua, 35100 Padua, Italy

During the last decade selective percutaneous thermocoagulation of the gasserian ganglion has become the treatment of choice for trigeminal neuralgia (22,25). This technique, in comparison to other traditional neurosurgical procedures, is more simple, noninvasive, requires only a short hospitalization, carries a lower incidence of complications, and has no contraindications (18,23–26). The most interesting characteristic of this procedure is the abolition of pain symptomatology with a good preservation of the facial tactile sensibility (20,24). Moreover, the risk of troublesome anesthesia is spared.

The neurophysiological basis for this procedure lies in the relatively higher resistance to thermic lesioning of the large myelinated fibers that mediate tactile sensibility in comparison to those unmyelinated or small myelinated fibers, in particular A-delta and C fibers (3,8,24). For this reason, an adequate thermal lesion affects the fibers that mediate pain while more or less preserving tactile sensibility.

One of the most important problems is the correct evaluation of results. In fact, the clinical evaluation of tactile sensibility is based in every case on a "subjective" response of the patient as, for example, the skin is touched. For this purpose, sophisticated techniques have been employed such as the test of Von Frey, modified by Semmes (21), with a set of nylon wires of different diameter. Although this technique may be accurate and reliable, it needs a subjective patient response. For this reason, we tried to utilize an evaluation as "objective" as possible, in which subjective components of the response are abolished, by studying the somatosensory evoked potentials (SEP).

In patients with spinal injury, evoked responses have been employed for objective evaluation of the anatomic lesion and as a prognostic tool (5,7,19). Similarly, to evaluate the extent of the damage after thermocoagulation, we applied an adequate electrical stimulus to the cutaneous areas of the corresponding trigeminal branch and registered the evoked responses at the scalp. Evoked responses have previously been employed by many authors, both to investigate the electrical conductivity of trigeminal branches in normal subjects (1) and in patients suffering from trigeminal pain (14) and to evaluate the results of microsurgical section of the trigeminal roots (16).

The purpose of the present work, on the other hand, was to evaluate the surgical lesion after percutaneous thermorhizotomy.

CLINICAL MATERIAL AND METHODS

Twenty-five patients, 15 male and 10 female, mean age 51, all affected by essential trigeminal neuralgia and who had previously undergone only pharmacological treatments, were studied by SEP before and after selective gasserian ganglion thermocoagulation. All the patients were informed about the purpose of the research and accepted it spontaneously.

Trigeminal branches were stimulated by a coaxial subcutaneous needle applied near the point of emergence of the respective peripheral nerve. Stimuli used were square waves, 0.1 msec in duration, at a random rate about 1.5 per second. The intensity was adjusted until a tingling sensation was evoked, this level being individually set for each patient (about 10–15 mA at 24 V).

Somatosensory EPs were registered at the scalp by two needle electrodes applied in the parietal region 7 cm from midline bilaterally, on the vertex–meatal line. Another indifferent electrode was placed at the vertex. In the presence of great stimulus artifacts, another indifferent cutaneous electrode of large diameter was placed in the middle frontal, and stimulus polarity was inverted after 60 sweeps. Responses were analyzed by an OTE Biomedica Neuroaverager. Analysis time was 100 msec, upper cutoff at 30 Hz, and 120 responses were summated. The whole gain of the system also remained unchanged during the subsequent controls.

Components of the SEP were indicated by their surface polarity and mean peak latency. Adopting the electrode distribution and the analysis time cited above, the most evident component is a positive wave with a mean latency of about 50 msec (P50) (6,15); other clearly recognizable components are P20 and N30 (Fig. 1).

The main characteristics of the P50 component are that it has maximal amplitude of the parietal regions (4,9,10,12), can be recorded over a relatively wide area, and appears with relatively low peripheral stimulation. In this manner, stimulus artifacts can be reduced in the majority of cases (2). When the responses obtained from each trigeminal division were judged acceptable and easily repeatable, they were recorded and photographed by a Hewlett Packard camera.

RESULTS

In all of our patients, tactile and pain sensibility before surgery appeared completely normal as they did by the test of Von Frey. The SEPs obtained from the affected branches were completely normal when compared to contra-

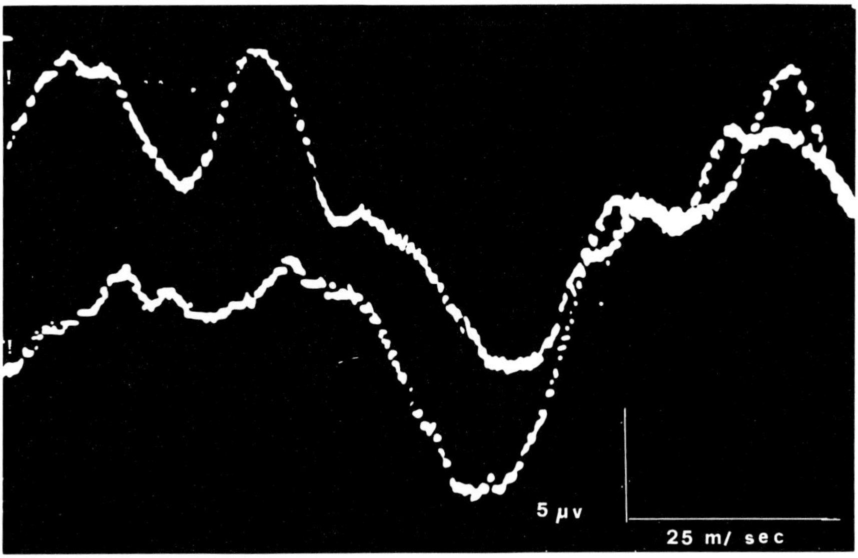

FIG. 1. Essential trigeminal neuralgia. Analysis time, 100 msec; 120 responses; biparietal registration. Preoperatively, no difference is detectable between the morphology of the two responses obtained from the first left (affected) trigeminal branch (top trace) and the opposite (unaffected) one, first right (bottom trace). Main components detectable are P20, N30, and P50 (negative up).

lateral, unaffected areas; the threshold of stimulation was the same bilaterally (Fig. 1).

The examination was then repeated 24 to 36 hr after trigeminal percutaneous thermocoagulation. The results found on subsequent testing, which appear to be related to the temperature of lesion, are as follows.

1. With a lesion temperature ranging from 60° to 70°C (15 cases), a moderate but clear hypoalgesia with immediate regression of pain symptomatology was noted. Tactile sensibility remained practically unchanged as judged by subjective responses. No clear change in the postoperative SEP was observed in this group of patients (Fig. 2).

2. In eight cases where the thermic lesion had been carried out at a temperature ranging from 70 to 75°C, the patients presented analgesia with constant and clear disturbances of tactile sensibility; this was also confirmed by the test of Von Frey. In these cases, SEPs were consistently altered; in particular, the whole response had increased latencies and was reduced in amplitude compared to the unaffected side. In these cases, the SEP reflected disturbances of tactile sensibility (Fig. 3).

3. Two patients who received a lesion at more than 75°C presented analgesia with a marked tactile hypesthesia. This observation was also confirmed by the test of Von Frey. The SEP was found markedly altered (Fig. 4).

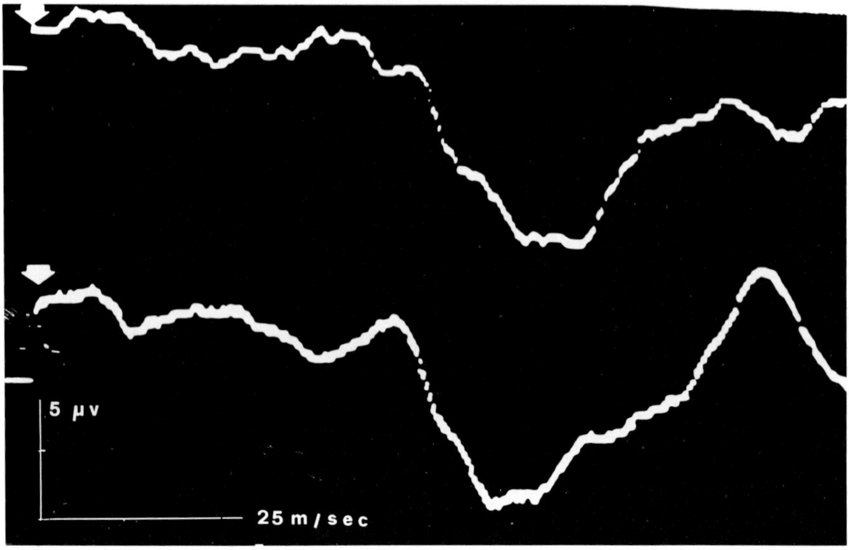

FIG. 2. Essential trigeminal neuralgia before (A) and after (B) thermocoagulation of the third right branch. Analysis time, 100 msec; 120 responses; biparietal registration. The morphology of the response obtained from the same branch (third right) before (top trace) and after (bottom trace) surgery is unchanged. The P20 and N30 components are not clearly detectable. By the technique of Von Frey, a slight disturbance of pain sensibility with no alteration of tactile sensibility has been demonstrated. (Negative up.)

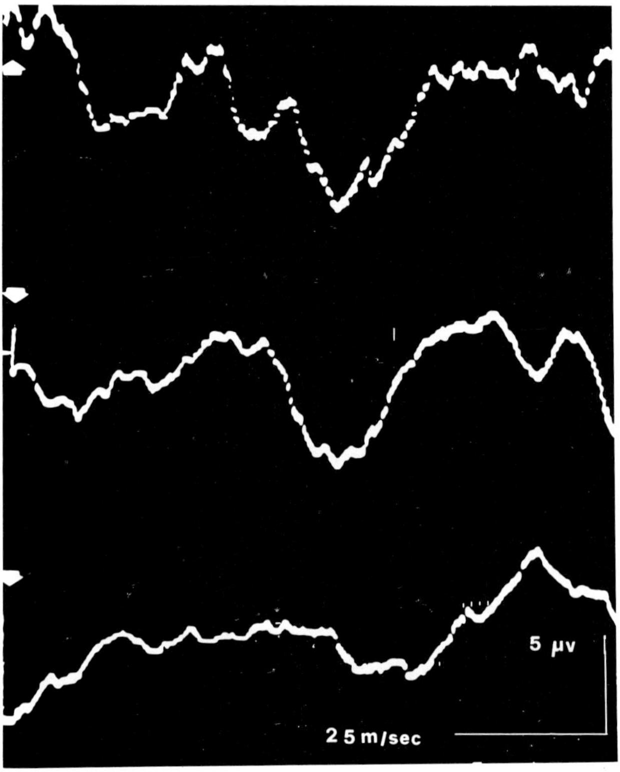

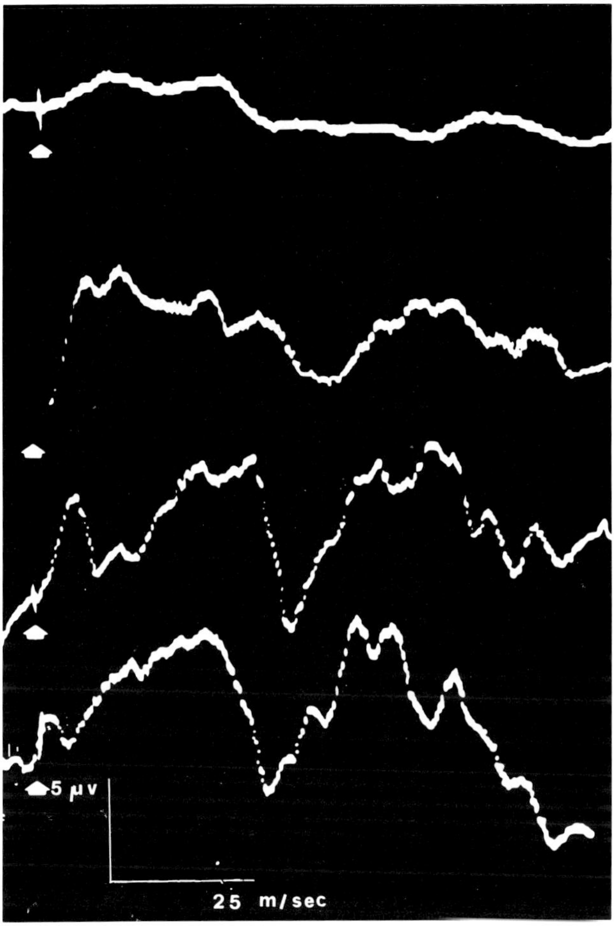

FIG. 4. Essential trigeminal neuralgia of the first and second left branches. Analysis time, 100 msec; 120 responses; biparietal registration. Postoperatively, the responses obtained from the first (third trace) and second (bottom trace) right trigeminal division (normal) are compared with the SEP obtained from the first (top trace) and second (second trace) branch of the opposite side (affected). The surgical procedure provoked a mild disturbance of tactile sensibility in the second left branch (second trace) with a marked disturbance in the first (top trace). The morphology of the SEP follows the degree of somatosensory loss. (Negative up.)

FIG. 3. Essential trigeminal neuralgia of the third left branch. Analysis time, 100 msec; 120 responses; bilateral registration. The SEP obtained after thermocoagulation of the third branch (bottom trace) shows decreased amplitude and increased latencies of P50; other components are not detectable. A slight disturbance of tactile sensibility with marked hypoalgesia is detected here. First and second branches (top and middle traces) are normal. (Negative up.)

CONCLUSIONS

By comparing clinical results obtained by the test of Von Frey with the SEP, it is possible to observe that the latter are correlated to impairment of tactile sensibility. In fact, we have found the evoked responses to be altered in the presence of disturbances of the tactile sensibility, and this alteration was proportional to the sensory loss. In contrast, the SEPs were quite unaffected in the presence of alterations only of pain sensibility.

Thus, it seems possible to hypothesize that the afferent volley of the SEP travels mainly along the pathways of tactile sensibility similarly to what has been suggested in spinal injury cases (11,13). In particular, section of the spino-thalamic tract as provoked during cordotomy does not affect the SEP (17); in contrast, experimental surgical lesions of the posterior columns in primates *do* cut off SEPs (5).

Finally, the SEP permits an objective evaluation to be made of the tactile facial sensibility.

REFERENCES

1. Bennett, M. H., and Jannetta, P. J. (1980): Trigeminal evoked potentials in humans. *Electroencephalogr. Clin. Neurophysiol.,* 48:517–526.
2. Bergamini, L., Bergamasco, B., Fra, L., and Gandiglio, G. (1965): Somatosensory evoked cortical potentials in subjects with peripheral nervous lesions. *Electromyography,* 5:121–130.
3. Broggi, G., and Siegfried, J. (1977): The effect of graded thermocoagulation on trigeminal evoked potentials in cat. *Acta Neurochir. (Wien)* [*Suppl.*], 24:175–178.
4. Broughton, R., Rasmussen, R., and Branch, C. (1968): Cortex and scalp recorded somatosensory evoked potentials in man. *Electroencephalogr. Clin. Neurophysiol.,* 24:285
5. Cusick, J. F., Myklebust, J. B., Larson, S. J., and Saunces, A. J. (1979): Spinal cord evaluation by cortical evoked responses. *Arch. Neurol.,* 36:140–143.
6. Debeker, J., and Desmedt, J. E. (1964): Les potentiels évoqués cérébraux et les potentiels de nerf sensible chez l'homme et l'utilisation de l'ordinateur numérique Mnemotron 400-B. *Acta Neurol. Belg.,* 64:1212–1248.
7. Dorfman, L. J., Perkash, I., Bosley, T. M., and Cummins, K. L. (1980): Use of cerebral evoked potentials to evaluate spinal somatosensory function in patients with traumatic and surgical myelopathies. *J. Neurosurg.,* 52:654–660.
8. Frigyesi, T. L., Siegfried, J., and Broggi, G. (1975): The selective vulnerability of evoked potentials in the trigeminal root to graded thermocoagulation. *Exp. Neurol.,* 49:11–21.
9. Giblin, D. R. (1964): Somatosensory evoked potentials in healthy subjects and in patients with lesions of the nervous system. *Ann. N.Y. Acad. Sci.,* 112:93–142.
10. Goff, W. R., Rosner, B. S., and Allison, T. (1962): Distribution of cerebral somatosensory evoked responses in normal man. *Electroencephalogr. Clin. Neurophysiol.,* 14:697–713.
11. Halliday, A. M. (1967): Changes in the form of cerebral evoked responses in man associated with various lesions of the nervous system. *Electroencephalogr. Clin. Neurophysiol.,* [*Suppl.*], 25:178–192.
12. Halliday, A. M. (1975): Somatosensory evoked responses. *Electroencephalogr. Clin. Neurophysiol.,* 8:60–66.
13. Halliday, A. M., and Wakefield, G. S. (1963): Cerebral evoked potential in patients with dissociated sensory loss. *J. Neurol. Neurosurg. Psychiatry,* 26:211–219.
14. King, R. B., and Meagher, J. N. (1955): Studies of trigeminal nerve potentials. *J. Neurosurg.,* 12:393–402.
15. Larsson, L. E., and Prevec, T. S. (1970): Somatosensory response to mechanical stimulation as recorded in the human. *Electroencephalogr. Clin. Neurophysiol.,* 28:162–172.

16. Ley, A., Montserrat, L., Bacci, F., and Ley, A., Jr. (1975): Clinical and electrophysiological studies on sensory conduction mediated by the accessory rootlets of the human trigeminal nerve. *J. Neurosurg.,* 42:513–521.
17. Namerow, N. S. (1969): Somatosensory evoked responses following cervical cordotomy. *Bull. Los Angeles Neurol. Soc.,* 34:184–189.
18. Nugent, G. R., and Berry, B. (1974): Trigeminal neuralgia treated by differential percutaneous radiofrequency coagulation of the gasserian ganglion. *J. Neurosurg.,* 40:517–523.
19. Perot, P. L., Jr. (1973): The clinical use of somatosensory evoked potentials in spinal cord injury. *Clin. Neurosurg.,* 20:367–381.
20. Salar, G., and Mingrino, S. (1979): Facial touch sensation before and after the treatment of trigeminal neuralgia by percutaneous electrocoagulation of the gasserian ganglion. In: *Proceedings of XVIII Congreso Latino Americano de Neurocirurgia,* Edited by J. Benaim, pp. 202–204. JMA S.A., Buenos Aires.
21. Semmes, J., Weinstein, S., Ghent, L., and Teubner, H. L. (1960): *Somatosensory Changes After Penetrating Brain Wounds in Man.* Harvard University Press, Cambridge.
22. Siegfried, J. (1977): 500 percutaneous thermocoagulations of the gasserian ganglion for trigeminal pain. *Surg. Neurol.,* 8:126–131.
23. Siegfried, J., and Vosmansky, M. (1975): Technique of controlled thermocoagulation of trigeminal ganglion and spinal roots. *Adv. Tech. Standards Neurosurg.,* 2:199–209.
24. Sweet, W. H., and Wepsic, J. G. (1970): Relation of fiber size in trigeminal posterior root condition of impulses for pain and touch: Production of analgesia. *Trans. Am. Neurol. Assoc.,* 95:134–137.
25. Sweet, W. H., and Wepsic, J. G. (1974): Controlled thermocoagulatoin of trigeminal ganglion and rootlets for differential destruction of pain fibers. Part I: Trigeminal neuralgia. *J. Neurosurg.,* 40:143–156.
26. Turnbull, I. M. (1974): Percutaneous rhizotomy for trigeminal neuralgia. *Surg. Neurol.,* 2:385–389.

Clinical Applications of Evoked Potentials in Neurology,
edited by J. Courjon, F. Mauguiere, and M. Revol.
Raven Press, New York © 1982.

Intraoperative Somatosensory Evoked Response Monitoring During Spinal Cord Surgery

*Robert M. Worth, **Omkar N. Markand, †G. Paul DeRosa, and **Carroll H. Warren

**Division of Neurosurgery, **Department of Neurology, and †Department of Orthopedic Surgery, Indiana University School of Medicine, Indianapolis, Indiana 46223*

One of the most distressing problems haunting the spinal surgeon is the development of a sometimes profound increase in neurological deficits in patients during the intraoperative period when the functional status of the spinal cord cannot be ascertained by direct clinical examination. A number of methods have been described in the attempt to monitor spinal cord function including the so-called "wake-up test" in which patients are actually awakened from anesthesia and a rudimentary clinical examination is performed. The inconvenience of this test, however, led Nash and others (8) to investigate the use of evoked potential techniques for monitoring in this situation. Our laboratory has developed a standardized protocol which can be quickly and dependably utilized to provide information about the functional status of the somatosensory conducting pathways during surgery in patients undergoing corrective operations for scoliosis. This chapter communicates our experience with this monitoring technique and makes a preliminary attempt to quantitate the changes seen.

MATERIALS AND METHODS

Out of 21 patients undergoing intraoperative monitoring of somatosensory evoked potentials (SEP), 12 were selected on the basis of completeness of stored data. This was the only criterion for inclusion, and no cases were eliminated on the basis of the results themselves.

Any patient to be monitored received an evaluation a day before the operation to ascertain baseline SEPs. The sites of both stimulating and recording electrodes were also marked on the skin with indelible crayon for subsequent stimulation and recording during the operation. The preoperative assessment allowed the entire monitoring set-up procedure to be accomplished within a few minutes of the patient's placement on the operating table.

Stimulation was carried out by applying square-wave electrical pulses to the posterior tibial nerve at both ankles individually. Surface electrodes were used for the base-line preoperative recording, but during the operation, once the patient was anesthetized, needle electrodes were implanted over the nerve to provide better contact and to minimize the danger of dislodgement by the drapes. Recording was obtained from a vertex electrode placed 2 cm behind the C_Z (10–20 system) position and connected to a reference electrode placed at F_Z position. Stimulation was carried out at a rate of 2 Hz with 0.1 msec pulse duration and constant current amplitude of less than 20 mA. Stimulus strength was adjusted to a level that produced good, but not maximal, distal motor response. The analysis time was 250 msec after the stimulus, and a total of 200 stimuli were used for each record. The scalp response was amplified 100,000 times and summed and stored in an averaging computer (Nicolet Med-80). The results were then graphed with an X–Y plotter and transferred to a disk for permanent storage. Results were analyzed by inspection of the graphed records, and statistical analysis of the latencies and amplitudes were provided by direct cursor readout from the computer. The Student's *t*-test for paired comparison was performed in most cases to evaluate statistical significance.

The method of anesthesia used was a balanced narcotic technique avoiding the use of agents such as halothane and enflurane that degrade the cortical evoked responses (2). Interestingly, in the few cases where anesthesia was instituted with these agents, the study had to be abandoned because of total failure to record the evoked response. In all patients, the surgical procedure consisted of a standard spinal straightening operation using Harrington rod instrumentation. Hypotension was used in all cases to reduce blood loss.

Somatosensory evoked potentials were recorded at frequent intervals throughout the case in response to the requests of the operating surgeon; the two legs were generally tested alternately. Regardless of other periods tested, SEPs were always obtained at the following five stages: during skin opening or preoperative preparation of the skin, immediately prior to distraction of the spine, immediately after distraction, 15 min after distraction, and at closing. These five records were selected for analysis as the basis for this report.

RESULTS

The base-line SEPs obtained in the laboratory preoperatively were in all cases normal and consisted of a multiphasic potential with alternating positve–negative peaks. The individual peaks are designated as P_1, N_1, P_2, N_2 in our laboratory, and the mean latencies of these peaks are 38, 48, 58, and 74 msec, respectively. The initial intraoperative recording had the same general configuration in a given patient but tended to be less well defined and generally lower in amplitude (Fig. 1). The early components P_1 and N_1 of the SEPs were often low in amplitude and therefore difficult to identify and quantitate. For this reason, the larger second negative peak (N_2) was used to perform the numerical evaluation, although the form of the entire SEP was always considered when the surgeon was advised about the status of the spinal cord function. We initially anticipated

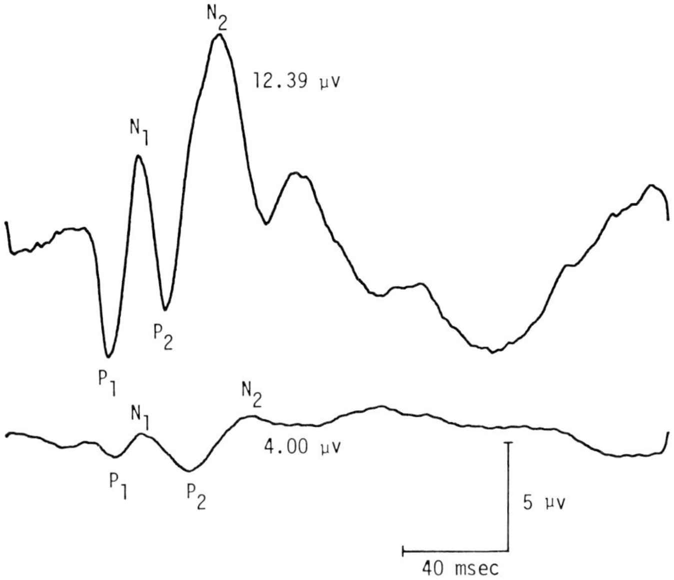

FIG. 1. Comparison between a laboratory recorded SEP in an alert patient and an intraoperative study in the same patient in the prone position under general anesthesia. Note the lower amplitude and loss of definition in the intraoperative study. Amplitude values refer to the amplitude of N_2.

that in addition to the amplitude, the latency of N_2 would also be a satisfactory parameter for evaluation, but this proved not to be the case. The latency seemed to respond to hypotension and distraction in an unpredictable manner, sometimes increasing and sometimes decreasing in response to the operative stresses. Therefore, only the amplitude of this wave was used as the most important parameter for comparison. The amplitude of N_2 was obtained by measuring the height (microvolts) between the trough of P_2 and peak of N_2. There was no difference between the SEPs obtained from right- and left-sided stimulation, and the two values were thus combined to calculate a mean value of 5.44 ± 2.83 μV for the amplitude of this peak.

Figure 2 and Table 1 illustrate graphically the changes that occurred in the amplitude of N_2 at various points during the operation. The induction of hypotension alone produced a statistically significant effect, the amplitude of N_2 dropping to 84.4%. When distraction was applied, the potential decreased further to 76.9% of the original amplitude. This value was also statistically different from the posthypotension result at the $p < 0.05$ level. After about 15 min following distraction, the amplitude had begun to increase and had returned to 82% of the base-line value, and by the time of closing, when the hypotension had also been reversed, the potential height had increased to 86.9% of its original level. Figure 3 illustrates these changes in the tracing obtained in a typical case at

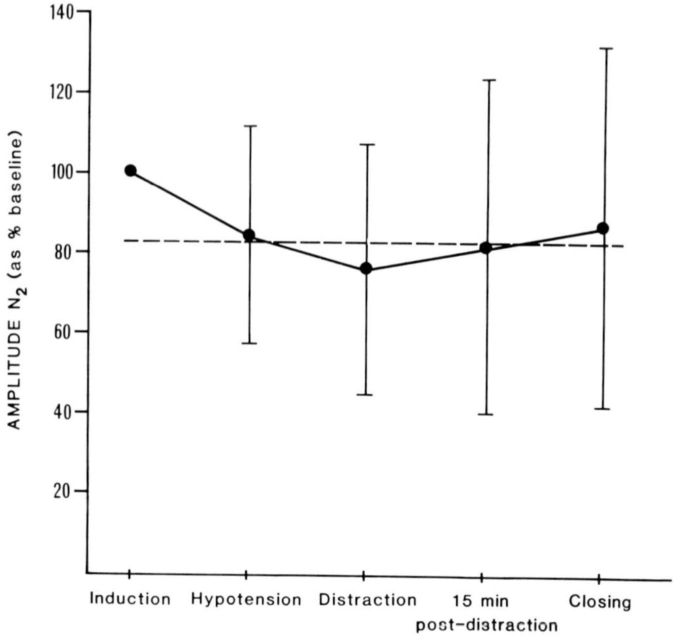

FIG. 2. Graphic representation of the amplitudes of N_2 expressed as a percent of base line for various stages in the operation. The *dashed line* represents the $p < 0.001$ significance level computed by the method of paired comparisons.

the specific periods during the operation. The changes, in general, were symmetrical for the SEPs obtained from right- and left-sided stimulation.

Although the standard deviation for the mean amplitude of N_2 was high relative to the actual value itself, the use of the method of paired comparison permitted the detection of significant changes in wave amplitude within a given patient in response to the various surgical manipulations affecting the spinal cord. With this means of analysis, 11 of the 12 patients in this report showed a statistically significant decrease in potential amplitude associated with hypoten-

TABLE 1. *The amplitude of N_2 expressed as a percentage of the base-line amplitude[a] at different stages of the operation[b]*

Hypotension	Distraction	15 min postdistraction	Closing
84.4% $p < 0.001$	76.1% $p < 0.001$	82.0% $p < 0.001$	86.9% $p < 0.001$

[a] Base-line mean amplitude of N_2 is 5.44 μV.

[b] Difference between hypotension and distraction effects has a significance level, $0.02 < p < 0.05$.

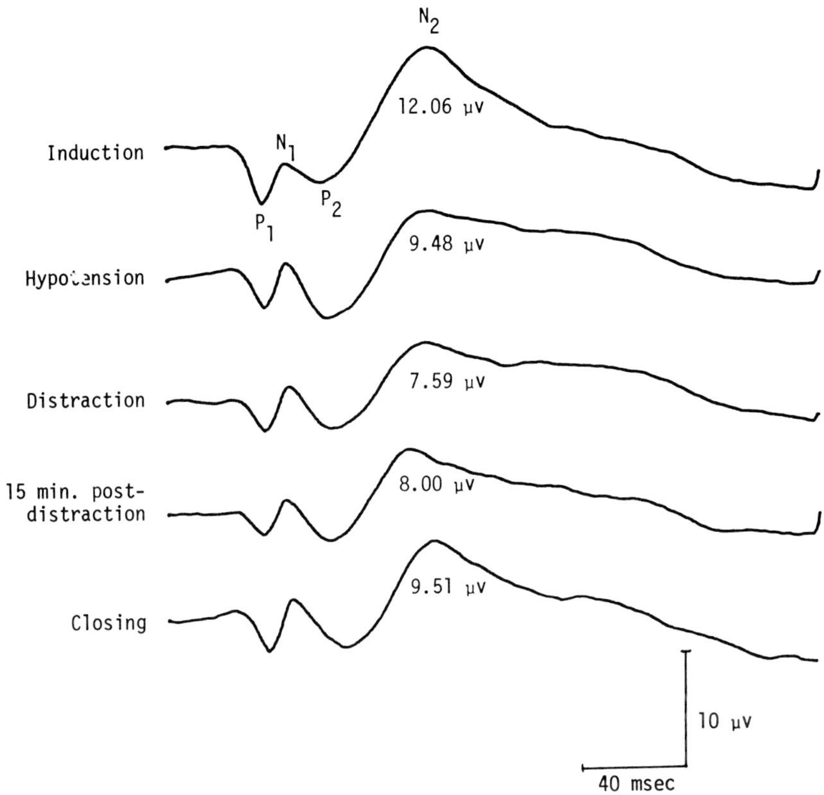

FIG. 3. The SEPs are recorded at specific periods during the operation in response to right posterior tibial stimulation. The amplitude values refer to the amplitude of N_2. Note the decreased amplitude after hypotension and the further decrease with distraction. The SEP then tends to recover as steady state distraction is maintained.

sion and distraction. None of these patients suffered an increase in neurological deficit postoperatively.

DISCUSSION

More than 30 years ago, Dawson (3) recorded for the first time evoked potentials from the scalp in response to stimulation of the peripheral nerves. It was not until 1969 that Donaghey and Numoto (4), from animal experiments, suggested that SEPs may provide prognostic information in spinal cord injuries. Perot (10) in 1972 applied the technique of SEPs as a predictive tool for impending injury to the spinal cord during spinal operations. More recently several workers (1,5,8) have used this technique to monitor the physiological integrity of the spinal cord during scoliosis operations.

The incidence of partial or complete paraplegia in scoliosis correction procedures has been quoted as 0.56%. Despite the fact that postoperative neurological deficits are thus uncommon, they are nonetheless distressing in a given patient, particularly since many of these patients are neurologically intact preoperatively. A technique for the clinical assessment of the effect of intraoperative distraction has been reported in which the anesthesia is actually partially reversed and the patient is awakened to a state where he can follow commands while the surgical procedure is still in progress (6). He is then asked to move his toes, and when this is accomplished, general anesthesia is reintroduced and the operation is completed. In addition to the inconvenience for the anesthesiologist and the surgeon and the possible risk and discomfort to the patient, one must be concerned by the rare but well-documented reports of patients who were already paraparetic when awakened. For these reasons, the evoked response monitoring of the status of the spinal cord during the spinal operation is being progressively applied in place of the "wake-up test."

The technical details and the parameters of the SEPs that are most relevant in providing information regarding spinal cord status are yet to be fully worked out. Some workers have attempted to record spinal evoked responses (rather than the scalp responses as reported here) by placing epidural electrodes (7) or electrodes inserted into the spinous processes (9). The direct spinal recording techniques are more difficult to set up and do not lend themselves well to pre- and postoperative evaluation of the patient. On the other hand, recording the evoked potentials from the scalp is a noninvasive technique and can be rapidly set up in both the laboratory and operating room.

The present work confirms the qualitative studies of Nash et al. (8) that showed that hypotension alone could induce a significant change in the SEP. The decrease in the amplitude produced by hypotension in the present report is significant at the $p < 0.001$ level. Our data, in addition, suggest that the distraction procedure is also capable of producing a further degree of SEP attenuation which is significant at the $p < 0.05$ level. All SEP changes revert towards normal as soon as the distraction has reached a steady state and the blood pressure approaches normotensive levels, although the amplitude of the SEP may still remain somewhat decreased even at the completion of the operation.

As none of our patients sustained any increase in neurological deficit postoperatively, we have no information as to the extent of SEP alterations that can be tolerated without permanent injury to the spinal cord. Our data, however, do indicate that a decrease of at least 24% in amplitude of N_2 component of the SEP is well tolerated provided the response shows a trend towards progressive normalization by the end of the operation. We observed changes in the amplitude of 50% or greater (one patient had 80% decline which quickly reverted to normal) with untoward effects on the patient's neurological status. Nevertheless, if such a patient failed to show the prompt reversal to normal pattern expected, measures to alleviate the spinal cord embarrassment would seem indicated.

Somatosensory responses are believed to be caused by the activity of the pathway going through the posterior columns. There is, therefore, a theoretical possibility that a major motor deficit could develop during the operation without being detected by the evoked response technique. However, it seems that the technique is extremely sensitive and reveals significant electrical alterations in response to surgical stresses and manipulation of the spinal cord, even in the majority of patients who remained neurologically intact following the operation.

We conclude that the technique of scalp recording of evoked responses elicited by peripheral nerve stimulation is a convenient, reliable, and sensitive method of monitoring spinal cord function during surgical manipulation of this structure. Set-up time is short and is greatly facilitated by the preoperative recording and marking session. Besides using the SEP waveform as others have done, we believe that utilization of the amplitudes of certain SEP components in evaluation of the responses may provide some quantification for comparison. The results reported here are still preliminary because these are based on a small series of patients. However, more experiences with the analysis of the SEP data will provide more insight into the degree of tolerable alteration of these parameters and will allow more accurate prediction of the results not only in the operative cases but in all types of spinal cord lesions.

REFERENCES

1. Brown, L. H., and Nash, C. L., Jr. (1979): Current status of spinal cord monitoring. *Spine,* 4:466–470.
2. Clark, D. L., and Rosner, B. S. (1973): Neurophysiologic effects of general anesthetics: I. The electroencephalogram and sensory evoked responses in man. *Anesthesiology,* 38:564–582.
3. Dawson, G. D. (1947): Cerebral responses to electrical stimulation of peripheral nerves in man. *J. Neurol. Neurosurg. Psychiatry,* 10:137–140.
4. Donaghey, R. N., and Numoto, M. (1969): Prognostic significance of sensory evoked potential in spinal cord injury. *Proceedings of the Seventeenth Spinal Cord Injury Conference,* pp. 251–257. Veterans Administration Hospital, Bronx, New York, September 1969.
5. Engler, G. L., Spielholz, N. I., Bernhard, W. N., Danziger, F., Merkin, H., and Wolff, T. (1978): Somatosensory evoked potentials during Harrington instrumentation for scoliosis. *J. Bone Joint Surg.,* 60A:528–532.
6. Hall, J. E., Lavine, C. R., and Sudhir, K. G. (1978): Inoperative awakening to monitor spinal cord function during Harrington instrumentation and spine fusion. *J. Bone Joint Surg.,* 60A:533–536.
7. Hattori, S., Saiki, K., and Kawai, S. (1979): Diagnosis of the level and severity of cord lesion in cervical spondylotic myelopathy. *Spine,* 4:478–485.
8. Nash, C. L., Lorig, R., Schatzinger, L. A., and Brown, R. H. (1977): Spinal cord monitoring during operative treatment of the spine. *Clin. Orthop.,* 126:100–105.
9. Nordwall, A., Axelgaard, J., Harada, Y., Valencia, P., McNeal, D. R., and Brown, J. C. (1979): Spinal cord monitoring using evoked potentials recorded from feline vertebral bone. *Spine,* 4:486–494.
10. Perot, P. L., Jr. (1972): The clinical use of somatosensory evoked potentials in spinal cord injury. *Clin. Neurosurg.,* 20:367–381.

Clinical Applications of Evoked Potentials in Neurology,
edited by J. Courjon, F. Mauguiere, and M. Revol.
Raven Press, New York © 1982.

Evoked Potentials as Objective Parameters for the Analgesic Response of Weak Analgesics

*P. Rohdewald, *H. Derendorf, **C. E. Elger, and †O. Knoll

**Institute for Pharmaceutical Chemistry, **Physiological Institute, and †Medical Polyclinic, Westfalische Wilhelms University of Münster, D-4400 Münster, Federal Republic of Germany*

In several studies, it has been demonstrated that painful electrical stimulation of the tooth pulp results in an evoked potential in the EEG the amplitude of which was found to parallel the subjective sensation of pain (2). The aim of the present investigation was to test whether a measurement of a nociceptive evoked potential may be a valid method for determining the analgesic potency of weak analgesics. This is of special interest because subjective methods such as pain rating and threshold discrimination have often failed to detect the effect of weak analgesics (1,6). In our study, we compared the subjective parameters and the amplitude of the nociceptive evoked potential in human volunteers. The following experimental series were performed: (a) two different weak analgesics with different analgesic potencies; (b) two mild analgesics with identical content but different bioavailabilities; and (c) an analgesic for which comparative data from dental patient studies were available.

METHODS

The studies were performed on 14 healthy volunteers aged 21 to 36 years. The electrical painful stimulation (duration 0.3 msec) was applied stochastically to one of the upper incisors during bipolar conductive rubber disks mounted in an individually formed impression of the teeth. The stimulation current was monitored on an oscilloscope.

Averaged evoked potentials (SEP) were taken from EEG recordings between C_z and F_8 (sweep number: 64). Although the SEP showed a considerable interindividual variability, the intraindividual variability was found to be small (Fig. 1). The negative peak of the SEP that occurred with a latency of 170 to 260 msec proved to be the most reproducible component of the evoked potential. Therefore, the amplitude of this peak was measured [for further details see (7)].

The rating of pain and the threshold of sensation were used as subjective parameters of sensory quality. Pain ratings given immediately after the stimula-

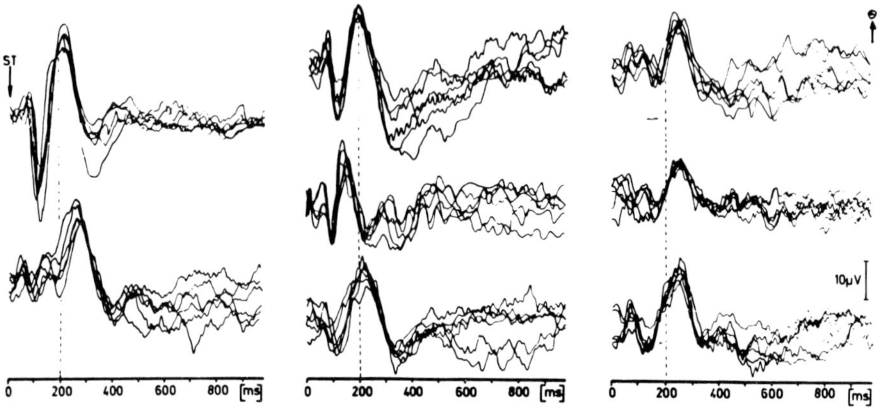

FIG. 1. Records of SEPs of eight volunteers after painful stimulation of the tooth pulp (ST) with the doubled individual threshold of sensation measured on six different days.

tion were based on eight categories: 0, no sensation; 1, threshold of sensation; 2, distinct sensation; 3, unpleasant sensation; 4, pain threshold; 5, weak pain; 6, distinct pain; 7, strong pain. The threshold of sensation was defined as the lowest current necessary to evoke sensation.

The tablets were given with 200 ml water 3 hr after a light meal. The amount of salicylic acid and paracetamol was measured in saliva to determine bioavailability. This is accepted as suitable and more convenient than blood level monitoring (3,4). All drugs (Table 1) were tested on each of the volunteers in a randomized double-blind study with intervals of at least 2 days between experiments.

TABLE 1. *List of drugs*

Tablet	Drug dose	Manufacturer
A	Salicylamide 0.17 g Phenacetin 0.15 g Caffeine citrate 0.02 g	Romigal-Werk 8000 München
B	Phenazone 0.50 g Caffeine 0.048 g	Hoechst AG 6230 Frankfurt 80
C	ASA 0.25 g Paracetamol 0.20 g Caffeine 0.05 g	Thomae GmbH 7950 Biberach
D	Aluminum acetylsalicylate 0.25 g Paracetamol 0.20 g Caffeine 0.05 g	Mack Chem. Pharm. Fabrik 7918 Illertisse
E	Propyphenazone 0.09 g Paracetamol 0.20 g Caffeine 0.05 g Metamizole 35 mg Bucetin 30 mg	Dr. G. Mann GmbH 1000 Berlin 20

The measurement was performed as follows: 5 min before drug intake, the sensation threshold was determined. The stimulation current was then doubled, and the resulting painful stimulus was used during the whole testing period. The measurements were performed at 20, 40, 60, 90, 120, and 150 min after drug intake. Because of the interindividual variability, the absolute values for the threshold current and the SEP peak amplitude as well as the pain ratings were calculated as percentages of the value determined before drug intake.

RESULTS AND DISCUSSION

In a first series, the effect of a mild-acting analgesic drug (substance A) was compared with a more effective one (substance B). As demonstrated in Fig. 2, the diminuation (%) of the peak amplitude of the SEP and of the pain rating

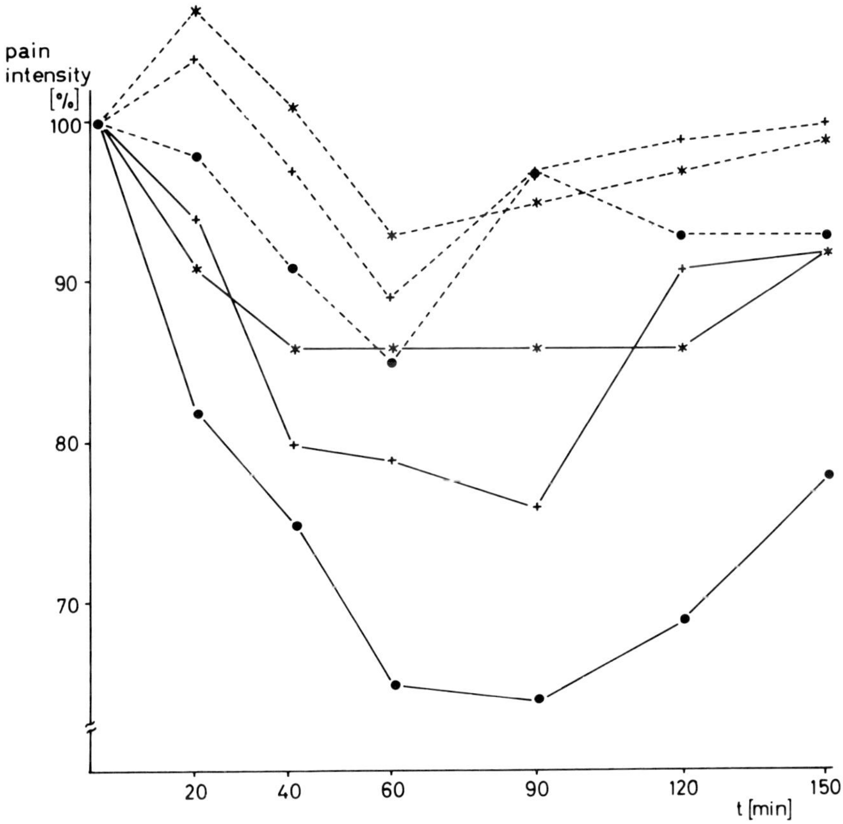

FIG. 2. Attenuation of pain after administration of the analgesics A and B (means of 14 subjects). *, subjectively determined by pain rating (%); +, subjectively determined by the threshold of sensation (%); ●, determined by the decrease of the SEP (%). *Dashed lines,* Tablet A; *solid lines,* Tablet B.

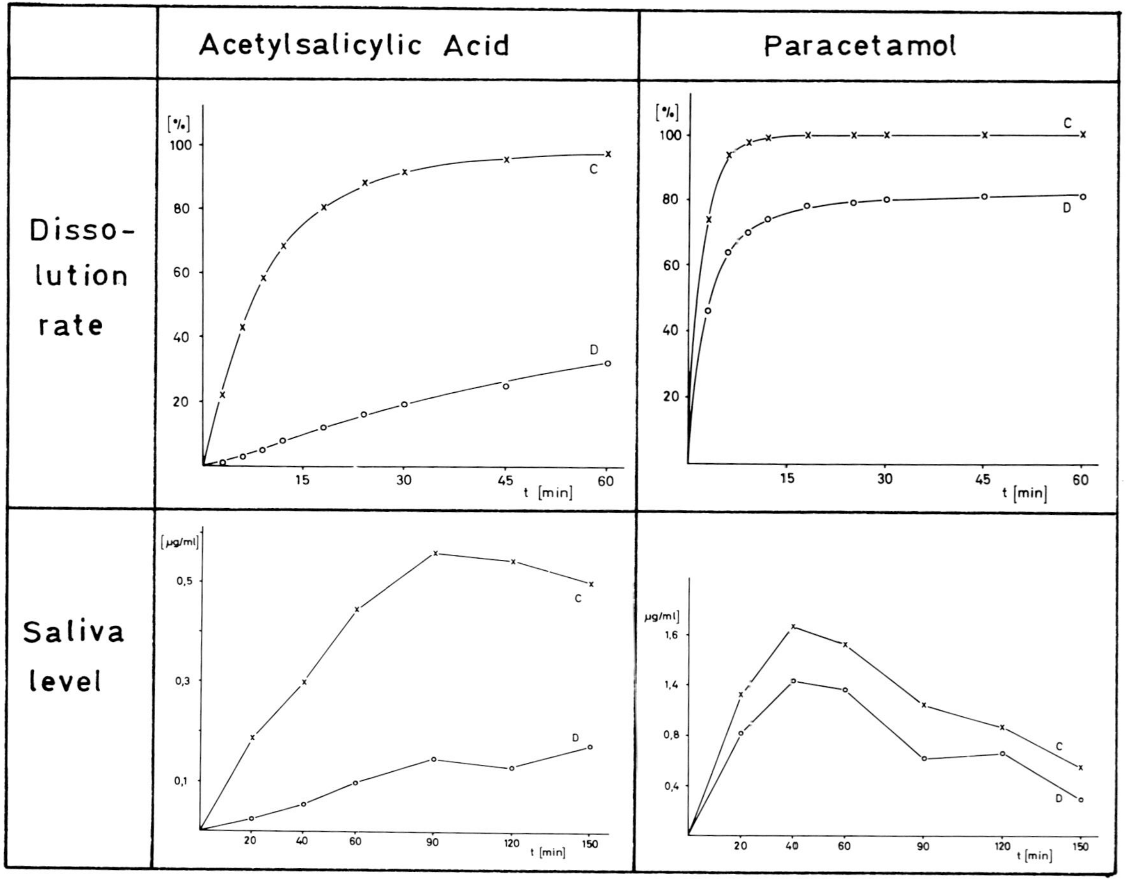

Fig. 3. Dissolution in gastric juice and the concentration in saliva of salicylic acid and paracetamol for the tablets C (×) and D (○).

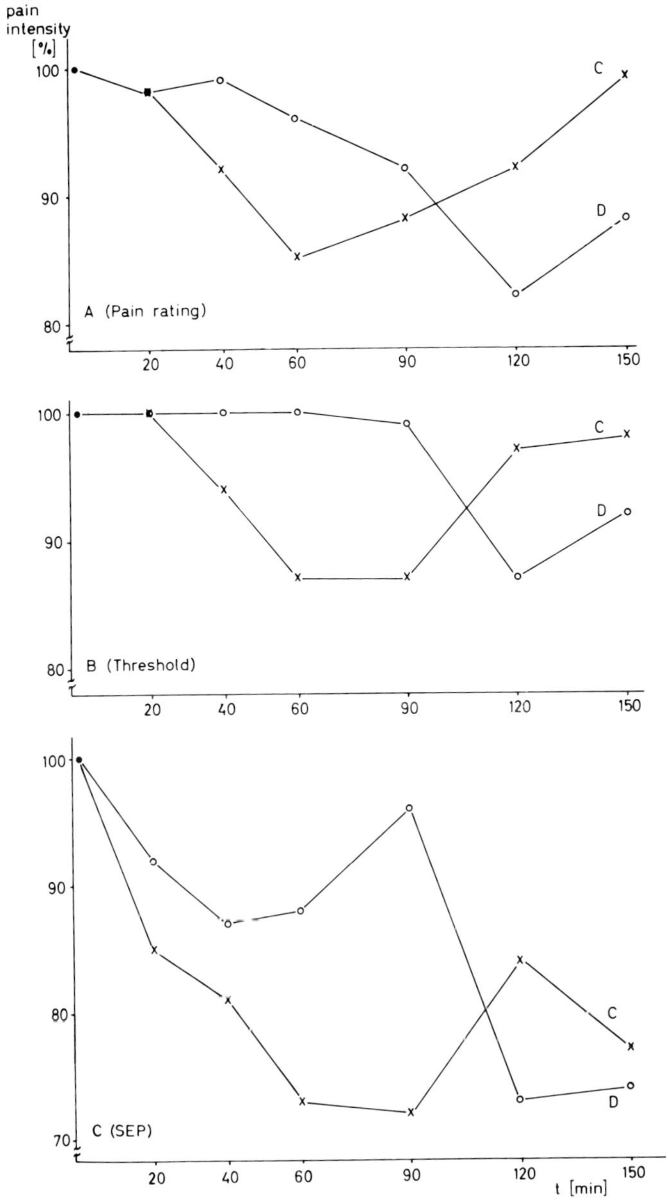

FIG. 4. Attenuation of pain after oral administration of the analgesics C and D (means of 14 subjects). **A:** Subjectively determined by pain rating (%). **B:** Subjectively determined by the threshold of sensation (%). **C:** determined by the decrease of the SEP (%). ×, Tablet C; ○, Tablet D.

as well as the threshold increase (%) were similar. After we could differentiate between the effects of 500- and 1,000-mg doses of acetylsalicylic acid (7), we tested in another series, the sensitivity of the method with two drugs with the same active ingredients (acetylsalicylic acid, paracetamol) but with different formulations (C,D) that lead to a difference in their bioavailability. The dissolved amounts of acetylsalicylic acid and paracetamol in gastric fluids determined *in vitro* as a function of time for the different formulations C and D are shown in the upper part of Fig. 3. These differences in the dissolution rate lead to similar differences in the bioavailability measured *in vitro* as the amount of salicylic acid and paracetamol in saliva (Fig. 3, lower part). The differences in bioavailabiltiy are reflected by SEP amplitude reduction as well as by the subjective pain measurements (Fig. 4). Tablet C gave a relatively quick attenuation of pain measured by all three parameters, whereas tablet D showed the maximum analgesic action only after 120 to 150 min.

In a third series, we compared the effect of the analgesic E using all parameters. During the first 60 min, all of these parameters showed similar changes (Fig. 5) At later times, the data of the subjective measurements indicated a return

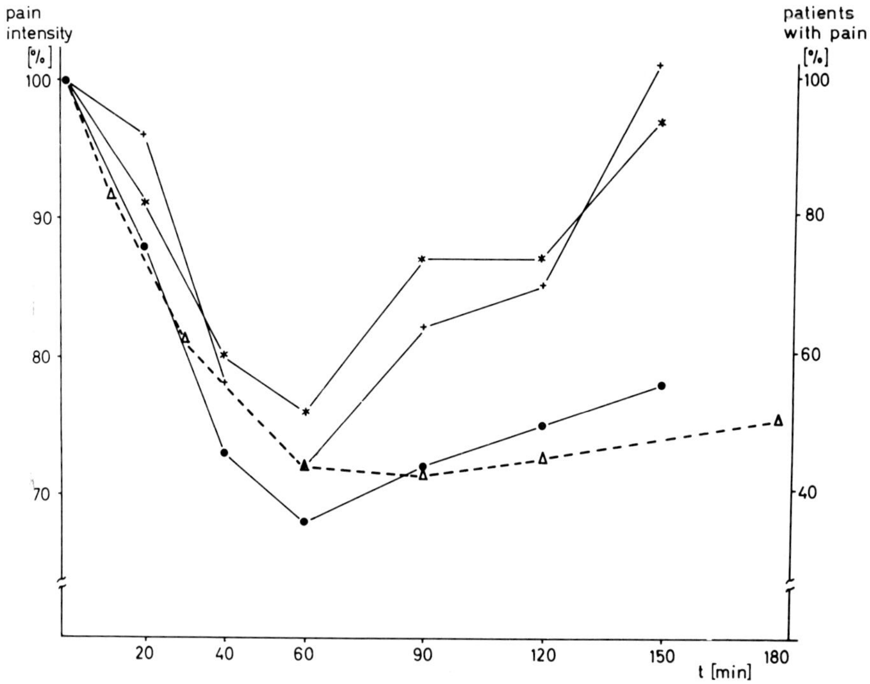

FIG. 5. Attenuation of pain after oral administration of the analgesic E (comparison between laboratory and clinical pain). *, subjectively determined by pain rating (%); +, subjectively determined by the threshold of sensation (%); ●, determined by the decrease of the SEP (%); △, determined by diminution of the number of patients with postoperative pain (%).

to the initial values, whereas the amplitude of the SEP remained reduced. This difference, often found as a trend in other experimental series, requires further study. However, a clear parallelism is obvious between this behavior of the SEP and data from measurements of the attenuation of postoperative tooth pain after application of the same drug, as done by Lincke and Harnisch [(5); dashed line in Fig. 5].

The data presented indicate that measurements of a SEP after painful tooth pulp stimulation together with subjective methods may be a useful aid for the determination of the analgesic potency of weak analgesics.

REFERENCES

1. Benjamin, F. B. (1958): Effect of aspirin on suprathreshold pain in man. *Science,* 128:303–304.
2. Chapman, C. R., Chen, A. C. N., and Harkins, S. W. (1979): Brain evoked potentials as correlates of laboratory pain: A review and perspective. In: *Advances in Pain Research and Therapy, Vol. 3,* edited by J. J. Bonica, J. C. Liebeskind, and D. G. Albe-Fessard, pp. 791–803. Raven Press, New York.
3. Glynn, J. P., and Bastein, W. (1973): Salivary excretion of paracetamol in man. *J. Pharm. Pharmacol.,* 25:420–422.
4. Graham, G., and Rowland, M. (1972): Application of salivary salicylate data to biopharmaceutical studies of salicylates. *J. Pharm. Sci.,* 61:1219–1222.
5. Lincke, U., and Harnisch, H. (1975): Doppelblindstudie über Wirkungsvergleich von Phenacetin und Paracetamol in einer Analgetika-Kombination. *ZWR,* 84:318–323.
6. Meyer, F. P., Grecksch, G., and Walther, H. (1977): Zur experimentellen Prüfung von Analgetika am Menschen. *Zentrabl. Pharm.,* 116:645–647.
7. Rohdewald, P., Derendorf, H., Elger, C. E., and Knoll, O. (1980): Quantifizierung der Dämpfung eines Schmerzreizes nach Gabe schwacher Analgetika mit Hilfe evozierter Potentiale. *Z. EEG EMG,* 11:199–204.

Clinical Applications of Evoked Potentials in Neurology,
edited by J. Courjon, F. Mauguiere, and M. Revol.
Raven Press, New York © 1982.

Relationship Between Somatosensory Evoked Potential Components and Cutaneous Pain Threshold: Effects of Transcutaneous Electrical Nerve Stimulation

*Fabio Francini, **Marco Maresca, **Paolo Procacci, and **Massimo Zoppi

* *Cattedra di Fisiologia Generale and ** Cattedra di Terapia Medica Sistematica, Università di Firenze, Florence, Italy*

Transcutaneous electrical nerve stimulation (TENS) has been largely used in recent years for relief of pain in patients suffering from various chronic pain syndromes (1,6–11). However, the mechanism of the analgesic effect of electrical stimulation is still a matter of discussion (1,7).

In previous research (3,4,8) we observed that TENS induced changes of cutaneous tactile, tingling, and pain thresholds determined with electrical stimuli. These changes were observed not only in the distribution area of the stimulated nerve but also in other parts of the body. In the distribution area of the stimulated nerve, the thresholds became higher in all subjects; outside this area, the thresholds became higher in subjects in whom, before TENS, they were low and became lower in the subjects in whom, before TENS, they were high. That is, TENS induced a reset of sensory thresholds to intermediate values, so that the differences among the various subjects decreased.

In the present investigation, we studied the effects of TENS on cortical somatosensory evoked potentials (SEP) in order to relate the data obtained with a neurophysiological objective method to the results observed with the psychophysical evaluation of sensory thresholds.

It is well known that the characteristics of SEP may be different in different subjects and may be modified in the same subject by different psychologic conditions (2,5). Therefore, we investigated: (a) the possible relationship between SEP components and cutaneous pain threshold in different psychologic conditions (novelty versus habituation); and (b) the possible variations of SEP components induced by TENS and their relation to changes of cutaneous pain threshold.

MATERIAL AND METHOD

The investigation was performed in 19 healthy subjects, 13 males and six females, between 24 and 40 years of age. All subjects were members of the laboratory staff or volunteer undergraduates, and all were right-handed. In all subjects, we determined pain thresholds and induced SEP before, during, and after transcutaneous electrical nerve stimulation.

Transcutaneous Electrical Nerve Stimulation

In every subject, TENS was applied with Ag/AgCl/KCl rectangular surface electrodes 3 × 7 cm. The cathode was applied on the volar surface of the wrist over the median nerve, the anode on the back of the hand. The pulses were constant-current square waves of 1 msec at a frequency of 50 Hz. The intensity of the current was raised until the subject felt a well-detectable tingling sensation radiating to the distribution area of the nerve. During the stimulation, the intensity of the current was changed in order to maintain a constant tingling sensation. The stimulation lasted 25 min.

Pain Threshold

The pain threshold was measured with 20-msec trains of 1-msec constant-current square waves at a frequency of 250 Hz applied to the skin of the forearm contralateral to TENS by means of two circular nonpolarizable electrodes (Ag/AgCl/KCl) of 8 mm diameter. The pain threshold, expressed in milliamperes, was evaluated by the method of limits: i.e., the stimulus strength was successively increased with notation of the value when the subject perceived pricking pain; then the stimulus strength was successively decreased with notation of the value when pain disappeared. This procedure was repeated at least three times. The mean of all readings was used to denote the threshold (3,8).

Somatosensory Evoked Potentials

In order to induce SEP, in every subject electrical stimuli were applied on the dorsal surface of the second finger of the left hand by means of two circular nonpolarizable electrodes (Ag/AgCl/KCl) of 8 mm diameter. The stimuli were single electrical 0.5-msec constant-current square waves repeated every 4 sec; the intensity of the current was regulated in order to induce a well-detectable nonpainful sensation.

The cortical potentials evoked by the stimuli were recorded from the right parietal scalp focus in the projection area of the hand (3 cm behind C3–C4) (2). The indifferent electrode was placed on the right ear lobe.

Somatosensory evoked potentials were averaged with the aid of a digital averager. The analysis time was 20 msec before and 440 msec after the stimulus with a digital sampling rate of 0.9 msec. The system bandpass extended from 0.2 to 1 kHz. The responses corresponding to each run of 150 stimuli were averaged. The rest period between runs was 2 min. The following components of SEP were analyzed: P25, N60, P95, N130, P190, N230, P280, and N360.

The mean latency values of the different components were the following (msec ± SE): P25, 24.4 ± 0.3; N60, 61.8 ± 0.9; P95, 96.1 ± 2.2; N130, 127.2 ± 2.5; P190, 186.2 ± 3.0; N230, 234.1 ± 3.8; P280, 282.3 ± 5.2; N360, 364.3 ± 7.0

General Procedure

In every experimental session the general procedure was two runs of 150 evoking stimuli delivered before, during, and after TENS applied at the side ipsilateral to the evoking stimuli and two runs of 150 evoking stimuli delivered during and after TENS applied at the side contralateral to the evoking stimuli. Pain threshold was measured at the beginning of the experimental session (before inducing SEP), immediately before TENS, just before the end of TENS, and 22 min after TENS.

During the first threshold test and the first run of evoking stimuli, the subjects were considered "naive." During the second threshold test and the second run of evoking stimuli, they were considered "habituated."

RESULTS

In naive subjects with pain threshold lower than 1.2 mA (low threshold), habituation induced an increase of the threshold; TENS induced a further increase. In naive subjects with pain threshold higher than 2.0 mA (high threshold), habituation induced a lowering of the threshold; TENS induced a further lowering. In naive subjects with pain threshold ranging from 1.2 to 2.0 mA (middle

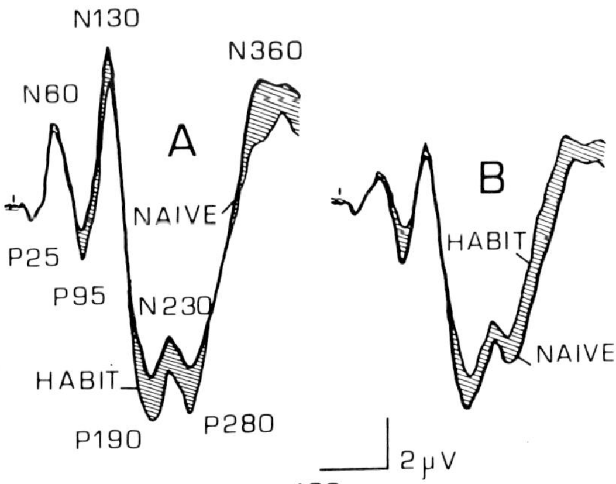

FIG. 1. Somatosensory evoked potentials recorded in naive subjects (first run of stimuli) and during habituation (second run) (HABIT). Two examples are represented. **A:** Subject with low pain threshold (i.e., less than 1.2 mA). **B:** Subject with high pain threshold (i. e., more than 2 mA). The averages of a run of 150 responses are represented.

threshold), neither habituation nor TENS induced any significant change of the threshold. These results are in agreement with our previous studies on sensory threshold changes induced by TENS (3,4,8).

Before TENS, in the subjects with low cutaneous pain threshold, the amplitude of the positive late SEP components (i.e., components with latency longer than 60 msec) was lower, and the amplitude of the negative late components was higher than in the subjects with high pain threshold. Such differences were more evident in "naive" subjects than in habituated subjects. In the subjects with middle threshold, the amplitude of negative and positive SEP components was intermediate (Figs. 1 and 3).

During TENS, the amplitude of positive late SEP components decreased in all subjects, both when TENS was ipsilateral to the evoking stimuli and when TENS was contralateral. The amplitude of negative components was correlated with the pain threshold during TENS (Figs. 2 and 3).

After TENS, the amplitudes of all late components, both positive and negative, changed again in all the subjects. The changes in amplitudes of all of the components correlated to pain threshold after TENS (Fig. 3): in the subjects with low basal pain threshold, the amplitude of the positive components after TENS was greater, and the amplitude of the negative components was smaller than before TENS; in the subjects with high basal pain threshold, the amplitude of the positive components was smaller, and the amplitude of the negative components was greater than before TENS. Consequently, the differences in SEP component amplitudes among the various subjects were smaller than before TENS; i.e., a resetting of SEP component amplitudes was evident.

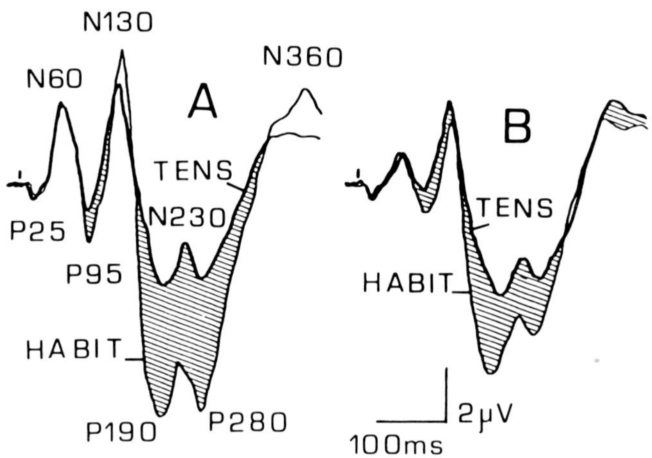

FIG. 2. Somatosensory evoked potentials recorded in habituated subjects (second run of stimuli) and during TENS (second run during TENS). Same subjects as in Fig. 1. The averages of a run of 150 responses are represented. Symbols as in Fig. 1.

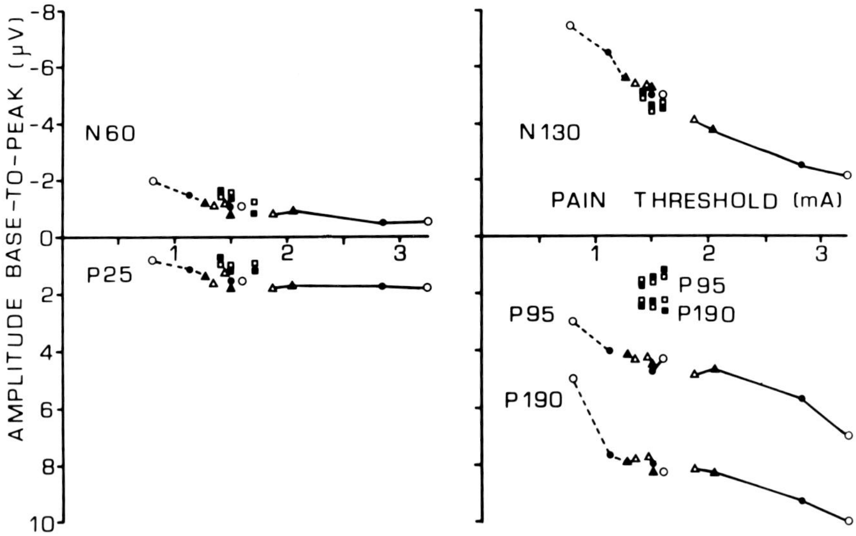

FIG. 3. Relationship between pain threshold and SEP component amplitudes (amplitude base to peak) in different conditions in the three groups of subjects (mean values). ○, naive; ●, habituated ; ■, during TENS, ipsilateral; ▲, after TENS, ipsilateral; □, during TENS, contralateral; △, after TENS, contralateral. The points corresponding to the subjects with low pain threshold (six subjects) are connected by a *broken line;* the points corresponding to the subjects with high pain thresholds (eight subjects) are connected by an *unbroken line;* the points corresponding to the subjects with middle thresholds (five subjects) are not connected.

In Fig. 3, we can observe an inverse relationship between SEP components and pain thresholds determined before and after TENS, significant at test of linear regression for late components (P95 and N130: $p < 0.001$; P190: $p < 0.005$), not significant for early components (P25: $p < 0.2$; P60: $p < 0.1$).

DISCUSSION

The data indicate that: (a) an inverse relationship between cutaneous pain threshold and late SEP components is present in naive subjects, in habituated subjects, and after TENS; and (b) TENS induces changes of the amplitude of late SEP components, and such effects are independent of the site of application of TENS.

It may be deduced that the changes of SEP components induced by TENS result from an action of TENS on general mechanisms that control sensory integration. This action during TENS induces a reduction of the amplitude of the positive components and a reset of the negative components, as illustrated in Fig. 3. After TENS, the amplitudes of all the late components are reset at intermediate values.

REFERENCES

1. Andersson, S. A. (1979): Pain control by sensory stimulation. In: *Advances in Pain Research and Therapy, Vol. 3,* edited by J. J. Bonica, J. C. Liebeskind, and D. G. Albe-Fessard, pp. 569–585. Raven Press, New York.
2. Desmedt, J. E., Robertson, D., Brunko, E., and Debecker, J. (1977): Somatosensory decision tasks in man: Early and late components of the cerebral potentials evoked by stimulation of different fingers in random sequences. *Electroencephalogr. Clin. Neurophysiol.,* 43:404–415.
3. Francini, F., and Maresca, M. (1978): Local and generalized changes of the cutaneous sensory thresholds during transcutaneous electrical stimulation (TES) in healthy subjects and in patients with chronic pain. In: *Pain Abstracts, Vol. 1,* p. 127. International Association for the Study of Pain, Seattle.
4. Francini, F., Procacci, P., Zoppi, M., and Maresca, M. (1978): Mechanisms of action of transcutaneous electrical stimulation (TES) for relief of pain (electroanalgesia). *Neurosci. Lett.* [*Suppl.*], 1:S431.
5. Ivanitsky, A. M., and Strelets, V. B. (1977): Brain evoked potentials and some mechanisms of perception. *Electroencephalogr. Clin. Neurophysiol.,* 43:397–403.
6. Long, D. M., and Hagfors, N. (1975): Electrical stimulation in the nervous system: The current status of electrical stimulation of the nervous system for relief of pain. *Pain,* 1:109–123.
7. Procacci, P., and Maresca, M. (1979): Traitements de la douleur par les stimulations périphériques. In: *La Douleur (Rapports Présentés au XLIIe Congrès Français de Médecine),* pp. 59–70. Masson, Paris.
8. Procacci, P., Zoppi, M., Francini, F., Maresca, M., and Bernardini, U. D. (1979): Variazioni locali e generalizzate delle soglie sensitive cutanee durante stimolazione elettrica transcutanea in soggetti normali e in pazienti con dolore cronico. In: *Il Dolore: Problemi di Fisiopatologia e Terapia,* edited by C. A. Pagni, P. Procacci, and V. Ventafridda, pp. 135–146. Edizioni Cortina, Verona.
9. Procacci, P., Zoppi, M., and Maresca, M. (1975): La terapia delle sindromi dolorose con stimolazione elettrica (elettroanalgesia). *Clin. Ter.,* 73:465–474.
10. Procacci, P., Zoppi, M., Maresca, M., and Francini, F. (1977): Hypoalgesia induced by transcutaneous electrical stimulation. *J. Neurosurg. Sci.,* 21:221–228.
11. White, J. C., and Sweet, W. H. (1969): *Pain and the Neurosurgeon.* Charles C Thomas, Springfield, Illinois.

Clinical Applications of Evoked Potentials in Neurology,
edited by J. Courjon, F. Mauguiere, and M. Revol.
Raven Press, New York © 1982.

Human Pain and Evoked Potentials: Possible Assessment of Headache with Endogenous Brain Potentials Triggered by the R Wave of EKG in Pain Patients

*Andrew C. N. Chen and **Samuel F. Dworkin

*Departments of *Anesthesiology, **Psychiatry and Behavioral Sciences, and **Oral Medicine, University of Washington, School of Medicine, Seattle, Washington 98195*

Accumulated evidence has identified a late component of the evoked potential (EP) occurring on the average 160 to 260 msec after stimulation as a major pain-related EP component (2). Research has confirmed that this N_{160}–P_{260} late component reflects subjective perceptual processes induced by external painful stimulation (1,3). We sought to explore whether or not the N_{160}–P_{260} late component arises endogenously during clinical pain states and to determine if the N_{160}–P_{260} component is a pain-related EP that can arise even without external or artificial stimulation.

To more closely approximate the study of brain activity during a pain state, we chose to explore the clinical state of chronic recurrent headache. Further, we sought to measure the EP during the presence and absence of clinical headache pain without introducing an exogenous, hence perhaps artificial, stimulus into the study of pain-related EP. We replaced the external signal, typically a painful electric shock, with a natural stimulus to trigger the accumulation of averaged EP data. The naturally occurring stimulus we chose was the subject's own heartbeat, specifically, the EKG R wave. Brain activity related to pain triggered by the EKG, already shown to be quantifiable, might, we felt, provide a convenient index for evaluating clinical pain. In this chapter, we present some preliminary observations using the EKG R wave to trigger computerized averaging of brain activity for patients during both headache states and nonheadache states. Again, we hypothesized that naturally triggered EP during headache states might reveal some patterns of endogenous brain activity associated with clinical states of subjective painfulness that were absent in the same individuals when they were clinically pain-free.

METHODS AND PROCEDURES

Subjects

Nine female subjects ranging from 19 to 29 years in age (mean, 25; SD, 3.8) were studied, thus controlling for sex and age variations in brain activity.

Inclusion criteria for "recurrent headache" included a history of periodic headaches extending over at least 4 years.

Sessions

Recordings were made during both headache state (headache session) and nonheadache state (control session). A medical history was taken at the beginning of the first session, and subjects were asked not to use any drugs on days when recordings were obtained.

Subjective Measures

Headache Status

The intensity and aversity of headaches were described using a Visual Pain Analog Scale (0–100 mm), and each subject was asked to rate her headache on a scale of 0 to 10. Only headaches rated greater than 6 out of 10 were studied during a headache session.

Anxiety and Depression Measures

Subjects completed a psychometric battery during control and headache sessions consisting of Speilberger's state and trait anxiety scales and Zung's depression questionnaire.

Electrode Placement and System Configuration

Each subject sat comfortably in a reclining dental chair. Standard EKG leads were attached to the right arm, left arm, and left leg. Electroencephalogram leads in Ag–AgCl disks were affixed to the scalp bilaterally at F_3–P_3 and F_4–P_4 montage. The EEG ground consisted of a linked reference to the mastoid bone. The equipment configuration for recording and integrating EEG data triggered by EKG is illustrated in Fig. 1.

Evoked Potential Recording and Measurement

Each recording session lasted 1 to 1.5 hr. The EEG was amplified (via a Model 278J analog isolation unit), and the signal from the operational amplifier was fed directly into a Nicolet 1072 signal averager. Input range on the Nicolet digitizer (SD-72/4A) was set to a time constant of 20 msec, resulting in an effective bandwidth of 0.2 to 100 Hz. The Nicolet computer of averaged transients was in turn triggered by the QRS complex of the EKG from the subject. A custom-made signal-conditioning module was designed for EKG triggering of stimulus pulses in the Grass S-44 stimulator and was installed in the system

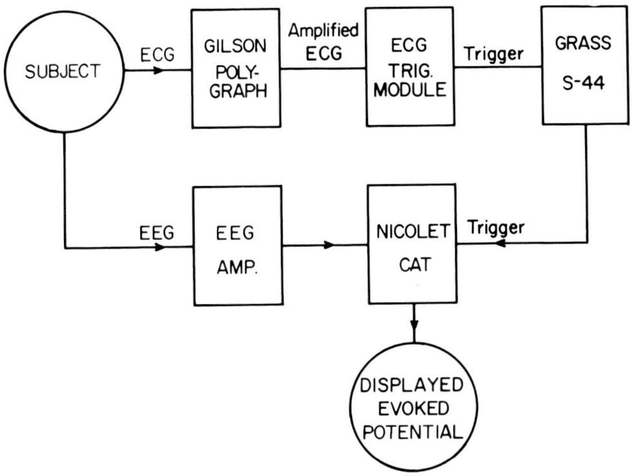

FIG. 1. Schematic representation for EKG R-wave triggering of evoked potentials in the human pain study.

described in Fig. 1. This EKG triggering module consisted of a low-pass filter of 0 to 20 Hz which shaped the QRS complex into a single pulse to trigger the S-44 stimulator.

An overall average of 192 trials of EP was obtained from the sum of three averagings of 64 brain responses to stimulus presentations triggered by the EKG. The stability of the three 64-trial averages was assessed to guard against possible artifacts caused by neck muscle tension, eyeblinks, or ocular rotation. Peak latency and peak-to-peak amplitude were digitized and submitted to analysis in accordance with the 1974 Brussels and 1977 Basel conventions. Evoked potentials were measured first in the left hemisphere (LH) and then the right hemisphere (RH).

Statistical Analysis

A set of planned contrasts was performed, and analysis of repeated measures with mixed design was employed to assess the laterality effect, pain state effect, and laterality–pain state interaction.

RESULTS

Subjects

Nine subjects selected for study report had a range of headache history from 4 to 20 years (mean, 11.2; SD, 6.2). Most are still under a primary physician's care for chronic, recurrent headache. Medications for headache relief were reported to be fair to poor in effectiveness. A few had tried biofeedback or relaxation training, and these results were also equivocal.

Pain Status

Patients reported experiencing headaches once or twice a week. During the headache session, the mean headache rating on the 10-point scale was 7.3. Results from a visual analog scale obtained during the headache session were consistent, indicating an overall mean pain intensity of 70.66 and mean pain aversity of 69.11 out of a possible 100.

Anxiety and Depression

Neither the mean Spielberger trait anxitey nor Zung depression scores changed from control to headache sessions (mean, 38.0 for trait anxiety and 43 for depression, both sessions). However, the state anxiety score showed a significant increase during the headache session compared to the control session (mean, 47.00 versus 36.3, respectively; $t = 4.03$, $p < 0.001$), suggesting that subjects become more anxious while experiencing headache.

Evoked Potentials

Morphology

With averaging techniques used, the EP triggered by the EKG R wave of the subjects did not show consistent morphology across the nine subjects in either control or headache sessions. However, there was relative consistency between left hemisphere (LH) and right hemisphere (RH) under both the control and headache sessions within each subject (see Fig. 2 for a typical subject).

Latencies

Although many negative and positive peaks showed considerable variability in latencies, it is significant to note that all subjects showed a major late component with a negative peak latency at about 160 msec and a positive peak latency at about 240 msec on both LH and RH under both control and headache conditions.

Analysis of variance for the control session and headache session of these N_{160}–P_{240} latencies across LH and RH indicates that there was no laterality effect ($F_{1,8} = 4.91$ for N_{160}; $F_{1,8} = 0.04$ for P_{240}), no pain state effect ($F_{1,8} = 1.73$ for N_{160}; $F_{1,8} = 0.04$ for P_{240}), and no laterality-by-pain-state interaction ($F_{1,8} = 2.28$ for N_{160}; $F_{1,8} = 0.13$ for P_{240}). These results show that the latencies of the late components are relatively stable.

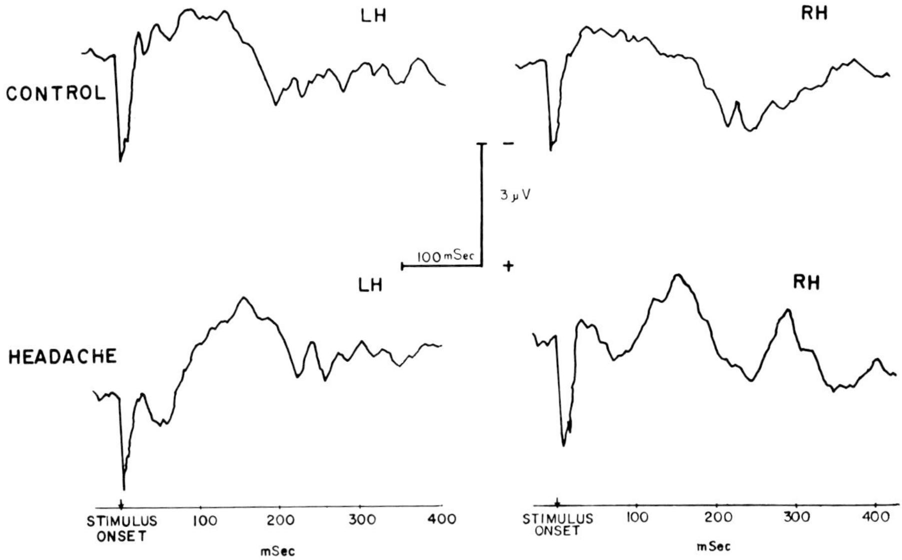

FIG. 2. Examples of endogenous EP in a headache subject.

Amplitudes

The mean peak-to-peak amplitude of the N_{160}–P_{240} component, across all subjects, for both LH and RH, under control and headache conditions is shown in Fig. 3. Analysis of variance indicates that there was a significant laterality-by-pain-state interaction effect ($F_{1,8} = 14.31$; $p < 0.005$), indicating that ampli-

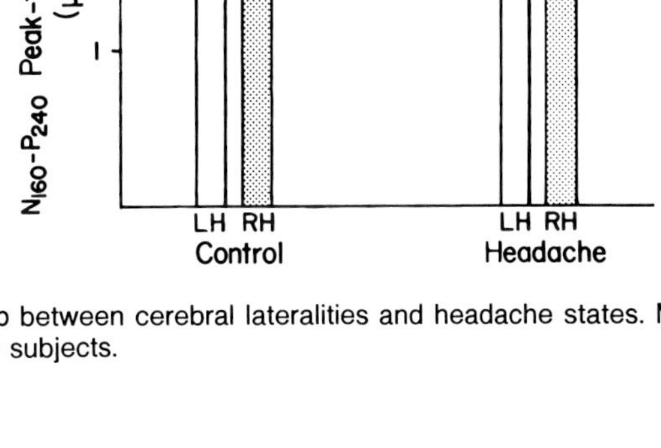

FIG. 3. Relationship between cerebral lateralities and headache states. Mean N_{160}–P_{240} peak amplitudes for nine subjects.

tude of the EP in the RH differed significantly from the LH as a function of pain state during control and headache sessions. This interaction of EP amplitude with the presence or absence of headache is also illustrated in Fig. 3. A Student's *t*-test shows that the amplitude of the N_{160}–P_{240} component in the LH was bigger than the comparable RH component during the control session ($t_{1,8} = 3.36$; $p < 0.01$). However, this EP component in the LH showed no change from the control session to the headache session ($t_{1,8} = 0.09$; $p > 0.75$). In contrast, there was a significant increase in amplitude of RH activity during the headache session ($t_{1,8} = 3.29$; $p < 0.01$), suggesting that there was more endogenous brain activity in the RH during headache states than during nonheadache states.

DISCUSSION

The observation that RH yields significantly larger discharge during headache is consistent with our previous study (4) demonstrating that the RH is associated with the control of pain by hypnosis during surgery. Even so, the relationship between brain laterality and pain remains sketchy and incomplete.

The type of EP studied is obviously distinct from the more conventional exogenously induced EP which is modality specific (e.g., auditory, somatosensory, etc.). In this study, nevertheless, there is a clear and consistent N_{160}–P_{240} component in every subject, in both hemispheres, which varies with control versus headache conditions. Components other than this late major one were also sometimes measurable but showed great variability in terms of their distributions, peak latencies, and waveforms. This may raise issues of reliability and stability of such endogenous brain potentials. Obviously, further analyses of all possible peaks and troughs, using larger sample populations, are required for more valid statistical inference.

This preliminary report focused on the consistent and reliable late major N_{160}–P_{240} component. The latency of this EP component easily falls in the latency range of the major late components associated with EP produced by a painful exogenous stimulus as reported by several pain laboratories around the world (2). The confirmation of this late endogenous EP component as pain related may stimulate new explanations of brain mechanisms for headaches, specifically, and for the clinical neurology of pain, more generally. Three mechanisms are suggested for understanding our observation that an EKG-triggered late EP is larger during headache than nonheadache states: (a) nonspecific differential hyperexcitability of the cortex during headache state; (b) certain pulsating vascular changes associated with heartbeat and headache pain; (c) neurologic events regulating heart rate and associated with headache pain. If the late EP component we observed proves to reflect brain activity unique to pain processes, we may have uncovered an objective measure for the subjective experience of pathologic pain.

ACKNOWLEDGMENTS

This research was supported by NIDR grant DE-05130 from the National Institutes of Health.

REFERENCES

1. Carmon, A., Friedman, Y., Coger, R., and Kenton, B. (1980): Single trial analysis of evoked potentials to noxious thermal stimulation in man. *Pain,* 8:21–32.
2. Chapman, C. R., Chen, A. C. N., and Harkins, S. W. (1979): Brain evoked potentials as correlates of laboratory pain: A review and perspective. In: *Advances in Pain Research and Therapy, Vol. 3,* edited by J. J. Bonica, J. C. Liebeskind, and D. G. Apbe-Fessard, pp. 791–803. Raven Press, New York.
3. Chen, A. C. N., Chapman, C. R., and Harkins, S. W. (1979): Brain evoked potentials are functional correlates of induced pain in man. *Pain,* 6:305–314.
4. Chen, A. C. N., Dworkin, S. F., and Bloomquist, D. S. (1981): Cortical power spectrum analysis of hypnotic pain control in surgery. *Int. J. Neurosci.,* 13:127–36.

Clinical Applications of Evoked Potentials in Neurology,
edited by J. Courjon, F. Mauguiere, and M. Revol.
Raven Press, New York © 1982.

Visual and Somesthetic Potentials in Neurolipidosis

A. M. d'Allest, P. Laget, and J. Raimbault

Laboratoire d'Electroencéphalographie et de Neurophysiologie, Clinique de l'Enfant, Hôpital Trousseau, Paris, 75012, France

In recent years, modifications of the evoked cortical potentials in infantile neurolipidosis have given rise to various publications (1). With regard to the aspects of the visual evoked potentials (VEP) in these encephalopathies, the results described by Harden and Pampiglione are the best known and the most significant (3–5).

However, few data are encountered on the progressive evolution of these electrophysiological events or on comparison between evoked potentials of various origins (somesthetic and visual potentials, for instance).

We report here the results obtained in 28 cases of neurolipidosis clearly established by the biochemical, neurohistological, and clinical signs and evolution and on one case in which the clinical and electrophysiological symptoms strongly suggested the diagnosis of Jansky–Bielchovsky disease but without histochemical probes at the time when the recordings were performed.

These observations concern six cases of Tay-Sachs' gangliosidosis, eight cases of sphingomyelinosis (Nieman–Pick disease), and 15 cases of neuronal ceroid lipofuscinosis.

The eight cases of sphingomyelinosis included the four forms described in children (2). We examined two precocious A forms (acute neuropathic form with precocious clinical signs and drastic involvement of the nervous system), one C form (subacute or juvenile form), one D form (Nova Scotia variant with important but belated nervous manifestations), and four B forms (hepatosplenomegalic form with sphingomyelin storage but without nervous involvement).

In our series of neuronal ceroid lipofuscinosis, we recorded one case of the precocious form (Santavuori–Hagberg disease), 10 cases of the infantile form (Bielchovsky–Hagberg disease), and four cases of the juvenile form (Spielmeyer–Vogt disease).

METHODS

The VEP and ERG were recorded in all patients, and the SEP in nine patients.

VEP and ERG Recording

An electrode was placed on each occipital scalp at 2 cm from the midline, and the VEP was derived between each occipital electrode and a frontal or sometimes earlobe reference electrode in order to avoid the artifact caused by eye blinking.

The stimulus was a conventional blue–white flash of 20-μsec duration and an energy of 0.3 joule. The flash lamp was set in front of the subject's eye at a distance of 20 cm. The stimulus frequency was 1/sec. A hundred flashes were used for each recording. The amplifying device had a band-pass from 0.5 to 1,000 Hz. After appropriate amplification, the cortical signals were fed into a computer of average transients (Tracor 1700), and the VEP transcribed on an X–Y plotter. Each response was recorded for 620 msec after the onset of the stimulus.

The ERG was derived between a contact lens electrode and a reference electrode put on the frontal midline. The stimulating, amplifying, and recording devices were the same as in the case of the VEP, but 50 flashes were used at the frequency of 1/sec.

SEP Recording

Eight electrodes were placed on the scalp, four over each hemisphere, in a line starting just above the ear and running up and backwards to overlie the postcentral parietal convolution. Their placement was considered to be optimal when the early positive surface main deflection was high and its morphology steady, in accordance with our previous experience with normal patients in the same age groups. The responses were derived between each of the four electrodes on a hemisphere and a reference electrode put on the frontal skull of the opposite side. The contralateral median nerve was stimulated at the wrist. We used electric rectangular pulses of 0.5 msec duration, and the intensity of stimulation was just strong enough to produce a slight contraction of the thenar muscles, for it was impossible to use subjective threshold appreciation in deeply mentally deficient patients.

Each evoked potential was produced by the summation of the effects of 100 repeated stimuli at the frequency of 1/sec. The responses of both hemispheres were always recorded and compared.

The amplifying and recording devices were the same as in the case of the VEP. During the VEP and SEP recordings, the spontaneous cortical activity was observed in order to verify the level of consciousness of the patient and the importance of the alterations. All recordings were made in awake children with open eyes. Prior to our examinations, routine EEG recordings had been performed in all patients, but except for some cases, the results will not be systematically reported here.

RESULTS

Tay–Sachs' Disease

In the six cases of Tay–Sachs' disease, various results were observed. In all cases, the VEP were modified, but the importance and the type of the alterations were different from one to another patient. In two children, the VEP had nearly disappeared, and in three, the responses were present. Their peak-to-peak amplitude was in the range of the normal, but the morphology was grossly abnormal, and various deflections had disappeared. In one case, the VEP did not exhibit significant modifications.

Alterations of ERG were present in three cases, and no correlation was found between alterations of the retinal and cortical activity.

This conservation of ERG in Tay–Sachs' gangliosidosis has been already observed, but it does not appear to be as constant as it has been reported by some authors (3).

Nieman–Pick's Disease

In the A form, the modifications of the evoked potentials were important and rapid.

In this respect, the case of the child El. G.N. . . . was representative. Because, in her family, a first child had died from Nieman–Pick's disease, diagnosis in N. . . . was precocious. The girl was born at term and without complication. At 3½ months of age, important splenohepatomegaly was observed. Two weeks later, a myelogram showed a significant increase in sphingomyelin and a marked decrease in sphingomyelinase. The psychomotor development was very poor, and the eye fundus showed typical alterations: grayish decoloration and reddish aspect of the macula.

The evolution of the neurophysiological signs paralleled the course of the illness (Fig. 1).

Three VEP and ERG (at 4, 8, and 11 months of age) and two SEP (at 5 and 8 months of age) were recorded. The amplitude of the first VEP was in the range of normal, and its morphology and its maturation were not very disturbed, but the ERG was strongly assymetrical, and the response of the left eye was smaller than the ERG of the right eye.

The second and third VEP showed a progressive decrease in amplitude and simplification. Similarly, the amplitude of the ERG diminished.

The SEP were asymmetrical, and their latency was longer (26 msec) than that of a normal subject of the same age (20 ± 1.2 msec). However, a certain degree of maturation could be observed in the second SEP.

In the D form (Nova Scotia variant), the results were rather similar, but the evolution was belated. In the only patient of this sort, two VEP, ERG, and SEP were recorded at 3½ months and 3 years, 5 months of age. The

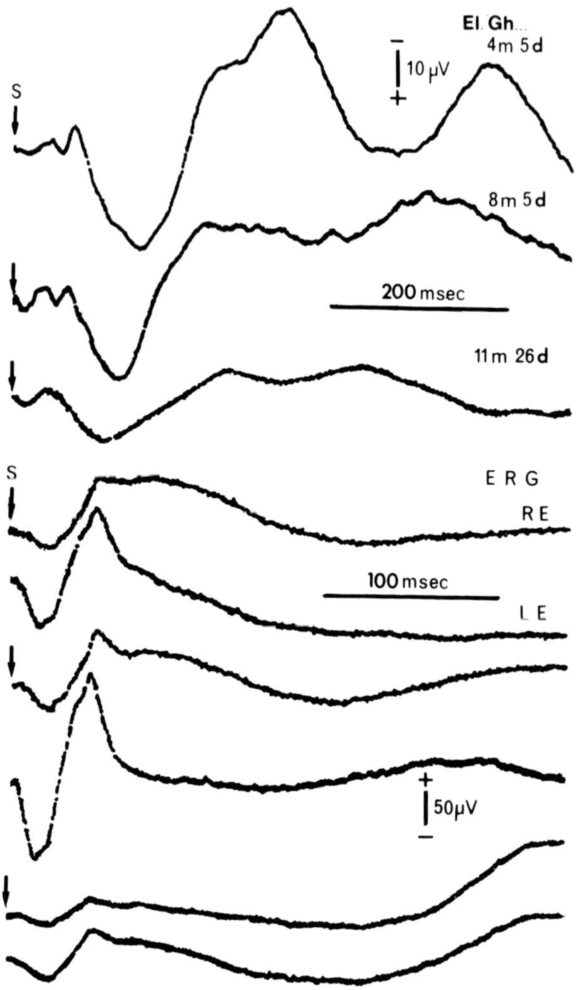

FIG. 1. Evolution of the VER and ERG in a girl suffering from Nieman–Pick disease (form A). The first, second, and third *traces* show the progressive alterations, simplification, and decrease of the VER. The first ERG is asymmetrical, and the response of the right eye is alterated. The third has nearly disappeared. Note the persistent asymmetry.

first VEP and SEP were normal, but the ERG exhibited a low amplitude and lengthening of the latency peak of the "b" wave. The second VER was deeply abnormal. Intermediary deflections had disappeared and were replaced by a late positive deflection. The ERG remained abnormal, but no evolution was observed. The second SEP exhibited alterations and marked asymmetry.

The results were comparable in the case of the C form.

In the B form, some discrete and nonspecific modifications of the VEP were observed, but the ERG were normal.

Neuronal Ceroid Lipofuscinosis

In the only case of Santavuori–Hagbert disease, our results are similar to other cases described by the authors (10,11), and in this 2-year, 11-month-old child, VER, ERG, and SEP had fully disappeared.

In the infantile form, our results were in good agreement with those of the authors, but complementary data could be cited.

VER

In all but one case of Jansky–Bielchovsky (J.B.) disease with obvious clinical signs and typical histological and histochemical aspects, VER exhibited characteristic features. The most conspicuous sign consisted in the presence of a very large positive surface deflection with latency to peak between 42 and 108 msec (see Table 1). This wave was followed by two to four intermediary deflections and a constant late negative deflection. In four cases, the first positive component was preceded by a feeble early negative wave.

The peak-to-peak amplitudes were always greatly increased (eight to ten times) compared to the mean amplitude in normal subjects of the same age.

ERG

In all patients, ERG were present but deeply altered. The main pathological features were an important decrease of amplitude (six cases), an increase of latency (seven cases), and a polyphasicity of the "b" wave (eight cases).

SEP

In three children, SEP were recorded on both hemispheres. They exhibited normal morphology, latency, and symmetry, but the voltage peak to peak was

TABLE 1. *Latencies to peak of the successive VEP deflections in 10 patients suffering from Jansky–Bielchovsky disease*

Subjects		Latency to peak of the successive deflections (msec)						
Name	Age	N	P	N	P	N	P	N
BE . . . M.F.	5 y	32	43	72	108	236		
CA . . . A	4 y 4 m		60	90	135			
CO . . . S.	3 y 10 m		42	50	56	80	130	
GE . . . L.	5 y 2 m		56	66	82	250		
GE . . . P.	3 y 4 m		70	110	160	280		
LA . . . A.	5 y 1 m	34	60	84	140	300		
MA . . . D.	4 y 10 m	42	54	66	72	90	130	
DU . . . A.	5 y 8 m		90	110	146	280		
VI . . . F.	4 y 7 m		108	120	140	184		
BE . . . M.	7 y 10 m	51	61	64	73	91	121	305

drastically increased (about eight times in relation to the SEP of the normal children of the same age and obtained with identical parameters of stimulation and recording).

Evolution

In one patient, it was possible to follow the evolution of VER when the first clinical signs appeared from the age of 3 years up to the age of 9½ years (5 months before death). Four recordings of VER and ERG were performed (at 3 y 2 m, 5 y 11 m, 8 y 3 m, and 9 y 6 m). The first showed VER and ERG near normal. In the third, the characteristic alterations of the state period were present. The SEP as early as 5 years, 1 month of age were symmetrical, normal in morphology and latency, but already exhibited an important increase of amplitude (about eight times in relation to the normal) (Fig. 2).

Juvenile Form (Spielmeyer–Vogt Disease)

Four children suffering from Spielmeyer–Vogt disease could be studied. All cases showed very deep alterations of the VEP and ERG, but the modifications were different from the infantile form and much less specific.

In siblings (a boy and a girl, respectively, 6 y 9 m and 9 y 11 m old), the morphology of the VEP was strongly altered (especially in the girl), but their amplitude was near normal. In contrast to the presence of the cortical responses, the ERG was completely extinguished.

In the third case (11 y 5 m old boy), the alterations of the VEP were very significant, but ERG was present, the "a" wave was normal, and the "b" wave showed a marked decrease (amplitude about half of normal).

In the fourth child, it was possible to follow the patient for 3 years. In the first recording (boy aged 10 years), the VEP was already very deeply altered, and ERG had completely disappeared (Fig. 3).

In two other recordings (at 11 and 13 years of age), VEP had vanished and were replaced by aleatory deflections without physiological significance.

DISCUSSION

Our results concerning evoked potentials in neurolipidosis generally fit those of other publications (1,3).

In Tay–Sachs illness, the alterations of the VEP are variable and have no morphologic specificity. It is the same for ERG, and its modifications are not firmly correlated with those of cortical responses. We can remark that a similar variability has been observed in the EEG (6).

In the Nieman–Pick disease, alterations of the evoked potentials and ERG are always observed in the forms in which the nervous involvement is important but failed in the B form. This good parallelism between the electrophysiological

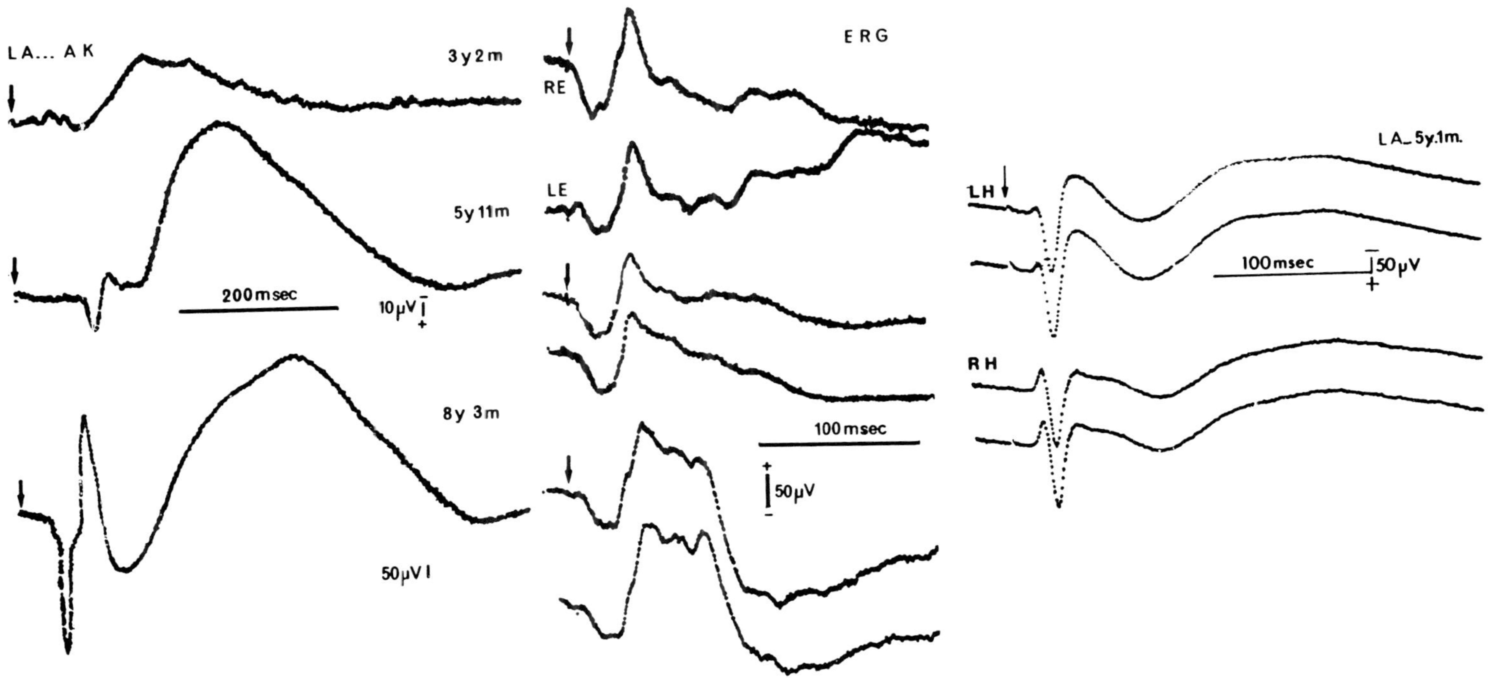

FIG. 2. Left column: Evolution of the VEP in a boy suffering from Jansky–Bielchovsky disease. The first response is near normal. In the *third recording,* a typical aspect is observed: simplification and high amplitude. **Middle column:** Progressive alterations of the ERG. In the *third recording* a significant lengthening and increase of the "b" wave is observed. **Right column:** SEP in the same child. Observe the normal morphology and latency but the significant increase of amplitude.

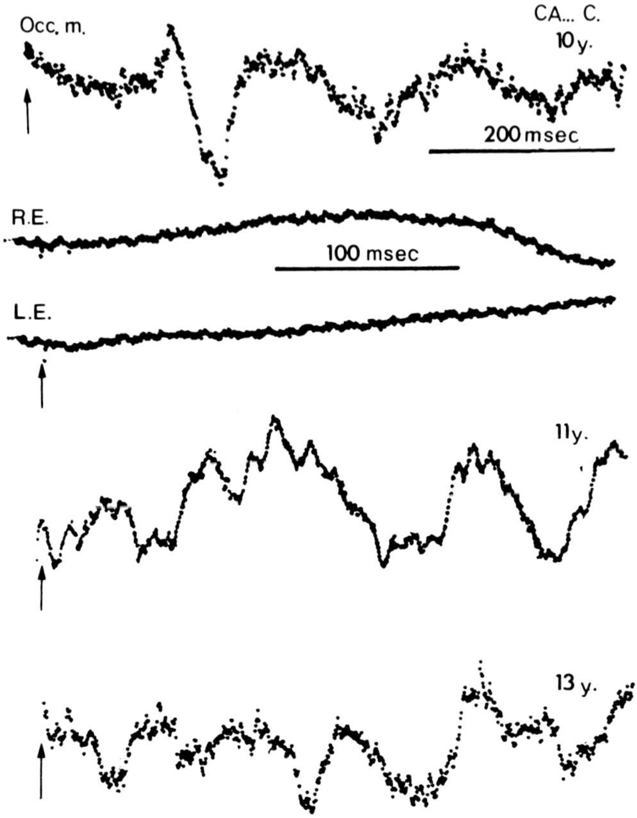

FIG. 3. Evolution of the VEP in a boy suffering from Spielmeyer–Vogt disease. In the *first recording* the occipital response is reduced to a late and atypical potential, and ERG has disappeared. In the *second* and *third recordings,* it is no longer possible to clearly identify the VEP.

and clinical signs is also encountered in the evolution of the illness. In addition, in this neurolipidosis, the latencies of the SEP are increased, and this phenomenon, which reflects a slowing of the condution velocities in the peripheral and central pathways, does not appear in the other neurolipidoses that we reported here.

The findings on the neurolipofuscinosis deserve further consideration. The most obvious feature is the very characteristic alterations of the VEP in the J.B. disease. We have reported that in nine out of 10 cases a very conspicuous positive wave is present. It is probable that it could result from different positive deflections of the normal response, for the latencies to peak are different in the various patients, and, on the whole, the visual evoked potentials have a less simplified morphology than appears on superficial examination (Table 1). It is possible that the simplification of the response would be correlated with the duration of the evolution.

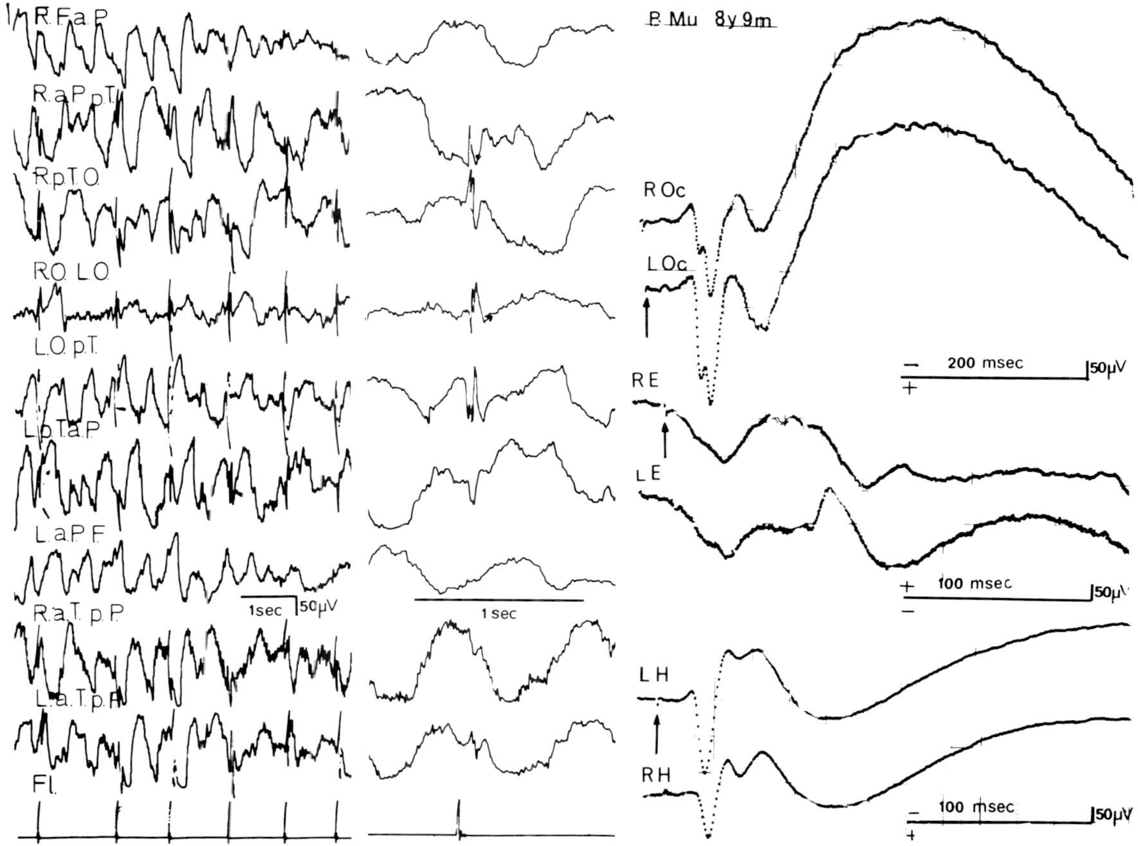

FIG. 4. In **a** and **b:** EEG of an 8-year, 9-month-old boy exhibiting all clinical and electrophysiological signs of Jansky–Bielchovsky disease although the histological evidence had not been available at the time of the recordings. In the **b** column, it is possible to observe that the paroxysms (see the *fourth trace*) are more or less distorted VEP. In **c:** VEP, ERG, and SEP showing characteristic alterations. Abreviations of the leads: R.F.a.P., right frontal–anterior parietal; R.a.P.p.T., right anterior parietal–posterior temporal; R.p.T.O., right posterior temporal–occipital; R.O.L.O., right occipital–left occipital; L.p.T.a.P., left posterior temporal–anterior parietal; L.a.P.F., left anterior parietal–frontal; R.a.T.p.P., right anterior temporal–posterior parietal; L.a.T.p.P., left anterior temporal–posterior parietal.

A very important voltage increase but without morphologic simplification is also observed in the SEP, but this feature does not seem to concern the auditory evoked cortical potentials (AEP). Indeed, in one patient with obvious clinical and electrical signs of J.B. disease but before the anatomopathological evidence could be brought, cortical AEP were performed and did not exhibit noticeable alterations.

This discrepancy between the evoked potentials relating to different sensory systems would justify complementary studies and recordings in more numerous cases of J.B. disease.

Another remark concerns the relation existing between the features of VEP in this illness and the EEG alterations already described by various authors (5) and produced by intermittent light stimulation (ILS) of low frequency. In three patients showing typical VEP and characteristic electroencephalographic responses by ILS, a careful observation of the tracings showed that the apparent spike waves synchronously produced by the flashes were, in fact, VEP, the morphology of which and especially the rapid and high positive deflection were disturbed by the pass band of the amplifying devices used in routine EEG (Fig. 4). Furthermore, in three patients with massive alterations of the EEG, this response produced by ILS was not clearly observed although the VEP exhibited characteristic morphology.

We do not have at present a valuable hypothesis or precise physiopathological theories to explain the special aspects of the evoked potentials in the infantile form of the lipofuscinosis. Indeed, if distinctive alterations of the neurons (meganeurites and deep modifications of the dendritic trees and synaptic locations) have been described in GM2 gangliosidosis in animals and in Tay–Sachs disease in man (7,8), up to now these typical aspects have not been encountered in ceroid lipofuscinosis (9). Moreover, it appears that in this group, considered by some authors as a single disease entity with a variety of clinical expression (12), the neurophysiological findings show that each form exhibits a very distinct pattern of evolution. Even the disappearance of ERG claimed by Harden and Pampiglione as a common feature is available only in a certain phase of evolution, and in J.B. disease, this phase is preceded by alterations (polyphasicity) that are not encountered in two other forms and that give them a complementary special aspect to this type of nervous disorder.

REFERENCES

1. Aicardi, J., Plouin, P., and Goutieres, F. (1978): Les céroïdes-lipofuscinoses. *Rev. Electrencephalogr. Neurophysiol., Clin.,* 8:149–160.
2. Fredrickson, D. S., and Sloan, H. R. (1972): Sphingomyelin lipidoses: Nieman–Pick disease. In: *The Metabolic Basis of Inherited Disease,* edited by J. B. Stanbury, J. B. Wyngxarden, and D. S. Fredrickson, pp. 783–807. McGraw Hill, New York.
3. Harden, A., and Pampiglione, G. (1977): Visual evoked potential, electroretinogram and electroencephalogram studies in progressive neurometabolic "storage" diseases of childhood. In: *Visual Evoked Potentials in Man. New Developments,* edited by J. E. Desmedt, pp. 470–480. Clarendon Press, Oxford.

4. Harden, A., Pampiglione, G., and Picton-Robertson, N. (1973): Electroretinogram and visual evoked responses in a form of "neuronal lipidosis" with diagnostic E.E.G. features. *J. Neurol. Neurosurg. Psychiatry,* 36:68–74.
5. Pampiglione, G., and Harden, A. (1974): An infantile form of neuronal "storage" disease with characteristic evolution of neurophysiological features. *Brain,* 97:355–360.
6. Pampiglione, G., Privett, G., and Harden, A. (1974): Tay–Sachs' disease: neurophysiological studies in 20 children. *Dev. Med. Child. Neurol.,* 16:201–208.
7. Purpura, D. P., and Baker, H. J. (1978): Meganeurites and other aberrant processes of neurons in feline G M_1-gangliosidosis: A Golgi study. *Brain Res.,* 143:13–26.
8. Purpura, D. P., Pappas, G. D., and Baker, H. J. (1978): Fine structure of meganeurites and secondary growth processes in feline G M_1-gangliosidosis. *Brain Res.,* 143:1–12.
9. Purpura, D. P., and Suzuki, K. (1976): Distortion of neuronal geometry and formation of aberrant synapses in neuronal storage disease. *Brain Res.,* 116:1–21.
10. Santavuori, P. (1973): E.E.G. in the infantile type of so-called neuronal ceroid lipofuscinosis. *Neuropaediatrie,* 4:375–387.
11. Santavuori, P., Haltia, M., Rapola, J., and Raita, C. (1973): Infantile type of so-called neuronal ceroid lipofuscinosis. Part I. Clinical study of 15 patients. *J. Neurol. Sci.,* 18:257–267.
12. Zeman, W., and Dyken, P. (1969): Neuronal ceroid-lipofuscinosis (Batten's disease). Relationships to amaurotic familial idiocy. *Pediatrics,* 44:570–583.

Clinical Applications of Evoked Potentials in Neurology,
edited by J. Courjon, F. Mauguiere, and M. Revol.
Raven Press, New York © 1982.

Multimodality Evoked Responses in Leukodystrophies

*O. N. Markand, *W. E. DeMyer, **R. M. Worth, and *C. Warren

**Department of Neurology and **Division of Neurosurgery, Indiana University School of Medicine, Indianapolis, Indiana 46223*

Recent advances in the recording of somatosensory, brainstem auditory, and visual evoked responses provide relatively noninvasive techniques for the evaluation of different afferent pathways from the periphery to the cerebral cortex. We recently reported dramatic changes in the brainstem auditory evoked potentials (BAEP) in leukodystrophies (5) and found that correlation of the findings of EEG and BAEPs is very helpful in differentiating progressive white matter diseases of childhood from progressive gray matter disorders (4). In this chapter, we extend our studies on more patients with leukodystrophy and report abnormalities seen also with the somatosensory and visual evoked potentials (SEP and VEP).

MATERIALS AND METHODS

Fifteen patients with leukodystrophies were subgrouped as follows: Pelizaeus–Merzbacher disease (PMD), 10; adrenoleukodystrophy (ALD), 3; and metachromatic leukodystrophy (MLD), 2.

Patients with PMD belonged to four different families. In three families, more than one sib was affected, and the disorder was transmitted as a sex-linked recessive trait. Only one patient, a 2½-year-old male, the only child of his parents, had no history of affected males in the same or previous generation. This patient had characteristic clinical features of PMD, consisting of nystagmoid eye movements noted from early infancy, progressive spastic quadriparesis, entire lack of speech, and requirement for total care. In the second family, there were two brothers aged 38 and 34 years, respectively. Two of their sisters were carriers of the abnormal gene, and each had one affected male child, 10 and 8 years old. The disease had a slower course in this family, but all showed rotary nystagmus from birth, poor head control, and hypotonia in infancy and subsequently developed spastic paralysis with limb contractures. All of them had significant intellectual deficits. In the third family, there were two brothers aged 3½ years and 7 years. Their mother's sister had an affected child, a 6-year-old male. In the remaining family, two male sibs who were 12 years and 16 years old had PMD. Patients belonging to the last two families had very severe disease. All showed quadriplegia, rotary nystagmus, entire lack of speech and mental functions.

In the two patients with MLD, the diagnosis was established by the absence of aryl-sulfatase-A in the urine. Progressive psychomotor decline from late infancy resulted in a severe hypotonic quadriplegia, absence of muscle stretch reflexes, and bilateral Babinski signs.

All patients diagnosed as ALD had evidence of decreased adrenal cortical function by decreased blood levels of cortisol and decreased responsiveness to ACTH stimulation. Of the three patients, two were brothers (13 and 7 years old) and the other (13 yeard old) was an isolated patient from a different family. Of the two brothers, the older was more severely affected, had increased skin pigmentation, unresponsiveness, and spastic quadriplegia. His younger brother had a milder disorder characterized by skin pigmentation, behavior problems, and mild intellectual impairment, but no long-tract signs. The third patient had progressive intellectual deficit, behavior disorder, bilateral pyramidal signs, and widespread translucencies of the subcortical white matter in his CT scan.

Brainstem auditory evoked potentials were obtained in response to clicks of 100 μsec delivered monoaurally at a rate of 10/sec. An intensity of 70 dB above the hearing threshold was used. When hearing threshold could not be determined, clicks of 80 to 103 dB were employed; the higher intensities were used if the responses were poorly delineated. For right monoaural stimulation, the recording was obtained between the right ear (A_2) and the vertex (C_Z) electrodes, with the left ear electrode (A_1) used as a ground electrode. The A_1 and C_Z derivation was used for the left ear stimulation, with A_2 serving as a ground electrode. Evoked responses of 2,000 to 4,000 click stimuli were summated, and at least two trials for each ear were made. The frequency response of the system was 300 to 3,000 Hz (−3 dB), and the analysis time was 12 msec following the stimulus.

Visual evoked potentials with pattern reversal and flash stimuli were recorded from the midoccipital electrode (5 cm above the inion) connected to the midfrontal electrode (F_Z). For pattern reversal VEPs, a black–white checkerboard pattern on a TV screen reversing every 0.5 sec was employed at 1 m from the patient's eyes. For flash-induced VEPs, medium- or high-intensity flashes (setting 4 or 16 on the Grass Model PS-2) were delivered at 2/sec from a stroboscope placed 30 cm in front of the eyes. Monocular stimulation was carried out, and the other eye was covered with a black eye patch. In patients where no VEP could be obtained, both eyes were simultaneously exposed to flashes. Analysis time of 250 msec was used, and responses of 200 to 500 stimuli were summated. The frequency response of the recording apparatus was 1 to 100 Hz (−3 dB).

Short-latency SEPs were obtained in response to stimulation of the median nerves at the wrist and/or elbows. Recordings were obtained from the electrodes placed at the ipsilateral Erb's point and the contralateral parietal area (2 cm behind C_3 or C_4 of the International 10–20 System). In some patients, additional recordings were also obtained from the midline electrode placed over the second cervical spine. A midfrontal electrode (F_Z) was used as the reference. Stimulation was carried out with square-wave pulses 100 to 200 μsec in duration and of intensity sufficient to produce nonpainful twitch of the thenar muscles. Responses of 200 to 500 stimuli delivered at 5/sec were summated, and at least two trials were obtained for each median nerve. The frequency response of the recording apparatus was 1 to 3,000 Hz (−3 dB), and the analysis time was 35 msec. In patients who showed no consistent early components over the scalp, long-latency SEPs were attempted by stimulating the median nerves with electrical pulses of 2/sec and increasing the analysis time to 250 msec. In some patients, long-latency SEPs from the scalp were similarly recorded following stimulation of the posterior tibial nerves at the ankle. The recording electrode for the posterior tibial study was placed 2 cm behind C_Z, and F_Z was used as a reference.

The evoked responses were considered abnormal if one or more major components were absent or if the latencies of the major peaks were delayed over two standard deviations (SD) from the mean. In the case of BAEP, I–III, III–V, and I–V intervals correlate better with conduction along the auditory pathways through the brainstem than do the absolute latencies of individual peaks. For short-latency SEPs (median), the intervals between the peak of the Erb's potential (N_{10}) and the two scalp peaks (N_{19} and P_{22}) provide a measure of central somatosensory conduction (cervical cord to cortex). These intervals were considered prolonged if they were longer than 2 SD beyond the mean. For the pattern reversal VEP, the latency of P_{100} and for the flash VEP, the latency of the major positivity (which we designate wave 4) were evaluated.

RESULTS

Brainstem Auditory Evoked Potentials

All of the major components of the BAEPs were well delineated in only two patients who had a milder form of ALD. The BAEPs were, however, abnormal in both, showing an increased I–III interval in one and III–V interval in the other.

The remaining 13 patients showed gross abnormalities of the BAEPs because of an entire absence of the wave III and IV/V complex which normally are the most prominent of the BAEP components. In four patients (three PMD, one MLD) only wave I was recorded, and all subsequent components were entirely absent, except in one where a markedly attenuative wave V may have been present at a severely prolonged latency. In six patients (four PMD, one ALD, and one MLD), a low-amplitude and inconsistent wave II followed a well-delineated wave I. In the remaining three patients (all with PMD), both waves I and II were well delineated, but subsequent components were entirely absent (Fig. 1).

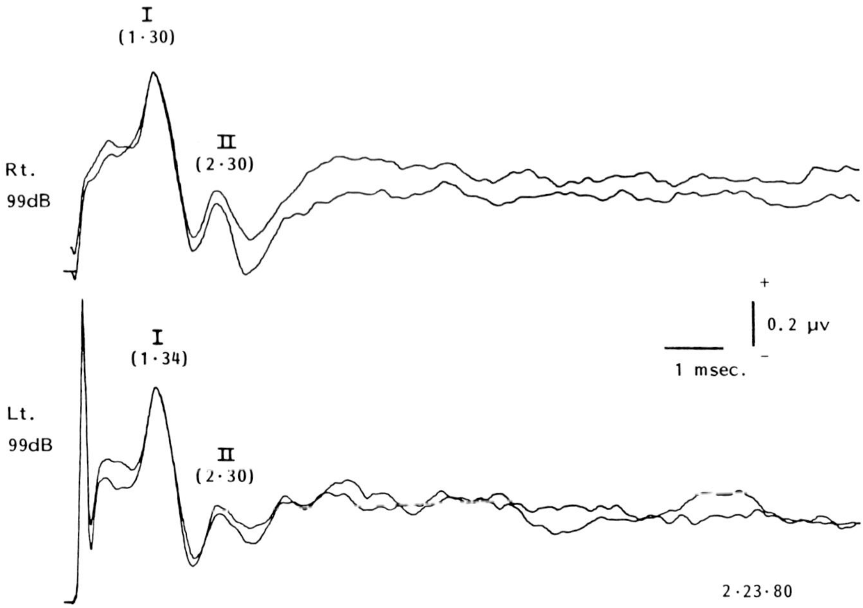

FIG. 1. Brainstem auditory evoked potentials of a 10-year-old patient with PMD showing waves I and II of normal latencies. All subsequent components are entirely absent. Values in brackets are latencies (msec).

Wave I, which was recorded in all patients, was of normal latency in eight. Both patients with MLD had severe prolongation of the latency of wave I. Four patients of PMD and one of ALD also had slight delays in the latency of wave 1.

Visual Evoked Potentials

Pattern Reversal

Of the seven older patients who could cooperate for adequate study, only one patient (mild ALD) had a normal pattern reversal VEP. In four patients (all with PMD), no VEP could be recorded with pattern reversal stimuli. In one patient with PMD, the pattern reversal VEP was absent on left-sided stimulation. Right monocular stimulation resulted in a consistent response, but P_{100} was markedly delayed. In the remaining patient (PMD), consistent pattern reversal VEPs were recorded both with right and left monocular stimulation, but the VEPs were abnormal because of prolongation of the latency of P_{100}.

Flash

These were attempted in 13 of the 15 patients. The VEP was entirely normal in only one patient, again the patient in the early stage of ALD. In two patients (one each of PMD and MLD), consistent VEPs could not be recorded in response to flash stimuli. In one additional patient (PMD), a low-amplitude VEP was recorded only when simultaneous binocular stimulation was carried out, and the major positivity (wave 4) was markedly delayed. In the remaining nine patients (seven PMD, one ALD, one MLD), the flash VEPs were well delineated both with right and left monocular stimulation, but the wave 4 was prolonged (Fig. 2). In all of these patients, the latency of the major positivity was symmetrical for the two eyes, varying 6 msec or less between the VEPs obtained from right and left monocular stimulation.

Somatosensory Evoked Potentials

Short-latency SEPs following left- and right-sided stimulation of the median nerves were obtained from the ipsilateral Erb's point and contralateral parietal area in 12 patients and following stimulation only of the left median nerve in two additional patients. A well-defined Erb's potential (N_{10}) at a normal latency was recorded in 12 patients (nine PMD, three ALD). Although well defined, this potential was significantly delayed in one patient with MLD. In the remaining patient who had severe MLD and with whom only left-sided stimulation was carried out, a consistent potential was recorded neither at the Erb's point nor over the right parietal region. In the 13 patients in whom a well-defined N_{10} could be obtained, so that it was certain that an adequate volley of stimuli did enter the central nervous system (CNS), the contralateral parietal response

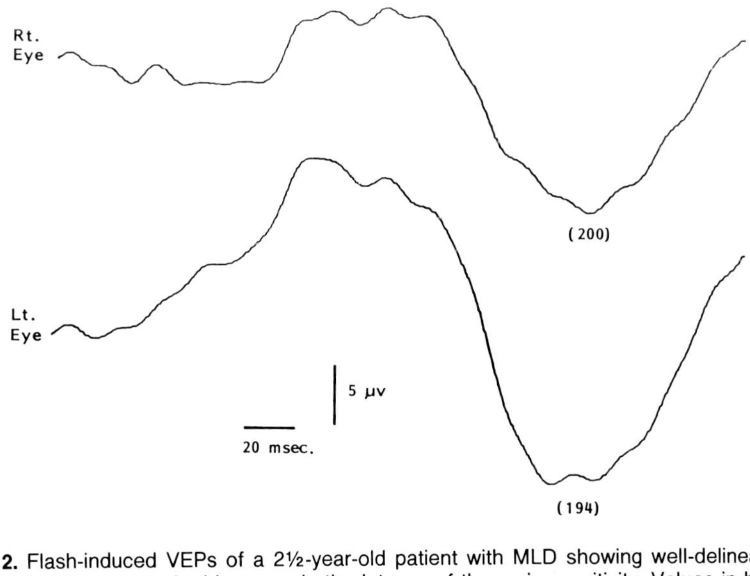

FIG. 2. Flash-induced VEPs of a 2½-year-old patient with MLD showing well-delineated responses but with a marked increase in the latency of the major positivity. Values in brackets are latencies (msec).

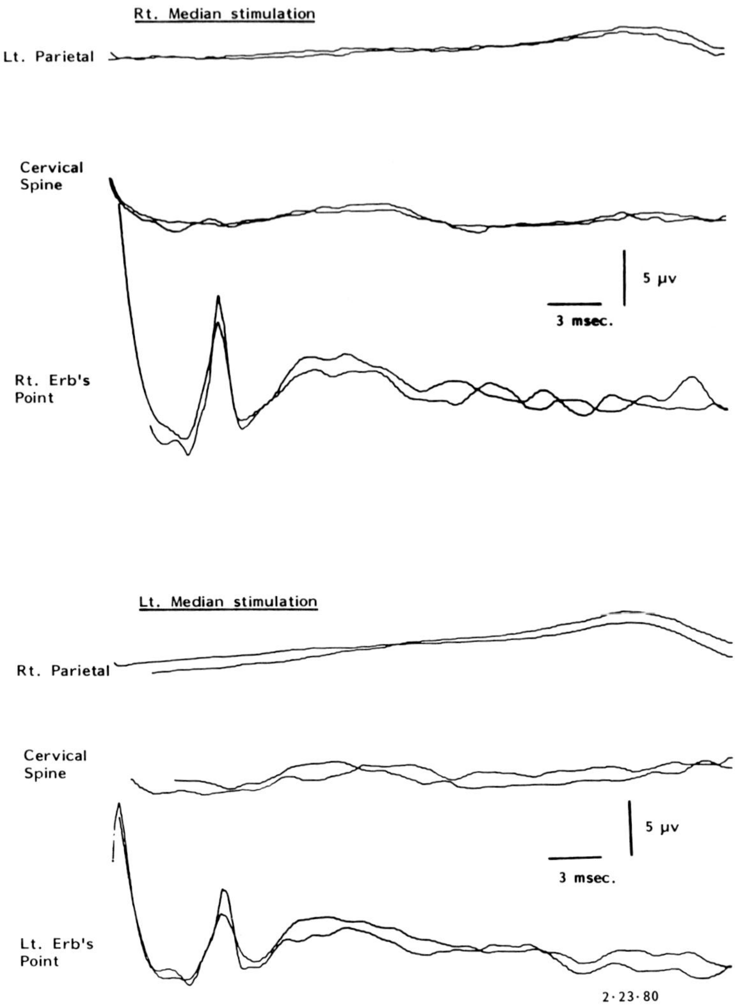

FIG. 3. Median nerve SEPs of a 10-year-old patient with PMD showing well-defined Erb's potential but entirely absent cervical (N_{14}) and early scalp potentials (N_{19} and P_{22}).

was abnormal in all. In nine (eight PMD, one MLD), early components (N_{19} and P_{22}) over the scalp were not recorded (Fig. 3), whereas in four (one PMD, three ALD), although N_{19} and P_{22} were recorded, one or both of these components were prolonged in latency and so also the N_{10}–N_{19} and N_{10}–P_{22} intervals. Of the eight patients who had recordings from cervical spine, five (PMD) had no identifiable cervical potential (N_{14}), and the remaining three (ALD) had normal N_{14}.

Seven of the nine patients who did not show short-latency scalp components had long-latency components recorded with median nerve stimulation. Three showed no responses at all. In the remaining four, long-latency SEPs were identified, but these were low in amplitude, poorly delineated, and showed prolongation of the latencies of different components. Only in six patients were SEPs attempted with posterior tibial stimulation. These were abnormal in all. In three patients (two PMD, one ALD), no identifiable scalp response could be recorded. In two (one PMD and one ALD), the initial positive peak (P_{40}) was prolonged in latency, whereas in the remaining patient (ALD), although the P_{40} was normal, the subsequent peaks (N_{50}, P_{60}) were significantly delayed in latency.

DISCUSSION

Leukodystrophies are genetically determined disorders characterized by abnormal synthesis or degradation of myelin with resultant widespread demyelination. Lesions are extensive in subcortical white matter, but subsequently, brainstem and spinal cord become progressively involved. The peripheral nervous system is affected only in MLD, whereas in PMD and ALD the demyelination is essentially confined to the CNS.

Demyelination involving several afferent systems in the CNS was apparently responsible for the severe alterations of the evoked responses seen in this series on leukodystrophy. All three evoked responses studied by us were abnormal in all patients except a normal VEP seen in the patient with early ALD. In most patients, wave I with or without a wave II were the only elements of the BAEP that remained; wave III and the IV/V complex, which are the most consistent components in normal subjects, were entirely absent. The effects of focal brainstem lesions in both animals and man (1,7,8) suggest that wave I of the BAEP originates from eighth nerve, wave II from the region of the cochlear nucleus, wave III from the region of the superior olive and trapezoid body, and waves IV and V from the midbrain. The severe abnormalities of BAEPs observed in our patients probably reflect severe demyelination of the ponto-mesencephalic regions of the brainstem.

Similarly, VEPs were severely altered; either no identifiable responses to flash or pattern reversal stimuli could be recorded or the major components were significantly delayed in latency. The abnormalities were usually symmetrical for the responses observed from right and left monocular stimulation. Such symmetrical abnormalities are usually seen with lesions at any level posterior to the optic chiasm (6). The abnormalities of VEPs in our patients probably resulted from cortical or subcortical white matter lesions involving inputs to the visual cortices.

Short-latency SEPs usually showed a well-preserved Erb's potential (N_{10}) which is supposed to arise from the activity of the median nerve fibers in the brachial plexus (3). The entire absence of cervical (N_{14}) and early scalp components (N_{19} and P_{22}) or the occurrence of scalp potentials with a significant delay following median nerve stimulation, as noted in all of the patients studied, would reflect lesions of somatosensory pathways in the region rostral to midcervical cord.

In MLD, where demyelination also occurs in the peripheral nervous system, one would expect to observe alterations in those evoked responses that are generated in the peripheral nervous system. Wave I of the BAEP and the Erb's potential (N_{10}) on median nerve stimulation are the components generated peripherally. In both patients with MLD, wave I of the BAEP was severely delayed in latency, occurring over 2 msec following stimulation of either ear, the mean and SD for this wave being 1.5 ± 0.11 msec. Similarly, the Erb's potential was entirely unrecordable in one patient with MLD and markedly delayed in latency in the other.

There have been only a few studies of the evoked responses in patients with CNS degenerative diseases (2,4,5), but none have utilized more than one modality of stimulation. The results of our study indicate that multimodality evoked responses provide more information regarding the functional integrity of several afferent systems in their course from peripheral nerves through spinal cord and brainstem to cerebral cortex. These findings, when correlated with the results of other conventional tests such as EMG, nerve conduction velocities, EEG, and CT scan, are helpful in the diagnosis and total assessment of the nervous system in patients suspected to have degenerative CNS disorder.

REFERENCES

1. Buchwald, J. S., and Huang, C.-M. (1975): Far-field acoustic responses, origins in the cat. *Science,* 189:382–384.
2. Cracco, J. B., Bosch, V. V., and Cracco, R. Q. (1980): Cerebral and spinal somatosensory evoked potentials in children with CNS degenerative disease. *Electroencephalogr. Clin. Neurophysiol.,* 49:437–445.
3. Jones, S. J. (1977): Short latency potentials recorded from the neck and scalp following median nerve stimulation in man. *Electroencephalogr. Clin. Neurophysiol.,* 43:853–863.
4. Markand, O. N., Ochs, R., Worth, R. M., and DeMyer, W. E. (1980): Brainstem auditory evoked potentials in chronic degenerative central nervous system disorders. In: *Evoked Potential,* edited by C. Barber, pp. 367–374. MTP Press, Lancaster.
5. Ochs, R., Markand, O. N., and DeMyer, W. E. (1979): Brainstem auditory evoked responses in leukodystrophies. *Neurology (Minneap.),* 29:1,089–1,093.
6. Shahrokhi, E., Chiappa, K. H., and Young, R. R. (1978): Pattern shift visual evoked responses in two hundred patients with optic neuritis and/or multiple sclerosis. *Arch. Neurol.,* 35:65–71.
7. Starr, A., and Hamilton, A. E. (1976): Correlation between the confirmed sites of neurological lesions and abnormalities of far field auditory brainstem responses. *Electroencephalogr. Clin. Neurophysiol.,* 41:595–608.
8. Stockard, J. J., and Rossiter, V. S. (1977): Clinical and pathologic correlates of brainstem auditory response abnormalities. *Neurology,* 27:316–325.

Clinical Applications of Evoked Potentials in Neurology,
edited by J. Courjon, F. Mauguiere, and M. Revol.
Raven Press, New York © 1982.

Pattern Evoked Potential Diagnosis of Multiple Sclerosis: A Comparison of Various Contrast Stimuli

*F. C. C. Riemslag, *H. Spekreijse, and **H. van Walbeek

**The Netherlands Ophthalmic Research Institute, 1005 EK Amsterdam, The Netherlands; and* ***The Alexander van der Leeuw Clinic, 1054 JN Amsterdam, The Netherlands*

Previous investigations have shown that the latency of the contrast-evoked potential (EP) is increased in many MS patients including those without any history of optic neuritis or visual impairment (4,5). Latency estimation typically is performed with recording techniques that measure either the transient reversal response or the steady-state reversal response. In the reversal stimulus conditions, the elements of a pattern (e.g., black and white checks) are interchanged abruptly. When recording the transient reversal response, the visual system is stimulated repetitively at a rate that is low enough to allow the system to recover prior to the next stimulus presentation. The evoked response obtained under these conditions generally contains a negative–positive–negative (NPN) wave complex. Latency estimation is obtained by measuring the peak latency of the major positive peak. However, peak latency measurement can be hampered by uncertainty of the response shape and by the presence of additional components.

This problem is not as evident when estimating apparent latency from the slope of the phase characteristic of the steady-state reversal EPs. In the steady-state condition, the system is stimulated at such a high rate that no recovery can take place within one stimulus period. As seen in Fig. 1, the response becomes more sinusoidal as stimulus rate increases and thus contains fewer higher harmonic components at higher rates. By Fourier analysis, the phase and amplitude of the first harmonic can be determined and plotted as a function of frequency, and the amplitude and phase characteristic as depicted in Fig. 1 is obtained. From the slope of the phase characteristic, an apparent latency can be calculated using the formula:

$$\tau = \frac{\text{phase shift [degrees]}}{\text{frequency interval [Hz]}} \times \frac{1{,}000}{360} \quad \text{[msec]}$$

Apparent latency also is reported to be increased in many MS patients (2,10).

Although the simplicity of the waveform of the steady-state response obviates uncertainty in estimating peak latency, reliable apparent latency estimates can

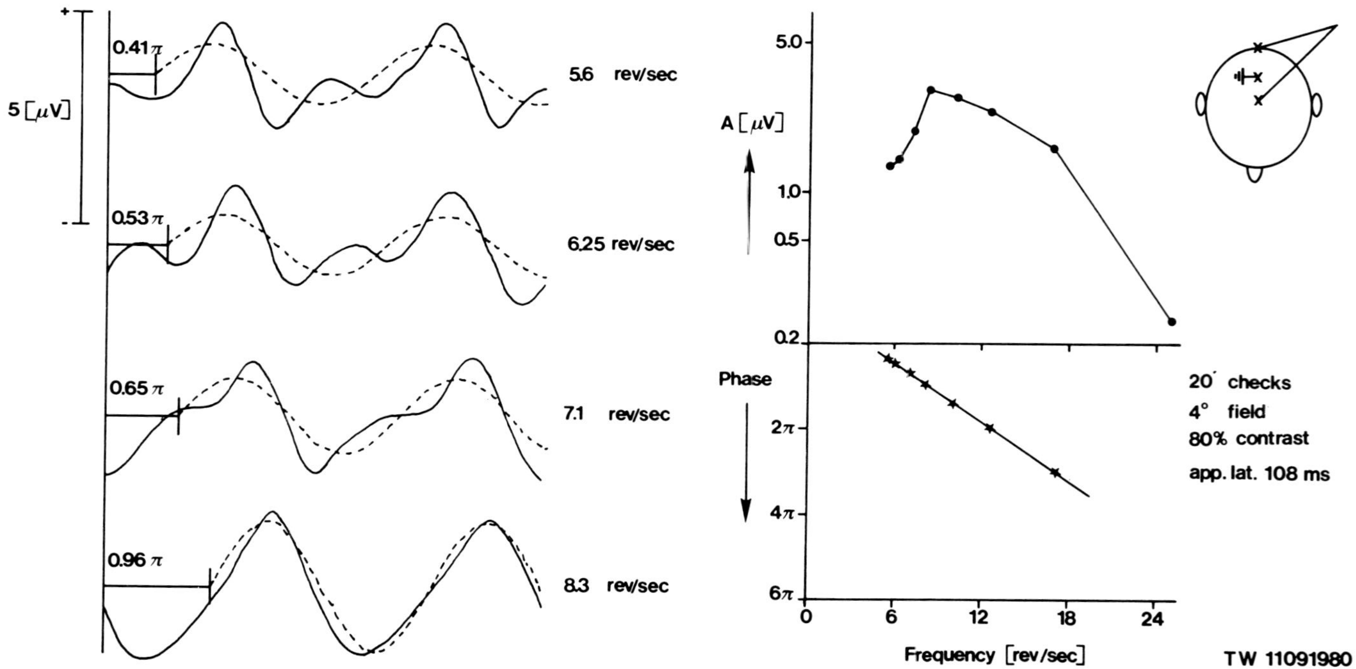

FIG. 1. Analysis of steady-state reversals. On the **left side,** responses to four different frequencies are shown. The *dotted lines* represent the first harmonic of the responses. The amplitudes and phases of these responses and of those to higher reversal rates are plotted on the **right side** to give an amplitude and phase characteristic. The phase is seen to vary proportionally to frequency, and from the slope of this phase characteristic, an apparent latency is obtained.

only be obtained by measuring the phase of the response at several temporal frequencies. More rapid latency estimates may be obtained with the transient method. To circumvent uncertainty of peak latency measurements. Fourier analysis may also be applied directly to the transient response (see Fig. 2). On theoretical grounds, it has been suggested that transient and steady-state recording techniques may give complementary information about the nonlinear system generating the EP (10). To evaluate this suggestion, we compared the apparent latency obtained under steady-state conditions to the apparent latency obtained from the phase spectrum of the Fourier-transformed transient response. On the basis of this analysis, we are able to design a new stimulus form that combines

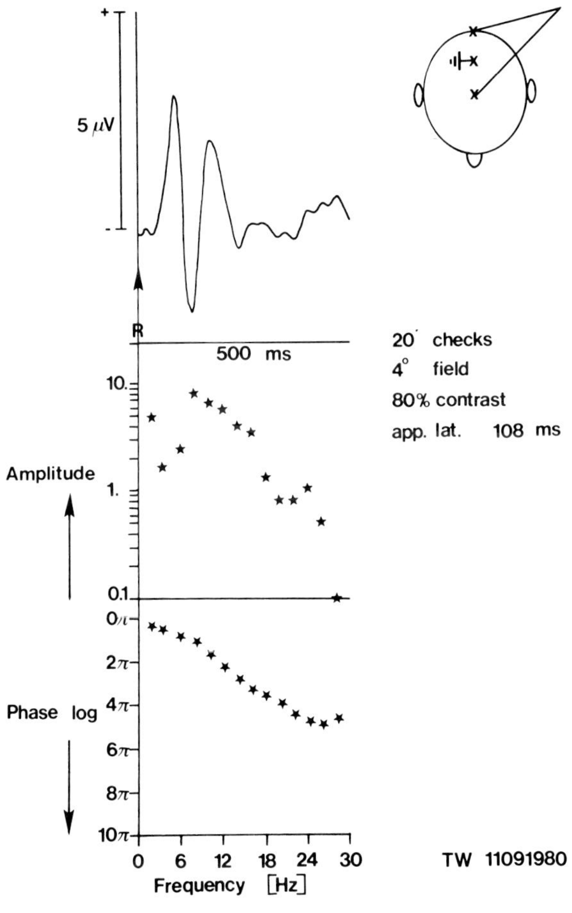

FIG. 2. Transient reversal response and its amplitude and phase spectrum. For the calculation of an apparent latency from this phase spectrum, only that region can be used within which the amplitudes are significant. According to our experience, this is in the interval from about 6 to 20 Hz.

the simplicity of the steady-state analysis and the speed of recording only a single transient response.

Although the reversal response is generally used in the differential diagnosis of MS, positive diagnosis is also possible on the basis of the peak latency of the major negative component of the pattern onset response. The onset response can be evoked by the replacement of a homogeneous field by the appearance of a pattern without change in mean luminance level. The evoked response obtained under this condition generally consists of a positive–negative–positive (PNP) (7) wave complex to the onset of the pattern and a positive component to the offset of the pattern. There is probably no relation between the onset EP and the reversal EP (11); however, a correlation seems to exist between the offset and the reversal response (3). Thus, by providing a second independent wave complex, i.e., the onset response, the onset–offset stimulus might be expected to give additional, clinically useful information. With the pattern onset–offset stimulus becoming readily available through the development of low-cost microprocessors, an appraisal of both methods seems indicated.

METHODS

Stimulus

A TV screen (Sony CVM-1810 E, 50 Hz) subtending 6° × 4° was used to display at a mean luminance of 200 asb a black-and-white checkerboard pattern with either 20′ or 55′ checks of nearly 100% contrast. To record the transient reversal responses, pattern reversals were presented at a rate of 2 reversal (rev)/sec. For the steady state intervals, stimulus rates ranged from 5.6 to 25 rev/sec. Note that for proper latency estimation, the reversal instants have to be locked to the frame rate of the TV (1). In the onset–offset condition, the pattern was presented for 300 msec every 800 msec. This long presentation time was chosen to insure that the onset responses would not be contaminated by the offset responses. The recording was performed with Ag–AgC1 electrodes positioned on the midline 2.5 cm above the inion and referenced to either linked ears or a midline electrode placed 9 cm above the inion. The bandwidth of the EEG amplifiers (Van Gogh) was set to 0.5 to 75 Hz. The EEG was also fed through a low-pass fourth-order Butterworth filter (Barr and Strout EF; cut-off frequency, 70 Hz). This low-pass filtering introduces an increase of peak latency of 9 msec in the records. The latency data presented in this paper are corrected for this artificial latency increase. A combined HP 21MX–HP 2100 computer system was used for data processing.

Subjects

For comparison of the transient and the steady state responses, 14 healthy subjects and 43 MS patients were tested under both conditions. For comparison of the onset–offset responses versus the reversal responses, a control group of 24 healthy subjects from 14 to 68 years of age and a group of 65 MS patients classified according to the McAlpine criteria (9) were tested with both stimuli. All subjects with reduced visual acuity were optimally refracted.

RESULTS

Twenty-five healthy eyes tested with transient and steady state pattern reversal conditions yielded an apparent latency for the steady state reversals of 102 + 10 msec as a normal value. The normative value of the apparent latency estimated from the phase spectrum of the Fourier-transformed transient reversal was 102 + 11 msec.

Table 1 summarizes the results of an evaluation of these apparent latencies obtained from 43 MS patients on the basis of a 3-SD criterion. From this table, it can be seen that, for most of the eyes tested (91%), both techniques give the same classification. The test results were not the same in only eight of 86 eyes, and in six of these, it was because no significant response could be obtained with one of the two methods.

Table 2 summarizes the incidence of latency increases in the three groups (McAlpine criteria) of MS patients as measured in the transient reversal and the onset–offset condition. It can be seen from this table that in the definite MS group, the onset–offset condition gives a much higher detection rate (63% versus 49%) than the reversal stimulus condition. Note that all patients except one (definite) with an increased latency for the reversal response also have an increased onset–offset latency. The lower detection rate for the reversal condition is because often no significant reversal response could be recorded (see Fig.

TABLE 1. *Classification of apparent latencies*

Steady-state reversals	Transient reversals		
	normal	increased	not significant
Normal	43	0	0
Increased	2	35	5
Not significant	1	0	0

TABLE 2. *Detection of increased latencies*

3SD criterion	Pattern reversal	Pattern on/offset	Both outside normal range	Both inside normal range
Definite (41)	20	26	19	10
Probable (15)	9	10	9	4
Possible (12)	4	4	4	5

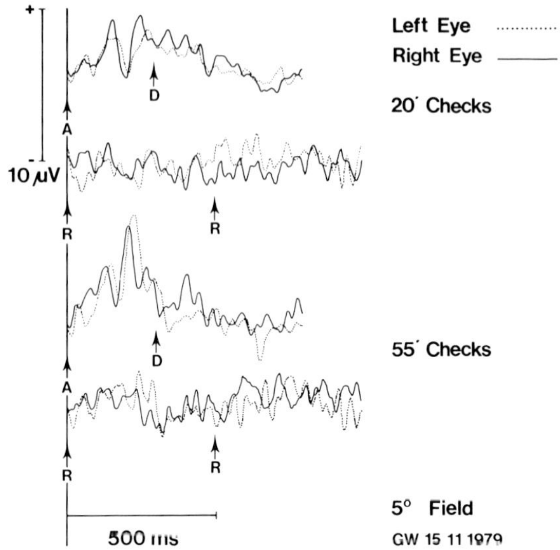

Fig. 3. Onset–offset **(A–D)** and reversal **(R)** *(traces)* responses as obtained from a definite MS patient. In the reversal condition, no significant resonses could be obtained for both check sizes. The onset responses, however, were clearly distinguishable from the background activity, although comparable (80–100) average counts were used.

3). Reversal responses could not be obtained for either 20′ or 55′ checks in this definite MS patient. The onset stimuli, however, yielded clear responses (upper and third traces). These were increased in latency from 50 to 70 msec, thus confirming the MS diagnosis.

Apart from the six definite MS patients showing nonsignificant reversal responses and increased latency onset responses, we observed three other possible MS patients who showed nonsignificant reversal responses although they had large normal onset responses. Two patients showed nonsignificant responses for one eye to both stimuli while showing normal responses for the other eye. Two patients in our sample did not give significant responses to either stimulus.

DISCUSSION

The similarity of the phase and amplitude spectra obtained with the transient and the steady state reversals favors a concept of the human contrast EP system in which every reversal triggers the same signal independent of whether the events are following each other at a slow or a fast rate. To test this hypothesis, we stimulated a healthy subject not only with the methods described above but also with a stimulus in which the reversal events followed each other in a random time sequence. The intervals between the reversal instants were equally distributed in a range from 100 to 1,000 msec. If each reversal is used as a trigger to store the subsequent 500-msec EEG signal, summation of these signal parts also results in a transient reversal response.

Figure 4 shows the averaged response of this experiment, its amplitude spectrum, phase spectrum, and coherence spectrum. The coherence spectrum is a measure of signal-to-noise ratio, and the solid line represents a 95% significance level. In the frequency region (see arrows) above this level, there is less than a 5% chance that the signals are incorrectly interpreted as response. Within this region, the phase changes proportionally with frequency, and an apparent latency can be calculated.

In the final figure (Fig. 5), the data obtained with all three methods are plotted. The amplitude spectra are shifted along the vertical logarithmic axis to overlap at the frequency of the maximal amplitude. It is seen from the figure that all amplitude and phase spectra (shifted multiples of 2π for clarity) have comparable shapes and therefore contain equivalent information. Since in the random reversal method, photic driving does not occur, this method seems to be the most efficient one to evoke a transient reversal response. At present, this stimulus method is being implemented with a low-cost microprocessor for a high-frame-rate TV monitor to test its clinical applicability.

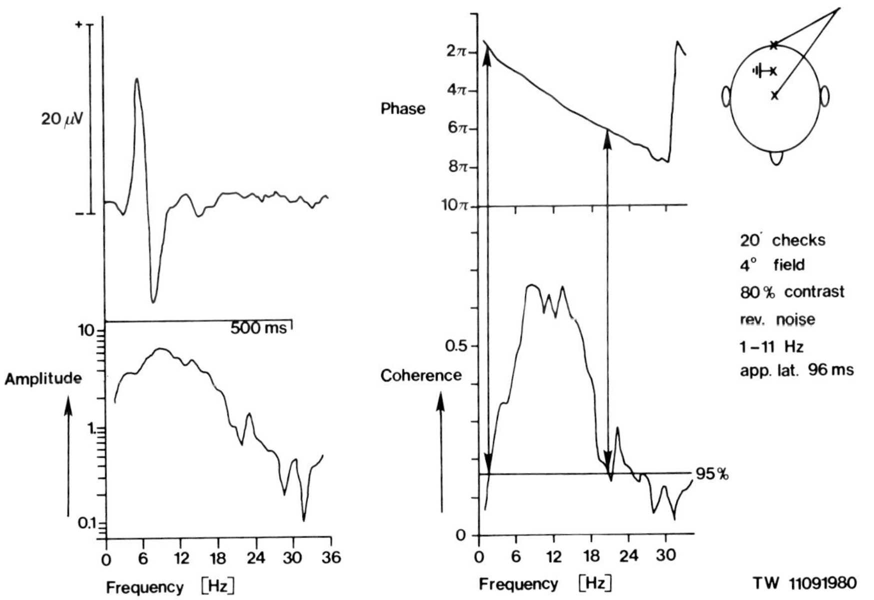

FIG. 4. Transient reverse response as obtained with the random presentation method. The averaged signal **(upper left)** its amplitude **(lower left),** phase **(upper right)** and coherence **(lower right)** spectrum. The coherence spectrum is a measure of signal-to-noise ratio, and a 95% significance level is presented by the *solid line.* In the part of the spectrum above this level *(arrows),* the phase is seen to vary linearly with frequency. Again, an apparent latency can be calculated.

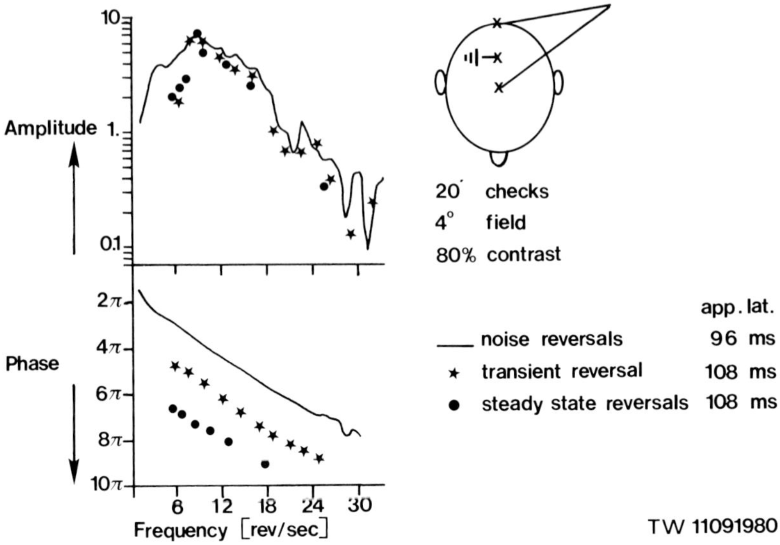

FIG. 5. Amplitude and phase spectra of the reversal response obtained, respectively, with the random presentation method *(solid line)*, the transient presentation method *(stars)*, and the steady-state method *(dots)*. The amplitude spectra are shifted along the vertical axis to overlap at the frequency of maximal amplitude. The phase spectra are shifted multiples of 2π for clarity. The amplitude and phase spectra of all three methods have the same shape and thus represent equivalent information.

In the data on the transient reversal versus the onset–offset stimulus, no support is found for either the presumed independence of the onset and the reversal response or the correlation between the reversal and the offset. On the one hand, all patients except one who showed an increased reversal latency also showed an increased onset latency. On the other hand, the absence of a significant reversal response does not imply the absence of the offset response.

However, in literature on EP diagnosis of MS, no special attention was drawn to the absence of significant reversal responses. It may be argued that the differences between our reversal stimulus conditions and those of other investigators account for our higher percentage of nonsignificant reversal responses. For instance, we used a field of 6° to 4° instead of the 32° of e.g., Halliday et al. (4). Our data show, however, that stimulation of this small field yields a detection rate comparable to the rates reported in literature (Cf. e.g., 12). Even Hennerici et al. (6), who stimulated with a single check of only 45′, obtained detection rates of the same order. It is difficult to interpret these data in the context of the characteristic patchy nature of the visual field loss in MS (9).

Furthermore, Matthews et al. (8), in their 1977 study of a large sample (156) of MS patients, mention patients showing nonsignificant reversal responses although they stimulated a large field of 16°. One possible explanation for the relatively high percentage of nonsignificant reversal responses may be the high incidence of nystagmus in MS (9). In the presence of nystagmus, good onset–offset responses can be obtained, and the reversal responses can be attenuated. (D. Creel, D. Reits, and H. Spekreijse, *unpublished results*). The finding of three possible patients showing nonsignificant reversal and normal latency onset–offset responses and of the two patients showing nonsignificant responses to the one eye and normal latency responses to the other indicate immediately that positive diagnosis of MS cannot be based on the absence of a significant reversal response.

CONCLUSIONS

1. The transient and steady-state reversals seem to give equivalent information.
2. Random presentation of pattern reversals evokes the same response as conventional repetitive stimulation. Since random stimulation abolishes rhythmic activity, it is the most efficient stimulus form to generate a reversal response.
3. The pattern onset–offset stimulus is preferred for clinical application, since this stimulus is more efficient in evoking a contrast-evoked potential.
4. The absence of an evoked potential should never be used as a positive diagnostic criterion in MS.

ACKNOWLEDGMENTS

We should like to thank Dr. D. Reits for providing the system-analytical tools necessary to run this study and Dr. P. Apkarian for the many critical suggestions she made when this text was prepared. Finally, we thank Mr. T. van Wessem and Miss I. Braamhaar for their helpful technical assistance in running the experiments.

REFERENCES

1. Arden, G. B., Faulkner, D. J., and Mair, C. (1977): A versatile television pattern generator for visual evoked potentials. In: *Visual Evoked Potentials in Man: New Developments,* edited by J. Desmedt, pp. 90–109. Clarendon Press, Oxford.
2. Duwaer, A. L., and Spekreijse, H. (1978): Latency of luminance and contrast evoked potentials in multiple sclerosis patients. *Electroencephalogr. Clin. Neurophysiol.,* 45:244–258.
3. Estevez, O., and Spekreijse, H. (1974): Relationship between pattern appearance–disappearance and pattern reversal responses. *Exp. Brain Res.,* 19:233–238.
4. Halliday, A. M., McDonald, W. I., and Mushin, J. (1972): Delayed visual evoked response in optic neuritis. *Lancet,* 1:982–985.
5. Halliday, A. M., McDonald, W. I., and Mushin, J. (1973): Visual evoked response in diagnosis of multiple sclerosis. *Br. Med. J.,* 4:661–664.
6. Hennerici, M., Wenzel, D., and Freund, H. J. (1977): The comparison of small-size rectangle and checkerboard stimulation for the evaluation of delayed visual evoked responses in patients suspected of multiple sclerosis. *Brain,* 100:119–136.
7. Jeffreys, D. A., and Axford, J. G. (1972): Source locations of pattern specific components of human visual evoked potentials. I and II. *Exp. Brain Res.,* 16:1–40.
8. Matthews, W. B., Small, D. G., Small, M., and Poutney, E. (1977): Pattern reversal evoked visual potential in the diagnosis of multiple sclerosis. *J. Neurol. Neurosurg. Psychiatry,* 40:1009–1014.

9. McAlpine, D., Lumsden, C. E., and Acheson, E. D. (1972): *Multiple Sclerosis: A Reappraisal.* Churchill-Livingstone, Edinborough.
10. Milner, B. A., Regan, D., and Heron, J. R. (1974): Differential diagnosis of multiple sclerosis by visual evoked potential recording. *Brain,* 97:755–772.
11. Shagass, C., Amadeo, M., and Roemer, R. A. (1976): Spatial distribution of potentials evoked by half-field pattern-reversal and pattern-onset stimuli. *Electroencephalogr. Clin. Neurophysiol.,* 41:609–622.
12. Spekreijse, H., Duwaer, A. L., and Posthumus-Meyjes, F. E. (1979): Contrast evoked potentials and psychophysics in multiple sclerosis patients. In: *Human Evoked Potentials, Applications and Problems,* edited by D. Lehman and E. Callaway, pp. 363–381. Plenum Press, New York.

Clinical Applications of Evoked Potentials in Neurology,
edited by J. Courjon, F. Mauguiere, and M. Revol.
Raven Press, New York © 1982.

Visual Evoked Potentials by Central Foveal and Checkerboard Reversal Stimulation in Multiple Sclerosis

G. Oepen, C. Brauner, M. Doerr, and U. Thoden

Neurologische Universitätsklinik mit Abteilung für Neurophysiologie, 7800 Freiburg, West Germany

In the diagnosis of multiple sclerosis (MS), recording of visual evoked potentials (VEP) may help to detect subclinical lesions in the visual pathway, which are among the earliest and most frequently involved sites for plaques in MS (7,10).

Normal values of pattern-evoked potentials as well as the percentage of positive VEP findings reported by different authors vary considerably (1–6,8,9,11,12). These reported differences are probably caused by differences in equipment and the incongruent selection of patients. Therefore, the need of individual reference values for each laboratory has been stressed in all reports.

This study was performed to compare the diagnostic value of VEPs elicited by two different methods in patients suspected of MS, because one of the techniques has been reported to be more sensitive in detection of optic nerve demyelination (3).

PATIENTS AND METHODS

Visual evoked potentials of 200 patients suspected of MS were evaluated. With the criteria of McAlpine, they were classified into definite (79), probable (23), and possible MS (98) through their clinical documents. Ages ranged between 11 and 73 years; the duration of the disease varied between several days and 38 years.

Forty healthy subjects in a similar age range served as controls. In all subjects, visual acuity was normal or corrected by glasses.

For checkerboard reversal stimulation, a black-and-white pattern on a television monitor subtending 20° of the visual field was reversed by a time pulse generator. At constant overall luminance, the luminance of the white squares was 51.3 cd/m^2, that of the black ones was 0.3426 cd/m^2.

Central foveal stimulation was performed by offering a bright, small-sized rectangle in the visual axis subtending 45′, alternating with a black rectangle and changing every 800 msec while the background luminance remained constant.

Sixty-four responses from each eye were averaged over 500 msec for at least two series successively; in cases of doubt, several times. The details of recording VEPs are described elsewhere (11).

RESULTS

Control Subjects

Checkerboard Reversal Stimulation

The major positive potential appeared after 98 ± 8.3 msec with a mean interocular difference of 2.93 ± 3.28 msec. A peak latency longer than the normal mean values plus twice the standard deviation (115 msec), an intereye latency difference over 10 msec or absence of reproducible potentials were defined as abnormal. If potentials were not detectable despite prolonged searching for them and technical reasons were excluded, this was also considered as abnormal, because it never occurred in controls.

Foveal Stimulation

The mean latency of the major positive potential was 128 ± 13.1 msec with an upper limit of 155 msec ($\bar{x} + 2$ SD) (Fig. 1). In 20% of controls (32.5% of eyes), foveal VEPs were not detectable.

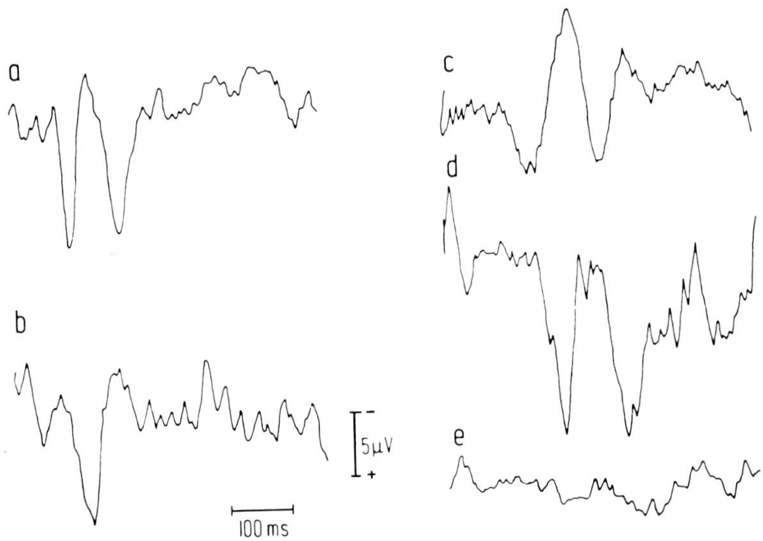

FIG. 1. a: Normal VEP (checkerboards). **b:** Normal foveal VEP. **c:** Pathologic VEP (checkerboard). **d:** Pathologic foveal VEP. **e:** "Absent" foveal VEP. For further details, see text.

Patients Suspected of MS

One or more periods of visual impairment were reported by 31 patients with definite MS, by nine with probable, and by seven with possible MS, totally by 47 out of the 200 patients. In three of seven patients with repeated VEP examination, latencies improved and reached normal values; in one it improved but still remained prolonged. Out of 47 patients with a history of retrobulbar neuritis, 37 showed pathologic checkerboard responses, and 36 abnormal foveal responses; in four patients, both methods gave normal results.

Checkerboard Reversal Stimulation

Pathologic responses (Fig. 1) were found in 72% of definite, 44% of probable, and 40% of possible MS, totally in 54% of all 200 patients. No potential could be discriminated in 6.5% of all patients. A pathologic interocular difference was seen in 34.2% in definite, 21.7% in probable, and 50.3% in possible MS. Prolonged latencies were observed in 48% in definite, 32.6% in probable, and 22% in possible MS.

Central Foveal Stimulation

Sixty-five percent of all 200 patients, 75% of definite, 74% of probable, and 54% of possible MS patients showed abnormal responses. From this group, in 37% the main peak could not be detected in one or both eyes, in 8% of patients foveal potentials of only one side could not be found (Fig. 1). A pathologic interocular difference was seen in 11.4% in definite, in 21.7% in probable, and in 9.2% in possible MS. Prolonged latencies were observed in 24.7% in definite, in 22.9% in probable, and in 19.4% in possible MS.

The pathologic results of both methods were not congruent. Abnormal checkerboard responses with normal foveal responses were seen in nine patients; pathological foveal responses in spite of normal checkerboard responses appeared in 11 patients.

DISCUSSION

The results obtained confirm, in general, the validity of VEP examination in the diagnosis of MS, but the assumed high diagnostic sensitivity of foveal elicited VEPs should be considered with reserve. There is no significant difference in diagnostic value of checkerboard versus foveal stimulation for most of the parameters except the nonrecognizable responses. As even 20% of normal subjects had foveal responses absent, the 37% of absent responses in patients have to be evaluated with caution. When only prolonged latencies in pathologic interocular differences are compared, foveal VEPs are not superior to checkerboard reversal stimulation. The higher sensitivity of central foveal stimulation as reported by Hennerici et al. (3) may be explained by a smaller standard deviation of mean values in the controls, which might have resulted from technical reasons and differences in equipment. But no absence of foveal VEPs observed in 20% of our controls and 37% of all patients was described.

The difficulty of fixating the small stimulus over the time of recording might be a possible explanation, as the amplitude of P_{100} decreases rapidly with increasing laterality of fixation points as during small eye movements, even for checkerboard stimulation (3).

The spontaneous nystagmus occurring in 38% of patients with undetectable foveal potentials can explain the negative results at least partially.

Although we were unable to confirm the very high incidence of pathologic central VEPs in MS, the technique provides a reliable method for detection of asymptomatic lesions of the visual pathways (7). The checkerboard reversal stimulation can be complemented by recording of central foveal responses but seems to be superior, more stable, and less influenced by attention.

Nevertheless, both methods overlap, and the percentage of abnormal responses increases if both methods are combined. Therefore, in cases of normal checkerboard response, central foveal stimulation may give an additional diagnostic hint.

SUMMARY

In 200 patients with suspected MS, the diagnostic value of VEP elicited by checkerboard reversal and central foveal stimulation was compared. No significant difference was evident, but both methods overlap. The more stable checkerboard reversal stimulation should be preferred as a diagnostic method. Only in suspected MS with normal checkerboard responses, additional foveal responses may give supplementary information. Normal VEPs cannot exclude a prior retrobulbar neuritis.

REFERENCES

1. Chain, F., Mallecourt, J., Leblanc, M., and Lhermitte, F. (1977): Apport de l'enregistrement des potentials évoqués visuels au diagnostic de la sclérose en plaques. *Rev. Neurol. (Paris),* 133(2):81–88.
2. Halliday, A. M., McDonald, W. I., and Mustin, J. (1973): Delayed pattern evoked response in optic neurites in relation to visual acuity. *Trans. Opthalmol. Soc. U.K.,* 93:315–324.
3. Hennerici, M., Wenzel, D., and Freund, H. J. (1977): The comparison of small-size rectangle and checkerboard stimulation for the evaluation of delayed visual evoked responses in patients suspected of multiple sclerosis. *Brain,* 100:119–136.
4. Kayed, K., Røsjø, Ø., and Kåss, B. (1978): Practical application of patterned visual evoked responses in multiple sclerosis. *Acta Neurol. Scand.,* 57:317–324.
5. Lehmann, D., and Mir, Z. (1976): Methodik und Auswertung visuell evozierter EEG-Potentiale bei Verdacht auf Multiple Sclerose. *J. Neurol.,* 213:57–103.
6. Lowitzsch, K., Kuhnt, V., Sakmann, C., Maurer, K., Hopf, H. C., Schott, D., Thäter, K. (1976): Visual pattern evoked responses and blink reflexes in assessment of MS diagnosis. A clinical study of 135 multiple sclerosis patients. *J. Neurol.,* 213:17–32.
7. Lumsden, C. E. (1970): The neuropathology of multiple sclerosis. In: *Handbook of Clinical*

Neurology, Vol. 9, edited by P. J. Vinken and G. W. Bruyn, pp. 217–309. North-Holland, Amsterdam and American Elsevier, New York.
8. Mastaglia, F. L., Black, J. C., and Collins, D. W. (1979): Quantitative studies of saccadic and pursuit eye movements in multiple sclerosis. *Brain,* 102:817–834.
9. Matthews, W. B., Small, D. G., Small, M., and Pounthey, E. (1977): Pattern reversal evoked visual potential in the diagnosis of multiple sclerosis. *J. Neurol. Neurosurg. Psychiatry,* 40:1009–1014.
10. McAlpine, D., Lumsden, C. E., and Acheson, E. D. (1972): *Multiple Sclerosis: A Reappraisal.* Livingstone, Edinburgh.
11. Oepen, G., Brauner, C., Doerr, M., Thoden, V. (1981): Visual evoked potentials (VEP) elicited by checkerboard versus foveal stimulation in multiple sclerosis. *Arch. Psychiatr. Nervenkr.,* 229:305–313.
12. Sharokhi, F., Chiappa, K. H., and Young, R. R. (1978): Pattern shift visual evoked responses. Two hundred patients with optic neuritis and/or multiple sclerosis. *Arch. Neurol.,* 35:65–71.

Clinical Applications of Evoked Potentials in Neurology,
edited by J. Courjon, F. Mauguiere, and M. Revol.
Raven Press, New York © 1982.

A Modification of the Visual Evoked Response Method Involving Small Luminance Decrements for the Diagnosis of Demyelinating Diseases

*Michael Hennerici and **Eugene R. Wist

**Department of Neurology and **Institute of Psychology, University of Dusseldorf, D-4000 Dusseldorf 1, Federal Republic of Germany*

The diagnostic value of recording visual evoked responses (VER) in patients suspected of suffering from MS has been established since 1972 when Halliday et al. first recommended the use of a checkerboard pattern-reversal stimulus (10). The percentage of abnormally delayed major positive potentials indicating an optic nerve lesion, even in the absence of a history of visual impairment or visual abnormalities seen in full ophthalmological investigation (8), has been found to range between 75 and 97% in patients with definite MS (Table 1). According to the diagnostic criteria of McAlpine, Lumsden, and Acheson (17), the incidence of pattern-evoked VER abnormalities was, however, considerably smaller in patients with probable and possible diseases.

Theoretical considerations suggested that small demyelinating lesions mainly affecting the slowly conducting fibers originating from foveal ganglion cells could be overlooked by the large-size checkerboard stimulation because of the preferential stimulation of the faster conducting axons arising from the retinal periphery (for references, see 13). Central vision, however, is commonly affected in MS, possibly because of the large number of foveal fibers and their extensive cortical projection.

The additional use of a small-size foveal stimulus resulted in a higher incidence of VER abnormalities, particularly in patients classified as "probable" or "possible" MS (Table 2). This method of stimulation thus appeared to be more sensitive in the detection of optic nerve lesions because the incidence of false positives in a healthy control population is negligible (7,13). However, as Table 2 shows, the incidence of abnormal foveal evoked potentials remains smaller in patients with probable and particularly in those with possible MS. The question thus arises as to whether the cases with normal VERs have no involvement of the optic nerve or whether the sensitivity of both stimulation methods is not adequate to reveal it.

In an earlier investigation involving a comparison of foveally and peripherally elicited VERs with a psychophysical method, it was found that MS patients

TABLE 1. *Incidence of abnormal evoked potentials in clinically definite MS (checkerboard pattern-reversal stimulation)*

Reference	No. of patients	% Abnormal
Asselman et al.(1)	31	84
Collins et al.(6)	37	78
Halliday et al.(11)	34	97
Hennerici et al.(13)	16	81
Lowitzsch(14)	81	83
Matthews et al.(16)	61	75

TABLE 2. *Incidence of abnormal VERs in clinically definite, probable, and possible MS patients for different methods of stimulation* (N = 480)

	Definite	Probable	Possible
No. of patients	168	183	129
Abnormal checkerboard pattern (%)	81	60	39
Abnormal foveal rectangle (%)	93	84	72

were very sensitive to a small reduction of luminance for the latter method (20). We therefore hypothesized that the diagnostic sensitivity of the two VER methods could be improved by reducing luminance. Our reasoning was that, under normal luminance conditions, fibers that are just able to conduct normally are sufficient to produce normal VER latencies. However, with a small reduction in luminance, the VER latencies become longer because the conduction velocities of these fibers can no longer be maintained.

The results to be presented show that the incidence of delayed VERs can in fact be increased by luminance decrements for the foveal stimulation method only, whereas no change in the sensitivity for conventional checkerboard-pattern stimulation could be demonstrated.

METHODS

For both stimulus conditions, the averaged VERs were recorded in a uniformly dimly lit room. A television screen producing 625 lines and 50 fields per sec was placed 150 cm in front of the patient who was instructed to fixate on a spot in the center of the monitor throughout each run. Sixty-four responses were averaged from each eye for both series successively. In the first series, a black-and-white checkerboard pattern was produced on the monitor which subtended 20° of the visual field (peripheral stimulation). Reversals of the checkerboard were performed by a time pulse generator. At intervals of 1 sec, the black squares became white and the white black. This resulted in a rectangular pattern moving one square to the right or left, alternately. The pulse triggering each movement was also used to trigger a computer to average the EEG recorded from the scalp during the following 320 msec. The overall luminance did not change. The luminance of the white squares was approximately 51 cd/m², that of the black ones was 0.5 cd/m². Check size was 1°10′.

In a second series, a bright, small-size rectangle (130 cd/m²) was applied on a diffuse monitor illumination providing a background luminance of about 3 cd/m². This stimulus was placed in the visual axis subtending 45′ of the patient's central visual area (foveal stimulation). Triggered by a time-pulse generator, this spot lasted for 1 sec. The interval between two successive spot displays was 1 sec.

The VERs recorded from scalp electrodes were high-pass filtered. Recordings were made with the electrodes placed 6 cm above the inion.

Additionally, each patient suspected to suffer from MS and normal subjects were both tested with the foveal and checkerboard VER methods under conditions that involved 0, 0.2, 0.5, and 1.0 log units of luminance attenuation.

In a few control experiments, repeated examinations of VERs in 30 healthy subjects at intervals of about 2 weeks after both stimulation with the large-size checkerboard pattern reversal and the small-size rectangle stimulus showed only minor latency variations intraindividually (SD, 1.7 msec for both stimulation procedures) (Fig. 1). The upper limit of normal (mean + 3SD) within this control population was not exceeded by any of the subjects retested. These data show a high repeat reliability for both methods. (For further details, see 13.)

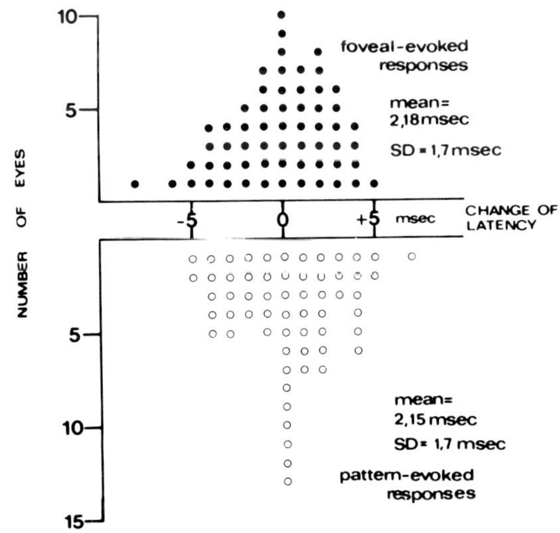

FIG. 1. Distribution of test–retest latency differences of the major positive potential of VERs evoked by a small-size rectangle stimulus (foveal-evoked responses: *dark circles*) and a large-size checkerboard pattern reversal (pattern-evoked responses: *open circles*) from both eyes of 30 healthy subjects.

Patients and Control Subjects

Four hundred eighty patients (aged from 17 to 59 years of age) were examined because of a suspected diagnosis of MS (168 definite, 183 probable, and 129 possible). From this initial group of patients, 14 were selected whose checkerboard VERs were normal though their foveal VER latencies were in the borderline region (mean + 3 SD). Only the data of this subgroup, consisting of three "definite," six "probable," and five "possible" MS cases on the basis of the criteria of McAlpine et al. (17) and of 13 healthy control subjects ranging between 21 and 29 years of age (26 eyes) will be presented in detail.

RESULTS

Normal Subjects

Checkerboard pattern and foveal small-size rectangle evoked responses were recorded monocularly in 13 healthy control subjects under conditions that involved 0, 0.2, 0.5, and 1.0 log units of luminance attenuation. With zero luminance attenuation, a large positive wave with a peak latency of 100 to 120 msec could generally be evoked from both eyes with checkerboard stimulation, whereas for the foveal stimulus, the amplitudes of the VERs were generally smaller, and the latency of the major positive potential was always larger. From

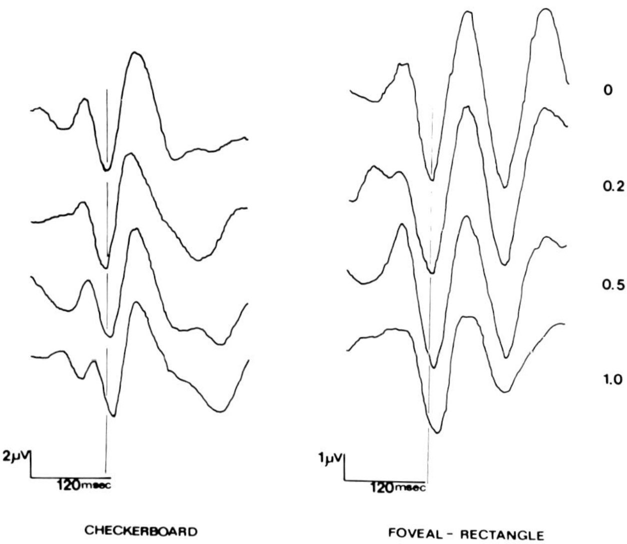

FIG. 2. Normal VERs elicited monocularly by checkerboard pattern–reversal **(left)** and foveal small-size rectangle stimulation **(right)** under conditions involving 0, 0.2, 0.5, and 1.0 log units of luminance attenuation (Positivity down).

these experiments, the upper limit of normal latencies was defined as the mean + 3 SD = 120 msec for checkerboard and 130 msec for foveal stimulation. As shown in Fig. 2, the latencies of the major positive potentials slightly lengthened, and the amplitudes decreased modestly with increasing luminance attenuation for both stimulation conditions. However, the upper limit of normal latencies was not significantly exceeded in any of the control subjects as shown in Fig. 3, even with 1 log unit of luminance attenuation.

Patients

Similarly, 14 patients suspected of MS and whose "0" filter foveal VER latencies were in the borderline region were tested. Since their checkerboard VER latencies were in the normal range both with and without luminance decrements, they could not be classified as abnormal with either stimulus.

In contrast, a considerable change in the foveal VERs could be observed with luminance attenuation: as shown in the lower portion of Fig. 4, the amplitudes of the foveal major positive potential decreased; they showed a slight broadening, and their latencies exceeded the upper normal limit. The VERs for the normals (upper portion) were hardly affected by luminance decrements.

Figure 5 summarizes the latency results of normal controls and MS patients and reflects the relationships shown in the previous figure. It should be emphasized here that all these patients showed pathological foveal latencies with luminance attenuation, although their checkerboard latencies were within the normal

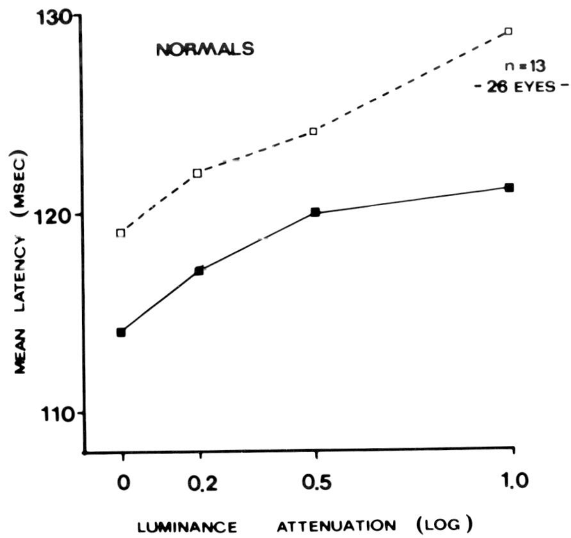

FIG. 3. Comparison of the mean peak latencies of the major positive potentials elicited by checkerboard pattern–reversal *(dark squares)* and foveal small-size rectangle stimulation *(open squares)* for luminance attenuations as in Fig. 2 in 13 healthy control subjects.

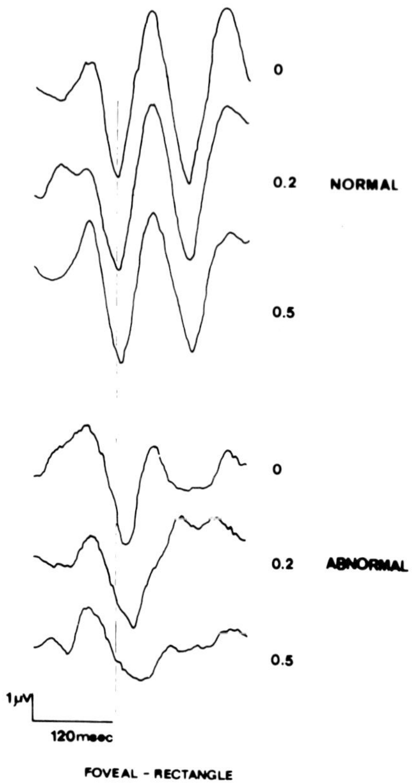

FIG. 4. Typical monocular VERs elicited by foveal stimulation of a normal control subject (NORMAL) and a patient suffering from "definite" MS (ABNORMAL) involving luminance attenuation as in Fig. 2. Note the small latency delay of the major positive potential of the patient in contrast to the normal subject (0 attenuation) which just reaches the borderline region (mean + 3 SD = 130 msec). With small luminance reductions (0.2 log units), the potential of this patient slightly broadens, and the latency increases. At 0.5 log units of attenuation, a marked flattening of the VER is visible. (Positivity down.)

range and although the foveal latencies without luminance attenuation were only borderline. In contrast to the normals, it was not possible to obtain measurable foveal latencies at 1 log unit for most MS patients. This was because of the marked reduction in VER amplitudes as shown in Table 3.

As can be seen from the upper portion of Fig. 5, luminance decrements failed to reveal a marked delay of the checkerboard-elicited major positive potential within the patient group. Their latencies did not exceed the upper normal limit (mean + 3 SD = 120 msec).

CONCLUSION

Evoked potential tests provide a very sensitive means of detecting second lesions in patients suspected of MS but in whom the diagnosis is not yet clinically definite. Although a substantial delay of the major positive visually evoked potential is not specific to MS (2–4,18), its incidence is often useful in making an early diagnosis in light of the clinical picture. The reliability and the diagnostic value of VER examination are known to depend substantially on the stimulus parameters used (5,7,12,13,19). Although the actual site of generation of the

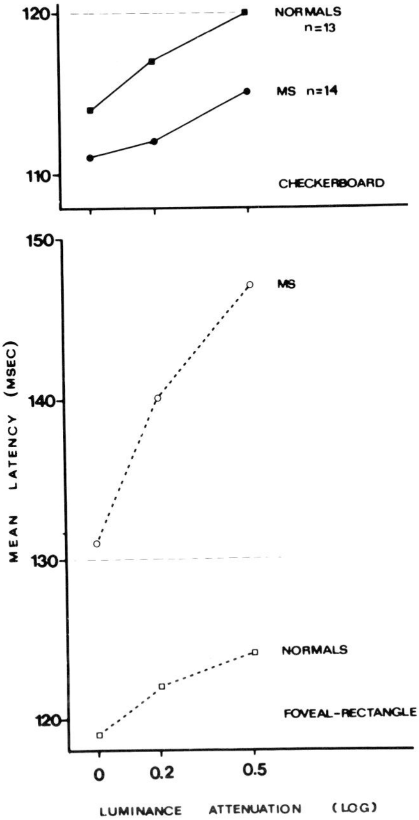

FIG. 5. Comparison of the mean peak latencies of the major positive potentials elicited by checkerboard pattern reversal **(upper half)** and foveal stimulation **(lower half)** for different luminance attenuations in 13 healthy control subjects and 14 MS patients. Luminance decrements failed to induce a marked delay for the checkerboard VERs in both groups. Therefore, the latency did not exceed the upper normal limit *(horizontal dashed lines)*. For the foveal stimulus, the patients' latencies clearly exceeded the upper normal limit with luminance attenuation.

major positive potential of the VER is as unknown as the exact nature of its changes (9,15), the varying incidence of abnormalities detected by different stimulation procedures seems to indicate a selective encroachment on distinct parts of the afferent visual input.

Based on the present data, we propose the use of diverse visual stimuli for VER examination. The shape and peak latencies of the standard checkerboard pattern reversal have been shown to be largely free of inter- and intraindividual variations and hence are most appropriate for routine clinical use. Yet, its effi-

TABLE 3. *Foveal rectangle VER amplitude reduction expressed as percentage of original amplitude (no filter)*

Luminance	Attenuation (log)	Normal	MS patients
	0.2	85	79
	0.5	79	40
	1.0	65	10

ciency for detecting clinically silent lesions, particularly in patients with "probable" and "possible" MS, is restricted. In order to improve the EP discrimination of optic nerve lesions in the early diagnosis of MS, we recommend the additional use of a stimulus preferentially stimulating the slowly conducting fibers originating from foveal ganglion cells, since central vision is commonly affected in MS. This can effectively be achieved by the use of a small rectangular stimulus placed in the visual axis of the patient (7,13). The major difficulty of this method is that the patient's cooperation in fixating is absolutely required, since the amplitude of the VER is markedly reduced with increasing eccentricity of the stimulus from the visual axis (13). The necessity of strict fixation also applies to the extended procedure involving commonly available neutral density filters. As a result of using luminance attenuation with the foveal method, patients whose optic nerve involvement would have remained undetected under normal luminance show pathological VERs, as indicated by the data presented here: for all these patients, the existence of an optic nerve lesion was revealed only with foveal luminance reduction.

REFERENCES

1. Asselman, P., Chadwick, D. W., and Marsden, C. D. (1975): Visual evoked responses in the diagnosis and management of patients suspected of multiple sclerosis. *Brain,* 98:261–282.
2. Cappin, J. M., and Nissim, S. (1975): Pattern visual evoked response in the detection of field defects in glaucoma. *Arch. Opthalmol.,* 93:9–18.
3. Carroll, W. M., Kriss, A., Baraitser, M., Barrett, G., and Halliday, A. M. (1980): The incidence and nature of visual pathway involvement in Friedreich's ataxia. *Brain,* 103:413–434.
4. Carroll, W. M., and Mastaglia, F. L. (1979): Leber's optic neuropathy: A clinical and visual evoked potential study of affected and asymptomatic members of a six generation family. *Brain,* 102:559–580.
5. Celesia, G. G., and Daly, R. F. (1977): Visual electroencephalographic computer analysis: A new electrophysiological test for the diagnosis of optic nerve lesions. *Neurology,* 27:637–641.
6. Collins, D. W. K., Black, J. L., and Mastaglia, F. L. (1978): Pattern-reversal visual evoked potential. *J. Neurol. Sci.,* 36:83–95.
7. Diener, H. C. (1980): Methodik und klinische Anwendung visuell evozierter Potentiale in der Neurologie. *Nervenarzt,* 51:159–167.
8. Feinsod, M., and Hoyt, W. F. (1975): Subclinical optic neuropathy in multiple sclerosis. *J. Neurol. Neurosurg. Psychiatry,* 38:1109–1114.
9. Halliday, A. M., and McDonald, W. I. (1977): Pathophysiology of demyelinating disease. *Br. Med. Bull.,* 33:21–27.
10. Halliday, A. M., McDonald, W. I., and Mushin, J. (1972): Delayed visual evoked responses in optic neuritis. *Lancet,* 1:982–985.
11. Halliday, A. M., McDonald, W. I., and Mushin, J. (1973): Visual evoked responses in diagnosis of multiple sclerosis. *Br. Med. J.,* 4:661–664.
12. Harter, M. R. (1971): Evoked cortical responses to checkerboard patterns: Effect of check-size as a function of retinal eccentricity. *Vision Res.,* 10:1365–1376.
13. Hennerici, M., Wenzel, D., and Freund, H. -J. (1977): The comparison of small-size rectangle and checkerboard stimulation for the evaluation of delayed visual evoked responses in patients suspected of multiple sclerosis. *Brain,* 100:119–136.
14. Lowitzsch, K. (1980): Pattern-evoked potentials in 251 MS patients in relation to ophthalmological findings and diagnostic classification. In: *Progress in Multiple Sclerosis Research,* edited by H. J. Bauer, S. Poser, and G. Ritter, pp. 571–577. Springer-Verlag, Berlin, Heidelberg, New York.
15. MacKay, D. M., and Jeffreys, D. A. (1973): Visually evoked potentials and visual perception

in man. In: *Handbook of Sensory Physiology,* edited by R. Jung, pp. 647–678, Springer-Verlag, Berlin, Heidelberg, New York.
16. Matthews, W. B., Small, D. G., Small, M., and Poutney, E. (1977): Pattern reversal evoked visual potential in the diagnosis of multiple sclerosis. *J. Neurol. Neurosurg. Psychiatry,* 40:1009–1014.
17. McAlpine, D., Lumsden, C. E., and Acheson, E. D. (1972): *Multiple Sclerosis: A Reappraisal.* Livingstone, Edinburgh.
18. McDonald, W. I. (1980): The role of evoked potentials in the diagnosis of multiple sclerosis. In: *Progress in Multiple Sclerosis Research,* edited by H. J. Bauer, S. Poser, and G. Ritter, pp. 564–568. Springer-Verlag, Berlin, Heidelberg, New York.
19. Richey, E. T., Kooi, K. A., and Tourtelotte, W. W. (1971): Visually evoked responses in multiple sclerosis. *J. Neurol. Neurosurg. Psychiatry,* 34:275–280.
20. Wist, E. R., Hennerici, M., and Dichgans, J. (1978): The Pulfrich spatial frequency phenomenon: A psychophysical method competitive to visual evoked potentials in the diagnosis of multiple sclerosis. *J. Neurol. Neurosurg. Psychiatry,* 41:1069–1077.

Clinical Applications of Evoked Potentials in Neurology,
edited by J. Courjon, F. Mauguiere, and M. Revol.
Raven Press, New York © 1982.

Delayed Visual Evoked Potentials in Multiple Sclerosis: Interpretation of VEP Latencies for Follow-up Studies

*F. Mauguière, *F. Brudon, *E. Challet, **G. Maraval, and *J. Courjon

**EEG Department Hôpital Neurologique, Lyon, France; and **C.E.M.I., Lyon, France*

Since the pioneer work of Halliday et al. (4,5), the latency of the P100 potential evoked by checkerboard reversal is considered to be a reliable means to detect subclinical demyelinating lesions of the optic pathways in patients with multiple sclerosis (MS). In most published series, increased P100 latencies up to 200 msec have been reported; in these cases, the VEP latency is usually evaluated by measuring the peaking time of the maximal positivity, with an analysis time that varies between 200 and 500 msec according to different authors. However, one does not know whether some of these very long delays may be wholly accounted for by a slowing of conduction in the optic tracts (9,10); it is therefore possible that such late positivities are not to be interpreted, in all cases, as delayed P100 potentials. For diagnostic purposes this question may seem speculative, since this type of response is obviously abnormal, but a correct interpretation becomes crucial for follow-up studies using repeated VEP recording in MS patients.

In this study, checkboard-reversal VEPs were studied in normals and MS patients with different sizes and contrasts of squares in order to investigate whether the modifications of VEPs induced by changing the stimulus parameters could be of any help for the analysis of abnormal responses in MS patients.

METHODS

Recording Procedure

Monocular stimulation by checkerboard pattern reversal was produced on a commercially available black-and-white television set by a pattern generator as previously described by Arden et al. (1). The size of the whole stimulus field was of 15° horizontally and 12° vertically, the subject being seated at a distance of 150 cm from the screen in a dark, sound-treated room.

The following stimuli were used: stimulus A, squares of 44′, luminance, 40 cd/m² for bright squares, 2.5 cd/m² for dark squares; stimulus B, squares of 22′, luminance, 40 cd/m² for bright squares, 2.5 cd/m² for dark squares; stimulus C, squares of 22′, luminance, 24 cd/m² for bright squares, 8.5 cd/m² for dark squares; stimulus D, squares of 5.5′, luminance, 40 cd/m² for bright squares, 2.5 cd/m² for dark squares.

The fixation point was a 24′ red target placed in the middle of the TV screen; the pupils were not dilated.

The VEPs were recorded simultaneously from a horizontally chain of six scalp disk electrodes placed over the occipital region at 3-cm intervals with the two medial ones at 1 cm from the middle and 5 cm above the inion. All six channels were referred to the interconnected earlobes. The ground electrode was placed on the forehead. The EEG was amplified through six Grass 7P5 amplifiers with a band-pass of 1 to 35 Hz (6 dB down). The averaging was conducted on line by means of a LABO 16 computer (7) triggered by the visual stimulator; 100 sweeps were averaged with an analysis time of 360 msec (1,024 samples). When necessary, a larger number of sweeps (up to 400) were used to obtain the response. The EEG was continuously recorded during visual stimulation; artifacted sweeps were rejected by the computer. The frequency of the pattern reversal was 1 Hz; peak latencies were automatically measured by the computer.

In the subjects whose VEPs were made of two positive peaks (see Fig. 1),

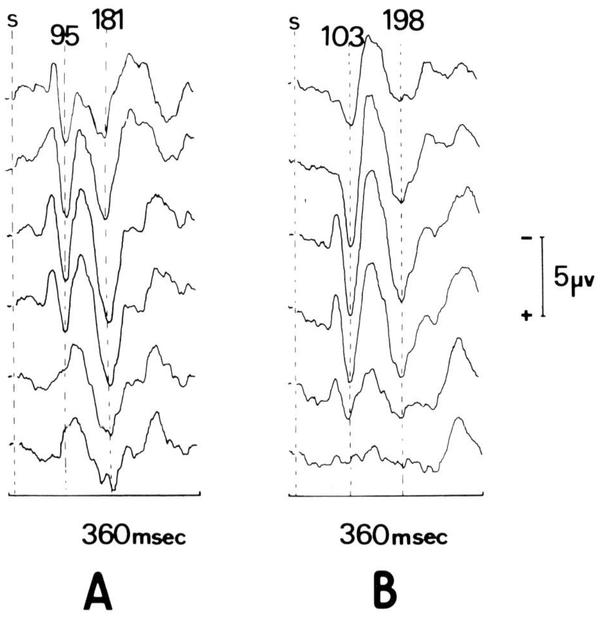

FIG. 1. Normal VEPs with two positive peaks. This type of response was observed in normals and in MS patients. With type B stimulus (22′ squares), the P100 component is better defined than with type A stimulus (44′ squares). The six occipital leads are represented: **top,** two right occipital leads; **middle,** two medial occipital leads; **bottom,** two left occipital leads.

the culmination latency of the first positive component was chosen providing that this component was recorded with its maximal amplitude in the medial occipital region, even though it was not the major positive wave. The use of different types of stimuli was found to be helpful in most of the cases to identify the P100 as demonstrated in Fig. 1.

The Student's test for paired data and *r* coefficient for regression line were used for statistics.

Normal Subjects

Normative data were obtained in 31 subjects (18 males and 13 females) aged 29 ± 6 years (mean ± SD), members of the medical staff of the hospital. All had normal visual acuity (10/10 for both eyes) with refraction correction when necessary.

Patients

One hundred and fifty patients (73 males, 77 females) aged 39 ± 12 years (mean ± SD) with definite (63 cases) or probable/possible (87 cases) multiple sclerosis were selected for this study. The McAlpine's criteria (8) were used for classification of patients. Twenty patients had suffered from unilateral (11 cases) or bilateral optic neuritis; two patients had unilateral or bilateral (one case) acute optic neuritis. In the 128 remaining cases, no history of optic neuritis was noted.

When the VEP recording was carried out, the visual acuity was normal for both eyes in 128 patients (256 eyes); the complementary ophtalmological examination (28-hues Farnsworth test, Goldmann campimetry, optic fundi) was normal in 110 of these subjects (220 eyes) and showed unilateral (six cases) or bilateral (12 cases) abnormalities in the 18 remaining patients. Twenty-two patients had low visual acuity (less than 6/10) for one eye (14 cases) or both eyes (8 cases) at the time of the VEP study.

RESULTS

Normative Data

In normal subjects (Fig. 2), a N70–P100–N140 complex was constantly observed in the median–occipital leads except for the highest spatial frequency stimulus (5.5′). This complex could, in some instances, be followed by a later positive wave the amplitude of which could be higher than that of the P100 component itself (Fig. 1). With the 5.5′ squares, the P100 potential was inconstant and, when observed, of much lower amplitude than with other types of stimulation (see Fig. 2). For this reason, the 5.5′ squares were considered as unsuitable for diagnostic purposes in patients with MS; thus, although this type of stimula-

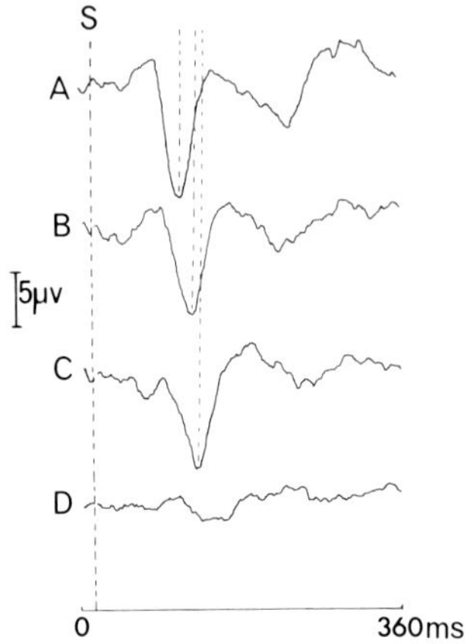

FIG. 2. Normal VEPs (medial occipital lead). The decrease of the angular size of the squares from 44′ to 22′ (A and B, respectively) does not modify the amplitude of the P100 potential but delays the peaking latency of P100. With 5.5′ squares (stimulus D), the amplitude of the response is lowered and the latency delayed. When decreasing the contrast with a constant square size (B and C) the latency of P100 is delayed without significant morphological change.

tion has been performed in all normals and patients, the results of this investigation will not be detailed in this paper.

As shown in Table 1, a significant increase of the P100 latency was observed when either the size or the contrast of squares decreased. This increase of P100 mean latency was much more significant for contrast decrement with a constant square size ($t = 7.72$; $p = 1.2 \times 10^{-7}$) than for square size decrement with a constant contrast ($t = 2.315$; $p = 2.4 \times 10^{-2}$). The amplitudes of the P100 potential and the interocular latency differences did not vary significantly with size or contrast. A high degree of linear correlation was found between the P100 latencies for left and right eyes for all types of stimulus. For each type of stimulation, the upper normal limit of P100 latency was calculated by adding 2.5 SD to mean value.

TABLE 1. *Normative data in controls*

	Stimulus A	Stimulus B	Stimulus C
P100 latency (msec) (mean value)	100.2	102.2	107.2
Upper normal Limit of P100 latency (msec) (mean + 2.5 SD)	115.8	118.0	125.0
Linear correlation Between right and left eye P100 latencies	$r = 0.705$ $p = 9.6 \times 10^{-6}$	$r = 0.695$ $p = 1.38 \times 10^{-5}$	$r = 0.87$ $p = 1.2 \times 10^{-7}$
Mean interocular difference of P100 latencies +2.5 SD (msec)	3.4 + 8.3	3.3 + 9	3.0 + 7
Mean amplitude of P100 ±SD (μV)	5.4 ± 2	5.1 ± 2	5.0 ± 2
Linear correlation Between right and left eyes P100 amplitudes	$r = 0.68$ $p = 3.04 \times 10^{-5}$	$r = 0.78$ $p = 4.8 \times 10^{-7}$	$r = 0.70$ $p = 1.38 \times 10^{-5}$

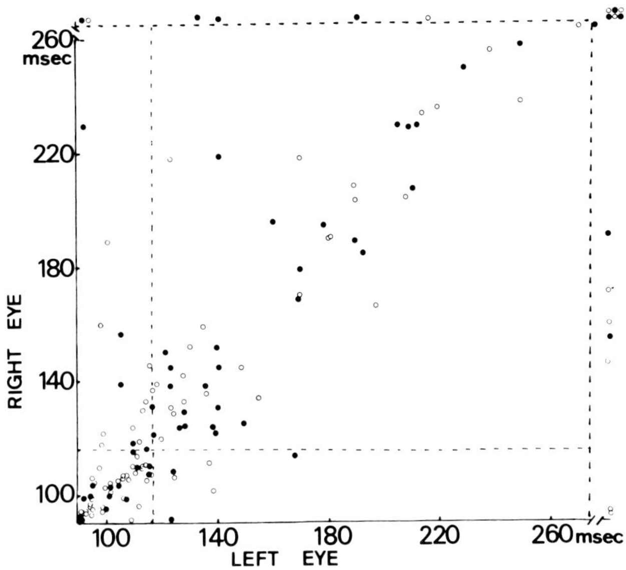

FIG. 3. VEP latencies in 150 MS patients (stimulus, 44′ squares; contrast, 40/2.5 cd/m²). *Black dots,* definite MS; *circles,* possible or probable MS. Absent responses are represented out of the frame. The upper limits of normal latencies (mean + 2.5 SD) are indicated by *dotted lines.*

Patients

As shown in Figs. 3–5, in which latencies for left and right eyes are plotted for each patient, the distribution of VEP latencies was found to be grossly bimodal. This was observed with the three types of stimulus studied in patients (stimuli A, B, and C). The first group corresponds to well-defined negative–positive negative VEPs with a normal or delayed P100 component (Fig. 6). In this group, the P100 latency was not over 170 msec in almost all cases. The second group is made of late and morphologically abnormal positive peaks with a latency over 180 msec in most instances (Fig. 7) and of responses for which the measurement of a latency was not possible because of a very poor definition and low amplitude.

In 70% of eyes, the VEPs were found to be the same with the different types of stimulus, the only modification being a slight increase of the P100 latency when changing from stimulus A to B or C. These shifts of latencies were of the same order as those observed in controls and occurred only when the N70, P100, N140 complex was well defined with stimulus A (Fig. 6). In 30% of cases, clear changes of VEPs occurred when the size of the squares was decreased and or the contrast of the checkerboard lowered. These changes of stimulus parameters decreased the amplitude of the responses and altered the morphology of the potentials so that the number of absent responses and of late and morphologically abnormal VEPs was higher with stimulus B or C

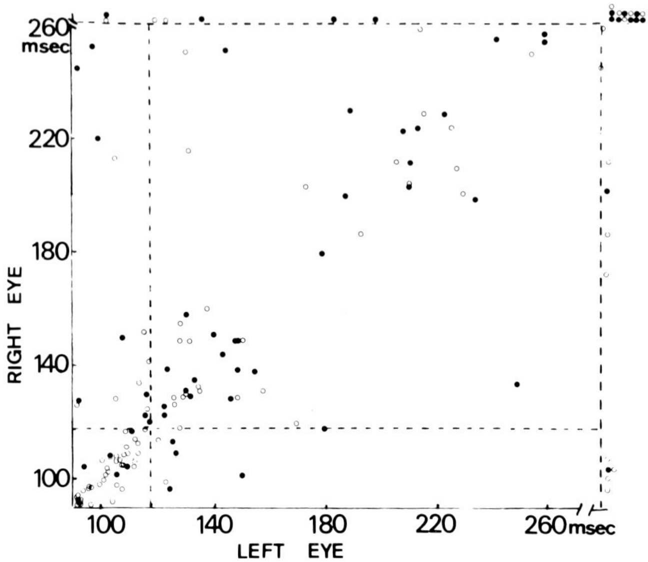

FIG. 4. VEP latencies in 150 MS patients (22′ squares; contrast, 40/2.5 cd/m²). Same symbols as in Fig. 3.

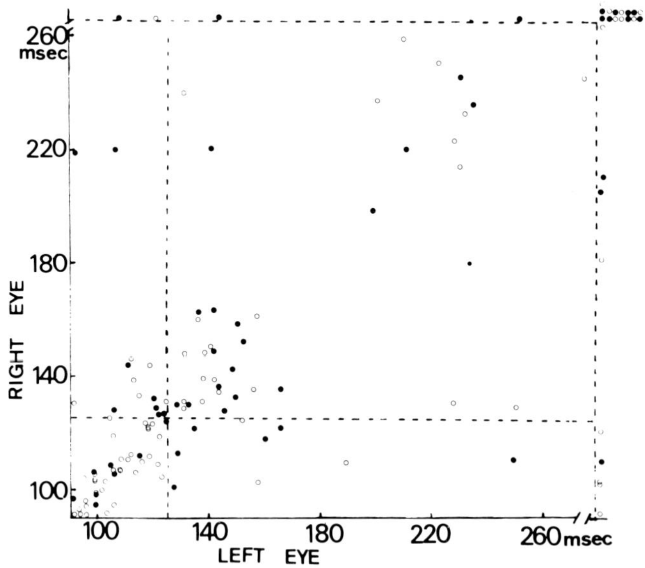

FIG. 5. VEP latencies in 150 MS patients (22′ squares; contrast, 24/8.5 cd/m²). Same symbols as in Fig. 3.

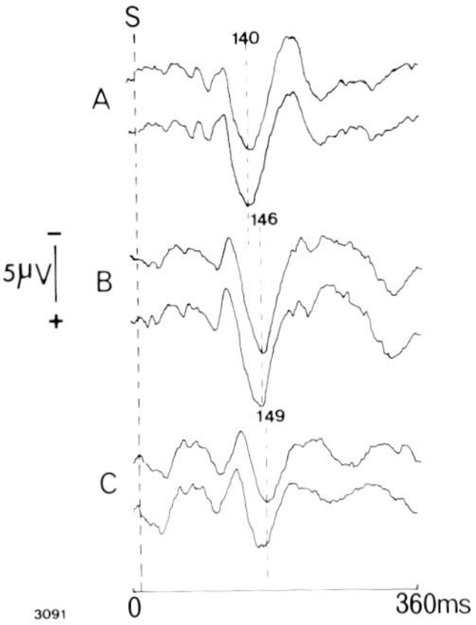

FIG. 6. Delayed P100 potential (unaltered morphology). The two medial occipital leads are represented for each type of stimulus, A, B, and C.

than with stimulus A (Figs. 3, 4, and 5). When using stimulus B or C, we observed in only a few instances a shift of the P100 latency out of the normal range for eyes with normal VEP latencies following type A stimulation. This occurred for 15 eyes with stimulus B and for 16 eyes with stimulus C (Fig. 8).

The percentages of patients with abnormal VEPs (i.e., delayed P100 or late positive morphologically abnormal peak or absent responses for one eye at least) according to the different types of stimulus are given in Table 2. It appears that the checkerboard made of 22′ squares of 20% contrast (stimulus C) was the most efficient stimulus; however, this increment of efficiency was mainly the result of a higher percentage of absent and of poorly defined VEPs

DISCUSSION AND CONCLUDING REMARKS

In normal subjects, the P100 latency was found to be significantly increased by lowering either the size or the contrast of squares; this result is in agreement

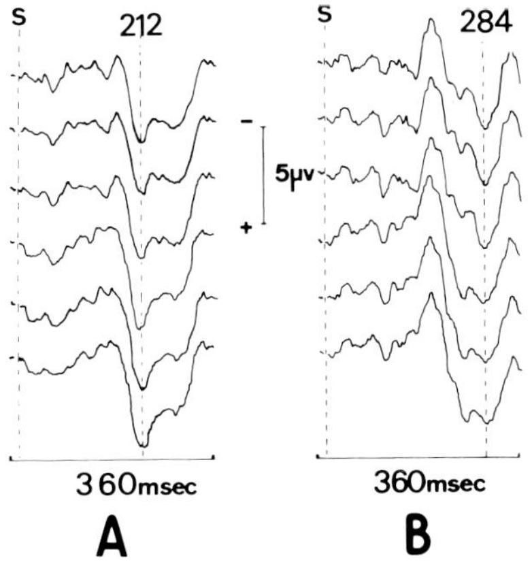

FIG. 7. Late positive response (abnormal morphology). Traces as in Fig. 1.

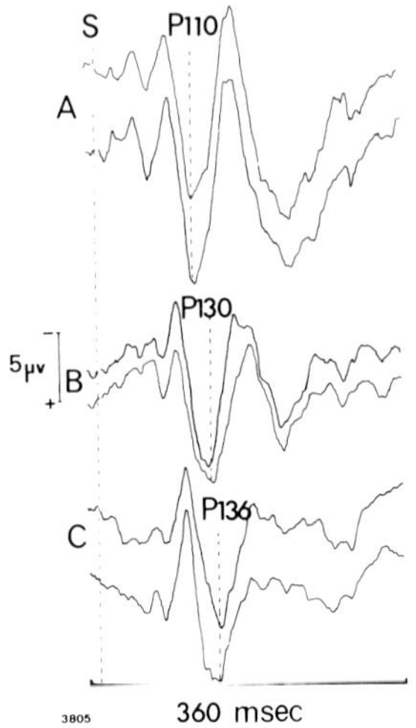

FIG. 8. Normal P100 latency with type A stimulus **(A)** becoming abnormally delayed with B and C stimuli **(B,C)** in a patient with possible MS (no history of optic neuritis, normal ophthalmological investigations). Only the two medial occipital leads are represented.

with those of Meienberg et al. (11) who described a similar phenomenon with a TV pattern. However, these authors compared two stimuli that differed with respect to size of stimulated field and size and contrast of squares all together. Our data suggest that the contrast of squares is certainly the most important factor in the variability of the P100 latency. Duwaer and Spekreijse (3) did not observe a significant increase of P100 latency when comparing 20′ and 50′ squares (TV set) in 11 normal subjects. However, the mean latency with the small-sized squares was a little longer; with a larger population of subjects, this difference might have become significant. The amplitude of P100 was found to be unmodified when comparing 44′ and 22′ squares with a constant contrast or 22′ squares with two different contrasts. Arden et al. (1) and Spekreijse et al. (12) reported that the amplitude of the P100 potential reaches its maximal value with a 20% contrast between bright and dark squares and with square sizes of 15′ to 20′.

As previously shown by Leserve and Remond (6) for pattern appearance and by Bartl et al. (2) for pattern reversal, 5.5′ squares evoked a low-amplitude potential in our normal subjects and were found unreliable in MS patients. Our data demonstrate that the diagnostic value of VEPs in MS patients may

TABLE 2. *Frequency of MS patients with abnormal VEPs according to stimulus parameters*

	Stimulus A		Stimulus B		Stimulus C	
	N	%	*N*	%	*N*	%
Definite MS (63 cases)	48	76	53	84	52	83
Possible or probable MS (87 cases)	52	60	56	64	60	69
Total No. of patients (150 cases)	100	66	109	73	112	75

be slightly increased by combining the three types of stimulus rather than using any one stimulus alone, the lowest percentage of VEP abnormalities (66%) being obtained with the largest and highest contrast squares (stimulus A), and the highest abnormality percentage with the smallest and lowest contrast squares (75%). Meienberg et al. (11) reported a certain degree of variability on repeated stimulation with a constant stimulus, but they never observed a shift of P100 latency beyond the upper normal limits in normals. Thus, the VEP changes observed in our patients when the stimulus parameters were changed were probably not consequences of the repetition of stimulation during the same recording session.

With any of the stimuli we used, we observed a gap between the latencies of delayed P100 potentials with normal morphologies (i.e., N70–P100–N140 complex) and the latencies of late positive abnormally shaped responses. Our opinion is that for this latter type of response, the P100 potential is to be considered as absent. Thus, it seems more reliable for a quantitative follow-up study based on repeated and comparative measurements of VEP latencies to select patients with a well-defined N70–P100–N140 complex on the first recording.

ACKNOWLEDGMENTS

Thanks are due to Ms. B. Demarcq and Ms. M. Piccolo for their invaluable help in the preparation of the manuscript.

REFERENCES

1. Arden, G. B., Faulkner, D. J., and Mair, C. (1977): A versatile television pattern generator for visual evoked potentials. In: *Visual Evoked Potentials in Man, New Developments,* edited by J. E. Desmedt. pp. 90–109. Clarendon Press, Oxford.
2. Bartl, G., Van Lith, G. G. M., and Van Marle, G. W. (1978): Cortical potentials evoked by a TV pattern reversal stimulus with varying check sizes and stimulus fields. *Br. J. Ophthalmol.,* 62:216–219.
3. Duwaer, A. L., and Spekreijse, H. (1978): Latency of luminance and contrast evoked potentials in multiple sclerosis patients. *Electroencephalogr. Clin. Neurophysiol.,* 45:244–258.
4. Halliday, A. M., and McDonald, W. I. (1972): Delayed visual evoked response in optic neuritis. *Lancet,* 1:982–985.
5. Halliday, A. M., McDonald, W. I., and Mushin, J. (1973): Visual evoked responses in diagnosis of multiple sclerosis. *Br. Med. J.,* 4:661–664.
6. Lesevre, N., and Remond, A. (1972): Potentiels Evoques par l'apparition de pattern, Effets de la dimension du pattern et de la densite des contrastes. *Electroencephalogr. Clin. Neurophysiol.,* 32:593–604.
7. Maraval, G., Pernier, J., Peronnet, F., Echallier, J. F., Gerin, P., and Mauguiere, F. (1980): EVØQ: Systeme configurable de stimulation automatique et d' enregistrement des potentiels evoques moyens sur miniordinateur, *Int. J. B. Comput.,* II:225–239.
8. McAlpine, D., Lumsden, C. E., and Acheson, E. D. (1972): *Multiple Sclerosis, a Reappraisal.* Livingstone Press, Edinburgh.
9. McDonald, W. I. (1974): Pathophysiology in multiple sclerosis. *Brain,* 97:179–196.
10. McDonald, W. I. (1977): Pathophysiology of conduction in central nerve fibres. In: *Visual Evoked Potentials in Man: New Developments,* Edited by J. E. Desmedt, pp. 427–437. Clarendon Press, Oxford.

11. Meienberg, O., Kutak, L., Smolenski, C., and Ludin, H. P. (1979): Pattern reversal evoked cortical responses in normals. A study of different methods of stimulation and potential reproductibility. *J. Neurol.,* 222:81–93.
12. Spekreijse, H., Estevez, O., and Reits, D. (1977): Visual evoked potentials and the physiological analysis of visual processes in man. In: *Visual Evoked Potentials in Man: New Developments,* edited by J. E. Desmedt, pp. 16–89. Clarendon Press, Oxford.

Clinical Applications of Evoked Potentials in Neurology,
edited by J. Courjon, F. Mauguiere, and M. Revol.
Raven Press, New York © 1982.

A Comparison of Clinical Neuroophthalmological Findings and Pattern Shift Visual Evoked Potentials in Multiple Sclerosis

Elizabeth B. Brooks and Keith H. Chiappa

The Robert S. Schwab Computer Facility of the Clinical Neurophysiology Laboratory, Department of Neurology, Massachusetts General Hospital, and Harvard Medical School, Boston, Massachusetts 02114

The relative sensitivity of the clinical neuroophthalmological examination as compared with pattern shift visual evoked potentials (PSVEPs) has been disputed in light of the cost of the latter. In 198 patients with multiple sclerosis (MS), we compared PSVEP results with those elements of the routine ophthalmological examination that pertain to optic nerve function (visual fields by confrontation and/or Goldmann perimetry, pupillary responses, funduscopic examination, absence or presence of red color desaturation, and history). When the PSVEP was normal, the clinical examination was always normal. Even when the PSVEP was abnormal, the clinical examination was normal to a surprising degree. Thus, the PSVEP provides a significant extension of the clinical neuroophthalmological examination.

PATIENTS AND METHOD

One hundred ninety-eight patients (121 females and 77 males; age range 13–74 years) who had MS according to the McAlpine diagnostic criteria (11) were studied.

The stimulus, a black-and-white checkerboard pattern, was projected onto a translucent screen using a commercial slide projector and a mirror. The pattern was shifted horizontally across one square's width by movements of a rotating mirror at a rate of 2/sec. The entire checkerboard subtended 8.8°, and each check was 16′. The difference in luminance between the black and white squares was 1.7 log foot lamberts at 1 m. The responses were recorded from midline scalp electrodes at C_z, mP_z (a location one-half the distance between P_z and O_z), and O_z (international 10–20 system for electrode placement), using a linked-ears reference (see Fig. 1). The differential amplifiers had a bandpass of 1 to 100 Hz (half-amplitude frequency). A poststimulus analysis time of 512 msec was used with a sampling rate of at least 500 samples per second per channel. The patient was seated in a chair 1 m from the screen and was instructed to

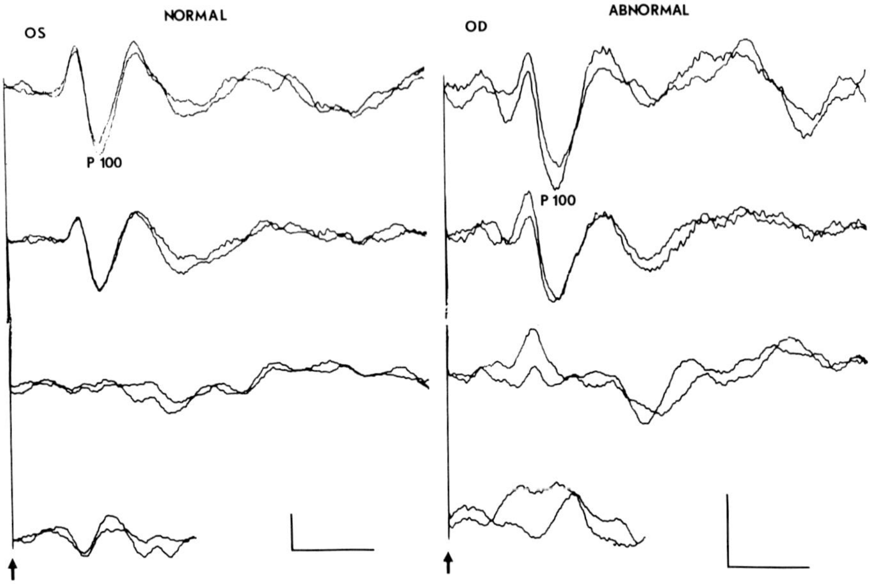

FIG. 1. Pattern shift visual evoked potential recorded from one patient following stimulation of each eye individually. The pattern shift occurred at the *arrow,* and analysis time was 512 msec. Left eye response is normal at 115 msec. Right eye response is abnormal, as the P100 peak is delayed in latency at 135 msec. The montage, from top to bottom, is O_z–C_z, O_z–ref, mP_z–ref, and C_z–ref (reference is linked-ears). Relative positivity at O_z produces a downwards trace deflection. Calibration marks are 100 msec and 5 μV.

fixate on a red dot placed in the center of the screen. Following stimulation of each eye individually, 128 responses were averaged; the nonstimulated eye was covered with an eye patch. Room luminance was held constant during testing.

The results of the clinical neuroophthalmological examination were tabulated retrospectively for the 198 patients. Not all patients had comments on all portions of the examination pertaining to optic nerve function (visual fields, pupillary responses, funduscopic examination, absence or presence of red color desaturation, and history).

We have previously studied normal subjects using this equipment (12). The normal value for peak latency of the major positive peak (P100) was 102.3 $\pm$ 5.1 msec (mean $\pm$ SD), and the intereye latency difference was 1.3 $\pm$ 2.0 msec. The mean + 3 SD was used as the upper limit of normal; thus, the upper limit for normal absolute peak latency of the P100 peak was 118 msec and for intereye difference was 8 msec. Figure 1 illustrates a normal and abnormal response from the left and right eye of a patient with multiple sclerosis.

RESULTS

Of the 198 patients studied, 60 (30%) had normal PSVEPs. Their neuroophthalmological examinations were always normal in all elements except for history. Of the 138 patients with abnormal PSVEPs, 96% had normal visual fields by confrontation, and 55% had normal fields by Goldmann perimetry. Pupillary responses were normal in 74%, and the funduscopic examination was normal in 39%. There was no red color desaturation in 27% of these patients; however, testing was done on only a small number of cases. The ophthalmological examination was normal in 33% of the patients with an abnormal PSVEP, and in 30% both the clinical examination and the history were negative, although the PSVEP was abnormal. Detailed results of the PSVEP relative to the findings of the clinical neuroophthalmological examination for the definite, probable, and possible MS groups are given in Table 1. In the table, the patients are divided into two groups depending on whether their PSVEP was normal or abnormal. The percentages given are the number of patients in that group (normal or abnormal PSVEP versus MS category versus clinical element) who had no abnormality found in that clinical element.

DISCUSSION

The patients were chosen because they had had a PSVEP as part of their work-up for MS, not because they had had a special, detailed neuroophthalmological examination. The intent was to see how PSVEP results compared with the findings of the routine clinical neuroophthalmological examination as the average neurologic or ophthalmologic clinician performed it. Thus, not all patients had comments on all portions of the examination.

Asselman et al. (1) and Halliday et al. (5) discussed the relationship between various elements of the neuroophthalmological examination and the PSVEP. They found that 46% and 43% of their patients, respectively, had normal funduscopic examinations but abnormal PSVEPs, consistent with our value of 39%. Asselman et al. (1) also found that 28% of their patients with a normal complete eye examination had abnormal PSVEPs, consistent with 33% of ours.

However, most authors reporting on PSVEPs in MS have concerned themselves primarily with the relationship between PSVEP results and the presence or absence of a history pertaining to optic neuritis. The percentage of patients with an abnormal PSVEP and no history of optic neuritis has varied widely from 93% as reported by Halliday et al. (5) to 36% as reported by Shahrokhi et al. (12; see also 1–3,6–10,14,15).

In the present study, we found that 30% of our patients with a normal eye examination and no history of optic neuritis had an abnormal PSVEP. Presumably, the variability between studies is caused by many factors including diagnostic and historical criteria and rigor, patient population and type, and presentation of the stimulus.

Swart and Millac (13) compared PSVEPs and the flight of colors (FOC) test (based on the number of colors and the duration for which they are seen with eyes closed after a bright light is shined in one eye). In 21 patients, they found that PSVEP and FOC results were the same, either both normal or both abnormal, for all except two. In one of these, the PSVEP was normal

TABLE 1. *PSVEPs and clinical neuroophthalmological findings in patients with MS*

Neuroophthalmological finding		MS classification			
	PSVEP	Definite	Probable	Possible	Total
Normal fields (clinically)	Abnormal	41/43 (95%)	23/24 (96%)	11/11 (100%)	75/78 (96%)
	Normal	10/10 (100%)	16/16 (100%)	30/30 (100%)	56/56 (100%)
Normal fields (formal)	Abnormal	17/30 (57%)	11/19 (58%)	3/7 (43%)	31/56 (55%)
	Normal	5/5 (100%)	4/4 (100%)	11/11 (100%)	20/20 (100%)
Normal pupillary responses	Abnormal	48/71 (68%)	33/40 (83%)	14/18 (78%)	95/129 (74%)
	Normal	11/11 (100%)	16/16 (100%)	30/30 (100%)	57/57 (100%)
Normal fundi	Abnormal	21/75 (28%)	19/42 (45%)	12/17 (71%)	52/134 (39%)
	Normal	11/11 (100%)	17/17 (100%)	28/28 (100%)	56/56 (100%)
No red color desaturation	Abnormal	1/10 (10%)	2/6 (33%)	3/6 (50%)	6/22 (27%)
	Normal	—	1/1 (100%)	1/1 (100%)	2/2 (100%)
Normal eye exam (all above)	Abnormal	18/78 (23%)	16/43 (37%)	11/17 (65%)	45/138 (33%)
	Normal	11/11 (100%)	18/18 (100%)	31/31 (100%)	60/60 (100%)
Normal eye exam plus no history of optic neuritis	Abnormal	16/78 (21%)	16/43 (37%)	10/17 (59%)	42/138 (30%)
	Normal	10/11 (91%)	16/18 (89%)	31/31 (100%)	57/60 (95%)

and the FOC was abnormal, and in the other the PSVEP was abnormal and the FOC was normal. In their study, however, the only diagnostic criterion used was absolute latency of the P100 peak. The fact that they did not use intereye latency difference decreased the sensitivity of the PSVEP.

It is apparent that the PSVEP reveals a significant proportion of abnormalities in the visual system that have not been revealed by the routine neuroophthalmological examination and/or history. The PSVEP, therefore, is a very sensitive adjunct to the routine clinical neuroophthalmological examination.

ACKNOWLEDGMENT

This study was supported in part by the Edwin Minot Fund for Research in Electroencephalography.

REFERENCES

1. Asselman, P., Chadwick, D. W., and Marsden, C. D. (1975): Visual evoked responses in the diagnosis and management of patients suspected of multiple sclerosis. *Brain,* 98:261–282.

2. Celesia, G. G. (1978): Visual evoked potentials in neurological disorders. *Am. J. EEG Technol.,* 18:47–59.
3. Collins, D. W. K., Black, J. L., and Mastaglia, F. L. (1978): Pattern-reversal visual evoked potential: Method of analysis and results in multiple sclerosis. *J. Neurol. Sci.,* 36:83–95.
4. Halliday, A. M., McDonald, W. I., and Mushin, J. (1972): Delayed visual evoked response in optic neuritis. *Lancet,* 1:982–985.
5. Halliday, A. M., McDonald, W. I., and Mushin, J. (1973): Visual evoked response in diagnosis of multiple sclerosis. *Br. Med. J.,* 4:661–664.
6. Hennerici, M., Wenzel, D., and Freund, H. J. (1977): The comparison of small-size rectangle and checkerboard stimulation for the evaluation of delayed visual evoked responses in patients suspected of multiple sclerosis. *Brain,* 100:119–136.
7. Hoeppner, T., and Lolas, F. (1978): Visual evoked responses and visual symptoms in multiple sclerosis. *J. Neurol. Neurosurg. Psychiatry,* 41:493–498.
8. Hume, A. L., and Cant, B. R. (1976): Pattern visual evoked potentials in the diagnosis of multiple sclerosis and other disorders. *Proc. Aust. Assoc. Neurol.,* 13:7–13.
9. Mastaglia, F. L., Black, J. L., and Collins, D. W. K. (1976): Visual and spinal evoked potentials in diagnosis of multiple sclerosis. *Med. J.,* 2:732.
10. Matthews, W. B., Small, D. G., Small, M., and Pountney, E. (1977): Pattern reversal evoked visual potential in the diagnosis of multiple sclerosis. *J. Neurol. Neurosurg. Psychiatry,* 40:1009–1014.
11. McAlpine, D., Lumsden, C. E., and Acheson, E. D. (1972): *Multiple Sclerosis: A Reappraisal.* Churchill Livingstone, Edinburgh.
12. Shahrokhi, F., Chiappa, K. H., and Young, R. R. (1978): Pattern shift visual evoked responses. 200 patients with optic neuritis and/or multiple sclerosis. *Arch. Neurol.,* 35:65–71.
13. Swart, S., and Millac, P. (1980): A comparison of flight of colors with visually evoked responses in patients with multiple sclerosis. *J. Neurol. Neurosurg. Psychiatry,* 43:550–551.
14. Trojaborg, W., and Petersen, E. (1979): Visual and somatosensory evoked cortical potentials in multiple sclerosis. *J. Neurol. Neurosurg. Psychiatry,* 42:323–330.
15. Zeese, J. A. (1977): Pattern visual evoked responses in multiple sclerosis. *Arch. Neurol.,* 34:314–316.

Clinical Applications of Evoked Potentials in Neurology,
edited by J. Courjon, F. Mauguiere, and M. Revol.
Raven Press, New York © 1982.

Improved Diagnostic Yield in Evaluation of Multiple Sclerosis Using Critical Frequency of Photic Driving with Pattern Reversal-Evoked Potentials

*Stanley N. Cohen, *Karl Syndulko, *Edward C. Hansch, *Eugene Gilden, *Kenneth Phillips, *Wallace W. Tourtellotte, and **Alfred R. Potvin

**Neurology and Research Services, VA Wadsworth Medical Center, Los Angeles, California, 90073 and Department of Neurology, University of California at Los Angeles School of Medicine, Los Angeles, California 90024; and **Biomedical Engineering Program, University of Texas at Arlington, Arlington, Texas 76019*

Pattern reversal-evoked potentials (PVEP) have been shown to be effective diagnostic tools in the evaluation of patients suspected of having multiple sclerosis (MS) (1,5,6,8). The diagnostic yield is greater in patients with definite MS than with probable and possible MS. The percentage of abnormal results is also higher in patients with a history of optic neuritis than in those with no history of optic neuritis (4,8). Prior reports suggest that adding the critical frequency of photic driving (CFPD) can increase the sensitivity of the test to visual abnormalities in MS (2,3). We are reporting on our experience testing 100 consecutive patients with definite, probable, and possible MS using both PVEP and CFPD.

METHODS

The PVEP and CFPD were tested in each eye separately by methods described by Cohen et al. (3). The upper limit of normal for P100 was 117 msec (mean plus 2 standard deviations). Normal CFPD was defined as the presence of averaged photic driving at flash stimulus rates of 41 Hz or higher.

Patients were referred for testing from the MS Research Ward and general neurology ward at Wadsworth VA Hospital. Some patients were referred from neurologists in the community. Patients were classified as either definite MS or probable or possible MS by their referring neurologist using the criteria of Rose et al. (7). Historical data regarding optic neuritis as well as physical examination including funduscopic examination and visual acuity tests were taken from information provided by the referring neurologist. Cerebrospinal fluid testing was performed in the laboratory of Dr. Tourtellotte. Abnormality was defined as an IgG synthesis of greater than 3.0 mg/day (9). Normative data were obtained from hospital personnel and healthy male volunteers.

RESULTS

Results of the testing are presented in Table 1. The difference in percentage of patients showing abnormal responses between PVEP used alone and PVEP used concomitantly with CFPD was statistically significant in the "all MS patients" category ($p < 0.02$) and in the "possible and probable MS" category ($p < 0.05$). Although the other clinical categories did not show a significant difference between the use of pattern alone and both tests concomitantly, each category showed the trend of increased percentage of abnormal results for concurrent use of the two tests.

DISCUSSION

Our PVEP results are similar to those reported by other EP laboratories (1,4,6,8). The PVEP demonstrated the highest percentage of abnormalities in patients with definite MS and in patients with symptoms and/or signs of a

TABLE 1. Percentages of MS patients showing abnormal responses on PVEP, CFPD, and both tests

	PVEP	CFPD	Both
All MS patients (*N*=100)	82	74	92
Normal funduscopic exam and visual acuity (*N*=48)	82	67	94
Negative history for optic neuritis (*N*=41)	84	70	97
Negative ophthalmic history and exam (*N*=35)	89	70	97
Negative ophthalmic history and exam and CSF exam (*N*=9)	77	56	89
Definite MS (*N*=75)	89	78	99
Normal funduscopic exam and visual acuity (*N*=31)	93	82	100
Negative history for optic neuritis (*N*=28)	93	86	100
Negative ophthalmic history and exam (*N*=25)	96	83	100
Possible and probable MS (*N*=25)	64	55	71
Normal funduscopic exam and visual acuity (*N*=17)	61	41	77
Negative history for optic neuritis (*N*=13)	64	46	91
Negative ophthalmic history and exam (*N*=10)	70	40	90
Negative ophthalmic history and negative CSF exam (*N*=7)	75	43	88

history of optic neuritis. The CFPD results are similar to results reported by Celesia and Daly (2). They found 56% abnormality in possible and probable MS and 42% abnormal in the group of all MS patients. Our data for possible and probable MS correspond very well to theirs. Our percentage of abnormality was greater for all MS patients (74% versus 42%). This difference could be caused by a number of factors. First, criteria for abnormality was different. Celesia and Daly used a sliding scale dependent on age. We chose an arbitrary cutoff at 41 Hz to define normal. Second, technique differed slightly in that we placed the photic stimulator further from the patient. Third, the patient population may have differed. Many of our patients with definite MS were referred from a population with a longstanding disease. The chronicity of the disease may increase the possibility of an abnormal result. In analyzing their PVEP data, Celesia and Daly used interocular latency asymmetry and latency of an N1 wave as well as P100 latency to define normalcy. Thus, their PVEP data are not directly comparable to ours. However, they too found that the use of CFPD with PVEP increases the percentage of abnormal results in MS patients as compared to the use of PVEP alone.

Testing of CFPD can be conducted in most laboratories currently performing VEP testing by simply adding a photic stimulator. The test requires about 10 min per eye of additional testing time in a patient already "wired" for testing PVEP. The test requires minimal patient cooperation. In addition, CFPD seems to be valid in patients whose best corrected vision is too poor for proper assessment of PVEP.

We conclude that CFPD is of value in the diagnostic assessment of patients with MS. It should be routinely examined in patients being evaluated for MS with visual evoked potentials.

ACKNOWLEDGMENT

The authors would like to thank Ms. Karen Cohen for editorial support and Ms. Diane Guntrip and Ms. Diane Varnas for secretarial support.

REFERENCES

1. Asselman, P., Chadwick, D. W., and Marsden, C. D. (1975): Visual evoked responses in the diagnosis and management of patients suspected of multiple sclerosis. *Brain,* 98:261–282.
2. Celesia, G. G., and Daly, R. F. (1977): Visual electroencephalographic computer analysis (VECA). *Neurology,* 27:637–641.
3. Cohen, S. N., Syndulko, K., Tourtellotte, W. W., and Potvin, A. R. (1980): Critical frequency of photic driving in the diagnosis of multiple sclerosis. *Arch. Neurol.,* 37:80–83.
4. Halliday, A. M., McDonald, W. I., and Mushin, J. (1972): Delayed visual evoked response in optic neuritis. *Lancet,* 1:982–985.
5. Halliday, A. M., McDonald, W. I., and Mushin, J. (1973): Visual evoked response in diagnosis of multiple sclerosis. *Br. Med. J.,* 4:661–664.
6. Hennerici, M., Wenzel, D., and Freund, H.-J. (1977): The comparison of small-size rectangle and checkerboard stimulation for the evaluation of delayed visual evoked responses in patients suspected of multiple sclerosis. *Brain,* 100:119–136.

7. Rose, A. S., Ellison, G. W., Myers, L. W., and Tourtellotte, W. W. (1976): Criteria for the clinical diagnosis of multiple sclerosis. *Neurology,* 26:20–22.
8. Shahrokhi, F., Chiappa, K. H., and Young, R. R. (1978): Pattern shift visual evoked responses. *Arch. Neurol.,* 35:65–71.
9. Tourtellotte, W. W., Potvin, A. R., Fleming, J. O., Murthy, K. N., Levy, J., Syndulko, K., and Potvin, J. H. (1980): Validation of central nervous system IgG synthesis rate. *Neurology* 30:240–244.

Clinical Applications of Evoked Potentials in Neurology,
edited by J. Courjon, F. Mauguiere, and M. Revol.
Raven Press, New York © 1982.

The Pattern Visual Evoked Potential in the Clinical Assessment of Undiagnosed Spinal Cord Disease

*L. D. Blumhardt, **G. Barrett, and **A. M. Halliday

**University Department of Neurology, Radcliffe Infirmary, Oxford OX2 4HE, England; and **National Hospital for Nervous Diseases, London WC1 3BG, England*

A common problem in neurological practice is the typically middle-aged patient who presents with a slowly progressive spastic paraparesis with no signs of CNS disease outside the spinal cord. A proportion of these cases remains undiagnosed despite intensive investigations (8,10,15). If this group is followed for a period of 5 to 10 years, approximately one in five cases will develop features of multiple sclerosis (MS) (8,10). At autopsy, about one in three may be shown to have this disease (10).

The detection of clinically silent plaques in the optic pathways by pattern visual evoked potential (VEP) recording offers an objective and noninvasive method for distinguishing patients with demyelinating disease from the group of otherwise undiagnosed myelopathies. However, many published studies of the value of the VEP in patients with "possible" or "probable" MS have not identified those cases in whom disease is clinically limited to the spinal cord. Where this has been reported, the numbers of patients studied were small, and the proportion with abnormal VEPs varied widely from 0 to 78% (1,4,6,7,11–14).

In an attempt to clarify this situation, we report here our results in patients referred to our laboratory with undiagnosed spinal cord disease.

METHODS

Selection of Case Material

The hospital notes of all patients with undiagnosed spinal cord disease admitted to the National Hospitals for Nervous Diseases and referred for VEP recording during the 6-year study period, 1972 to 1977, were reviewed. The results of full clinical assessments by at least two staff neurologists were available in all cases.

The notes were searched for any objective or symptomatic evidence of involvement of the CNS outside the spinal cord. All patients with unequivocal evidence of previous optic neuritis or brainstem or cerebral hemisphere involvement were excluded. Also rejected were four patients with positive family histories of hereditary spastic paraplegia. Two patients who had first-degree blood relatives with MS were not excluded. Where there were inconsistencies between neurologists with respect to the presence of "soft" symptoms or signs above the neck of doubtful relevance, the decision to include or exclude the patient from the study was based on whether such features could be considered as unequivocal evidence of a pathological lesion elsewhere than the cord. There were 49 patients included in the study with one or more of these "soft" symptoms or signs. In no cases were there "appropriately associated" symptoms and signs, for example, vague blurring of the vision with possibly pale disks.

The clinical data, including the age at onset of symptoms, the progress of the disease up to the time of the VEP, neurological signs, results of investigations and VEP recording, and follow-up information, were entered into a computer for analysis. The results of routine hematology, biochemistry, tests for syphilis, serum B_{12}, X-rays of the spine, CSF protein, cells, and IgG/albumin ratio, and myelography were examined. The results of HLA tissue typing, oligoclonal banding of CSF protein, CAT scans, and sophisticated tests of brainstem and spinal cord function such as electronystagmography, AEP, SEP, and ESG were not available in sufficient cases to be analyzed.

One hundred and thirty-one patients satisfied the criteria for inclusion, their ages varying from 13 to 72 with a mean of 46 years. Ages varied with the clinical characteristics of the spinal disease (Table 1). The patients were divided into three groups according to the mode of presentation: acute or subacute cases; chronic relapsing cases; and chronic progressive cord syndromes. The first group contained 31 patients in whom cord symptoms developed over the course of hours or several days. It included nine cases of transverse myelitis. Thirty-six had a relapsing and remitting cord syndrome with an average of seven major relapses per patient. The remaining 64 chronic patients had a slowly progressive spinal cord syndrome of insidious onset. Ninety of the 131 patients

TABLE 1. *Clinical material: mean ages (years ± SD) at first symptom and VEP according to course of spinal disease*[a]

Clinical category	Age at first symptom	Age at VEP
Acute/subacute	37 ± 12	37 ± 12
(*N* = 31)	(13–61)	(13–61)
Chronic relapsing	35 ± 11	41 ± 12
(*N* = 36)	(14–54)	(19–64)
Chronic progressive	46 ± 12	52 ± 12
(*N* = 64)	(10–67)	(20–72)

[a] *N* = 131; ranges are shown in parentheses.

in the study had had at least one myelogram performed. Twenty were reported as showing abnormalities.

Stimulating and Recording Techniques

Detailed descriptions of our methodology have previously been published (6). The limits of the normal range in this study were based on the full-field (16° radius) monocular responses of 134 healthy subjects aged between 16 and 89 years. The upper limit of peak latency for the major full-field positive wave (P100) was defined as the mean + 2.5 SD. The upper limit (2.5 SD) for interocular latency differences was 8 msec. Amplitude criteria were not applied, but waveforms were deemed abnormal where there was such marked dispersion or attenuation of the responses that the P100 peak could not be reliably defined.

RESULTS

The overall proportion of patients with abnormal VEPs was 38/131 (29%), but the hit rate varied in the different clinical groups.

The 100 patients with chronic disease of more than 6 months' duration had a combined incidence of abnormalities of 35%. There was a slightly higher hit rate in the relapsing cases (36%) as compared with the progressive category (33%) (difference not significant). The chronic cases included 17 in whom symptoms or signs could be attributed, at least partly, to cord compression. Thus, the VEP abnormalities could be considered in relation to the results of myelography (Table 2).

The 16 chronic relapsing and 38 progressive cases with normal myelograms satisfy the criteria of the "early probable, or latent" and the "progressive probable" MS categories, respectively, of McDonald and Halliday's classification (9). Again, however, there was no significant difference in hit rate between the two subgroups, and the combined incidence was 28%. Further analysis was therefore carried out on all chronic patients with negative myelography.

When analyzed by time elapsed from first symptom to VEP, there appeared to be no significant differences among the three intervals (Table 3). However,

TABLE 2. *Proportion of abnormal VEP versus myelography result in clinical subgroups*

Clinical Category	Myelography			
	Not done	Normal	Abnormal	Totals
Acute/subacute ($N=31$)	1/13 (8%)	2/15 (13%)	0/3	3/31 (10%)
Chronic relapsing ($N=36$)	6/16 (38%)	5/16 (31%)	1/4	12/36 (33%)
Chronic progressive ($N=64$)	10/13 (77%)	10/38 (26%)	3/13 (23%)	23/64 (36%)

TABLE 3. *Proportion of cases with chronic undiagnosed spinal cord disease*[a] *(N = 54) with abnormal VEP versus interval from first symptom to VEP*

	≤3 years (*N* = 18)	3–6 years (*N* = 18)	More than 6 years (*N* = 18)
Abnormal/normal VEP	2/16 (11%)	7/11 (39%)	6/12 (33%)

[a] Normal myelograms.

there was a three fold increase in the hit rate when the VEP was recorded more than 3 years after symptoms began. Furthermore, this proportion of abnormal responses appeared to stabilize at approximately one-third despite the inclusion of some extremely long duration cases. The highest incidence of VEP abnormality was in those cases who did not have myelography (77%). This is likely to be an artifact of the clinical routine whereby some neurologists decided to perform myelography according to the VEP result. The alternative explanation, that the diagnosis of MS in this subgroup was possible on clinical grounds, seems unlikely on reviewing the clinical data.

Fifteen of the 20 patients with abnormal myelograms had normal VEPs. Myelography showed definite cervical cord compression in nine cases. Two further patients had narrow cervical canals with spondylotic changes but without definite evidence of cord compression. Four patients had compression of the thoracic cord from either a prolapsed disk (one case), angioma (one case), or meningioma (two cases). In two of these 15 cases, the CSF and follow-up information suggested the coexistence of MS (i.e., a possible false-negative rate of 13%).

Five patients had abnormal VEP and abnormal myelograms. In three of these cases, the evidence for cervical spondylotic myelopathy was equivocal, the X-rays showing only narrow cervical canals and spondylotic changes. Of these three cases, two have subsequently developed signs and symptoms suggestive of MS. In the remaining two cases, there was unequivocal evidence of cord compression caused, respectively, by a prolapsed cervical and thoracic disk. There was no clinical evidence of MS. After laminectomy, one patient (cervical compression) showed little change, but the other case made a marked recovery. Further follow-up data are awaited to confirm whether these two cases represent either VEP false positives or the coexistence of demyelination and cord compression.

The proportion of abnormal VEPs in patients with trivial symptoms or "soft" signs above the neck of doubtful significance was 14/49 (29%). Only one of 13 cases with visual symptoms that were deemed "insignificant" had an abnormal VEP. The incidence in the remaining cases without such "soft" signs and symptoms was also 29% (24/82).

Visual Evoked Potential Abnormalities

The majority of the abnormal responses were simple delays of the major positivity, but these were often associated with waveform changes. The major positivity was often broadened, and its peak was less well defined in the delayed responses which were also frequently reduced in amplitude. In a few patients, the waveform showed asymmetries or features similar to those recorded in patients with central scotomata (2,5). In a minority of responses, the potentials were so dispersed and attenuated that they could be considered abnormal on waveform grounds alone. There were no obvious differences between the pathological alterations of the VEP in this study and those recorded in patients after classical attacks of optic neuritis.

The 38 patients with abnormal responses included 17 with monocular and 21 with binocular abnormalities. The incidence of binocular abnormalities did not correlate with the duration of the disease. For example, bilateral delays could be found in patients with very short histories (Fig. 1) and monocular delays in cases with very longstanding spinal symptoms (Fig. 2). Responses of normal latency and waveform were on occasion recorded in spastic paraparesis

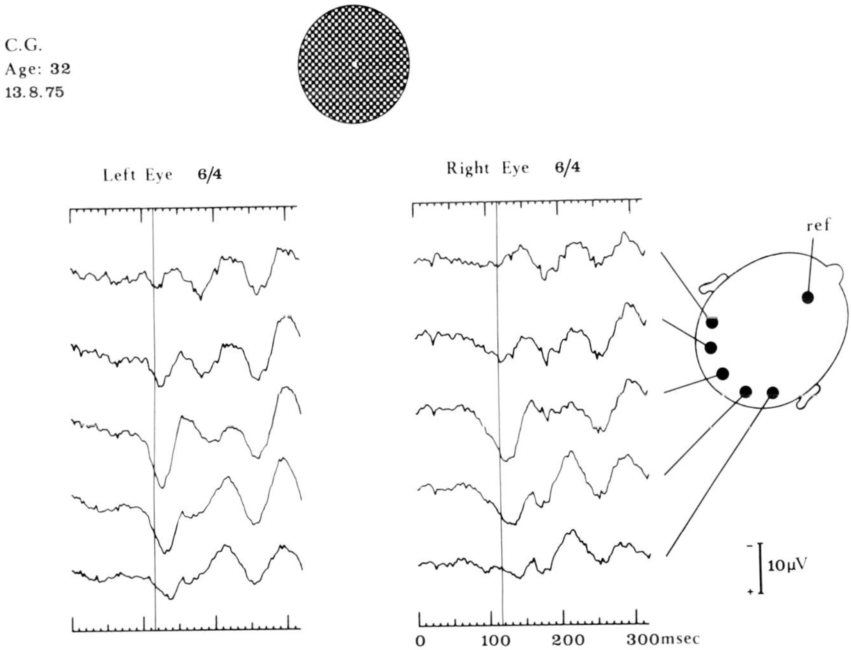

FIG. 1. Mild bilateral delays of VEP (126 and 125 msec) in a patient with a subacute (3-week) history of paraplegia. Note the broadened and blunted major positive wave from the right eye. The CSF contained abnormally increased cells and IgG. *Vertical lines* show upper limit for major positive peak.

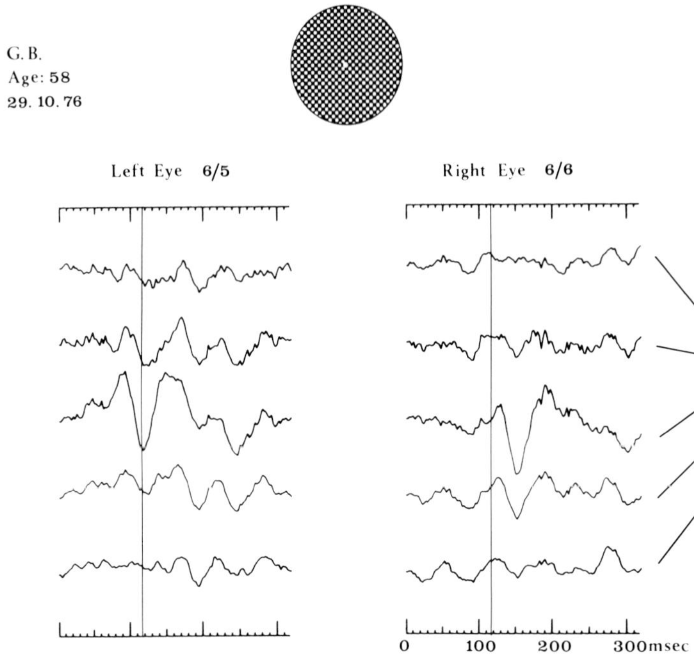

FIG. 2. Monocular delay (150 versus 117 msec) in a patient with a 15-year history of pure motor spinal cord syndrome (spastic quadraparesis). Both CSF and myelogram were normal.

of more than 25 years' duration (Fig. 3). In the 17 cases with normal myelograms and abnormal VEPs, there were seven monocular delays, eight binocular delays, and two cases with bilaterally abnormal waveforms. Two cases with monocular delays had associated waveform changes in the same or opposite eye. In 138 eyes of 69 patients with normal myelography, there were 133 recognizable major positive waves. The mean latency in the 30 affected eyes was 129.0 ± 12.4 msec compared with 106.3 ± 4.6 msec in the 103 unaffected eyes, a mean delay of 22.7 msec. The delayed responses were also smaller by an average of 3.5 μV for the left eyes and 2.0 μV for the right eyes, but these differences did not reach significance.

Acute/Subacute Clinical Category

Only three of the 31 patients in this category had abnormal responses, a detection rate of 10%. Of the 10 patients recorded within 1 month of the onset of symptoms, only one had an abnormal response (Fig. 1). No abnormalities were detected in the responses of the nine cases of transverse myelitis.

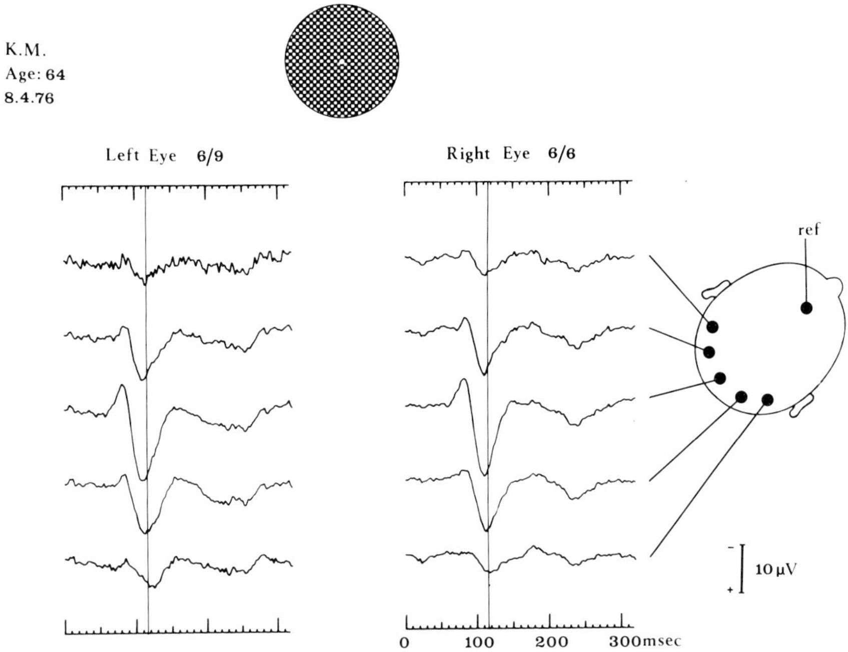

FIG. 3. Normal responses in a patient with a 25-year history of relapsing and remitting spastic paraparesis with episodic sensory disturbance and "questionably pale" optic disks. Both CSF and myelogram were normal.

DISCUSSION

The present study was primarily concerned with the value of the VEP in the diagnosis of patients with chronic paraparesis of unknown etiology. The results suggest an incidence of subclinical optic neuropathy of 29% in such patients. Of particular interest is the finding of a three-fold increase in optic nerve lesions in cases recorded more than 3 years after their first symptom as compared with those seen earlier in the course of the spinal cord lesion. This result suggests an increasing incidence of plaques in these patients in the early years of the disease after which the proportion with optic nerve damage stabilizes. This may indicate that the remaining majority of this group of patients do not have MS. The proportion of cases in the longest duration group with optic nerve damage (33%) correlated closely with the available autopsy data which suggests that about 34% of a similar patient population will have demyelinating disease (10). However, the autopsy data are limited, and the possibility of false negative VEP results, for which there was some evidence, perhaps suggests that the true incidence of MS in this group is higher. Such a conclusion will require confirmation from follow-up or autopsies.

A scrutiny of the previous literature suggests that in the acceptable spinal cases the accumulated hit rate is 60/144 (42%), a higher incidence than found in the present study. However, the incidence of abnormal VEPs in different studies varies widely from extremes of 0 to 78% (11,14). Although differences in methodology, for example, the use of steady-state (13) or light-emitting diode (4) stimuli, could account for some variability, the discrepancies among studies using similar techniques (1,6,7,11,14) imply that other factors are operating. The most important variable is probably selection of case material. Some reports of the VEP in "spinal MS" or in "chronic undiagnosed myelopathy" have included patients with brainstem or ocular involvement (4,13), whereas others appear to have varied in their inclusion of "early probable" cases (1,12,14). Some studies do not clearly distinguish patients with negative myelography in the analysis (4,13). As the clinical evidence of MS in these patients increases with time (8,10), the incidence of patients left undiagnosed with abnormal VEPs will steadily decline. Thus, large discrepancies would be expected between studies of populations with different average disease durations. The estimated proportion with MS, as based on the VEP data, will therefore depend on the stage of the disease at the time such a group is studied.

A further criticism of all reports to date, including the present study, is the possibility of the preselection of cases by variations in the referral of patients before or after myelography according to the diagnostic strategy of the clinicians. Such unknown factors in selection, for example, the high incidence of VEP abnormalities in the patients who did not have myelograms may markedly alter the results. Further, it is possible that a relatively small number of cases found to have abnormal myelograms would subsequently be referred for VEP recording.

The results also show that the VEP is less effective as an indicator of demyelination in the early stages of a spastic paraparesis. The hit rate in acute lesions was low (10%), parallelling the findings in other studies, particularly of patients with "suspected MS" who have acute single lesions at other sites in the CNS (1,11). The results suggest that the VEP cannot detect, during the first 3 years, approximately two-thirds of the patients with chronic spinal disease who may eventually be found to suffer from MS. This seems a serious limitation of the usefulness of the test.

This study also provides support for the association of mild cervical spondylotic myelopathy and MS in some patients (3). On the basis of CSF or VEP abnormalities or follow-up data, there appeared to be a possible correlation of the two conditions in six cases. The true incidence cannot be estimated, as the number of patients with cord compression not referred for VEP is unknown. Although the existence of the two conditions has been considered as a contraindication to surgical intervention (3), the patient with bilaterally delayed VEPs and dorsal cord compression who recovered after laminectomy indicates a need for caution in the use of the VEP result to exclude patients from myelography. Whether this patient will go on to develop signs of MS awaits further follow-up. It should also be noted in this context that delayed VEPs have been reported in association with the spastic paraparesis of an Arnold–Chiari malformation (9).

In conclusion, this study confirms that patients with undiagnosed myelopathy that satisfies the criteria for "progressive possible" MS have a low incidence of VEP abnormalities. The proportion of cases with apparent subclinical demyelination of their optic pathways on this test corresponds with the reported incidence of MS in similar groups coming to autopsy. This apparently high degree of sensitivity of the VEP to MS patients without significant symptoms or signs outside the spinal cord is striking, but it must be remembered that this result is subject to the errors inherent in a retrospective study and must await confirmation from follow-up clinical data and pathological correlation.

REFERENCES

1. Asselman, P., Chadwick, D. W., and Marsden, C. D. (1975): Visual evoked responses in the diagnosis and management of patients suspected of multiple sclerosis. *Brain,* 98:261–282.
2. Blumhardt, L. D., Barrett, G., Halliday, A. M., and Kriss, A. (1978): The effect of experimental 'scotomata' on the ipsilateral and contralateral responses to pattern-reversal in one-half-field. *Electroencephalogr. Clin. Neurophysiol.,* 45:376–392.
3. Brain, R., and Wilkinson, M. (1957): The association of cervical spondylosis and disseminated sclerosis. *Brain,* 80:456–478.
4. Bynke, H., Olsson, J., and Rosen, I. (1977): Diagnostic value of visual evoked response clinical eye examination and CSF analysis in chronic myelopathy. *Acta Neurol. Scand.,* 26:55–69.
5. Halliday, A. M., Barrett, G., Blumhardt, L. D., and Kriss, A. (1979): The macular and paramacular subcomponents of the pattern evoked response. In: *Human Evoked Potentials,* edited by D. Lehmann and E. Callaway, pp. 135–151. Plenum Press, New York.
6. Halliday, A. M., McDonald, W. I., and Mushin, J. (1973): Delayed visual evoked responses in progressive spastic paraparesis. *Electroencephalogr. Clin. Neurophysiol.,* 37:328.
7. Hennerici, M., Wenzel, D., and Freund, H. J. (1977): The comparison of small-size rectangle and checkerboard stimulation for the evaluation of delayed visual evoked responses in patients suspected of multiple sclerosis. *Brain,* 100:119–136.
8. Hubbe, P., and Mouritzen, A. (1973): Spastic paraplegia of unknown origin. *Acta Neurol. Scand.,* 49:536–542.
9. McDonald, W. I., and Halliday, A. M. (1977). Diagnosis and classification of multiple sclerosis. *Br. Med. Bull.,* 33:4–8.
10. Marshall, J. (1955): Spastic paraplegia of middle age. A clinicopathological study. *Lancet,* 1:643–646.
11. Matthews, W. B., Small, D. G., Small, M., and Pountney, E. (1977): Pattern reversal evoked visual potential in the diagnosis of multiple sclerosis. *J. Neurol. Sci.,* 40:1009–1014.
12. Paty, D. W., Blume, W. T., Brown, W. F., Jaatoul, N., Kertesz, A., and McInnis, W. (1978): Chronic progressive myelopathy: Investigation with C.S.F. electrophoresis, evoked potentials, and CAT scan. *Trans. Am. Neurol. Assoc.,* 103:110–112.
13. Regan, D., Milner, B. A., and Heron, J. R. (1976): Delayed visual perception and delayed visual evoked potentials in the spinal form of multiple sclerosis and in retrobulbar neuritis. *Brain,* 99:43–66.
14. Trojaborg, W., and Petersen, W. (1979): Visual and somatosensory evoked potentials in multiple sclerosis. *J. Neurol. Neurosurg. Psychiatry,* 42:323–330.
15. Ungar-Sargon, J. Y., Lovelace, R. E., and Brust, J. C. M. (1980): Spastic paraplegia–paraparesis, a reappraisal. *J. Neurol. Sci.,* 46:1–12.

Clinical Applications of Evoked Potentials in Neurology,
edited by J. Courjon, F. Mauguiere, and M. Revol.
Raven Press, New York © 1982.

Results of a Prospective Study on the Value of Combined Visual, Somatosensory, Brainstem Auditory Evoked Potentials and Blink Reflex Measurements for Disclosing Subclinical Lesions in Suspected Multiple Sclerosis

*P. Deltenre, *C. Van Nechel, **A. Vercruysse, *S. Strul, *A. Capon, and †P. Ketelaer

**Department for Rehabilitation of Neurological Disorders, Brugmann Hospital, B-1020 Brussels, Belgium; **Department of Neurology, Middelheim General Hospital, B-2000 Antwerpen, Belgium; and †Multiple Sclerosis Clinic, B-1910 Melsbroeck, Belgium*

The diagnosis of MS still depends on the demonstration of at least two distinct lesion sites in the CNS in addition to a compatible time course and exclusion of other possible conditions (10).

Numerous studies have already demonstrated the ability of evoked potentials to disclose subclinical lesions in MS patients (1–5, 7, 8, 10, 13–15). The present work has been designed as a prospective trial for assessing the diagnostic value of combined visual, auditory (brainstem), somatosensory evoked potentials, and blink reflex measurements at the stage of the differential diagnosis of a yet unidentified neurological disease which could have been MS.

SUBJECTS AND METHODS

For each type of measurement, normative data were established from at least 30 normal subjects chosen from the hospital staff and whose ages ranged from 17 to 50. In addition, 133 outpatients for whom the diagnosis of MS was being contemplated were submitted to the test battery. The complete examination included: recording of the pattern reversal VEP by the rotating mirror technique; recording of the BAEP using an unfiltered monaural click of 65 dB hearing level (HL) at a 10 Hz rate and a vertex to ipsilateral ear lobe derivation; simultaneous recording of the brachial plexus activity from Erb's point of the neck somatosensory potentials and of cortical potentials after electrical stimulation of the median nerve at the wrist—the cortical responses following stimulation of the peroneal nerves at the fibula head were also obtained; and recording of the electrically induced blink reflex as the surface EMG of both orbicularis palpebrae muscles after stimulation of the supraorbital nerve.

In view of the great amplitude variability encountered in the normative values, no amplitude data were used except when absence of a component was found or, for neck-evoked SEP, when amplitude was inferior to 0.8 μV, a significant value computed from normative data.

For pattern reversal VEP, absolute peak latencies and intereye latency differences of P_{100} were considered.

For BAEP data, only interpeak latencies were studied in order to avoid interference from possible middle or inner ear dysfunction.

Latency analysis for SEP data was also restricted to intercomponent values referred to N_9 in order to consider central conduction only.

Blink reflex data analysis was focused on R_1 latency, thought to reflect intrapontine conduction, provided the examination of the late components had not revealed a fifth or seventh nerve lesion pattern (6)

Absolute or relative latency values were considered abnormal if they exceeded three standard deviations above the mean computed from normal data. The occurrence of bilateral normal median nerve spinal SEPs with badly disturbed cortical potentials from lower limbs was interpreted as an evidence of a spinal lesion below the cervical level.

At the time of the EP recording, the patients were initially classified according to McDonald and Halliday's criteria (10) into four subgroups: suspected, progressive possible, progressive probable, and early probable or latent. After a follow-up period of up to 4 years, (mean value, 17.6 months; SD, 10.6 months; range, 2 to 51.6 months), the same patients were grouped under three headings on the basis of their clinical evolution or of the results of ancillary diagnostic procedures excluding EP data: definite MS; outstanding diagnosis; and other neurological diseases. Their initial EP data were then reviewed and analyzed in terms of the ability of the tests to reveal at least one subclinical distinct lesion in a given patient.

RESULTS

Definite MS Group

Forty-four patients eventually evolved to this diagnosis (Table 1). Typical abnormal VEP and BAEP obtained from patients of this group are illustrated by Figs. 1 and 2.

Thirty-five of these patients (79.5%) were classified as early probable or latent at the time of EP recording. At least one new localization was disclosed by the test battery in 30 out of these patients (87.5%). Nine (20%) of the eventual definite patients were initially considered as suspected. In six out of these nine cases (66.6%), subclinical lesions were disclosed by the EP battery. Among these 44 patients who were indeed suffering from MS at the time of testing, the combined EP thus disclosed subclinical lesions in 36 of them (81.8%).

Evoked potential results for the remaining seven patients (15.9%) merely confirmed the clinical data. Only one genuine MS patient exhibited a complete

TABLE 1. *Eventual definite MS patients (*N = *44)*

Initial Classification	EP results (+)[a]	+[b]	N[c]
Early probable or latent, 35/44 (79.5%)	30/35 (85.7%)	4/35 (11.4%)	1/35 (2.85%)
Suspected, 9/44 (20.5%)	6/9 (66.6%)	3/9 (33.3%)	

[a] The (+) indicates the proportion of patients for whom an abnormal EP disclosed at least one new localization.

[b] The + indicates the proportion of patients for whom an abnormal EP merely confirmed already known lesion sites.

[c] The *N* indicates the proportion of patients with completely normal EP results.

series of normal results when first seen after a previous attack of vision blurring. On retest following recurrent visual symptoms, the VEP alone was found abnormal. She later developed brainstem signs.

Outstanding Diagnosis Group

The proportion of patients for whom new localization(s) was disclosed was definitely lower in this group: 19.35% as compared with 81.8% for the definite

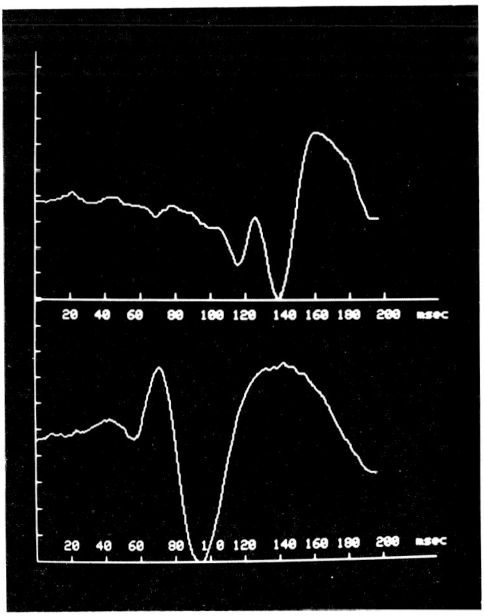

FIG. 1. *Upper trace:* Typical abnormal VEP disclosing an infraclinical optic neuritis. *Lower trace:* Typical normal result from a control subject.

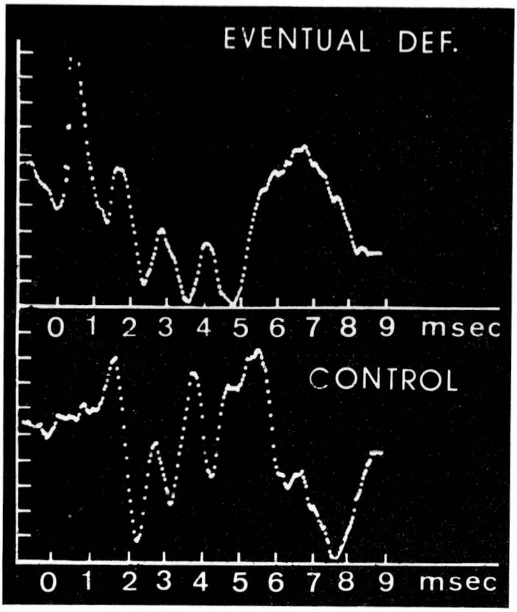

FIG. 2. A typical abnormal BAEP *(upper trace)* is compared to the usual normal potential *(lower trace).*

group (Table 2). It was among the initial early probable or latent subgroup that the highest proportion of occult lesions was found. The occurrence of fully normal results was much more frequent, with a proportion of 34.7%, even in the initial early probable or latent group.

Other Neurological Diseases

Twenty-seven patients could be diagnosed as suffering from neurological diseases other than MS (Table 3). Clinically unsuspected lesions were found in 18.5% of these patients.

It is already known from literature that EP alterations bear no specificity to MS (10). The present data underline the fact that the demonstration of discrete

TABLE 2. *Outstanding diagnosis group (N = 62)*

Initial classification	EP results (+)	+	N
Early probable or latent, 23/62 (37%)	6/23 (26%)	9/23 (39%)	8/23 (34.7%)
Progressive probable, 3/62 (4.8%)	1/3 (33.3%)	2/3 (66.6%)	
Progressive possible, 8/62 (13%)	2/8 (25%)	2/8 (25%)	4/8 (50%)
Suspected, 28/62 (45.2%)	3/28 (10.7%)	16/28 (57.1%)	9/28 (32.2%)

TABLE 3. *Other neurological diseases (N = 27)*

Eventual diagnosis	Test[a]
B_{12} deficiency	VEP
Friedreich's ataxia	VEP and SEP
Cervical disk prolapse	BAEP
Cervical spondylosis	BAEP
Frontal hygroma	BAEP and SEP

[a] Test column indicates which test disclosed an unsuspected lesion among the other neurological diseases patients.

multiple lesions must always be considered in the whole clinical context: subclinical optic nerve and dorsal column dysfunctions are not surprising in early cases of Friedreich's ataxia or B_{12} deficiency, and it can be speculated that cervical spine disease may impair the vertebrobasilar circulation to explain abnormal BAEPs in this condition.

DISCUSSION

The design of a prospective study was intended to evaluate the diagnostic yield of the EP battery at the stage of differential diagnosis. The analysis of the data from the eventual definite MS group is relevant in this respect.

It can be seen from Table 4 that the pattern reversal VEP was the best lesion detector, followed by SEP and then by BAEP and blink reflex. Applied alone, the VEP would have suggested the correct diagnosis in 56% of the genuine MS patients after a recording session of less than a half hour duration. The addition of the rest of the battery required a 3-hr recording session but increased the positive finding rate from 51 to 81.8%.

The blink reflex, which is a very rapid procedure (10 min), is the only test that can be omitted without decreasing the detection rate. Any other omission in order to reduce time consumption would also have reduced the diagnostic

TABLE 4. *Eventual definite MS patients: hit rate for each EP modality*[a]

Test	Hit rate
VEP	25/44 (56%)
SEP	11/44 (35%)
BAEP	7/44 (15.9%)
Blink reflex	6/44 (13.6%)
Combined tests	36/44 (81.8%)

[a] Hit rate is the proportion of cases in which a test, given alone, would have disclosed a new lesion.

yield. This reduction would have been of 25% for VEP omission, of 11.3% for SEP omission, and of 4.5% for BAEP omission.

A detection rate of 81.8% is very encouraging, but the possibility that the results are biased by a rather short follow-up period must be considered. It may be that a follow-up period of at most 4 years has selected patients with a rapidly evolving form of the disease, since analysis is restricted to those patients who developed clinical signs of definite MS during the follow-up period. If this selection has taken place, it may be that the high detection rate observed is a feature of this peculiar form of the disease. It will be necessary to await the long-term results from the actual outstanding diagnosis group to further elucidate the matter. With respect to the results from the other neurological diseases group, it must be further emphasized that the EP battery merely provides us with additional but nonspecific data which must be handled as such in the diagnosis-reaching process.

The occurrence of fully normal results in genuine MS patients has been rare (1/44 or 2.3%) in this series. The proportion of such results is, however, much higher (34.7%) in the group of patients classified as early probable or latent and whose diagnosis is still unsettled. It is likely that some of these will eventually develop evidence of MS. It must be kept in mind that the occurrence of fully normal results for the battery described cannot eliminate the diagnosis of MS. The risk that a given patient with entirely normal EP has MS seems low, but its precise quantification must await longer follow-up periods.

From the experience gained throughout this study and from some published reports, a modified strategy has been elaborated for future application to the early diagnosis of MS. Time could be saved or at least used more efficiently by restricting EP investigation to those regions in which no lesion has been proven to exist.

The search for an infraclinical optic neuritis could be improved by the addition of steady-state VEP. It is well known (11) that steady-state and transient EPs provide complementary information on CNS function. This complementary behavior has already been reported for the uncovering of optic neuritis in spinal MS patients (12)

The demonstration of an occult brainstem lesion is likely to be increased by the adoption of separate normative data for males and females (8).

It is not rare to find normal BAEP results in definite MS patients with unequivocal signs of brainstem lesion (C. Van Nechel and P. Ketelaer, *unpublished observations*). Electrophysiological testing of the brainstem white matter can be enriched by recording of the crossed acoustic response (3) and by electrooculographic movement analysis (9,16).

ACKNOWLEDGMENTS

We thank Drs. G. Monseu, M. Soeur, G. Beauherz, P. Khoubesserian, C. Coërs, N. Telerman-Toppet, C. Moerman, J. Retif, G. Hildebrand, and M. Gerard for having referred the patients.

REFERENCES

1. Asselman, P., Chadwick, D. W., and Marsden, C. D. (1975): Visual evoked responses in the diagnosis and management of patients suspected of multiple sclerosis. *Brain,* 98:261–282.
2. Bynke, H., Olsson, J. E., and Rosen, I. (1977): Diagnostic value of visual evoked response, clinical eye examination and C.S.F. analysis in chronic myelopathy. *Acta Neurol. Scand.,* 56:55–69.
3. Clifford-Jones, R. E., Clake, G. P., and Mayles, P. (1979): Crossed acoustic response combined with visual and somatosensory evoked responses in the diagnosis of multiple sclerosis. *J. Neurol. Neurosurg. Psychiatry,* 42:749–752.
4. Halliday, A. M., McDonald, W. I., and Mushin, J. (1973): Visual evoked responses in diagnosis of multiple sclerosis. *Br. Med. J.,* 4:661–664.
5. Hisako I., Tremain, K. E., and Sanders, M. D. (1978): Neurophysiological investigation in optic nerve disease: Combined assessment of the visual evoked response and electroretinogram. *Br. J. Ophthalmol.,* 62:227–239.
6. Kimura, J. (1973): The blink reflex as a test for brainstem and higher central nervous system function. In: *New Developments in Electromyography and Clinical Neurophysiology,* edited by J. E. Desmedt, pp. 682–691. Karger, Basel.
7. Kimura, J. (1975): Electrically elicited blink reflex in diagnosis of multiple sclerosis. *Brain,* 98:413–426.
8. Kjaer, M. (1979): Evaluation and graduation of brainstem auditory evoked potentials in patients with neurological diseases. *Acta Neurol. Scand.,* 60:231–242.
9. Mastaglia, F. L., Black, J. L., Cala, L. A., and Collins, D. W. K. (1979): The contribution of visual and somatosensory evoked potentials and quantitative electrooculography in the diagnosis of multiple sclerosis. In: *Evoked Potentials,* edited by C. Barber, pp. 559–565. MTP Press, Lancaster.
10. McDonald, W. I., and Halliday, A. M. (1977): Diagnosis and classification of multiple sclerosis. *Br. Med. Bull.,* 33(1):4–8.
11. Regan, D. (1977): Fourier analysis of evoked potentials; some methods based on Fourier analysis. In: *Visual Evoked Potentials in Man,* edited by J. E. Desmedt, pp. 110–117. Clarendon Press, Oxford.
12. Regan, D., Milner, B. A., and Heron, J. R. (1977): Slowing of visual signals in multiple sclerosis measured psychophysically and by steady state evoked potentials. In: *Visual Evoked Potentials in Man,* edited by J. E. Desmedt, pp. 461–469. Clarendon Press, Oxford.
13. Robinson, K., and Rudge, P. (1977): The early components of the auditory evoked potential in multiple sclerosis. In: *Progress in Clinical Neurophysiology, Vol. 2, Auditory Evoked Potentials in Man. Psychopharmacology Correlates of Evoked Potentials,* edited by J. E. Desmedt, pp. 58–67. Karger, Basel.
14. Robinson, K., and Rudge, P. (1977): Abnormalities of the auditory evoked potentials in patients with multiple sclerosis. *Brain,* 100:19–40.
15. Small, D. G., Matthews, W. D., and Small, M. (1978): The cervical somatosensory evoked potential (SEP) in the diagnosis of multiple sclerosis. *J. Neurol. Sci.,* 35:211–224.
16. Solingen, L. D., Baloh, R. W., Myers, L., and Ellison, G. (1977): Subclinical eye movement disorders in patients with multiple sclerosis. *Neurology,* 27:614–619.

Clinical Applications of Evoked Potentials in Neurology,
edited by J. Courjon, F. Mauguiere, and M. Revol.
Raven Press, New York © 1982.

Brainstem Auditory Evoked Potentials in Reclassification of 143 MS Patients

*K. Maurer and **K. Lowitzsch

*Departments of *Psychiatry and **Neurology, University of Mainz, D-6500 Mainz, Federal Republic of Germany*

The clinical MS diagnosis in the present study relies on three main criteria: the clinical course of the disease, the dissemination of the demyelinating process in space and time, and characteristic changes of the CSF (1). One-third of the diagnostic certainty is based on the fact of dissemination. In many cases, however, the clinical symptomatology does not reliably indicate more than one lesion. Therefore, cortical and subcortical evoked potentials are being investigated to detect clinically silent lesions. Thus, BAEP in MS were recorded using click stimulation by Starr and Achor (7), Chiappa et al. (2) and Stockard et al. (8). The report of Robinson and Rudge (6) included 88 MS patients, but these researchers applied binaural stimuli. Because of the importance of the stimulation modalities, we used a tone pip for monaural stimulation (3). The aim of this study was to confirm the involvement of the eighth cranial nerve and brainstem structures by abnormalities of latencies and amplitudes of waves I to V for reclassification of MS diagnosis in 143 MS patients.

PATIENTS, CONTROLS

Each of the 143 MS patients underwent a standardized neurological, otological, and CSF examination as well as VEP testing by pattern reversal (K. Lowitzsch and K. Maurer, *this volume*). The description of BAEP abnormalities concerned only 122 patients. The reclassification was done later, and 21 "supplementary" cases could be added to the possible category. For clinical classification, the documentation system developed by Poser et al. (5) was used. Normative data were gained in 40 healthy subjects with unimpaired hearing (4).

METHODS

Methods of recording have been published elsewhere (4). Patients were examined in supine position without sedation. The signal was obtained from electrodes applied at the vertex and the ipsilateral mastoid. The interelectrode impedance was kept below 3,000 ohms. The EEG activity amplified by a low-noise differential amplifier with filter settings of 300 and 3,200 Hz was summed by a signal averager (1,500 sweeps, 1,024 sampling points, automatic artifact rejection). Stimuli presented monaurally by Beyer DT 48 earphones were produced electrically by a half sine wave with a duration of 250 μsec; acoustically, a gaussian signal with sharp rise and short duration was obtained. Latency delays and

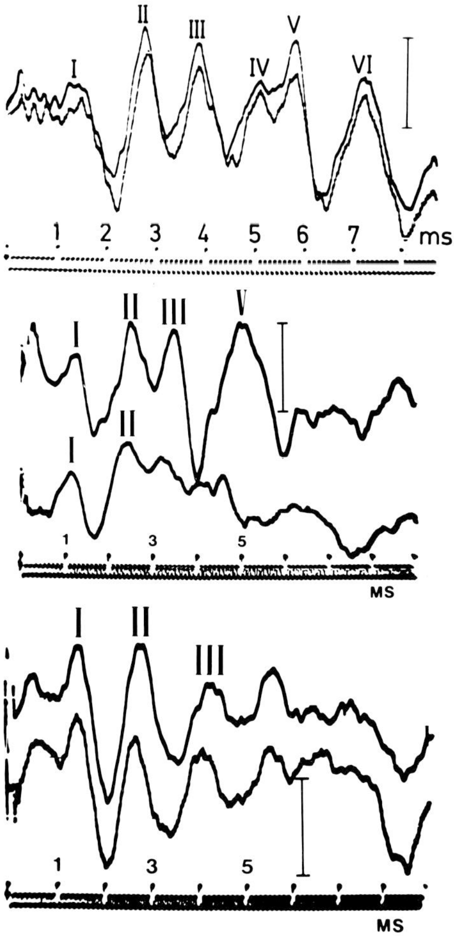

FIG. 1. Top: Scalp recordings of the auditory nerve (I) and brainstem evoked potentials (II to VI) in a neurologically and audiometrically normal person. Roman numerals indicate six vertex-positive potentials. Each of the two curves represents the average of 1,500 responses evoked by 10/sec 80 db HL tone pips. Calibration, 200 nV. **Middle:** Unilateral lesion. Normal potentials with a IV/V complex could be recorded on the left side *(upper trace).* Right stimulation *(lower trace)* revealed abnormalities affecting wave III and subsequent components. Calibration, 200 nV. **Bottom:** Traces are in response to 80 dB HL pips. *Upper trace* is from the left, and *lower trace* from the right ear. Example of a bilateral lesion at the same level. Calibration, 300 nV.

amplitude reductions were considered to be abnormal if the mean was exceeded by 2.5 SD.

RESULTS

Three types of abnormal responses were observed: increase of latency, decrease of amplitude, and combined changes of both parameters (Fig. 1). All MS patients were examined and classified as mentioned above; 10 patients were in the definite, 46 in the probable, and 66 in the possible group. The BAEPs were abnormal in nine of 10 patients of the definite MS group, in 63% of the probable, and in 41% of the possible category. In 31 patients, we found unilateral and in 34 bilateral abnormalities of the BAEP. For the bilateral abnormalities, wave alterations were observed at different levels of the brainstem in 32% of the patients. In the monaural stimulation mode, we could record BAEPs from each auditory pathway separately (Fig. 2). Of the ears tested, 144 showed a normal response; wave I was altered in 13, wave II in 22, wave III in 11, and waves IV and V in 53 ears.

It was not possible in every case to correlate brainstem symptoms (cranial nerve lesions) to a corresponding wave abnormality. Wave I was altered mostly

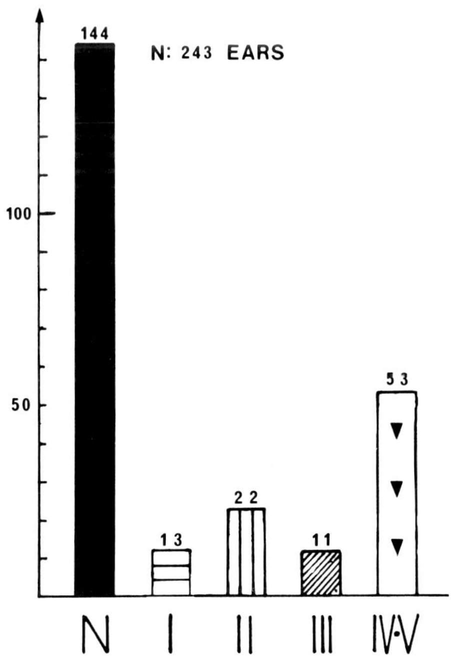

FIG. 2. A total of 243 ears (122 patients) was investigated (one ear had mumps in early childhood) with regard to abnormalities of waves I to V. N, normal BAEP; I–V, number of affected ears.

in patients with eighth nerve symptoms (acoustic and vestibular nerve). Waves II and III were mostly changed in lesions of cranials nerves V to XII, and waves IV and V in mesencephalic disturbances (Fig. 3).

For clinical reclassification, suspected MS patients (possible and probable groups) were taken into account, enlarging the possible group by another 21 cases. A reclassification could be done by BAEP in 36 of the 133 suspected cases; i.e., the diagnostic certainty could be shifted toward the next superior level in 27% of the cases (Fig. 4).

CONCLUSIONS

Wave abnormalities of BAEP could be observed at each level of the auditory pathway between cochlea and midbrain. The amount of BAEP change was greater than could be expected from clinical results, suggesting that clinically silent lesions can be detected in a high percentage. The overall prevalence of wave abnormalities in our patients without clinical brainstem signs is similar to that reported by Stockard et al. (8) and Robinson and Rudge (6).

Strictly unilateral changes prove that BAEPs are generated from different levels of the auditory pathway of only one side. It can be suggested that bilateral abnormalities at different levels are produced by at least two demyelinating processes. The validity of the method is reduced in brainstem lesions combined

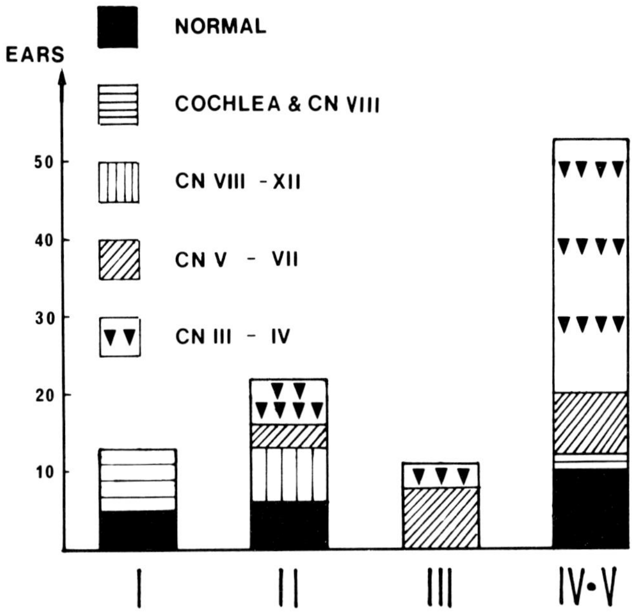

FIG. 3. Correlation between wave abnormalities and corresponding cranial nerve symptoms. CN, cranial nerve.

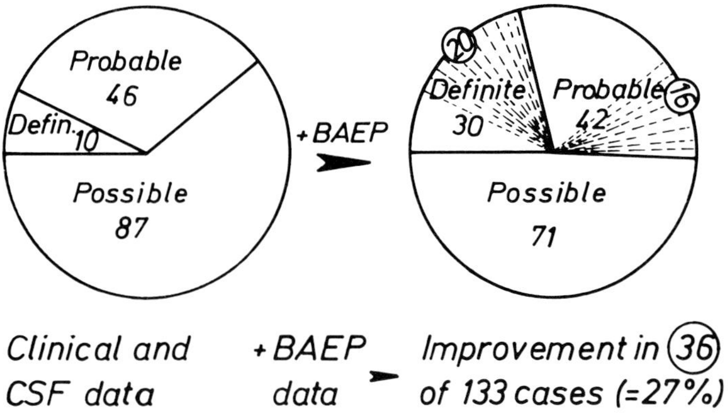

FIG. 4. Reclassification in 143 MS patients. *Dotted lines* mean sum of cases that underwent an improvement of diagnostic certainty ($N = 36$).

with long-tract symptoms. Clinically, the precise location of the demyelinating process can be very difficult. If the BAEP reveals a brainstem lesion, this cannot be interpreted as a sign of a second lesion in any case, since clinically observed symptoms may be caused by the lesion found in the BAEP. Thornton (9), in 1978, concluded from latency variance analysis that, for clinical purposes, "it is reasonable to regard the responses from one side as being due to the activity of nuclei of that side." The occurrence of a unilateral abnormal BAEP combined with a unilateral central motor paresis, both homolateral to the stimulated ear, cannot be explained by a single lesion (4).

With specific regard to the cases that showed no signs of a polytopic manifestation as far as physical examination and VEP are concerned, seven patients with normal VEP could be reclassified by considering BAEP in addition to the clinical findings. Five could be transferred from the probable to the definite category, and two from the possible to the probable group.

To summarize, BAEP provides a test that can be used to increase the level of diagnostic certainty in suspected MS cases. The BAEP completes the neurophysiological diagnostic procedure in detecting silent lesions, particularly if MS-independent ophthalmological disturbances prevent a VEP examination. A reclassification was possible in more than one-fourth of the presented 133 patients suspected of MS.

ACKNOWLEDGMENT

This study was supported by the Deutsche Forschungsgemeinschaft (MS-Schwerpunktprogramm, Dr. Fischer-Bosch-Stiftung).

REFERENCES

1. Bauer, H. (1974): Assessment of the validity of a clinical MS-diagnosis. *Acta Neurol. Scand.* [*Suppl.*], 50:58.

2. Chiappa, K. H., Norwood, A. E., and Young, R. R. (1977): Brainstem auditory evoked responses in clinical neurology, utility and clinicopathological correlations. *Electroencephalogr. Clin. Neurophysiol.,* 43:518.
3. Maurer, K., Leitner, H., Schäfer, E., and Hopf, H. C. (1979): Frühe akustisch evozierte Potentiale, ausgelöst durch einen sinusförmigen Reiz. *Dtsch. Med. Wochenschr.,* 104:546–550.
4. Maurer, K., Schäfer, E., Hopf, H. C., and Leitner, H. (1980): The location by early auditory evoked potentials (EAEP) of acoustic nerve and brainstem demyelination in multiple sclerosis. *J. Neurol.,* 223:43–58.
5. Poser, S., Hauptvogel, H., and Bauer, H. J. (1973): Methodik der maschinellen Erfassung von Daten bei einer multizentrischen Studie über die Multiple Sklerose. *Z. Neurol.,* 204:301–308.
6. Robinson, K., and Rudge, P. (1977): Abnormalities of the auditory evoked potentials in patients with multiple sclerosis. *Brain,* 100:19–40.
7. Starr, A., and Achor, L. J. (1975): Auditory brain stem responses in neurological disease. *Arch. Neurol.,* 32:761–768.
8. Stockard, J. J., Stockard, J. E., and Sharbrough, F. M. (1977): Detection and localization of occult lesions with brain stem auditory responses. *Mayo Clin. Proc.,* 52:761–769.
9. Thornton, A. R. D. (1978): Interpretation of cochlear nerve and brain stem responses. In: *Evoked Electrical Activity in the Auditory Nervous System,* edited by R. F. Naunton, and C. Fernandez, pp. 429–442. Academic Press, New York.

Clinical Applications of Evoked Potentials in Neurology,
edited by J. Courjon, F. Mauguiere, and M. Revol.
Raven Press, New York © 1982.

Pattern-Reversal Visual Evoked Potentials in Reclassification of 472 MS Patients

*K. Lowitzsch and **K. Maurer

*Departments of *Neurology and **Psychiatry, University of Mainz, D-6500 Mainz, Federal Republic of Germany*

The diagnosis of MS is based on clinical data concerning the symptomatology and the course of the disease (13). However, in many cases, it is difficult to decide whether the course is characteristic and the dissemination of the demyelinating process is definitely proven. For that reason, different gradation systems of diagnostic probability were established (1,11). Furthermore, since the Göteborg symposium in 1972, many European neurologists have become familiar with the criteria given by Bauer (3) including the clinical course of the disease, the dissemination of the process in time and space, and the CSF data. Nevertheless, very often, the diagnostic level remains within the "suspected" categories because of the lack of proven dissemination. Several attempts have therefore been made to support the clinical findings by neurophysiological methods in order to detect clinically silent lesions. In the present study of 472 MS patients, the value of pattern-reversal EPs in relation to ophthalmological findings and diagnostic classification as well as to reclassification will be demonstrated. Moreover, in a subgroup of 143 MS patients, BAEP were also done (K. Maurer and K. Lowitzsch, *this volume*) so that reclassification validity of both methods can be compared.

METHODS

Pattern-reversal stimulation was used to evoke cortical visual potentials according to the method given by Cobb et al. (4) in the modification by Halliday (5,6). A mirror system triggered by a digital stimulation unit displaced a checkerboard pattern twice per second. The reversal time was 5 msec. Single squares measured 50′ × 50. Luminosity and contrast data as well as the recording and averaging arrangements were described in detail in a previous paper (9). The BAEP method is presented elsewhere (K. Maurer and K. Lowitzsch, *this volume*).

MS Patients

A total of 472 unselected MS patients were examined. Neurological, ophthalmological, and CSF examinations were performed in all patients; moreover, in a subgroup of 135 patients color vision and visual field were also tested. The clinical classification was set up using the criteria stated by Bauer (3,9,12). The "possible" MS group comprised 240 patients, the "probable" group 139, and the "definite" group 93 patients.

RESULTS

Control Subjects

The control group consisted of 48 healthy subjects of both sexes and various ages (7,9). The mean value of P100 latency from all VEPs derived by monocular stimulation was 104.3 ± 4.5 msec, the interocular difference of latency being 2.05 ± 2.1 msec. Values have been classified as abnormally delayed if the normal mean plus 2.5 SD was exceeded, i.e., 115.5 msec for P100 latency and 7.5 msec for interocular difference (Fig. 1).

MS patients

Ophthalmological Findings

In the subgroup of 135 MS patients undergoing a sophisticated ophthalmological investigation (9), a history of RBN was present in 52%. Abnormally low visual acuity (<5/7) was found in 20% and visual field defects in Goldmann perimetry in 27%; color vision testing showed disturbances in 34%, and Friedmann perimetry in 41% of the total of 269 eyes. The VEP, however, was delayed in 63.5% (9).

VEP Abnormalities

A total of 289 patients (61%) showed an abnormally delayed VEP according to the figures given above on one or on both eyes (457 of 943 eyes = 48.5%).

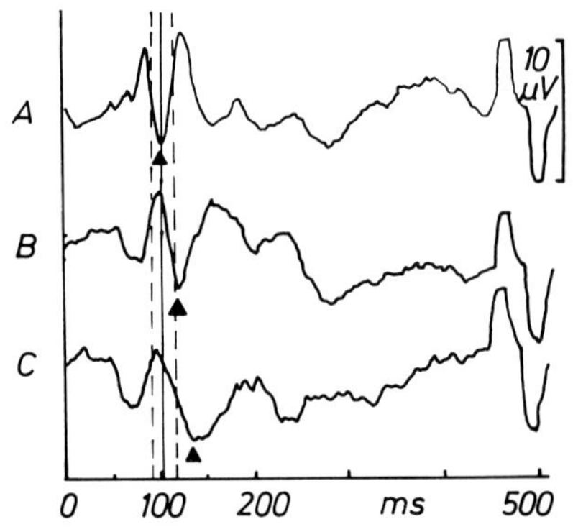

FIG. 1. Original traces of pattern reversal-evoked potentials (VEP) in a normal eye (A) and from a young female patient with suspected MS: B, left eye without any complaints; C, right eye with blurred vision. *Striped area:* mean ± 2.5 SD for P100 latencies of the control group. P100 is marked by a *filled triangle.*

In the "possible" group, the VEP was delayed in 113 patients (47%; 164 of 480 eyes = 34%). In the "probable" category, we found a delay in 103 patients (74%; 167 of 278 eyes = 60%) and in the "definite" group in 73 patients (78.5%; 126 of 185 eyes = 68%) (Fig. 2).

RECLASSIFICATION

In many "suspected" cases, the clinical symptomatology does not indicate more than one lesion in the CNS (12). Thus, by detecting a second lesion by neurophysiological methods, the proof of dissemination is established, and reclassification can be done. Concerning the group of 379 patients with "suspected"

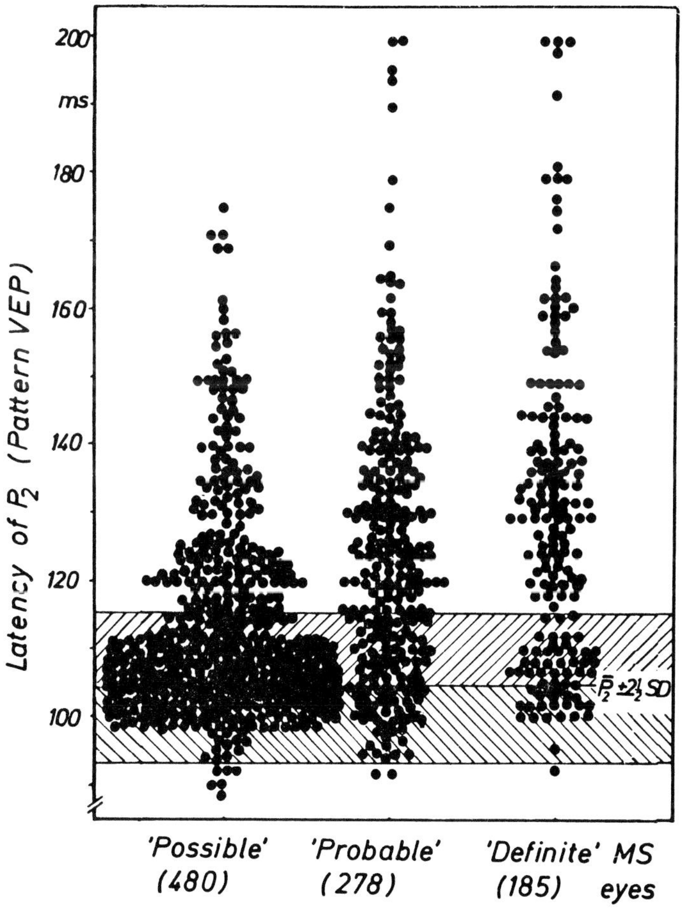

FIG. 2. Scatter plot, of P100 latencies of 943 eyes in relation to the clinical MS classification. *Hatched area,* normal range of the control group (mean ± 2.5 SD).

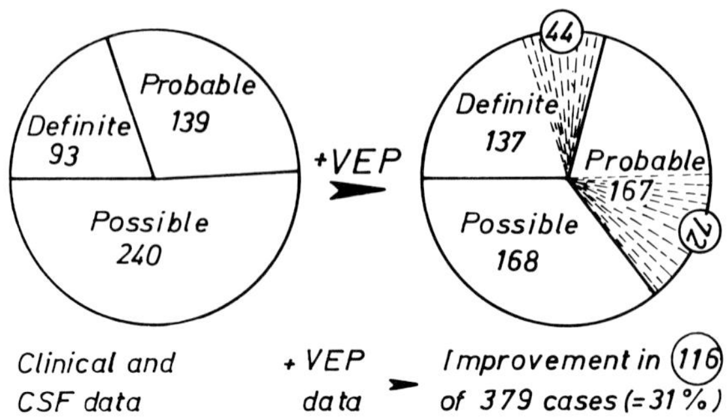

FIG. 3. Clinical MS classification **(left)** and reclassification including VEP data **(right)** of 472 MS patients. *Dashed sectors,* reclassified patients shifted toward the next superior classification degree. Figures indicate number of patients.

MS, i.e., patients from the "possible" and "probable" groups, in 116 cases (31%), a reclassification could be achieved by delayed VEPs indicating a second lesion in the visual system (Fig. 3). The VEP changes caused by MS-independent ophthalmological disturbances were carefully excluded from this series.

In a subgroup of 133 "suspected" MS patients, VEP as well as BAEP were recorded. As described elsewhere (K. Maurer and K. Lowitzsch, *this volume*), the reclassification by BAEP data was possible in 27%. On the other hand, when VEP data were taken into consideration, a reclassification in 36% could be done. Thus, the superiority of VEP in comparison with BAEP in detecting silent lesions in the CNS is demonstrated. Concerning VEP and BAEP data together, the reclassification quantity can further be improved to 45%.

CONCLUSIONS

The value of VEP investigation in MS diagnosis has been demonstrated in several publications (2,5,6,8–10). Although the VEP is not MS-specific, the test verifies clinically proven lesions as well as so-called "silent" lesions in the visual pathways in a high percentage of cases. Consequently, clinically assumed lesions can be confirmed by objective data, and subclinical lesions can be detected, indicating the dissemination of the process, especially in "spinal" MS.

The advantage of the VEP lies in the separation of the visual system from other brain structures so that superpositions of local and long-tract signs cannot be found as in brainstem lesions. Thus, because of the fact that there are two testable optic nerves independent from each other, the reliability of the VEP is the most pronounced of all EP procedures.

The reclassification quantity of suspected MS is more than 30% of the suspected cases taking VEP data into account; over that, this figure can be improved to more than 40% if additional BAEP data are applied (K. Maurer and K. Lowitzsch, *this volume*).

ACKNOWLEDGMENT

This study was supported by the Deutsche Forschungsgemeinschaft (MS-Schwerpunktprogramm, Dr. Fischer-Bosch-Stiftung; Az. Lo 228).

REFERENCES

1. Allison, R. S., and Millar, J. H. D. (1954): Prevalence of disseminated sclerosis in Northern Ireland. *Ulster Med. J.*, 23(Suppl. 2):5–27.
2. Asselman, P., Chadwick, D. W., and Marsden, C. D. (1975): Visual evoked responses in the diagnosis and management of patients suspected of multiple sclerosis. *Brain*, 98:261–282.
3. Bauer, H. J. (1974): Judgement of the validity of a clinical MS diagnosis. The international symposium on multiple sclerosis, Göteborg, 1972. *Acta Neurol. Scand.* [*Suppl.*] 58:71–74.
4. Cobb, W. A., Morton, H. B., and Ettlinger, G. (1967): Cerebral potentials evoked by pattern reversal and their suppression in visual rivalry. *Nature*, 216:1123–1125.
5. Halliday, A. M., McDonald, W. I., and Mushin, J. (1972): Delayed visual evoked response in optic neuritis. *Lancet*, 1:982–985.
6. Halliday, A. M., McDonald, W. I., and Mushin, J. (1973): Visual evoked response in diagnosis of multiple sclerosis. *Br. Med. J.*, 4:661–664.
7. Kuhnt, U., Lowitzsch, K., and Thäter, K. (1977): Pattern, flash and flicker evoked potentials. A comparison. *Electroencephalogr. Clin. Neurophysiol.*, 43:539.
8. Lowitzsch, K. (1980); Pattern-evoked visual potentials in 251 MS patients in relation to ophthalmological findings and diagnostic classification. In: *Progress in Multiple Sclerosis Research*, edited by H. J. Bauer, S. Poser, and G. Ritter, pp. 571–577. Springer-Verlag, Berlin, Heidelberg, New York.
9. Lowitzsch, K., Kuhnt, U., Sakmann, C., Maurer, K., Hopf, H. C., Schott, D., and Thäter, K. (1976): Visual pattern evoked responses and blink reflexes in assessment of MS diagnosis. A clinical study of 135 MS patients. *J. Neurol.*, 213:17–32.
10. Matthews, W. B., Small, D. G., Small, M., and Pountney, E. (1977): Pattern reversal evoked potential in the diagnosis of multiple sclerosis. *J. Neurol. Neurosurg. Psychiatry*, 40:1009–1014.
11. McAlpine, D., Lumsden, C. E., and Acheson, E. D. (1972): *Multiple Sclerosis. A Reappraisal.* Churchill Livingstone, Edinburgh, London.
12. Poser, S., and Hauptvogel, H. (1973): Clinical data from 418 MS patients in relation to the diagnosis. *Acta Neurol. Scand.*, 49:473–479.
13. Schumacher, G. A., Beebe, G. W., Kibler, R. F., Kurland, L. T., Kurtzke, J. F., McDowall, F., Nagler, B., Sibley, W. A., Tourtelotte, W. W., and Willmon, T. L. (1965): Problems of experimental trials of therapy in multiple sclerosis. *Ann. N.Y. Acad. Sci.*, 122:552–568.

Clinical Applications of Evoked Potentials in Neurology,
edited by J. Courjon, F. Mauguiere, and M. Revol.
Raven Press, New York © 1982.

Somatosensory Evoked Potentials Following Tibial Nerve Stimulation in Multiple Sclerosis and Space-Occupying Spinal Cord Diseases

B. Riffel, M. Stöhr, F. Petruch, H. Ebensperger, and K. Scheglmann

Department of Neurology, University of Tübingen, D-7400 Tübingen, Federal Republic of Germany

Somatosensory evoked potentials (SEP) following median nerve stimulation have become widely used for diagnosis in various neurological disorders, whereas SEP following stimulation of mixed or sensory nerves of the lower limb have been used more rarely (1,2,5–7). For the examination of spinal cord diseases, however, the latter stimulation site recommends itself because of the inclusion of the thoracic and lumbosacral sections of the spinal cord in the diagnostic procedure. This is also important for MS where involvement of the spinal cord is frequent, and, therefore, a higher incidence of pathological results can be expected when lower limb nerves are stimulated. To further clarify the usefulness of this method in differential diagnosis, we investigated SEP following stimulation of the posterior tibial nerve in 38 subjects with definite MS, in 32 subjects with space-occupying spinal cord diseases, and in a control group consisting of 38 healthy volunteers.

SUBJECTS

The control group consisted of 38 subjects without history, symptoms, or signs of nervous system diseases. They were 17 men and 21 women with a mean age of 34.4 years (range 20–56 years) and a mean height of 1.69 m. The MS group included 38 subjects (11 men and 27 women) with definite MS according to the criteria of McAlpine et al. (3). Their mean age was 35.8 years, ranging from 18 to 67 years. The mean height was 1.66 m. The group of patients with different space-occupying diseases of the spinal cord ("tumor group") comprised 15 subjects with spinal tumors, nine subjects with syringomyelia causing symptoms in the legs, and eight subjects with herniated cervical disk leading to medullary compression with an incomplete transverse lesion. Their mean age was 45.7 years with a range from 16 to 62 years; their mean height was 1.68 m. They were 16 men and 16 women.

METHODS

Stimulation of the posterior tibial nerve on the ankle was performed by rectangular pulses of 0.2 msec delivered regularly with a frequency of 2/sec via a bipolar surface electrode (cathode proximally). The stimulus strength was 4 mA above the motor threshold of the flexor halluxis brevis muscle.

Cortical potentials evoked by stimulation of the posterior tibial nerve were recorded with platinum needle electrodes (Disa, type 25 C 04). The recording electrode was placed 2 cm behind C_z, the reference electrode at F_z (10–20 system). The bandpass of the amplifier was set to 2 to 2,000 Hz, in some instances 5 to 2,000 Hz.

The signals were transferred from the amplifier to an averager using an analysis time of 100, sometimes 200, msec. From 128 to 1,024 sweeps were summed for each response. To confirm the reproducibility of the SEP, each measurement was repeated at least once. In all but six cases, both sides were investigated in an identical manner.

Latency measurements were performed on the screen by use of a system integrated marker to the first negative and to the first positive peak; if an initial negative peak was absent, the onset of the first positive deflection was measured instead. Amplitude measurements were taken from N_1 (N33) (respectively, the onset of the first positive peak) to P_1 (P40). From the results obtained, the side differences of latencies and amplitudes were calculated.

RESULTS

Normal Subjects

Seventy-five cortical responses in 38 subjects invariably exhibited a W shape with two (or three) negative and two positive peaks within the first 100 msec after the stimulus onset (Fig. 1). The normal values of the latency of N_1 and P_1 (N33 and P40, respectively) and the mean differences in latency between the two sides are shown in Table 1. Regarding the first positive peak (P40), the upper limit of normality was calculated to be 45.3 msec; the upper limit of the side difference was found to be 2.59 msec (mean value + 2.5 SD). Since the latency correlates with the height of the body (correlation coefficient, 0.75; $p < 0.001$), the latencies of P_1 were also corrected for the body height (Table 1, Fig. 2). The correlation of P40 with age ($r = 0.22$) is not significant ($p > 0.1$), and there are no significant sex-dependent differences if the different body height is taken into account.

MS Group

The analysis in the group of 38 patients with definite MS included 69 cortical responses. In all patients, bilateral stimulation was performed, but seven measurements gave no consistent SEP.

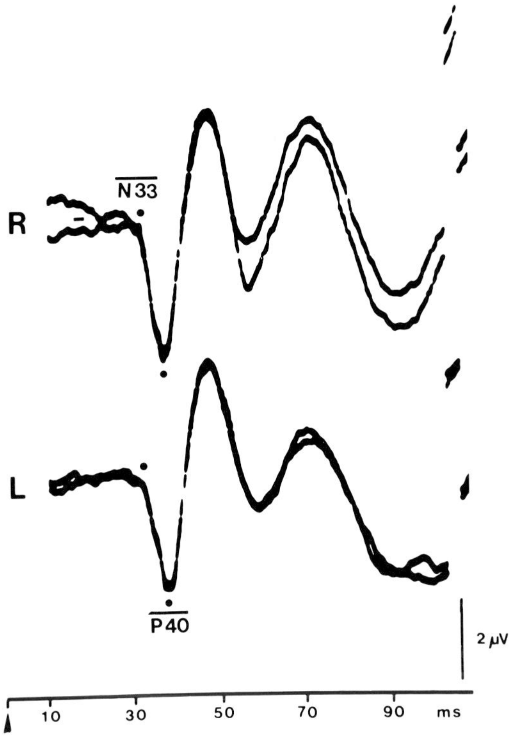

FIG. 1. A SEP following tibial nerve stimulation at the ankle in a healthy woman (22 years, 1.66 m). Latency P_1, 37.5 msec on the right, 38.5 msec on the left. (Sweep delay, 10 msec; negativity upwards in this and Figs. 3 and 4.)

The mean values of the latencies of N_1 and P_1 and of the amplitude (N_1/P_1) are displayed in Table 1. Pathological results were obtained in a total of 92%; 73% of the patients with a normal vibration and joint position sense on the legs (e.g., Fig. 3) and 100% of the patients with sensory impairment indicating uni- or bilateral involvement of the dorsal column showed a pathological increase in the latency of P40 or a pathological latency difference of P40 between sides.

Space-Occupying Lesions of the Spinal Cord

The analysis included 27 cortical responses in 15 patients with spinal tumors (3 unilateral, 12 bilateral measurements), 18 responses in 9 patients with syringomyelia, and 16 responses in 8 patients with cervical disk prolapse. The results are shown in Table 2. The main findings here are cortical responses with normal or relatively slightly prolonged latencies but reduced amplitudes (Fig. 4). Prolonged latencies and/or a pathological side difference were obtained in 18.7% of the patients (20.8% in the group with and 12.5% in the group without sensory disturbances). The mean latency of P40 is nearly identical in the three subgroups (Table 3).

TABLE 1. *Latencies and side differences in normal subjects and MS patients*

	N_1	P_1	ΔP_1	P_1/BH[a]	$\Delta P_1/BH$[a]	Amplitude N_1P_1	Δ Amplitude
Normal values[b]							
Mean	33.08	39.57	0.89	23.33	0.49	2.80	0.67
SD	2.06	2.28	0.68	0.95	0.46	1.41	0.78
Range	29.0–38.8	33.7–45.2	0–2.2	20.4–25.4		0.9–8.75	0–3.75
Upper limit (mean + 2.5 SD)	38.23	45.27	2.59	25.71	1.64		
MS patients[c]							
mean	45.97	54.38	4.73	32.77	2.83	1.52	0.56
SD	11.93	14.48	6.15	9.13	3.95	1.17	0.57
Range	31.4–87	37.3–102	0.1–34.4	23.6–60.4	0.1–21.4	2–5.5	0–2.6

[a] BH is body height (m).

[b] Seventy-five responses from 38 healthy volunteers.

[c] Sixty-nine responses from 38 patients with definite MS. Seven measurements gave no consistent SEP.

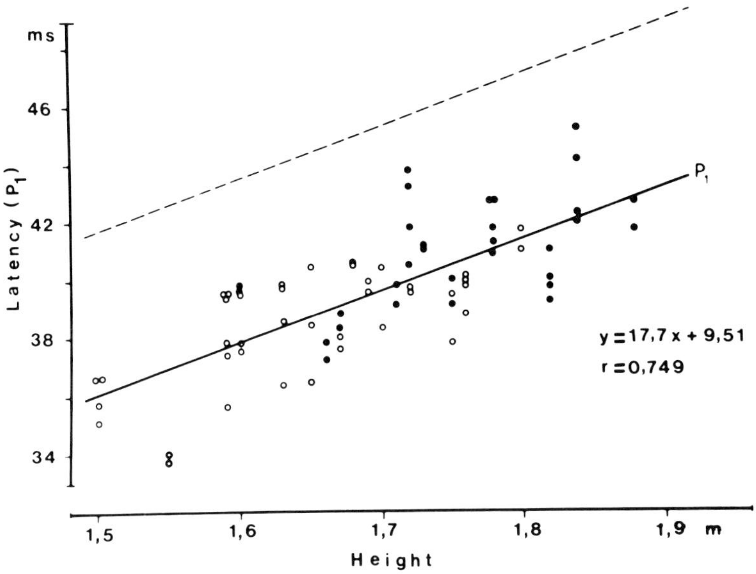

FIG. 2. Correlation between the latency P40 *(ordinate)* and the body height *(abscissa)* in 38 normal subjects (females, *open circles;* males, *filled circles*).

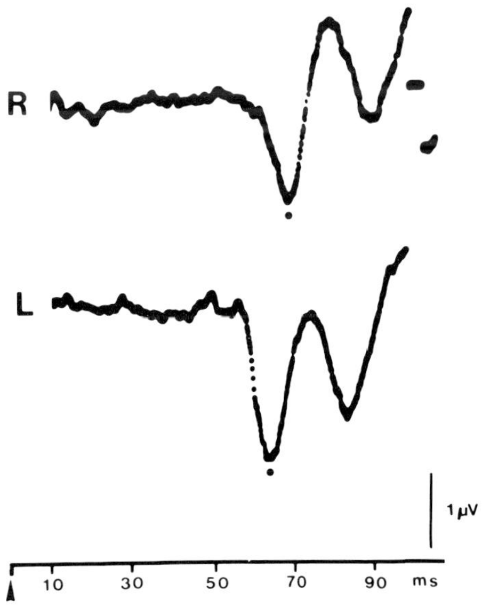

FIG. 3. Tibial nerve SEP in a 35-year-old man with definite MS. Normal joint position and vibratory sense on the legs. Latency of P_1, 68.5 msec on the right, 64.5 msec on the left. (Sweep delay, 10 msec.)

TABLE 2. *Latencies and side differences in patients with space-occupying spinal lesions*

	N_1	P_1	ΔP_1	P_1/BH	ΔP_1/BH	Amplitude N_1/P_1	Δ Amplitude
Mean	35.97	41.94	1.92	24.86	1.17	1.72	0.53
SD	3.79	3.34	1.98	2.02	1.21	1.14	0.72
Number	46	53	25	51	24	51	26
Range	29–43	36.3–53.2	0.1–9.6	22–31.67	0.06–5.71	0–6	0–3.5

DISCUSSION

MS Group

Focal or multifocal demyelination including the sensory pathway is known to produce some delay in sensory impulse conduction. Patients with a definite MS, as diagnosed on the basis of their history and their symptoms, show a prolonged latency of P40 in 75% and a pathologically increased side difference in 63%. The total frequency of abnormal tibial nerve SEP, resulting from combin-

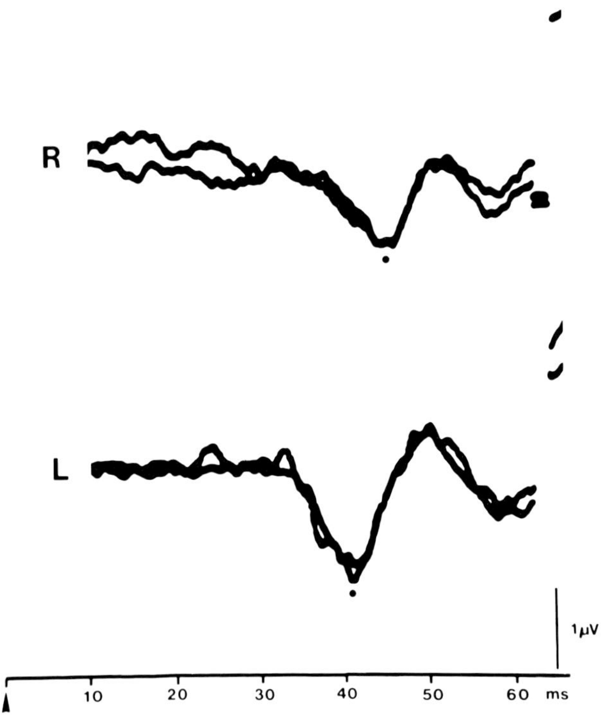

FIG. 4. Tibial nerve SEP in a 52-year-old woman with an intramedullary tumor extending from the fourth thoracic to the 10th thoracic level (case not included in the statistical analysis). Loss of vibratory sense on both legs, moderate impairment of joint position sense on the right leg. Latency of P_1, 41 msec on the right, 37.5 msec on the left.

TABLE 3. *Latency and amplitude of P_1 in various space-occupying spinal lesions*

	Spinal tumors	Syringomyelia	Cortical disk protrusion
P_1 latency	42.5	41.9	41.5
SD	3.47	4.6	2.09
Range	37.4–48.2	36.3–53.2	38.5–44.4
P_1 amplitude	1.19	1.1	1.75
SD	1.3	0.91	1.51
Range	0–6	0–3	0.5–6

ing this information, was 92%; in subjects without clinically impaired discrimination of vibratory and/or joint position from the legs, 73%. The proportion of abnormal responses is very similar to that in the study of Trojaborg and Petersen (6) who used median and (proximal) peroneal nerve stimulation and found an abnormal SEP in 86% of their patients with definite MS.

Space-Occupying Lesions of the Spinal Cord

Unifocal lesions of the dorsal columns caused by a tumor, a syrinx, or compression by a ruptured vertebral disk should mainly be accompanied by a partial or total disruption of sensory impulse conduction on the side of the lesion, resulting in corresponding diminution in amplitude or even loss of the SEP, but only slight or moderate delay (Fig. 4). In fact, significantly prolonged cortical responses to somatosensory stimulation of the leg are relatively rarely found with these diseases. Among the 32 patients investigated, we observed an increased latency of P40 only three times (twice together with an abnormal side difference) and an isolated pathological side difference in the latency of P40 in an additional three cases (18.7%, together). With the exception of one patient with a spinal gliosis extending from C5 to L4, the latency of P_1 did not exceed the upper limit of normality by more than 3 msec. The side difference never exceeded the upper limit of normality by more than 2 msec. These findings are in contrast to those of Noël and Desmedt (4) who invariably found delayed SEP latencies for the lower limb in seven patients with extrinsic compression of the cervical spinal cord.

In patients with a low-amplitude response, a sufficiently high number of averaged responses and one or two repetitions of each measurement are mandatory. Otherwise, a small P40 peak may be missed and P_2 (P58) may erroneously be taken for a prolonged P40.

Comparison Between the Two Groups of Patients

To differentiate between MS and other spinal cord diseases may be difficult without invasive diagnostic procedures. Space-occupying lesions of the spinal cord may be misdiagnosed as MS, and patients with MS may undergo unnecessary and potentially hazardous diagnostic methods such as myelography or spinal angiography. It would therefore be valuable to have a noninvasive diagnostic tool that could help to differentiate between demyelinating and nondemyelinating spinal cord diseases. The results obtained in the present study suggest that cortical responses to tibial nerve stimulation may help in such cases. Patients with spinal tumors, syringomyelia, or cervical disk protrusion show normal latencies in most cases. The comparatively small percentage of 18.7% of the subjects exhibiting increased latencies and/or side differences of P40 showed only a slight delay which never exceeded values of 3 and 2 msec, respectively (with one exception). In contrast, 92% of the patients with definite MS revealed an increased side difference and/or a prolonged latency of P40, which was moderate or marked in many cases.

A moderate or marked increase in the P40 latency in patients with a spinal cord disease of unknown origin favors the assumption of MS (or of one of the rare diseases leading to systemic demyelination of the lemniscal pathway). This is especially true if the clinical examination does not reveal an impairment of vibratory or joint position sense in the legs. Normal or only slightly increased latencies of P40—especially in addition to sensory impairment on the legs—favors a spinal cord disease of other origin and may lead to invasive diagnostic procedure.

REFERENCES

1. Dorfman, L. J., Bosley, T. M., and Cummins, K. L. (1978): Electrophysiological localization of central somatosensory lesions in patients with multiple sclerosis. *Electroencephalogr. Clin. Neurophysiol.,* 44:742–753.
2. Jones, S. J., and Small, D. G. (1978): Spinal and subcortical evoked potentials following stimulation of the posterior tibial nerve in man. *Electroencephalogr. Clin. Neurophysiol.,* 44:299–306.
3. McAlpine, D., Lumsden, C. E., and Acheson, E. D. (1972): *Multiple Sclerosis. A Reappraisal.* Churchill Livingstone, Edinburgh and London.
4. Noël, P., and Desmedt, J. E. (1980): Cerebral and far-field somatosensory evoked potentials in neurological disorders involving the cervical spinal cord, brainstem, thalamus and cortex. In: *Clinical Uses of Cerebral, Brainstem and Spinal Somatosensory Evoked Potentials,* edited by J. E. Desmedt, pp. 205–230. Karger, Basel, New York.
5. Terao, A., and Araki, S. (1975): Clinical application of somatosensory cerebral evoked response for the localization and the level diagnosis of neuronal lesions. *Folia Psychiatr. Neurol. Jpn.,* 29:341–354.
6. Trojaborg, W., and Petersen, E. (1979): Visual and somatosensory evoked cortical potentials in multiple sclerosis. *J. Neurol. Neurosurg. Psychiatry,* 42:323–330.
7. Tsumoto, T., Hirose, N., Nouaka, S., and Takahashi, M. (1972): Analysis of somatosensory evoked potentials to lateral popliteal nerve stimulation in man. *Electroencephalogr. Clin. Neurophysiol.,* 33:379–388.

Clinical Applications of Evoked Potentials in Neurology,
edited by J. Courjon, F. Mauguiere, and M. Revol.
Raven Press, New York © 1982.

Brainstem Auditory Evoked Potentials in Multiple Sclerosis: Influence of Body Temperature Increase

*G. Geraud, **J. Coll, †M. C. Arne-Bes, †L. Arbus,
**Y. Lacomme, and *A. Bes

*Services de *Neurologique, **ORL, and †Explorations Fonctionelles Neurologiques, C.H.U. Rangueil, 31054 Toulouse, France*

The diagnosis of multiple sclerosis (MS) initially depends on several clinical and paraclinical factors, chief among which is the notion of dissemination of lesions in the central nervous system. This dissemination is not always clinically evident in the early stages of the disease. By permitting detection of clinically silent lesions on the somatosensitive or sensorial pathways of the central nervous system, methods of evoked potential recording play an important role in identifying MS.

An increase in body temperature often provokes a transitory worsening of the clinical condition of MS patients (15). As early as 1951, Guthrie (7) proposed the hot bath test to help diagnose MS. At that time, the effects of the warming could only be clinically evaluated. In 1976, Jestico and Ellis (8) used electronystagmography to evaluate quantitatively the influence of heat on the appearance or the increase of a nystagmus.

The aim of this study is to evaluate the influence of body temperature increase on brainstem auditory potentials (BAEPs) in normal and pathological subjects.

MATERIALS AND METHODS

The BAEPs were obtained by monoaural stimulation. The subject lay down in a soundproof room. The clicks had a duration of 12 μsec, a frequency of 20 Hz, and an intensity of 90 db HL. A white noise is presented to the other ear at an intensity 20 db less than the click. The same procedure was repeated for each patient at 80, 70, and 60 db as an aid in recognizing wave V. The recording was made by means of electrode needles placed under the skin in the two earlobes and at the vertex. The activity was recorded in bipolar fashion between the earlobe homolateral to the stimulation and the vertex, with the controlateral ear serving as ground. Each measurement consisted of 2,048 clicks.

The potentials were recorded before and after the raising of body temperature. Warming was achieved by means of a thermostatically controlled hydraulic circuit blanket. Once the body temperature increase was deemed satisfactory, the heating blanket was removed, and the subject wrapped in a survival blanket. The second BAEP measurement was then immediately taken. Thus, recording before and after warming was effected in most cases on the same day; there was never more than a 24-hr interval. This technique was used on 18 patients diagnosed as definite MS cases (average age, 39 years), on 14 control subjects (average age, 37), and on eight patients suffering from other neurological diseases (average age, 55 years): three vertebro–basilar ischemic attacks, two Friedreich ataxias, two brainstem gliomas, one epidemic vertigo. These eight patients were chosen because they had exhibited transitory or definite signs of brainstem lesions. The increase of body temperature was on the average 0.7°C, ranging from 0.5°C to 1°C. In each case it was determined that the temperatures taken at the beginning and end of the recording period differed by no more than 0.1°C.

Only the latency and the amplitude of the wave V were retained among the measurable parameters. For the latencies, the upper limit considered normal was chosen at the mean + 3 SD of 49 control subjects; that is, 6.5 msec for the latency of the wave V and 4.8 msec for the interpeak I–V latency. The variability in wave V amplitude was so great in the control subjects that only the absence of wave V was considered pathological in patients. Also viewed as pathological were asymmetries between right and left ears of at least 0.4 msec for wave V latency and 0.5 μV for wave V amplitude.

RESULTS

Of the 18 MS patients studied before heating, 15 (83%) had abnormal BAEPs: in seven cases, there was an increase of wave V latency, three times unilaterally and four times bilaterally; in two cases, there existed an abnormal asymmetry of wave V latency between left and right ear, although latencies were normal or at the upper limit of normal; and in six cases, there was no wave V, once only on one side, five times on both sides.

Figure 1 shows the effects of increased body temperature on wave V latency. In each case the measurements taken on both ears were reported. With the 14 control subjects, the maximum variation in wave V latency between before and after warming was ±0.3 msec. We therefore considered abnormal those variations greater than ±0.3 msec. In the 36 latency measurements taken on the 18 MS patients, wave V latency showed no abnormal variation 16 times; 11 times, this latency could not be measured because of the absence of wave V; nine times, this latency varied beyond the limits of normal, four times as an increase, five times as a decrease.

Thus, the effects of raising body temperature on the 18 MS patients may be summed up as follows: in 10 cases, there was no abnormal change of wave V latency or amplitude; in four cases, there was wave V latency modification, but as often an increase as a decrease; and in four cases, there was amplitude modification, three times expressed as a decrease.

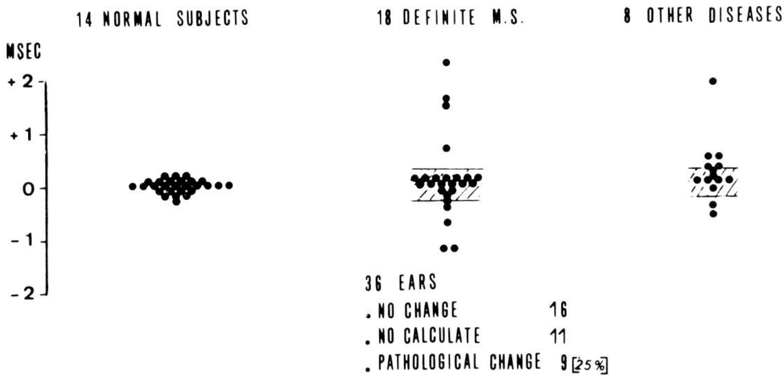

FIG. 1. Effects of body temperature increase on wave V latency in 14 normal subjects, 18 MS patients, and 8 other neurological patients (see text). *Ordinate axis* indicates the difference between latencies before and after warming. Tracings from each ear have been indicated for each subject.

Figure 2 presents an example of bilateral diminution of wave V amplitude. These modifications do not seem specific to MS, since with the eight other patients, 16 measurements of wave V latency revealed abnormal variations in seven cases (Fig. 1).

DISCUSSION

The influence of raising body temperature on MS patients has long interested many authors. Following the first clinical observations of Simons (15) and Collins (2), Guthrie (7) performed hot water immersion studies on MS patients and found that they experienced weakness, dysarthria, diminished visual acuity, and scotoma. Edmund and Fog (5) confirmed Guthrie's observations and reported exacerbations of nystagmus and changes in extraocular movements. Davis (3)

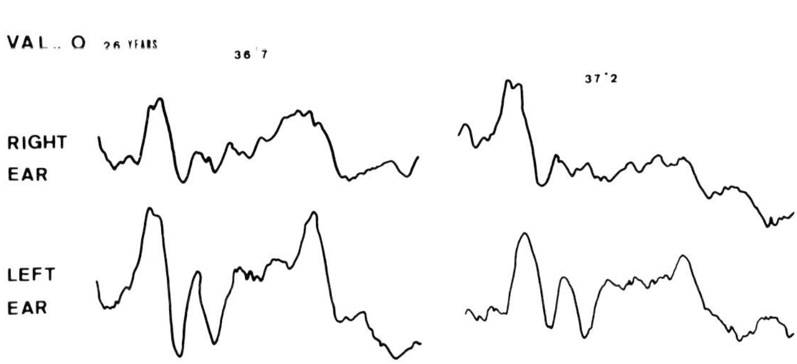

FIG. 2. Right and left BAEPs of a definite MS patient in basal conditions **(left)** and after 0.5°C body temperature increase **(right).** Both sides show wave V amplitude decrease after warming. Positivity up; calibration: 0.30 μV, 5 msec.

even employed the hot bath test as an aid in the diagnosis of this disease. Nelson et al. (11) submitted 100 normal or pathological subjects to this test: they observed that clinical modifications can occur in all patients, but changes in MS patients took place more frequently and at a smaller temperature increase. Inversely, it was found that cooling the body could transitorily decrease preexisting symptoms (1,17).

More recently, several authors have used instrumental tests to evaluate the effects of warming. Namerow (10) reported a dramatic fall in critical flicker fusion frequency on exposure to heat in 18 MS patients having a history of optic neuritis, whereas normal subjects showed a slight rise of this frequency. Galvin et al. (6) and Regan et al. (13) used double light flashes and visual evoked potentials: warming impaired double flash resolution, and cooling improved it. Results of VEPs were both more inconsistant and more contradictory. Jestico and Ellis (8), using electronystagmography, reported that after warming, nystagmus was increased or provoked in 21 out of 27 MS patients but in none of the control subjects. No positive results were obtained in 12 patients with other neurological diseases, even when nystagmus was part of the clinical picture.

The influence of temperature on the BAEPs has been minimally studied. Jones et al. (9) observed modifications of wave latency in cats with minimal temperature variations (less than 1°C), but these changes were very small, on the order of 0.1 msec. These findings correspond rather well to what we observed in our 14 control subjects, as the variations of wave V latency did not exceed 0.3 msec. In man, in situations of accidental hypothermia or hypothermia provoked during anesthesia, Stockard et al. (16) observed latency increases from 0.4 msec at 35°C to 0.9 msec at 32°C (interpeak I–V).

Results are quite different when there is demyelination in the auditory pathways of the brainstem. Neurophysiological studies of single axons have shown that raising the temperature of normal or partially demyelinated axons slightly increases conduction velocity until just below the temperature at which axonal conduction fails (the blocking temperature). Raising the temperature yet further produces a marked fall of conduction velocity. Demyelination can reduce the blocking temperature to such an extent that conduction fails at temperatures only slightly above normal body temperature (4,12,14).

Such neurophysiological observations can partly explain the transient deterioration experienced by MS patients while being warmed. These findings can also explain our own results with the BAEPs: in the nine cases in whom the wave V latency varied abnormally, four were increases, and five were decreases (Fig. 1); according to the relative percentages of normal fibers and demyelinated fibers in each patient, there could occur either an increase or a decrease in conduction velocity.

As Nelson et al. (11) clinically observed and in contrast to the conclusions drawn by Jestico and Ellis (8), we have not had the impression that the changes observed in the BAEPs were specific to MS, since we noticed them just as often in other neurological diseases. On the other hand, among the eight MS patients showing modifications after warming, two had normal BAEPs before warming. Thus, the practical interest of warming appears to lie, in our opinion, in the possibility of making pathological a BAEP that was not in basal conditions.

REFERENCES

1. Boynton, B. L. (1959): Observations on the effects of cool baths for patients with multiple sclerosis. *Phys. Ther. Rev.,* 39:297–299.
2. Collins, R. T. (1938): Transitory neurological changes during hyperthermia. *Bull. Neurol. Inst. N.Y.,* 7:291–296.
3. Davis, F. A. (1966): Hot bath test in the diagnosis of multiple sclerosis. *J. Mount Sinai Hosp.,* 33:280–282.
4. Davis, F. A. (1970): Axonal conduction studies based on some considerations of temperature effects in multiple sclerosis. *Electroencephalogr. Clin. Neurophysiol.,* 28:281–286.
5. Edmund, J., and Fog, T. (1955): Visual and motor instability in multiple sclerosis. *Arch. Neurol. Psychiatry,* 73:316–323.
6. Galvin, R. J., Regan, D., and Heron, J. R. (1976): A possible means of monitoring the progress of demyelination in multiple sclerosis: Effect of body temperature on visual perception of double light flashes. *J. Neurol. Neurosurg. Psychiatry,* 39:861–865.
7. Guthrie, T. C. (1951): Visual and motor changes in patients with multiple sclerosis. *Arch. Neurol. Psychiatry,* 65:437–451.
8. Jestico, J. V., and Ellis, P. D. M. (1976): Changes in nystagmus on raising body temperature in clinically suspected and proved multiple sclerosis. *Br. Med. J.,* 2:970–972.
9. Jones, T. A., Scharn, V., Siu, G., Stockard, J. J., Rossiter, V., and Bickfard, R. G. (1977): Effects of local and systemic cooling on brain stem auditory responses. *Electroencephalogr. Clin. Neurophysiol.,* 43:469–474.
10. Namerow, N. S. (1971): Temperature effect on critical flicker fusion in multiple sclerosis. *Arch. Neurol.,* 25:269–275.
11. Nelson, D. A., Jeffreys, W. H., and McDowell, F. (1958): Effects of induced hyperthermia on some neurological diseases. *Arch. Neurol. Psychiatry,* 79:31–39.
12. Raminsky, M. (1973): The effects of temperature on conduction in demyelinated nerve fibers. *Arch. Neurol.,* 28:287–292.
13. Regan, D., Murray, T. J., and Silver, R. (1977): Effect of body temperature on visual evoked potential delay and visual perception in multiple sclerosis. *J. Neurol. Neurosurg. Psychiatry,* 40:1084–1091.
14. Schauf, C. L., and Davis, F. A. (1974): Impulse conduction in multiple sclerosis: A theoretical basis for modification by temperature and pharmacological agents. *J. Neurol. Neurosurg. Psychiatry,* 37:152–161.
15. Simons, D. J. (1937): A note on the effects of heat and cold upon certain symptoms of multiple sclerosis. *Bull. Neurol. Inst. N.Y.,* 6:385 386.
16. Stockard, J. J., Sharbrough, F. W., and Tinker, J. A. (1978): Effects of hypothermia on the human brainstem auditory response. *Ann. Neurol.,* 3:368–370.
17. Watson, C. W. (1959): Effect of lowering of body temperature on the symptoms and signs of multiple sclerosis. *N. Engl. J. Med.,* 261:1253–1259.

Clinical Applications of Evoked Potentials in Neurology,
edited by J. Courjon, F. Mauguiere, and M. Revol.
Raven Press, New York © 1982.

The Value of a Multimodal Evoked Potential Approach in the Diagnosis of Multiple Sclerosis

Mogens Kjær

Department of Neurology, Municipal Hospital, DK 8000 Aarhus C, Denmark

Extensive literature exists on patients with definite multiple sclerosis (MS) examined by evoked potential (EP) techniques. The findings in these patients are of great methodological interest, but the techniques are more important as a diagnostic tool when used to examine patients with a less certain diagnosis, especially when the tests indicate abnormalities at a site in the CNS that do not give rise to clinical signs, such as abnormal recordings of VEPs in patients without signs of optic neuritis (2,7,12–15), of SEPs in patients without known sensory deficits (14,16,18), and of BAEPs in patients without clinically recognized brainstem lesions (5,6,11,17). Recently, diagnostic accuracy has been shown to improve when results of two or more techniques are combined (1,8,-10,11,13,14,16,18).

The tests are nonspecific, as is any sign in a clinical examination; therefore, results should always be interpreted in a clinical context, and other causes that might give rise to abnormalities should be considered.

Symptoms similar to those seen in MS patients might be caused by other diseases, including space-occupying lesions. Unless a MS diagnosis is made, such lesions must be excluded, and this will often necessitate invasive procedures such as myelographies or even exploratory operations. In contrast, the evoked potential (EP) techniques are quite harmless, less expensive, and give more positive information in MS patients than would mere elimination of other diseases.

This chapter presents my findings in MS patients examined by BAEP and combinations of VEP, SEP, and blink reflexes (BR) with a special reference to the diagnostic value of the tests.

TECHNIQUES

Normal subjects and patients were examined under equivalent conditions in the same room. Random interstimulus intervals were used, for BAEP around 230, and for VEP and SEP around 440 msec. Relatively wide frequency bands were used. Stimuli tested included BAEP [75-dB HL, 0.1-msec monaural clicks (3,9)], VEP [checkerboard pattern-reversal (rotatable mirror) (7)], SEP [0.2-

msec electrical pulses at the median nerve at the wrist (10)], and BR [0.1-msec electrical pulses at the supraorbital nerve (10)]. The leads were vertex to mastoid for BAEPs, occipital to vertex for VEPs, Erb's point, 6., 7., and 2. cervical level, contralateral parietal, all referred midfrontally, for SEPs, and bilaterally 1 cm inferior to the external orbital angle to the side of the nose for BRs.

NORMAL MATERIAL AND DATA

For BAEP 80 and VEP 70, normal subjects comprising both sexes and ages from 10 to 69 years were examined. Significant differences were found related to sex and age, and these were used in the evaluation of recordings (3,9). The BAEPs were considered abnormal if any of the waves I, III, or V were not reproduced, if wave V was delayed, if two or more of the components I to VI showed delay, absence, or highly reduced amplitudes (4). Abnormality in a VEP was assessed by a delay of P 100 or abnormal side difference in latencies or amplitude ratio (7).

The normal subjects for SEP and BR were 30 individuals aged 20 to 49 years. Only patients within these age limits were examined. The SEP criteria for abnormality were a delay of absolute and interpeak latencies of N 14, N 14–10, N 20, N 20–10, and N 20–14. The BR criteria were latencies of R_1 and R_2 and side difference in R_1 latencies (10). Sixteen normal subjects were examined by all four techniques.

PATIENTS

A total of 160 patients aged 14 to 69 years was examined by at least one technique. Sixteen patients appear twice in the BAEP and four in the VEP material because of a significant change in the clinical state between two recordings.

Definite and probable MS patients had signs indicating two or more lesions, and these were separated by history, age, and CSF findings. Possible MS patients had one lesion, and suspected MS patients had no signs but a history compatible with a MS diagnosis (10,11).

RESULTS AND DISCUSSION

The results obtained by the different techniques and combinations of these are shown in Tables 1 through 4.

The VEP test was the most sensitive, as it showed abnormal recordings in all patients with clinically recognized optic neuritis and in all but one of patients who had a history of optic neuritis. The BR technique was the least reliable, giving many false-negative results and only being abnormal when the BAEP also was so; the BAEP and SEP recordings were abnormal in 80% of patients

TABLE 1. *Brainstem auditory evoked potential results in groups of MS patients*

Classification	*N*	Abnormal *N*	Abnormal %	Clinically silent *N*
Definite	78	61	78	4
Probable	28	18	64	2
Possible	58	28	48	26
Suspected	9	2	22	2
Total	173	109	63	34

TABLE 2. *Visual evoked potential results in groups of MS patients*

Classification	*N*	Abnormal *N*	Abnormal %	Clinically silent *N*
Definite	58	57	98	20
Probable	18	15	83	10
Possible	41	27	66	25
Suspected	8	3	38	3
Total	125	102	82	58

TABLE 3. *Somatosensory evoked potential results in groups of MS patients*

Classification	*N*	Abnormal *N*	Abnormal %	Clinically silent *N*
Definite	3	3		0
Probable	3	2		0
Possible	19	11		3
Suspected	4	0		0
Total	29	16	55	3

TABLE 4. *Blink response results in groups of MS patients*

Classification	*N*	Abnormal *N*	Abnormal %	Clinically silent *N*
Definite	3	2		0
Probable	3	1		0
Possible	20	4		4
Suspected	4	0		0
Total	30	7	23	4

with clinical signs indicating lesions at levels of the CNS traversed by the pathways examined.

The number of false-positive results in patients can only be evaluated by a lengthy follow-up.

All examinations show a higher incidence of abnormalities in patients with probable and definite MS, but in these patients, the diagnostic value is most often limited to a confirmation of clinical signs.

If neurophysiological evidence is accepted as a reliable indicator of lesions, the demonstration of hitherto undiagnosed lesions in patients with only suspected or possible MS can lead to a reclassification to a more certain group, so further examinations become unnecessary.

The findings in the patients least affected are summarized in Table 5. Abnormal recordings were found in about 50% of these patients by either BAEP or VEP, and when the results were combined, subclinical lesions were evidenced in 71%, making a transfer to a more definite category possible.

Although the incidence of SEP abnormalities was high, the test only showed subclinical lesions in three patients. I have combined all four techniques in a group of young patients with special diagnostic difficulties, but the addition of SEP and BR only revealed one subclinical lesion that was not found by the BAEP/VEP combination.

Table 6 shows the results of this combination in the different groups of patients. A decrease in the incidence of abnormalities was found with decreasing diagnostic certainty, but a score of 78% abnormality in patients with only one clinically recognized lesion and 63% in patients without signs at all demonstrates the diagnostic value of the tests.

The incidences of EP abnormalities obtained in this study are among the highest described in MS patients. This might be explained by the evaluating criteria using differentiated normative data related to age and sex and perhaps by somewhat more sensitive techniques (7,9,11).

TABLE 5. *Incidence of findings indicating a reclassification of patients from suspected to possible and from possible to probable or definite MS*

Examinations		Transfer	
Type	*N*	*N*	%
BAEP	67	28	42
VEP	49	28	57
SEP	23	3	13
BR	24	4	17
BAEP + VEP	48	34	71
All four	23	17	74

TABLE 6. *Findings by combining BAEP and VEP*

		BAEP and VEP abnormalities				
					Either or both	
Classification	*N*	Both	Only BAEP	Only VEP	*N*	%
Definite	56	46	0	9	55	98
Probable	18	10	1	5	16	89
Possible	40	15	5	11	31	78
Suspected	8	0	2	3	5	63
Total	122	71	8	28	107	88

SUMMARY AND CONCLUSIONS

Evoked potential findings are nonspecific and can only bring new pieces to the diagnostic puzzle.

I have examined 160 patients covering all states of MS with one, two, or all of the BAEP, VEP, SEP, and BR techniques. In addition, a large number of normal subjects were examined, giving different sets of normative data related to age and sex.

All techniques show a high incidence of abnormal findings in probable and definite MS patients, but the diagnostic value is greatest when subclinical lesions are evidenced in patients with only suspected or possible MS. Either BAEP or VEP revealed such a lesion in about 50% of 48 patients of these categories, and the combination made a transfer to a more certain group possible in 71%. This figure increased to 74% when SEP and BR were added to the tests.

Because of these findings, a routine combination of BAEP and VEP examinations is now used in these patients, and SEP is added only in patients without spinal lesions; BR is considered superfluous.

ACKNOWLEDGMENTS

I wish to thank E. Pedersen, M.D., head of the department, for excellent working facilities, Mr. B. Klemar for skilled technical assistance, and Mrs. H. Kristensen for valuable help in the laboratory. Financial support was given by the Danish MS Society and G. Brøndsted's Legacy.

REFERENCES

1. Deltenre, P., Vercruysse, A., Van Nechel, C., Ketelaer, P., Capon, A., Colin, F., and Manil, J. (1979): Early diagnosis of multiple sclerosis by combined multimodal evoked potentials: Results and practical considerations. *J. Biomed. Eng.*, 1:17–21.
2. Halliday, A. M., McDonald, W. I., and Mushin, J. (1973): Visual evoked response in diagnosis of multiple sclerosis. *Br. Med. J.*, 4:661–664.

3. Kjær, M. (1979): Differences of latencies and amplitudes of brain stem evoked potentials in subgroups of a normal material. *Acta Neurol. Scand.,* 59:72–79.
4. Kjær, M. (1979): Evaluation and graduation of brain stem auditory evoked potentials in patients with neurological diseases. *Acta Neurol. Scand.,* 60:231–242.
5. Kjær, M. (1980): Variations of brain stem auditory evoked potentials correlated to duration and severity of multiple sclerosis. *Acta Neurol. Scand.,* 61:157–166.
6. Kjær, M. (1980): Localizing brain stem lesions with brain stem auditory evoked potentials. *Acta Neurol. Scand.,* 61:265–274.
7. Kjær, M. (1980): Visual evoked potentials in normal subjects and patients with multiple sclerosis. *Acta Neurol. Scand.,* 62:1–13.
8. Kjær, M. (1980): Brain stem auditory and visual evoked potentials in multiple sclerosis. *Acta Neurol. Scand.,* 62:14–19.
9. Kjær, M. (1980): Recognizability of brain stem auditory evoked potential components. *Acta Neurol. Scand.,* 62:20–32.
10. Kjær, M. (1980): The value of brain stem auditory, visual and somatosensory evoked potentials and blink reflexes in the diagnosis of multiple sclerosis. *Acta Neurol. Scand.,* 62:220–236.
11. Kjær, M. (1982): Evoked potentials in multiple sclerosis with special reference to the diagnostic value. *Acta Neurol. Scand., (in press).*
12. Lowitzsch, K. (1980): Pattern-evoked visual potentials in 251 MS patients in relation to ophthalmological findings and diagnostic classification. In: *Progress in Multiple Sclerosis,* edited by K. Triltsch. Springer-Verlag, Heidelberg.
13. Lowitzsch, K., Kuhnt, U., Sakmann, C., Maurer, K., Hopf, H. C., Schott, D., and Thäter, K. (1976): Visual pattern evoked responses and blink reflexes in assessment of MS diagnosis. A clinical study of 135 multiple sclerosis patients. *J. Neurol.,* 213:17–32.
14. Mastaglia, F. L., Black, J. L., Cala, L. A., and Collins, D. W. K. (1980): The contribution of visual and somatosensory evoked potentials and quantitative electro-oculography in the diagnosis of multiple sclerosis. In: *Evoked Potentials,* edited by C. Barber, pp. 559–565. MTP Press, Lancaster.
15. Mastaglia, F. L., Black, J. L., and Collins, D. W. K. (1976): Evoked potential studies in neurological disorders. *Proc. Aust. Assoc. Neurol.,* 13:15–23.
16. Small, D. G., Matthews, W. B., and Small, M. (1978): The cervical somatosensory evoked potential (SEP) in the diagnosis of multiple sclerosis. *J. Neurol. Sci.,* 35:211–224.
17. Stockard, J. J., Stockard, J. E., and Sharbrough, F. W. (1977): Detection and localization of occult lesions with brain stem auditory responses. *Mayo Clin. Proc.,* 52:761–769.
18. Trojaborg, W., and Petersen, E. (1979): Visual and somatosensory evoked cortical potentials in multiple sclerosis. *J. Neurol. Neurosurg. Psychiatry,* 42:323–330.

Clinical Applications of Evoked Potentials in Neurology,
edited by J. Courjon, F. Mauguiere, and M. Revol.
Raven Press, New York © 1982.

Brainstem Auditory Evoked Potentials: A Comparative Study of Monaural Versus Binaural Stimulation in the Detection of Multiple Sclerosis

D. K. Prasher and W. P. R. Gibson

Medical Research Council, Hearing and Balance Unit, Institute of Neurology, National Hospital, Queen Square, London WCIN 3BG England

Multiple sclerosis (MS) is a disorder characterized by multiple areas of demyelination in the central nervous system. The clinical diagnosis depends on the detection of two or more such discrete lesions. Evoked potential studies have proven to be of great value in the detection of such lesions in the visual sensory system (1,7,8,14) and also in the somatosensory system (5,10). In the auditory system, abnormalities of the brainstem auditory evoked potentials (BAEP) have been observed (15,16) despite the fact that there is rarely any significant auditory deficit that can be shown by routine audiometric tests. The frequent occurrence of plaques of demyelination in the brainstem may, however, account for the abnormal BAEP recordings. In the studies of Robinson and Rudge, binaural stimulation was employed to evoke the brainstem potentials. Although the binaural technique produces a greater amplitude response with greater intertest consistency in the normal subject (2), it raises the question of whether the clinically silent or unilateral lesions are being missed, as the response from the unaffected side might predominate on stimulation of both ears simultaneously.

In a recent study (13), it was shown that there are significant latency differences between ipsilateral and contralateral stimulation in normal subjects. The aim of the present investigation is to compare the latency differences between ipsilateral and contralateral stimulation in MS patients with a view to developing a more sensitive test criteria for the detection of BAEP abnormalities in MS.

METHOD

The BAEP from 25 patients (17 females; 8 males) were studied. Ages ranged from 17 to 65 years (mean 41.6 years). The patients were subdivided into clinically definite, probable, or possible MS according to the criteria of McAlpine et al. (11). The clinical classification consisted of 10 patients in the clinically definite MS category, 3 in the probable MS, and 12 in the possible MS categories.

A normal control group of subjects consisted of 15 females and eight males in the age range 17 to 60 years (mean 31.5 years). The BAEP were recorded as detailed elsewhere (13).

RESULTS

A representative selection of responses from patients with possible MS is shown in Fig. 1A where it can be seen that only the contralateral stimulation results in an abnormally late response. Both the responses from ipsilateral and binaural stimulation appear normal. In Fig. 1B are shown a typical set of responses from a patient in the clinically definite MS category. The responses from patients in this group were abnormally late for all conditions of stimulation. The latency of a particular wave was considered abnormal if it lay more than two standard deviations from the normal mean.

Table 1 shows the number of patients with abnormal BAEP wave latencies with ipsilateral or contralateral stimulation compared to those showing abnormal BAEP latencies with binaural stimulation. In the clinically definite MS category, the detection rate is improved from 70% with binaural stimulation to 90% with ipsilateral/contralateral stimulation.

With only one exception, patients categorized as "possible MS" according to McAlpine's criteria were found to have normal BAEP latencies to binaural stimulation but showed abnormal latencies on either ipsilateral or contralateral stimulation. In fact, the detection rate in this group was negligible with binaural stimulation compared to 67% with ipsilateral or contralateral stimulation. In a number of patients in the "possible MS" category, the response was only abnormally late with either ipsilateral or contralateral stimulation.

The mean latencies of waves III and V and interwave latency (III to V) are shown with their standard deviations in Table 2. A comparison of these figures with those from the normal subjects (also shown in Table 2) reveals a marked increase in latency of wave V in MS relative to that of wave III. In order to evaluate the statistical significance of the observed difference in the means of the latency of wave V between the MS patients and normal subjects, the Fisher–Behrens test ("*d*" statistic) was employed since the two groups exhibited unequal variances. The observed values of *d* with the associated significance level for the various comparisons are shown in Table 2. The difference in the mean latency of wave V and the interwave latency (wave III to V) between the normal and the patient group was of high statistical significance. Interwave latency (wave III to V) is prolonged in MS patients in comparison with normal subjects. The increase in interwave latency in MS patients is greater in the "clinically definite" group than it is in the "possible MS" group. The mean

FIG. 1. Top: BAEP recordings from a patient in the possible multiple sclerosis group. Note the abnormally late response on contralateral stimulation. **Bottom:** A typical set of responses from a patient in the clinically definite multiple sclerosis category. Wave V is late for all conditions of stimulation.

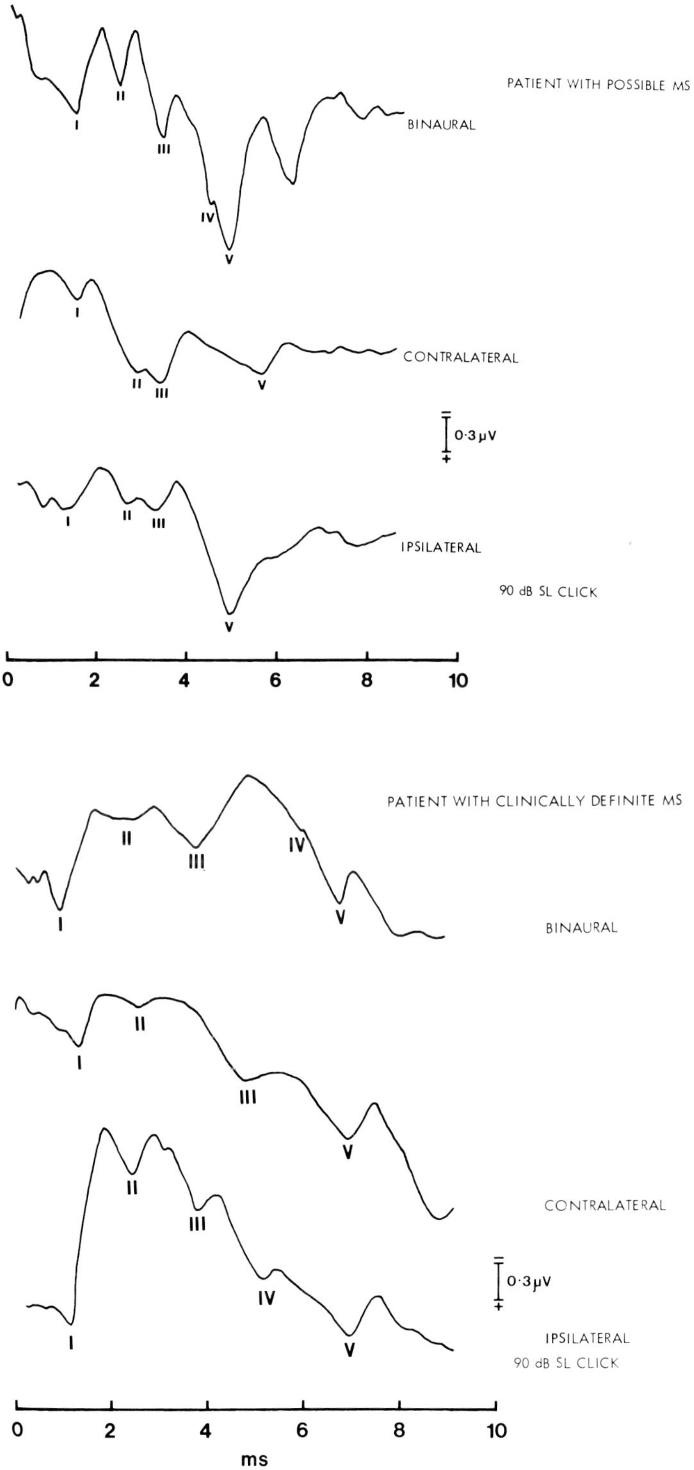
PATIENT WITH POSSIBLE MS
BINAURAL
CONTRALATERAL
IPSILATERAL
0·3µV
90 dB SL CLICK
I
II
III
IV
V
0
2
4
6
8
10
PATIENT WITH CLINICALLY DEFINITE MS
BINAURAL
CONTRALATERAL
IPSILATERAL
0·3µV
90 dB SL CLICK
ms

TABLE 1. *Comparison of ipsilateral or contralateral stimulation with binaural stimulation in the detection of MS*

Classification of patients according to McAlpine (11)	Clinically definite MS		Probable MS		Possible or suspected MS	
	Ipsilateral or contralateral	Binaural	Ipsilateral or contralateral	Binaural	Ipsilateral or contralateral	Binaural
Number of patients showing abnormal BAEP	9	7	2	0	8	1
Number of patients showing normal BAEP	1	3	1	3	4	11
Detection (%)	90%	70%	67%	0%	67%	8%

TABLE 2. *Means and standard deviations (SD) for waves III and V in normals and patients*[a]

	Wave III		Wave V		Waves III–IV	
	MS patients	Normals	MS patients	Normals	MS patients	Normals
Stimulus: L ear; recording: L side						
Mean (msec)	3.81	3.755	6.27	5.60	2.55	1.85
SD	0.270	0.161	1.129	0.186	1.102	0.173
d	1.16		2.92**		3.13**	
Stimulus: R ear; recording: L side						
Mean (msec)	3.83	3.68	6.24	5.71	2.42	2.03
SD	0.462	0.119	0.848	0.159	0.755	0.139
d	1.57		3.07**		2.54*	
Stimulus: R ear; recording: R side						
Mean (msec)	3.88	3.76	5.87	5.61	2.06	1.85
SD	0.216	0.141	0.537	0.163	0.543	0.152
d	2.30*		2.31*		2.11*	
Stimulus: L ear; recording: R side						
Mean (msec)	3.69	3.69	6.29	5.73	2.66	2.03
SD	0.318	0.122	1.04	0.196	0.993	0.159
d	—		2.64*		3.13**	
Stimulus: binaural; recording: R side						
Mean (msec)	3.80	3.70	6.18	5.62	2.45	1.95
SD	0.350	0.296	0.83	0.220	0.60	0.217
d	1.07		3.25**		3.89**	

[a] Significance levels of differences: *5% level; **1% level.

and standard deviation for the two groups are shown in Table 3, together with the observed values of *d* and their significance level. The difference in the mean interwave latency between the clinically definite MS group and the possible MS group was found to be statistically significant.

A particularly striking finding was the greater variance in latency of waves III and V in the patient groups compared to the normal subjects, especially with respect to the clinically definite group.

In a normal subject, a repeat test produces the same latency values (within measurement error), but in a patient with MS, a repeat test results in a difference in the latency of wave V of between 0.3 msec and 1.3 msec (with a mean of 0.57 msec) in the clinically definite group. In the "possible MS" category, the difference is less marked, with a range of 0 to 0.77 msec (mean 0.18 msec). A greater interpatient variability is to be expected, since the patients represent a heterogenous group with varying degree of severity of the disease. Nevertheless, the fact that the intrasubject variability in MS is also significantly higher than in normal subjects would appear to be a factor of some diagnostic importance.

DISCUSSION

In the "possible MS" group of patients, a large number showed normal latency BAEP wave forms on binaural stimulation but had abnormally late waves on ipsilateral or contralateral stimulation. In this group, a lateralized abnormality is suggested. The response, on binaural stimulation, from a patient with a lateralized abnormality appears to be masked by the response from the unaffected side and so provides seemingly normal latencies. Dobie and Berlin (6) have shown in the guinea pig that "the BAEP to binaural stimulation cannot be considered a linear summation of the monaural BAEPs." Their preliminary studies suggest a similar phenomenon in human BAEPs which supports our

TABLE 3. *Interwave latency (wave III to V): Comparison between the clinically definite MS group and possible MS*

	Ipsilateral or contralateral		Binaural	
	Clinically definite MS	Possible MS	Clinically definite MS	Possible MS
Mean interwave latency, wave III to V (msec)	3.69	2.58	2.87	2.10
SD	1.00	0.60	0.81	0.28
d	3.07		2.867	
Significance level	>1%		5%	

findings that in the human a unilateral lesion may not necessarily result in an abnormal BAEP wave form or latency on binaural stimulation.

Chiappa et al. (4) have also found marked asymmetries between the responses obtained from each ear by stimulating and recording monaurally. Thus, there is evidence to suggest that a large number of patients with possible MS "may have been missed" with binaural stimulation studies of BAEP abnormalities. Some recent studies (3,19) show much lower detection rate figures than those reported here, but before direct comparison among the different studies may be made, consideration must be given not only to the criteria for patient selection but also to the statistical limits imposed for the assessment of abnormality. Chiappa (3) has used three standard deviations from normal mean, and Stockard et al. (19) consider 90% tolerance limits, whereas we have chosen two standard deviations as our criteria for abnormality.

Our results show that the interwave latency (wave III to V) is prolonged in MS patients compared to normals. As the interwave latency represents conduction time between two discrete regions in the brainstem, any increase in this conduction time may be attributed to a defect in conduction caused by demyelination. In this connection, it is noteworthy that Shah et al. (17) have shown in rats with impaired myelination that there is an association between experimentally induced myelin deficiency and latency prolongation. There is further evidence (18,20) that the waves that manifest abnormally long latencies correspond to those brainstem and thalamic generator sources within the acoustic pathway that most commonly have a loss of myelin at postmortem examination. Longer interwave latency in long-standing MS cases suggests a link between interwave latency prolongation and progression of a demyelinating process.

The finding that the test repeatability was significantly poorer in MS patients might well have diagnostic implications. Our experience in patients with cerebello–pontine angle tumors is that such large differences in BAEP latencies are not apparent on test repetition. The intrasubject intertest variability shown in this study is in agreement with that reported by Lacquaniti et al. (9). Many of their patients categorized as clinically definite MS had BAEP recordings that showed little superimposition on consecutive repetition. They stated that this great variability did not depend on either stimulus intensity or the number of responses averaged.

Nodar (12) has observed a bizarre, unrepeatable BAEP tracing for at least one ear in 82% of his 38 patients.

The abnormally variable latencies in the BAEP wave form from test to test cannot simply be the result of desynchronization, as this would tend to alter the wave morphology, rendering the particular waves indistinguishable. Although this may happen in certain cases, in a large number of clinically definite cases, the BAEP waves are recognizable but show great variability in latency, suggesting a more complex underlying cause. Intermittent and defective conduction coupled with imprecise synchronization are obvious considerations that come to mind. However, before intrasubject variability can be considered to be pathognomonic of MS or even of a demyelinating process, further information on BAEP latency in other brainstem lesions is needed.

REFERENCES

1. Asselman, P., Chadwick, D. W., and Marsden, C. D. (1975): Visual evoked responses in the diagnosis and management of patients suspected of multiple sclerosis. *Brain,* 78:261–282.
2. Blegvad, B. (1975): Binaural summation of surface recorded electro–cochleographic responses. *Scand. Audiol.,* 4:233–238.
3. Chiappa, K. H. (1980): Pattern shift visual, brainstem auditory, and short latency somatosensory evoked potentials in multiple sclerosis. *Neurology (Minneap.),* 30:110–123.
4. Chiappa, K. H., Gladstone, K. J., and Young, R. R. (1979): Brainstem auditory evoked responses. Studies of wave form variations in 50 normal human subjects. *Arch. Neurol.,* 36:81–87.
5. Desmedt, J. E., and Noël, P. (1973): Average cerebral evoked potentials in the evaluation of lesions of the sensory nerves and of the central somatosensory pathway. In: *New Developments in Electromyography and Clinical Neurophysiology, Vol. 2,* edited by J. E. Desmedt, pp. 352–371. Karger, Based.
6. Dobie, R. A., and Berlin, C. I. (1979): Binaural interaction in brainstem evoked responses. *Arch. Otolaryngolo,* 105:391–398.
7. Halliday, A. M., McDonald, W. I., and Mushin, J. (1972): Delayed visual evoked response in optic neuritis. *Lancet,* 1:982–985.
8. Halliday, A. M., McDonald, W. I., and Mushin, J. (1977): Visual evoked potentials in patients with demyelinating disease. In: *Visual Evoked Potentials in Man; New Developments,* edited by J. E. Desmedt, pp. 438–449. Clarendon Press, Oxford.
9. Lacquaniti, F., Benna, P., Gilli, M., Troni, W., and Bergamasco, B. (1979): Brainstem auditory evoked potentials and blink reflex in quiescent multiple sclerosis. *Electroencephalogr. Clin. Neurophysiol.,* 47:607–610.
10. Matthews, W. B., and Esiri, M. (1979): Multiple sclerosis plaque related to abnormal somatosensory evoked potentials. *J. Neurol. Neurosurg. Psychiatry,* 42:940–942.
11. McAlpine, D., Lumsden, C. E., and Acheson, E. D. (1972): *Multiple Sclerosis. A Reappraisal, Second Edition.* Churchill Livingstone, Edinburgh, London.
12. Nodar, R. H. (1980): Brainstem auditory evoked potentials on individuals with multiple sclerosis. In: *Evoked Potentials,* edited by C. Barber, pp. 581–586. MTP Press, Lancaster.
13. Prasher, D. K., and Gibson, W. P. R. (1980): Brainstem auditory evoked potentials: Significant latency differences between ipsilateral and contralateral stimulation. *Electroencephalogr. Clin. Neurophysiol.,* 50:240–246.
14. Regan, D., Milner, B. A., and Heron, J. R. (1976): Delayed visual perception and delayed visual evoked potentials in the spinal form of multiple sclerosis and in retrobulbar neuritis. *Brain,* 99:43–67.
15. Robinson, K., and Rudge, P. (1975): Auditory evoked responses in multiple sclerosis. *Lancet,* 1:1164–1166.
16. Robinson, K., and Rudge, P. (1977): Abnormalities of the auditory evoked potentials in patients with multiple sclerosis. *Brain,* 100:19–40.
17. Shah, S. N., Bhargava, V. K., Johnson, R. C., and McKean, C. M. (1978): Latency changes in brain stem auditory evoked potentials associated with impaired brain myelination. *Exp. Neurol.,* 58:111–118.
18. Starr, A., and Hamilton, A. E. (1976): Correlation between confirmed sites of neurological lesions and abnormalities of far-field auditory brain stem responses. *Electroencephalogr. Clin. Neurophysiol.,* 41:595–608.
19. Stockard, J. J., Stockard, J. E., and Sharbrough, F. W. (1980): Brainstem auditory evoked potentials in neurology. Methodology, interpretation and clinical application. In: *Electrodiagnosis in Clinical Neurology,* edited by Aminoff, M. J., pp. 370–413. Churchill Livingstone, Edinburgh.
20. Wiederholt, W. C., Kobayashi, R. M., Stockard, J. J., and Rossiter, V. S. (1977): Central pontine myelinolysis. *Arch. Neurol.,* 34:220–223.

Clinical Applications of Evoked Potentials in Neurology,
edited by J. Courjon, F. Mauguiere, and M. Revol.
Raven Press, New York © 1982.

The Optically Evoked Blink Reflex in the Diagnosis of Multiple Sclerosis

*J.-P. Malin, **H. Müller, and *U. Patzold

**Neurologische Klinik and **Abteilung für Klinische Neurophysiologie und Experimentelle Neurologie, Medizinischen Hochschule, D-300 Hannover 61, Federal Republic of Germany*

The electrically elicited blink reflex is a well established method for detecting lower brainstem lesions in multiple sclerosis (3). In particular, cases with pontine lesions or internuclear ophthalmoplegia (IOP) have a high incidence of delayed reflex responses. Yet, even in cases with "definite MS" and IOP, the electric blink reflex may be normal (5). A supplementary method for detecting brainstem lesions at the mesencephalic level is the optically evoked blink reflex. There is some evidence that optic nerve fibers synapsing in the superior colliculus constitute the afferent link of the optic blink reflex (2).

METHOD

We used flashes from a stroboscope and evoked the reflex monocularly as well as binocularly after dark adaptation (luminosity below 3 cd/m^2). The stimuli were triggered manually, and at least five clear reflex responses were registered including eyes open, eyes closed, and each eye open and closed separately. Because of the rapid habituation of the optically evoked blink reflex, there was a pause of at least 30 sec before the next stimulus. The evoked muscle activity was recorded with silver surface electrodes (diameter, 5 mm) from the orbicularis oculi muscle. The signals were amplified and filtered with the Medelec MS 6 apparatus, using a filter with threshold frequency from 1.6 Hz to 8 kHz and a sensitivity of 200 to 500 μV/cm. Latency, amplitude, and duration of the reflex responses were evaluated and statistically treated. An extensive ophthalmological examination of all patients was part of the study.

Control Subjects

To establish normal values of the optically evoked blink reflex, 50 healthy volunteers (25 females and 25 males) were examined, all ophthalmologically and clinically normal subjects. The group of the healthy volunteers consisted of subjects from the laboratory staff, students, and ambulatory outpatients. Their ages ranged from 16 to 62 years. The mean age was 37 years (34 years in

TABLE 1. *Experimental program: 50 normal subjects, no reflex response: 6 from 50 (12%)*

Binocularly		
Eyes open: 10 reflex responses		
Eyes closed: 10 reflex responses		
Monocularly		
Right eye open: 10 reflex responses	(5 homolateral,	5 contralateral)
Right eye closed: 10 reflex responses	"	"
Left eye open: 10 reflex responses	"	"
Left eye closed: 10 reflex responses		
Total		
60 reflex responses per subject		
2640 reflex responses per 44 subjects		

females and 39 years in males). In six of the 50 healthy volunteers (12%), the optic blink reflex could not be evoked. These subjects were 46 to 62 years old with a male/female ratio of 2 : 1. Therefore, per subject 60 reflex responses were obtained, with a total of 2,640 responses (44 × 60). Table 1 shows the experimental program. Figure 1 shows a normal optically evoked blink reflex, and Table 2 presents the normal values. From this study, and optically evoked blink reflex was considered pathological if the latency exceeded more than 55 msec. There is a low variability within each individual and a remarkable variability among individuals. The interindividual range is 19 msec for binocular stimulation (34.0–53.0 msec) and 20.4 msec for monocular stimulation (32.6–53.0 msec).

A statistically significant difference between left and right eye during binocular stimulation could not be demonstrated (Wilcoxon matched-pairs signed rank test, 1% level of significance). Furthermore, the right–left difference of latencies after monocular stimulation was not statistically significant. However, the latencies on the left side were always shorter than those on the right side. A comparison between monocularly and binocularly derived reflex latencies does not show a significant difference. This conclusion, however, is not correct for the reflex duration: the statistical evaluation of this variable shows that there are significant differences between left and right eye stimulation during closed and opened eyes. The amplitudes of the reflex, which are quite variable in normal subjects, were not considered to be a reliable index of abnormality.

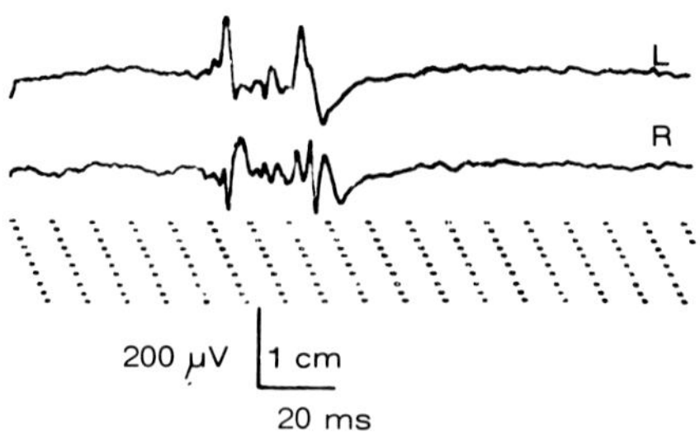

FIG. 1. Normal optically evoked blink reflex.

TABLE 2. *Binocular stimulation, eyes open* (N = 44)

	Mean	SD	$S_{\bar{x}}$	Min.	Max.
Latency (msec)					
Left	45.959	5.097	0.768	34.00	53.00
Right	46.014	5.103	0.769	34.80	53.00
Amplitude (μV)					
Left	171.227	84.924	12.803	76.00	434.00
Right	171.909	92.997	14.020	72.00	456.00
Duration (msec)					
Left	42.945	7.430	1.120	27.60	58.40
Right	43.677	7.766	1.171	28.40	59.40

MS Patients

The method of examination was the same as described in Table 1 for the control subjects. The MS group consisted of inpatients and ambulatory outpatients. Altogether, 145 patients (97 females and 48 males) were examined. The optically evoked blink reflex was recorded in 75 patients with "definite MS," in 30 patients with "probable MS," and in 40 patients with "possible MS," according to the criteria devised by McDonald and Halliday (7), McAlpine et al. (6), and Bauer (1). Twenty-five cases with an acute monosymptomatic retrobulbar neuritis were classified in the group "possible MS." The age in the MS group ranged from 18 to 62 years with an average of 37 years.

For comparative purposes the electric blink reflex was recorded in all MS patients by stimulation of the supraorbital nerve.

RESULTS

Table 3 summarizes the results by group. Altogether, 39% of the MS patients showed abnormal latencies. For the duration of the reflex response, we determined 60 msec (mean + 2 SD) to be the upper normal limit. Yet, consideration of this variable did not add further information. Among the MS group, each case with prolonged duration also showed abnormal latencies. The results in the subgroup with acute monosymptomatic retrobulbar neuritis were of special

TABLE 3. *Abnormal optically evoked blink reflex*

Definite MS (*N* = 75)	Probable MS (*N* = 30)	Possible MS (*N* = 40)	Possible MS monosymptomatic retrobulbar neuritis (*N* = 25)	Total (*N* = 145)
Both eyes: 38	6	3	—	47
One eye: 6	3	1	—	10
Total: 44(58%)	9(30%)	4(10%)	—	57(39.3%)
No response: 8(11%)	4(13%)	5(12.5%)	3(12%)	20(13.8%)

interest because none of the cases showed abnormal latencies. Even in patients with an actual visus of 0.5, the optically evoked blink reflex was normal. We obtain quite a different picture if we correlate the reflex measurements with the topography of the lesions. All patients with marked optic atrophy had delayed reflex responses. In this context, the word "marked" means with severe functional deficit, e.g., a visual acuity of 0.5 or less.

Similarly, among patients with mesencephalic signs (i.e., disturbances of the third and fourth or sixth cranial nerves as well as gaze paralysis) without optic atrophy 87.5%, had abnormal optic blink reflexes (Table 4). In a previous study, we demonstrated the diagnostic value of the electrically elicited blink reflex in MS diagnosis (5). We found an abnormal blink reflex in 50% of patients with "definite MS." Kimura (3) reported an incidence of 66%, and Lowitzsch et al. (4) of 60% of abnormal blink reflexes. In the study reported here, the electrically elicited blink reflex was abnormal in 50% of patients with "definite MS," and the optically evoked blink reflex was abnormal in 58%. In the group with "probable MS," 25% displayed an abnormally delayed electrically evoked blink reflex, and 30% of the patients had a delayed visual blink reflex on one or both sides. All patients with an acute monosymptomatic retrobulbar neuritis showed normal electrical and optical blink reflexes. The incidence of abnormal blink reflexes was only 10% for the optically evoked reflex and 15% for the electrically elicited reflex in the group with "possible MS." There was a particularly high incidence of delayed reflex responses in patients with pontomedullary signs (IOP). In such cases, we found delayed electrical blink reflexes in 81%. By contrast, patients with mesencephalic signs nearly always had normal electrical blink reflexes. In these cases the visual blink reflex was abnormal in 87.5%. In 36 cases with optic atrophy (marked functional deficit), the optically evoked blink reflex showed delayed latencies in 83%, but the electric blink reflex was delayed in only 32%. Alteration of the electric blink reflex in cases with optic atrophy was always associated with clinical signs suggesting pontine or medullary lesions.

In conclusion, the combination of optical and electrical blink reflex examina-

TABLE 4. *Delayed latencies of optically evoked blink reflexes in 145 MS patients related to topography of lesions*

Optic atrophy (marked functional deficit)	Optic atrophy (slight functional deficit)	Retrobulbar neuritis (no optic atrophy)	Mesencephalic signs	Pontine and medullary signs
No. of patients:				
36	51	25	48	102
Delayed latencies:				
30(83%)	13(25%)	—	42(87.5%)	43(42%)
(No response: 6)		(No response: 3)		

tion gives valuable information about the involvement of the brainstem in suspected MS. Whereas the electric blink reflex verifies lesions in the pons and medulla, the optic blink reflex indicates involvement of the optic nerve or the mesencephalic level.

REFERENCES

1. Bauer, H. J. (1974): Judgment of the validity of a clinical MS diagnosis. *Acta Neurol. Scand.* [*Suppl.*], 58:13–21.
2. Brodal, A. (1969): *Neurological Anatomy, Second Edition.* Oxford University Press, London.
3. Kimura, J. (1975): Electrically elicited blink reflex in diagnosis of multiple sclerosis. *Brain,* 98:413–426.
4. Lowitzsch, K., Kuhnt, U., and Sakmann, C. (1976): Visual pattern evoked responses and blink reflexes in assessment of MS diagnosis. *J. Neurol.,* 213:17–32.
5. Malin, J.-P., and Müller, H. (1980): Zum Stellenwert der Untersuchung des elektrisch ausgelösten Blinkreflexes in der Diagnostik der multiplen Sklerose. In: *Fortschritte der Technischen Medizin in der Neurologischen Diagnostik und Therapie,* edited by H. Reisner and G. Schnaberth, pp. 235–237. Neurologische Universitätsklinik, Vienna.
6. McAlpine, D., Lumsden, C., and Acheson, E. D. (1972): *Multiple Sclerosis. A Reappraisal, Second Edition.* Churchill Livingston, Edinburgh.
7. McDonald, W. I., and Halliday, A. M. (1977): Diagnosis and classification of multiple sclerosis. *Br. Med. Bull.,* 33:4–8.

Clinical Applications of Evoked Potentials in Neurology,
edited by J. Courjon, F. Mauguiere, and M. Revol.
Raven Press, New York © 1982.

Changes in Visual and Short-Latency Somatosensory Evoked Potentials in Patients with Multiple Sclerosis

A. W. de Weerd and E. J. Jonkman

T.N.O. Research Unit for Clinical Neurophysiology, Westeinde Hospital, 2512 VA The Hague, The Netherlands

In multiple sclerosis (MS) research, a need exists for parameters for quantitating the course of the disease (1). The Kurtzke scales (7) have proven to be useful as a clinical method for investigating the activity of the disease. Brown et al. (1) suggested the use of evoked potentials (EP) for follow-up studies of the spontaneous course of MS and the effect of therapy. Up to now, there have been only a few attempts to relate the clinical course to changes in the EP. In a small number of patients who had a relapse, Robinson and Rudge (13) found an instability of the BAEP in contrast to the highly consistent findings in control subjects and in patients who were clinically stable. Diener and Scheibler (4) found the most VEP changes in time in those patients who had an optic neuritis; the relation between changes in visual acuity and VEP was poor. After serial recording of EP in MS patients, Matthews and Small (9) concluded that no role for VEP and SEP as objective measures of the activity of MS could be demonstrated. Namerow (11), however, found improvement in the SEP after resolution of the sensory deficits in one MS patient.

In view of these inconsistent findings in the literature, a prospective study of the variability in EP in normal subjects and MS patients was planned as well as a study of the relation of these changes to the clinical condition of the patients.

MATERIAL AND METHODS

Subjects

In 27 normal volunteers (14 M, 13 F; range, 20–55 years) VEP and SEP were investigated. The recordings were done twice with an interval of 3½ months. Volunteers with a history of neurological or ophthalmological disease were excluded. Corrected refraction errors were allowed. No drugs were used. This group was used as controls for the study in MS patients.

Twenty-five patients were investigated (Table 1). The clinical diagnosis of MS was made according to the criteria of McDonald and Halliday (10). Only "clinically definite" cases and four MS patients with a progressive spinal dysfunction (progressive probable MS) were studied. Other causes of the signs and symptoms were excluded by blood assays, myelography, and computerized tomography. Cerebrospinal fluid assays included cell count, total protein, IgG index, and agarose electrophoresis (5). A relapse of the disease was defined by the criteria of Schuhmacher et al. (15). Visual acuity was measured with the Snellen method. A significant change was assumed when the visual acuity changed by more than 0.2. Sensory handicap and the disability of the patients were scored on the "functional system scale" and the "Disability Status Scale" (DSS) of Kurtzke (7). The MS group was investigated twice with an interval of 3½ months. Six patients who had had relapses and underwent a 2-week treatment with ACTH were studied three times: VEP and SEP were measured at the beginning and the end of the therapy as well; the investigation was repeated 3 months later.

Methods

The recordings were made in a room with a constant temperature of 22°C. Preparation of the subjects took place in the same room. The VEP was recorded with the subject comfortably seated approximately 60 cm from the screen. The SEP was recorded in supine position. The room was darkened during the recording of the VEP.

The stimulus for the VEP was a black-and-white checkerboard pattern projected onto a translucent screen via a rotatable mirror (Digitimer). The pattern was reversed twice a second. Two sizes of squares were used, subtending, respectively, angles of 1° and 0.5° of the visual field; the whole pattern measured 30 cm and 17 cm, respectively (26° and 15° in the visual field). The contrast from black and white was 78%. The person under study was asked to fixate on a spot in the center of the screen. Each eye was stimulated separatively with 256 stimuli. For the SEP, the right and left median nerves were separately stimulated at the wrist with a square pulse of 0.1 msec duration, and voltage adjusted to produce a twitch of the thumb. Two hundred fifty-six stimuli were given with an interval of 0.2 sec.

TABLE 1. *Multiple sclerosis patients in the present study*

Sex	
Male	11
Female	14
Age range (years)	24–59
Diagnosis	
Clinically definite	21
Progressive probable	4

Pattern reversal VEP were recorded from an active electrode at O_z (10–20 system) using a reference electrode at C_z. Electrode positions C_3 and C_4 were used for recording of the SEP at the scalp, and a midline point just above the seventh vertebra for the cervical SEP. A reference electrode was placed at F_z. The signals were led to Tektronix T_7A_{22} amplifiers and averaged by a Tektronix P_{7001} processor. In SEP studies, Medelec AA_6MK_{II} preamplifiers were used. Bandpass filters were set at 1 to 3,000 Hz (−3 dB). Measurements were taken from Polaroid pictures. Only the latencies of the VEP ($P_{\overline{100}}$), cervical ($N_{\overline{13}}$), and short-latency cortical SEP ($N_{\overline{20}}$) were studied.

Latency values for our laboratory as obtained in controls are given in Table 2. The variations of the EP across the time intervals mentioned above were calculated. The change of EP latencies in patients was considered significant when the calculated difference exceeded the mean difference as found in the normal subjects plus 2 SD (normal values: Table 3). Appearance or disappearance of EP was considered as improvement or deterioration, respectively.

TABLE 2. *Normal subjects* (N = 27)

	Latencies of evoked potentials (msec)		
	Mean	SD	Mean + 2 SD
VEP			
1° squares	120.9	8.2	137.3
0.5° squares	118.4	8.5	135.4
SEP (arm ≤ 70 cm)			
$N_{\overline{13}}$	12.3	0.9	14.1
$N_{\overline{20}}$	18.3	0.8	19.9
SEP (arm > 70 cm)			
$N_{\overline{13}}$	14.0	1.0	16.0
$N_{\overline{20}}$	19.7	1.1	21.9
All SEP			
$N_{\overline{20}} - N_{13}$	5.5	0.8	7.1

TABLE 3. *Variability of evoked potentials in normal subjects between tests*[a]

	Difference *(d)* in latencies (msec)		
	Mean	SD	Mean ± 2 SD
VEP			
1° squares	−0.1	6.3	$-12.7 < d < 12.5$
0.5° squares	−0.6	6.5	$-13.6 < d < 12.4$
SEP			
$N_{\overline{13}}$	0.2	0.7	$-1.2 < d < 1.6$
$N_{\overline{20}}$	0.4	0.6	$-0.8 < d < 1.6$
$N_{\overline{20}} - N_{\overline{13}}$	0.1	0.6	$-1.1 < d < 1.3$

[a] Average interval between tests was 106 days for VEP and 101 days for SEP. *N* = 27.

RESULTS

At the first EP recording, 76% of the patients had abnormal latencies of the VEP and 64% of the SEP. In all but two of the 25 patients, VEP and/or SEP were abnormal (Table 4).

The variation of the latencies of the EP found in successive measurements in normal subjects was small (Table 3). It did not exceed 10% of the absolute values used in our laboratory.

Before presentation of the compiled data, two typical cases will be given.

Patient A was a 20-year-old woman. In 1977, she had the first symptoms of MS. Two exacerbations occurred in 1979; during the second exacerbation, EP were obtained. At this time she had an internuclear ophthalmoplegia; there was a visual acuity of 4/300 of the right eye and a hypesthesia of the left side of the body. The SEP after stimulation of the left median nerve is shown in Fig. 1a. After 2 weeks of ACTH therapy, the latency of the cortical SEP had diminished (Fig. 1b).

Patient B, with MS, had normal vision at the first recording. Her VEP were normal (Fig. 2a). Three months later she complained of blurred vision in both eyes. The visual acuity in the right eye was 0.5. The latency of the VEP of this eye had increased by 70 msec to 185 msec (Fig. 2b).

Across the interval of 3½ months, VEP changes were noted in 23 eyes (16 patients). When Snellen letters were used, 19 eyes (12 patients) improved or deteriorated. There was a relationship between the changes in VEP and the changes in visual acuity. Significantly more changes (improvement or deterioration) were seen in VEP when visual acuity changed (Table 5).

The neurological reexamination revealed changes in sensory function in few patients, making an estimate of the correlation between the variations in SEP and sensory symptoms impossible. In most patients without changes in sensory function between the first and second recording, a stability of the SEP was demonstrated. In three patients, paradoxic results were seen. Two of them had an increase in the latency of the SEP contrasting to the improvement of sensory functions (Table 6).

In four patients, normalization of an abnormal VEP was seen. The SEP returned to normal in five cases. This improvement of EP was accompanied by a disappearance of clinical symptoms in visual and sensory function, respectively.

TABLE 4. *Evoked potentials in MS patients at first test*

Evoked potential	Patients with abnormal latency
VEP	19/25 (76%)
SEP	16/25 (64%)
VEP and/or SEP	23/25 (92%)

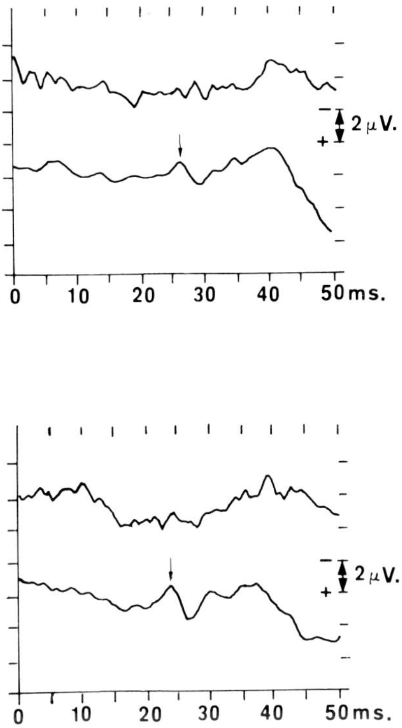

FIG. 1. a (top): Somatosensory evoked potentials before the beginning of ACTH therapy. $N_{\overline{20}}$ *(arrow)* at 27 msec. **b (bottom):** Somatosensory evoked potentials 2 weeks later at the end of ACTH therapy. $N_{\overline{20}}$ *(arrow)* at 23 msec. The $N_{\overline{13}}$ cannot be distinguished (cervical SEP in the *top traces*).

No correlation could be found between changes in the disability status scale (DSS), which gives a score of the overall disability of the patient, and the changes of EP in these patients.

Twenty-one patients underwent CSF assay at the time of the first EP recording. A high IgG index and oligoclonal IgG bands suggested active demyelination in 15 patients. Changes of EP in time were not more frequent in these patients than in those with normal CSF.

Nine of the 25 patients underwent a 2-week treatment with ACTH. Evoked potentials were recorded three times in six of them. This small number of patients

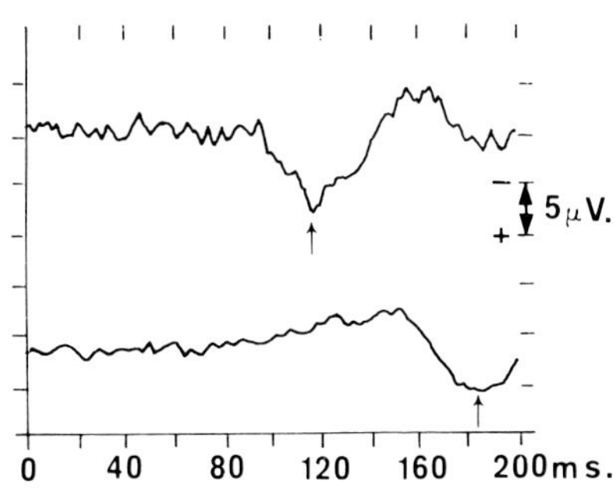

FIG. 2. a (top): Visual evoked potentials of the right eye at first recording. Normal VEP *(arrow);* visual acuity (Snellen letters), 1.0. **b (bottom):** Visual evoked potential of the right eye 3 months later. The latency of the VEP had increased by 70 msec; visual acuity, 0.5.

TABLE 5. *Changes in VEP latency compared with visual acuity*[a]

VEP latency	Visual acuity		
	Better	Same	Worse
Decrease (13)	8	4	1
Same (27)	2	22	3
Increase (10)	0	5	5

[a] More changes occurred in VEP (improvement or deterioration) when visual acuity changed ($x^2 = 9.6$ $p < 0.005$). Interval between tests was, on average, 104 days. $N = 25$.

TABLE 6. *Changes in SEP latency compared with sensory function*[a]

Latency of SEP	Sensory function		
	Better	Same	Worse
Decrease (12)	2	9	1
Same (27)	1	26	0
Increase (11)	2	6	3

[a] Interval between tests was, on average, 104 days. $N = 25$.

made statistical analysis impossible. However, our data suggest that after 3½ months no difference exists in the variability of EP between the treated patients and those who had no ACTH.

DISCUSSION

The use of EP for detection of demyelinating lesions in MS is now well established. Chiappa (2), Mastaglia et al. (8), and Paty et al. (12) found abnormal EP in nearly all of their patients in combined studies with VEP and SEP or with VEP, SEP, and BAEP. This has been confirmed in our study.

Diener and Scheibler (4) made serial recordings of the VEP in normal subjects with some weeks interval. They found only little variability of the latencies of VEP. In our study of normal subjects, it was shown that maximal changes in EP after an interval of 3½ months were about 10% of the latencies found at the first recording. This stability of EP in controls seems to allow detection with EP of changes within the visual and sensory systems of patients. Our follow-up study has demonstrated that changes in EP occurred over the long interval as well as in the interval of 2 to 3 weeks.

In the literature, a number of explanations have been given for the improvement in EP. It has been shown that apposition of a few new layers of myelin gives a considerable improvement of conduction in a demyelinated fiber in the CNS (6). The remyelination, however, takes some time and cannot account for the quick recovery seen in some of our patients. Possibly a diminution of edema in the MS plaques, which might be an effect of ACTH, could be an explanation of this phenomenon. Rogart and Ritchie (14) have demonstrated that conduction in an experimentally demyelinated CNS fiber can be restored even in the absence of remyelination. After demyelination, a change in the internodal axonal membrane was seen. The number of sodium channels in this membrane increased, transforming the inert membrane to an electrically excitable one. The time required for this improvement was several days to weeks. Possibly, the different mechanisms proposed by these three theories could offer an explanation of the decrease in latencies of EP. In the short interval in which ACTH was given, the recovery could be a result of the diminution of edema. Remyelination or increased permeability of the axonal membrane might be an explanation of the improvement over the long term.

The variability of EP in patients who had ACTH did not differ from the changes in time in the EP seen in patents who had no treatment. Thus, no role of ACTH in stabilizing or improving the conduction in CNS fibers could be demonstrated in this study.

In the patients who had an abnormal CSF with evidence of intrathecal production of IgG, changes in time in EP appeared comparable with the variability in EP in those patients who had normal CSF. It has been shown by Christensen et al. (3) that a high IgG index in the CSF cannot be used as a parameter of activity of MS. Evoked potentials might be more useful for this purpose (13).

In our study, changes in VEP and SEP had a certain relation to clinical parameters of the visual and sensory system. No correlation could be established with the most general parameter for activity of the disease, the DSS.

In conclusion, VEP and SEP seem to be useful for the study of changes in time in certain parts of the CNS in MS patients. Evoked potentials are probably more sensitive to variations in functions than is the clinical examination of the visual and sensory system.

The role of EP has been established in the diagnosis of MS; evoked potentials seem to be useful also as a parameter of the changes occurring in the CNS during the course of the disease.

REFERENCES

1. Brown, J. R., Beebe, G. W., and Kurtzke, J. F. (1979): The design of clinical studies to assess therapeutic efficacy in multiple sclerosis. *Neurology (Minneap.)*, 29:3–23.
2. Chiappa, K. H. (1980): Pattern shift visual, brainstem auditory and short latency somatosensory evoked potentials in multiple sclerosis. *Neurology (Minneap.,)* 30:110–123.
3. Christensen, O., Clausen, J., and Fog, T. (1978): Relationships between abnormal IgG index, oligoclonal bands, acute phase reactants and some clinical data in multiple sclerosis. *J. Neurol.*, 218:237–244.
4. Diener, H. C., and Scheibler, H. (1980): Follow-up studies of visual potentials in multiple sclerosis evoked by checkerboard and foveal stimulation. *Electroencephalogr. Clin. Neurophysiol.*, 49:490–496.
5. Johnson, K. P. (1980): Cerebrospinal fluid and blood assays of diagnostic usefulness in multiple sclerosis. *Neurology (Minneap.)*, 30(2):106–109.

6. Koles, Z. J., and Rasminsky, M. (1972): A computer simulation of conduction in demyelinated nerve fibres. *J. Physiol. (Lond.),* 227:351–364.
7. Kurtzke, J. F. (1965): Further notes on disability evaluation in multiple sclerosis with scale modifications. *Neurology (Minneap.),* 15:654–661.
8. Mastaglia, F. L., Black, J. L., Cala, L. A., and Collins, D. W. K. (1980): The contribution of visual and somatosensory evoked potentials and quantitative electro-oculography in the diagnosis of multiple sclerosis. In: *Evoked Potentials,* edited by C. Barber, pp. 559–566. MTP Press, Lancaster.
9. Matthews, W. B., and Small, D. G. (1979): Serial recording of visual and somatosensory evoked potentials in multiple sclerosis. *J. Neurol. Sci.,* 40:11–21.
10. McDonald, W. I., and Halliday, A. M. (1977): Diagnosis and classification of multiple sclerosis. *Br. Med. Bull.,* 33:4–9.
11. Namerow, N. S. (1968): Somatosensory evoked responses in multiple sclerosis patients with varying sensory loss. *Neurology (Minneap.),* 18:1197–1204.
12. Paty, J., Delia, P., Gioux, M., and Franqui-Zannettacci, M. (1980): An approach to diagnosis of multiple sclerosis with cerebral evoked potentials (visual, auditory, somatosensory). In: *Evoked Potentials,* edited by C. Barber, pp. 593–603. MTP Press, Lancaster.
13. Robinson, K., and Rudge, P. (1978): The stability of the auditory evoked potentials in normal man and patients with multiple sclerosis. *J. Neurol. Sci.,* 36:147–156.
14. Rogart, R. B., and Ritchie, J. M. (1977): Pathophysiology of conduction in demyelinated nerve fibres. In: *Myelin,* edited by P. Morell, pp. 353–382. Plenum Press, New York and London.
15. Schuhmacher, G., Beebe, G., Kibler, R., Kurland, L., Kurtzke, J., McDonnell, F., Nagler, B., Sibley, W., Tourtellotte, W., and Willmon, T. (1965): Problems of experimental trials in multiple sclerosis. Report by the panel on the evaluation of experimental trials in multiple sclerosis. *Ann. N.Y. Acad. Sci.,* 122:552–568.

Clinical Applications of Evoked Potentials in Neurology,
edited by J. Courjon, F. Mauguiere, and M. Revol.
Raven Press, New York © 1982.

Exacerbation Detection in Multiple Sclerosis by Clinical and Evoked Potential Techniques: A Preliminary Report

William Likosky and Robert S. Elmore

Kaiser Permanente Medical Center, Santa Clara, California 95051

Multiple sclerosis (MS) is characterized by clinical exacerbations and remissions. Until evoked potential (EP) studies became available, there had been no method of identifying asymptomatic disease. Although this test is becoming widely available in identifying subclinical lesions to help in the initial diagnosis of MS, little is known of long-term electrophysiologic changes detectable by this technique and whether subclinical exacerbations or remissions are detectable and occur in any frequency in these patients. Our studies with visual (VEP), auditory (AEP), and somatosensory (SEP) evoked potentials demonstrate a striking and unexpected prevalence of significant neurophysiologic changes in MS patients not reflected by clinical exacerbations. The neuropathologic correlate of these changes must be defined.

METHODS

Twenty MS patients from the Santa Clara, California Kaiser Foundation Hospital Multiple Sclerosis Clinic volunteered and were selected on the basis of a clinically typical exacerbation–remission form of the disease, the McDonald (3) clinical criteria, and the presence of oligoclonal bands in cerebrospinal fluid. The group consisted of 17 females and three males. Three were between the ages of 20 and 29, six between 30 and 39, and 11 between 40 and 49. The patients had an average of 2.5 exacerbations in the year before the study. Symptoms and signs of disease activity were monitored for each patient's participation during the study period from December, 1978 through June, 1980 by monthly phone calls, clinical examinations at the time of EP studies, and additional visits with any clinical exacerbation. Evoked potential studies were performed at regular intervals, usually 2 to 4 months but as infrequently as 10 months. Clinical exacerbations were classified on the basis of history and physical examination as involving visual system, brainstem, upper extremity, lower extremity, and/or other pathways. Visual exacerbations comprised retrobulbar neuritis. Brainstem exacerbations consisted of any clinical event best explained by disease in that location. Upper and lower extremity exacerbations comprised clinical events involving motor or any sensory dysfunction confined to a single or paired extremity. Some clinical exacerbations involved other systems, e.g., bladder, cerebellum.

The EP studies were performed using a Nicolet CA 1000 modular system. The VEP stimulus consisted of pattern reversal of 16×16 black-and-white checkerboard squares presented on a TV screen 1 m from the patient. Two runs of at least 100 reversals were recorded using O_Z–C_Z linkages and monocular stimulation. The patient wore glasses if he normally would do so at this distance. The AEP rarefaction click of 100 μsec duration was recorded at C_Z referred to a reference electrode on the ipsilateral mastoid. A minimum of 2,000 stimuli were presented monaurally in each of two runs at 60 dB above the patient's hearing level. The SEP were elicited by electrical stimulation of the median nerve at the wrist (MSEP) or posterior tibial nerve (PTSEP) posterior to the medial malleolus. Stimulation was adjusted to give an easy visible twitch of the thumb or great toe, respectively; current was increased rather than stimulation duration, if possible. At least 100 stimuli were recorded in C_3- or C_4-to-contralateral–mastoid derivations for right and left median studies, respectively, or in C_Z-to-contralateral–mastoid derivation for PTSEP studies.

Normative evoked potential data were obtained from well hospital employee volunteers. A significant VEP change was defined as loss of the P100 or a 2-SD increment of its latency. A significant AEP change was defined as a loss of wave V or a 2-SD increase in the I–V interval. In the infrequent instance where a clear wave I was not found, a 2-SD increase in the absolute latency of wave V was used. A significant change in the SEP was defined as a loss of the N1 wave or of a 2-SD increment in its latency. An abnormal test was defined as one whose major parameter was 2-SD above the mean of normal or was absent.

RESULTS

The 20 patients were studied over a total of 209 patient months comprising 76 study intervals. During this time, the 20 patients experienced 21 clinical exacerbations, some involving more than one clinical pathway. These exacerbations involved clinical pathways in the following frequency: one visual, four brainstem, three upper extremity, and 17 lower extremity. Fifty-five study intervals were without recognized clinical exacerbations. Visual EP, AEP, and MSEP recordings were obtained for each of the 76 intervals, but PTSEP for 50. Twenty-six PTSEP were excluded as technically unsatisfactory for comparative analysis. All 20 patients had at least one abnormal test. The VEP was abnormal on at least one occasion in 16 patients (80%), the AEP in seven (35%), the MSEP in 15 (75%), and the PTSEP in 13 (65%). Of 48 significant changes noted in any evoked potential study, the VEP demonstrated 11, the AEP 10, MSEP 17, and PTSEP 10.

The 21 clinical exacerbations were recognized in 209 study months comprising

76 intervals (Table 1). Thirty-three of these intervals were associated with significant EP changes. Eleven of 21 (52%) clinical exacerbations and 22 of 55 (40%) clinically quiescent periods were associated with significant EP changes.

Visual EP changes are tallied by type of exacerbation in Table 2. Of 21 clinical exacerbations, the VEP demonstrated a significant change in five (24%). Of 55 clinically quiescent periods, the VEP demonstrated a significant change is six (11%). The single visual clinical exacerbation was detected by VEP.

Auditory EP changes are tallied by exacerbation type in Table 3. Of 21 clinical exacerbations, the AEP was significantly changed in three (14%). Of 55 clinically quiescent periods, the AEP was significantly changed in seven (13%). Of four exacerbations clinically involving the brainstem, the AEP was not significantly changed.

Median nerve SEP changes are tallied by exacerbation type in Table 4. Of 21 clinical exacerbations, the MSEP was significantly changed in four (19.1%). Of 55 clinically quiescent periods, the MSEP was positive in 13 (24%). Of

TABLE 1. *Clinical exacerbations and evoked potential changes by study intervals*

	Clinical exacerbation/EP change				
	+/+	+/0	0/+	0/0	Total
No. of intervals	11	10	22	33	76

TABLE 2. *Clinical exacerbations by type and visual evoked potential changes for study intervals*

	Clinical exacerbation/VEP change				
	+/+	+/0	0/+	0/0	Total
Any clinical exacerbation	5	16	6	49	76
Visual exacerbation	1	0	10	65	76

TABLE 3. *Clinical exacerbations by type and auditory evoked potential changes for study intervals*

	Clinical exacerbation/AEP change				
	+/+	+/0	0/+	0/0	Total
Any clinical exacerbation	3	18	7	48	76
Brainstem exacerbation	0	4	10	62	76

TABLE 4. *Clinical exacerbations by type and median somatosensory evoked potential changes for study intervals*

	Clinical exacerbation/MSEP change				
	+/+	+/0	0/+	0/0	Total
Any clinical exacerbation	4	17	13	42	76
Arm exacerbation	0	3	17	56	76

TABLE 5. *Clinical exacerbations by type and posterior tibial somatosensory evoked potential changes for study intervals*

	Clinical exacerbation/PTSEP change				
	+/+	+/0	0/+	0/0	Total
Any clinical exacerbation	3	9	7	31	50
Leg exacerbation	2	6	8	34	50

three exacerbations involving fiber tracts related to the arms, the SEP was significantly changed in none.

Clinical exacerbations were tallied by PTSEP and study intervals in Table 5. Fifty study intervals were studied satisfactorily. Of 12 clinical exacerbations studied, the PTSEP was positive in three (25%). Of 38 quiescent intervals, the test was significantly changed in seven (18%). Of eight exacerbations involving pathways affecting the legs, two (25%) were positive. Of 42 intervals without leg symptoms, eight (19%) were associated with significant changes in PTSEP.

DISCUSSION

The application in the past decade of computerized averaging techniques to the study of CNS sensory tracts has provided a method to document neurophysiologic fiber tract function. Numerous studies have demonstrated the usefulness of the EP in documenting clinical and subclinical disease in the MS patient. The EP sensitivity to subclinical disease has suggested that it may be a useful adjunct to clinical evaluation in monitoring MS disease activity. We have recognized an unexpectedly high occurrence of EP changes and a complexity in evaluating the relationship among clinical events, EP changes, and presumed neuropathologic disease progression.

Poser (5) recently questioned the common practice of relating clinical symptoms to disease activity and cited the poor anatomic correlation between the patients' signs and symptoms and demonstrable areas of activity by radionucleotide and contrast-enhanced CT scans. A number of mechanisms may account for apparent disease progression and include the gliotic reparative process, fluctuations related to systemic illness (e.g., urinary tract infection), temperature fluctuations with intercurrent illness, and possibly psychogenic factors. Symptomatic progression and remission may then occur in patients whose basic underlying disease process is arrested, and fluctuations in symptoms or signs must not be equated with disease progression.

The relationship between EP parameter changes and the progression of MS is undefined. Matthews and Small (2) followed seven patients with MS an average of 18 months with VEP and SEP at 1- to 3-month intervals. A larger mixed group of definite, probable, and possible MS patients was also studied. They found a reasonable but not invariable association between clinical exacerbations and EP results. Some EP changes were noted in patients without clinical changes, and their significance was unclear. Robinson and Rudge (6) studied the AEP serially in 27 patients with clinically diagnosed MS over a 2.5-year period. They found a poor correlation between clinical and EP events. Some patients had abnormal tests occur and remit without clinical worsening. These studies using one or two EP parameters have suggested that EP fluctuations may be frequent and not closely related to clinical events.

The present study was undertaken to define further the relationship between clinical and EP events. The population was well defined as MS by clinical and spinal fluid techniques and was followed closely to compare prospectively clinical and EP changes. We confirmed earlier reports in demonstrating a high occurrence of abnormal tests in MS patients in clinically involved and uninvolved pathways. The EP changes associated with exacerbations were often in clinically uninvolved pathways, and clinically uninvolved pathways were often without significant changes. The findings are similar to those of Matthews and Small as well as those of Robinson and Rudge in that frequent fluctuations were found which were often without clinical correlation.

In other studies, clinical monitoring of MS patients indicates an exacerbation frequency of every 0.5 to 1.5 years (1,4,7). If the 40% of clinically quiescent intervals with significant EP changes represent pathologically active periods, then a marked upward revision in exacerbation frequency would need to be made. These fluctuations in EP wave forms and latencies may reflect pathologic MS activity involving these pathways or fluctuations in conduction in diseased fiber tracts from as yet undefined cause. The ultimate utility of EP monitoring of MS exacerbations will depend on the development of techniques to define what these fluctuations represent.

SUMMARY

The EP is well demonstrated as a useful indicator of subclinical demyelinating disease. Our study performed on patients well defined as MS and monitored closely for clinical exacerbations demonstrated an unexpectedly high occurrence of significant worsening in EP parameters. These changes occurred in the presence or absence of clinical worsening. The parameter changes may represent new demyelination or other pathologic or neurophysiologic changes in neuropathologically static lesions.

ACKNOWLEDGMENT

This study was supported by a grant from the Kaiser Foundation Research Institute. The authors wish to thank Eileen Long, Linda Sanchez, Eva Predac, Kathy Frazier, and Gayle Smothers for their technical aid.

REFERENCES

1. Alexander, L., Berkeley, A., and Alexander, A. (1943): Prognosis and treatment of multiple sclerosis. *J.A.M.A.*, 166:1943–1949.
2. Matthews, W., and Small, D. (1979): Serial recording of visual and somatosensory evoked potentials in multiple sclerosis. *J. Neurol. Sci.*, 40:11–21.
3. McDonald, W. (1978): What is multiple sclerosis? Clinical criterion for diagnosis. In: *Multiple Sclerosis Research,* edited by A. Davison, J. Humphrey, A. Liversedge, W. McDonald, and J. Porterfield pp. 1–8. Elsevier, New York.
4. Muller, R. (1949): Studies in multiple sclerosis. *Acta. Med. Scand.* [*Suppl.*], 222:1–214.
5. Poser, C. (1980): Exacerbations, activity, and progression in multiple sclerosis. *Arch. Neurol.*, 37:471–474.
6. Robinson, K., and Rudge, P. (1978): The stability of the auditory evoked potentials in normal man and patients with multiple sclerosis. *J. Neurol. Sci.*, 36:147–156.
7. Thygesen, P. (1953): *The Course Of Multiple Sclerosis.* Rosenkilde and Bagger, Copenhagen.

Clinical Applications of Evoked Potentials in Neurology,
edited by J. Courjon, F. Mauguiere, and M. Revol.
Raven Press, New York © 1982.

Course of Visual Evoked Potentials in Multiple Sclerosis: Electroclinical Correlations and Pathophysiological Considerations in 25 Patients

C. Confavreux, F. Mauguière, J. Courjon, G. Aimard, and M. Devic

Hôpital Neurologique, Lyon, France

The diagnostic contribution of VEPs in MS is largely accepted (7,8). They can demonstrate topographic dissemination of lesions that may otherwise be undetected for a long time. However, VEP alterations are not specific for demyelination.

Up to now, the only systematic study of the VEPs during the course of MS has been that of Matthews and Small (12). This type of study could determine the precocity of VEP abnormalities if performed from the early stages of the disease. Moreover, VEP recording could give new insight into the pathophysiology of the disease.

PATIENTS

Twenty-five MS patients were studied. They were not systematically selected but where the first patients in the neurological departments in Lyon to be studied with checkerboard-reversal stimulation. This technique has been operational since January, 1979. One year later, the same patients were invited to attend a second electrophysiological examination.

This group of 25 patients was a representative sample of our MS population (2) according to mean age at onset of the disease (31.4 ± 8.9 years) and distribution by sex (13 males, 12 females), symptomatology at onset, remittent or progressive type of onset, and severity classification (see Table 1).

We used our own diagnostic classification (2) which is based on McAlpine's (16) but takes into account the paraclinical data (acquired dyschromatopsia, retinal periphlebitis, CT scan, VEPs) for the "dissemination in space" criteria and CSF data. "Definite," "probable," and "possible" forms were respectively 11, seven, and seven cases without information about VEPs and 20, one, and four cases with this information.

The period of follow-up varied from 1 month to 33 years, with a mean at 6.3 ± 7.7 years and a median at 26 months.

TABLE 1. *Basic data on the disease course in the 25 patients studied*

First VEP:	Normal							Abnormal															NI		
Second VEP:	Normal				Abnormal			Improved			Not modified						Worsened								
Case No.:	1	2	3	4	5	6	7	8	9	10	11	12	13	14	15	16	17	18	19	20	21	22	23	24	25
Symptoms at the onset																									
Monosymptomatic LT[a]	+	+	+	+	+	+	+	−	−	−	−	+	+	+	−	+	−	+	+	−	+	+	−	−	+
BS[a]	−	−	−	−	−	−	−	+	−	−	−	−	−	−	−	−	−	−	−	−	−	−	−	−	−
ON[a]	−	−	−	−	−	−	−	−	−	−	−	−	−	−	+	−	+	−	−	+	−	−	+	+	−
Plurisymptomatic Without ON	−	−	−	−	−	−	−	−	+	−	+	−	−	−	−	−	−	−	−	−	−	−	−	−	−
With ON	−	−	−	−	−	−	−	−	−	+	−	−	−	−	−	−	−	−	−	−	−	−	−	−	−
Course at the onset																									
Remittent	−	−	+	+	+	+	−	+	+	+	+	−	−	+	+	−	+	+	+	+	+	+	+	+	−
Progressive	+	+	−	−	−	−	+	−	−	−	−	+	+	−	−	+	−	−	−	−	−	−	−	−	+
Disease severity classification																									
Benign	−	−	+	−	−	+	−	−	−	+	−	−	−	−	−	−	−	−	−	−	−	−	+	−	−
Not determinable	+	+	−	+	−	−	+	+	+	−	+	−	+	−	−	+	+	+	+	−	+	+	−	+	+
Hyperacute	−	−	−	−	+	−	−	−	−	−	−	−	−	−	−	−	−	−	−	−	−	−	−	−	−
Acute	−	−	−	−	−	−	−	−	−	−	−	+	−	−	+	−	−	−	−	−	−	−	−	−	−
Subacute	−	−	−	−	−	−	−	−	−	−	−	−	−	+	−	−	−	−	−	+	−	−	−	−	−
Intermediate	−	−	−	−	−	−	−	−	−	−	−	−	−	−	−	−	−	−	−	−	−	−	−	−	−

[a] Abbreviations: LT, long tracts (lower and or upper extremity dysfunction, sensory disturbances, sphincter disturbances); BS, brainstem; ON, optic neuritis.

Clinical and paraclinical data were fed into a standardized document used in our department since 1976 and brought up to date each time the subject was reexamined as an out- or inpatient.

METHODS

The VEP technique was the same in every case and at every examination. It has been described in detail elsewhere (14,15). Whenever possible, the second recording was performed after a period of 1 year. The mean interval between the two examinations was 12.7 ± 3.3 months, and the median was 13 months. This interval was 10 to 18 months for 22 patients but 5 to 7 months for the last three.

The latency of the major positive wave (P100) of the pattern-reversal response was studied, as it is the most significant parameter in multiple sclerosis (5). The normal value of P100 latency was found to be 103 ± 7 msec in 52 controls (14). The amplitude of the response was not plotted. However, when it was too reduced for accurate measurement, the response was labeled "nonidentifiable" (NI) to avoid an arbitrary latency figure.

The responses of the 25 patients were distributed among three electrophysiological forms according to the first recording: normal latencies for both eyes; abnormal latencies for both eyes (or not identifiable for one of them); not identifiable for both eyes. Each of these forms was subdivided according to the results of the second recording, compared to the previous one: improved—latencies shorter by 10% or more for both eyes or returned to the normal range for at least one eye; not modified—no shift of latencies within 10%; or worsened—latencies increased by 10% or more for both eyes or become abnormal for at least one of them. The figure of 10% is arbitrary and debatable but was considered to be suitable for comparison.

These various electrophysiological forms were established in ignorance of the clinical data. At a further stage of the study, they were related to several clinical parameters:

1. Basic data: sex, age, symptomatology, remittent or progressive course at the onset of the disease; disease's severity classification (see definition in 2); diagnostic classification.
2. Data at the first recording: duration of the disease; integrated symptomatology, i.e., all of the various symptoms since the onset of the disease; number of previous relapses; chronological connection with a relapse; remittent or progressive stage of the disease; nonreversible vision disability (none, unilateral amblyopia, bilateral amblyopia—none of the patients were amaurotic); functional score at the moment of the examination (which differs from the nonreversible disability classification in the case of a relapse); current treatment.
3. Data at the second recording: occurence of an optic neuropathy, of a new relapse, of a progressive stage; deterioration in the nonreversible locomotion and/or vision disability; therapeutic modifications.

RESULTS

The latencies of the two recordings are given in the Table 2, the 25 patients being distributed among the various electrophysiological forms. The basic data and the data assessed at the first and second recording sessions are given in the Tables 1, 3, and 4 according to the same classification. Only the most significant parameters are shown.

The first recording was normal for seven patients. For each of them, symptomatology was initially and subsequently related to long-tract lesions, but one of them also had had an optic neuritis. There were no visual complaints at the first recording. The majority of the patients were in the early stages of the disease (4/7 with duration of the disease less than 2 years), with none or moderate nonreversible disability (6/7). The recording was usually performed when no relapse was in evolution (5/7). One year later, the latencies were pathologic for the only three patients with occurrence of an optic neuritis and/or a relapse and/or an aggravation in the basic disability since the previous recording.

Fifteen patients had an abnormal first recording. Five of them had an optic neuritis in their symptomatology. In three patients, the second VEP was improved. They were remittent forms with no or moderate basic locomotion disability. There was no basic vision disability. For all of these patients, the first recording was performed during a relapse (one of which was visual), and there were no clinical events during the interval between the two VEPs. Case 10 was an exception, but the relapse occured 5 months after the first VEP and 13 months before the second VEP. In six patients, the second VEP was not modified. They were advanced forms at the progressive stage, with a clear nonreversible disability in locomotion and, sometimes, vision. The first test was usually performed when no relapse was in evolution, and no new clinical event occured between the two examinations. In six patients, the second VEP was worsened. They were mainly remittent forms at the early stages of the disease with no basic locomotion or vision disability. The first recording was performed during a relapse, and a new relapse, an optic neuritis, or a deterioration in the disability were observed during the interval between the two VEPs.

Finally, three patients had not identifiable first VEPs. Two among them had chronic optic neuropathy with definitive amblyopia, but the first test was performed during a transient visual relapse. Therefore, the second VEP showed some improvement. The third patient had a severe myopia and was affected by a progressive optic atrophy during the interval between the two tests.

DISCUSSION

The diagnosis of multiple sclerosis is still based on clinical and biological grounds. The VEPs are only valuable in support of the diagnosis. In our series, their contribution was noticeable: they were the only means to assess the lesional dissemination in nine patients. According to whether or not the VEPs are used

TABLE 2. *Latencies of VEPs at consecutive recording sessions for 25 patients*[a]

First VEP:	Normal							Abnormal															NI		
Second VEP:	Normal				Abnormal			Improved			Not modified						Worsened								
Case No.:	1	2	3	4	5	6	7	8	9	10	11	12	13	14[b]	15	16	17	18	19	20[c]	21	22	23	24	25[d]
Latencies of the first VEP (msec)																									
RE	105	105	109	106	99	105	107	132	180	175	188	157	145	220	154	140	190	150	131	176	175	165	NI	NI	NI
LE	105	110	112	100	99	95	107	124	180	150	187	159	149	140	NI	120	190	150	129	178	140	160	NI	NI	NI
Mean (both eyes)		106.56				102			157				160						161					—	
SD			3.7			5.0			25.1				28.1						21.4					—	
Interval between the 2 VEPs (months)	13	14	16	16	5	12	15	13	16	18	13	10	12	12	7	15	12	15	13	12	17	16	6	10	10
Latencies of the second VEP (msec)																									
RE	103	101	95	106	122	125	188	107	110	118	189	158	136	214	157	120	215	173	176	NI	248	181	235	127	NI
LE	102	99	101	100	99	130	229	125	97	113	189	150	138	127	NI	120	220	183	221	NI	235	190	NI	NI	NI
Mean (both eyes)		10[illegible]				149			112				154						204					—	
SD			3.2			49.2			9.6				31.2						26.8					—	

[a] Abbreviations: RE, right eye; LE, left eye; NI, nonidentifiable latencies; SD, standard deviation.
[b] Case 14 had a history of right congenital amblyopia.
[c] Case 20 had a history of right posttraumatic amblyopia.
[d] Case 25 had a history of a major myopic choroidosis.

TABLE 3. *Clinical data at time of first VEP*

First VEP:	Normal							Abnormal															NI		
Second VEP:	Normal				Abnormal			Improved			Not modified						Worsened								
Case No.:	1	2	3	4	5	6	7	8	9	10	11	12	13	14	15	16	17	18	19	20	21	22	23	24	25
Duration of the disease																									
≤5 months	−	−	−	−	−	−	−	−	+	−	+	−	−	−	−	−	−	−	+	−	−	−	−	−	−
6–11 months	−	−	−	−	+	−	−	−	−	−	−	−	−	−	−	−	−	−	−	−	−	−	−	+	−
12–23 months	+	+	−	−	−	−	+	−	−	−	−	−	−	−	−	−	+	+	−	−	+	−	−	−	−
2–4 years	−	−	−	+	−	−	−	−	−	−	−	−	+	−	−	−	−	−	−	−	−	+	−	−	−
5–9 years	−	−	+	−	−	−	−	−	−	−	−	−	−	−	+	+	−	−	−	−	−	−	−	−	+
≥10 years	−	−	−	−	−	+	−	+	−	+	−	+	−	+	−	−	−	−	−	+	−	−	+	−	−
Integrated symptomatology																									
Monosymptomatic LT	+	+	−	+	+	+	+	−	−	−	−	+	+	−	−	+	−	−	+	−	−	+	−	−	−
BS	−	−	−	−	−	−	−	−	−	−	−	−	−	−	−	−	−	−	−	−	−	−	−	−	−
ON	−	−	−	−	−	−	−	−	−	−	−	−	−	−	−	−	−	−	−	−	−	−	+	−	−
Plurisymptomatic Without ON	−	−	−	−	−	−	−	+	+	−	+	−	−	−	−	−	−	+	−	−	+	−	−	−	+
With ON	−	−	+	−	−	−	−	−	−	+	−	−	−	+	+	−	+	−	−	+	−	−	−	+	−
Number of previous relapses	0	0	4	2	3	1	0	3	1	>10	1	0	0	3	>5	0	4	2	1	>5	3	4	3	3	0
Relapse in evolution																									
Without ON	−	−	−	+	+	−	−	+	+	−	+	−	+	−	−	−	+	+	+	−	+	−	−	−	−
With ON	−	−	−	−	−	−	−	−	−	+	−	−	−	−	−	−	−	−	−	−	−	−	+	+	−
Phase of the disease																									
Remittent	−	−	+	+	−	−	−	+	+	+	+	−	−	−	−	−	+	+	+	−	+	+	+	−	−
Progressive	+	+	−	−	+	+	+	−	−	−	−	+	+	+	+	+	−	−	−	+	−	−	−	+	+
Nonreversible locomotion disability																									
None	−	−	+	−	−	−	−	−	+	+	+	−	−	−	−	−	+	+	+	−	+	+	+	−	+
Moderate	+	+	−	+	−	+	+	+	−	−	−	−	+	−	−	+	−	−	−	−	−	−	−	+	−
Severe	−	−	−	−	+	−	−	−	−	−	−	+	−	+	+	−	−	−	−	+	−	−	−	−	−
Nonreversible vision disability																									
None	+	+	+	+	+	+	+	+	+	+	+	+	+	−	−	+	+	+	+	−	+	+	−	−	+
1 eye	−	−	−	−	−	−	−	−	−	−	−	−	−	+	−	−	−	−	−	−	−	−	+	−	−
2 eyes	−	−	−	−	−	−	−	−	−	−	−	−	−	−	+	−	−	−	−	+	−	−	−	+	−

TABLE 4. *Modifications in symptomatology, course, and nonreversible disability during the interval between the two VEP recording sessions*

First VEP:	Normal							Abnormal															NI		
Second VEP:	Normal				Abnormal			Improved			Not modified						Worsened								
Case No.:	1	2	3	4	5	6	7	8	9	10	11	12	13	14	15	16	17	18	19	20	21	22	23	24	25
Occurrence of an optic neuropathy	−	−	−	−	+	−	+	−	−	−	−	−	−	−	−	−	−	−	−	−	−	−	−	−	+
New relapses Without ON	−	−	−	−	−	+	−	−	−	+	+	−	−	−	−	−	−	+	+	−	−	+	−	+	−
With ON	−	−	−	−	+	−	−	−	−	−	−	−	−	−	−	−	−	−	−	+	−	−	−	−	−
Deterioration in the nonreversible disability																									
Locomotion	−	−	−	−	−	+	−	−	−	−	−	−	−	+	−	−	−	+	−	+	−	−	−	−	+
Vision	−	−	−	−	−	−	+	−	−	−	−	−	−	−	−	−	−	−	−	−	−	−	−	−	+

in the diagnostic classification, the definite forms are 44 or 80% in our series.

The efficiency of this technique in demonstrating optic pathway involvement has been definitive in our series. All patients with a nonreversible amblyopia or studied during a relapse with an optic neuritis had abnormal or nonidentifiable VEP latencies. However, there was no clear relationship between the degree of abnormality of the VEPs on the one hand and the nonreversible locomotion disability score or the whole severity of the disease or the number of previous relapses on the other hand (see Tables 1 and 3). This is a further demonstration of the classic mutual independence of the plaques.

Finally, our results show a phenomenon so far rarely mentioned: the variability of the VEP latencies. Twelve of our patients had frankly different recordings at a 1-year interval. The widespread opinion since the work of Halliday et al. (7) is that when VEP latencies have become abnormal following a transient optic neuritis, it is definitive. However, other authors (1,6,13) have observed normal VEPs in patients with antecedent and reversible optic neuritis. It is impossible to state if these VEPs had ever been normal or if they have returned to normal.

More recently, Matthews and Small (12) have emphasized the variability of the VEP latencies in the course of the disease. This instability has also been noted by these authors in the case of somatosensory evoked potentials (SEP); similar observations have also been made by Namerow (17), by Robinson and Rudge (19), and, to a minor extent, by Kjaer (10) for the auditory evoked potentials (AEP), and by Kimura (9) for the blink reflex. In our series, the variability of latencies seems to parallel the remittent–progressive course of the disease, as already noted by Robinson and Rudge for the AEPs, and by Matthews and Small for the SEPs. Thus, latencies seem to increase during the relapse, *whether they concern the visual pathways or not,* and then return to a basal value, possibly normal, which, in any case, is stable for some time after the relapses. When the disease advances, becoming disabling and/or progressive, VEP latencies usually remain abnormal, even in the absence of a clinical optic neuropathy. If they are only slightly altered from one year to the next—but this interval is brief for such a disease—they probably tend to increase as the course of the disease is going on; this is not demonstrated in our series.

This nonreversible alteration of the neuronal conduction in the visual pathways at the advanced stages of the disease may easily be explained in terms of demyelination and "extenso-progressive gliosis" (see 4). However, the variability of latencies during the remittent phase needs further discussion. In our series (and even more in the Matthews and Small series), this phenomenon is not absolute: two of our patients, recorded from during a relapse, had normal VEPs; two other patients, each with a relapse during the interval between the two VEPs, had pathological but stable VEPs. These facts argue against the setting in action during relapses of factors able to induce a general slowing (even blocking) of nervous conduction.

This hypothesis was cautiously proposed by Robinson and Rudge (19) and would have been based on the "blocking factors" (see 20). It is more judicious to involve the development of limited lesions in the visual pathways simultaneously with those developed elsewhere in the neuraxis. Plaques without any clinical correspondence are frequently observed at autopsy (11) or with the CT scan (18). The actual nature of these lesions must be further defined. The exclusive participation of demyelination would prevent improvement or normalization of the latencies: remyelination is poor in multiple sclerosis. Furthermore, eventual rearrangements of the axolemma as described by Waxman (21,22) are not adequate to restore a normal conduction. Consequently, an *en plaque* edema mechanism may be suggested. In some cases, it is free of demyelination, so that *restitutio ad integrum* may occur. In that sense, the recent work of Dalakas, et al. (3) is of prime interest in experimentally demonstrating that an acute inflammation immunologically triggered is not necessarily coupled with demyelination.

SUMMARY

Twenty-five MS patients had VEPs recorded at 1-year interval. Abnormal VEPs were observed at least once in 21 patients. They were the only means of assessing the lesional dissemination in nine patients. Their contribution in the diagnositic classification is such that the proportion of "definite" cases rises from 44 to 80% of the 25 cases.

The degree of abnormality of the VEPs had no relation to the disability status or to the whole severity of the disease.

The main feature was the variability of the VEP latencies at a 1-year interval: they seem to follow the remittent progressive course of the disease whether visual pathways are clinically affected or not. These results are interpreted in light of the pathophysiological data of the disease. In the cases with improvement or normalization of the second VEPs, *en plaque* edema may be an important mechanism, sometimes free of demyelination so that perfect *restitutio ad integrum* may occur.

ACKNOWLEDGMENTS

We are grateful to Dr. J. J. Ventre for his help in the computerized data processing, to Mrs. Chalet for her technical assistance, and to Mrs. Droguet and Miss Christine Fernandez for the typescript.

REFERENCES

1. Asselmann, R., Chadwick, D. W., and Marsden, C. D. (1975): Visual evoked responses in the diagnosis and management of patients suspected of multiple sclerosis. *Brain,* 98:261–282.
2. Confavreux, C., Aimard, G., and Devic, M. (1980): Course and prognosis of multiple sclerosis assessed by the computerized data processing of 349 patients. *Brain,* 103:281–300.
3. Dalakas, M., Wright, R. G., and Prineas, J. W. (1980): Nature of the reversible white matter lesion in multiple sclerosis. Effects of acute inflammation on myelinated tissue studied in the rabbit eye. *Brain,* 103:515–524.

4. Fog, T., and Linnemann, F. (1970): The course of multiple sclerosis in 73 cases with computer designed curves. *Acta Neurol. Scand.* [*Suppl.*], 47:1–175.
5. Halliday, A. M. (1978): Clinical application of evoked potentials. In: *Recent Advances in Clinical Neurology, Vol. 2,* edited by W. B. Matthews and G. H. Glaser, pp. 47–73. Churchill Livingstone, Edinburgh, London, and New York.
6. Halliday, A. M., and McDonald, W. I. (1977): Pathophysiology of multiple sclerosis. *Br. Med. Bull.,* 33:21–27.
7. Halliday, A. M., McDonald, W. I., and Mushin, J. (1972): Delayed visual evoked response in optic neuritis. *Lancet,* 1:982–985.
8. Halliday, A. M., McDonald, W. I., and Mushin, J. (1973): Visual evoked response in diagnosis of multiple sclerosis. *Br. Med. J.,* 4:661–664.
9. Kimura, J. (1975): Electrically elicited blink reflex in diagnosis of multiple sclerosis. *Brain,* 98:413–426.
10. Kjaer, M. (1980): Variations of brain auditory evoked potentials correlated to duration and severity of multiple sclerosis. *Acta Neurol Scand.,* 61:157–166.
11. Lumsden, C. E. (1970): The neuropathology of multiple sclerosis. In: *Handbook of Clinical Neurology, Vol. 9, Multiple Sclerosis and Other Demyelinating Diseases,* edited by P. J. Vinken and G. W. Bruyn, pp. 217–309. North-Holland, Amsterdam.
12. Matthews, W. B., and Small, D. G. (1979): Serial recording of visual and somatosensory evoked potentials in multiple sclerosis. *J. Neurol. Sci.,* 40:11–21.
13. Matthews, W. B., Small, D. G., Small, M., and Pountney, E. (1977): Pattern reversal evoked visual potentials in the diagnosis of multiple sclerosis. *J. Neurol. Neurosurg. Psychiatry,* 40:1009–1014.
14. Mauguiere, F., Mitrou, H., Chalet, E., Pourcher, E., and Courjon, J. (1979): Interêt des potentiels évoqués visuels dans la sclérose multiloculaire (S.M.): Etude comparative des résultats obtenus en stimulation par éclair lumineux et inversion de damier. *Rev. Electroengephalogr. Clin.,* 9:209–220.
15. Mauguiere, F., Revol, M., and Courjon, J. (1980): Les potentiels evoqués visuels dans la sclérose en plaques. *Lyon Med.,* 6:301–310.
16. McAlpine, D., Lumsden, C. E., and Acheson, E. D. (1972): *Multiple Sclerosis. A Reappraisal,* Churchill Livingstone, Edinburgh.
17. Namerow, N. S. (1968): Somatosensory evoked responses in multiple sclerosis patients with varying sensory loss. *Neurology (Minneap.),* 18:1197–1204.
18. Poser, C. M. (1980): Exacerbations activity and progression in multiple sclerosis. *Arch. Neurol.,* 37:471–474.
19. Robinson, K., and Rudge, P. (1978): The stability of the auditory evoked potentials in normal man and patients with multiple sclerosis. *J. Neurol. Sci.,* 36:147–156.
20. Schauf, C. L., and Davis, F. A. (1978): The occurrence, specificity, and role of neuroelectric blocking factors in multiple sclerosis. *Neurology (Minneap.),* 28:34–39.
21. Waxman, S. G. (1977): Conduction in myelinated, unmyelinated and demyelinated fibers. *Arch. Neurol.,* 34:585–589.
22. Waxman, S. G., and Brill, M. H. (1978): Conduction through demyelinated plaques in multiple sclerosis: computer simulations of facilitation by short internodes. *J. Neurol. Neurosurg. Psychiatry,* 41:408–416.

Clinical Applications of Evoked Potentials in Neurology,
edited by J. Courjon, F. Mauguiere, and M. Revol.
Raven Press, New York © 1982.

Multimodal Evoked Potentials in Multiple Sclerosis: Basal and Follow-up Data

*D. Gambi, *P. M. Rossini, *L. Marchionno, *T. Iarlori, *A. Finarelli, and **M. Pirchio

**Institute of Neurology, University G. D'Annunzio, Chieti, Italy; and **Laboratory of Neurophysiology, C.N.R., Pisa, Italy*

In the last 10 years, the ability to disclose demyelinating lesions in the sensory pathways has been acquired by using averaging techniques.

The studies of Halliday et al. (2), Rosén et al. (7), and Paty et al. (4) have displayed delays of various evoked responses (particularly some components of VEPs, BAEPs, and SEPs) in subjects at different stages of multiple sclerosis and/or optic retrobulbar neuritis.

In the last 2 years, we have submitted 30 patients with multiple sclerosis to a series of electrophysiological tests with the following purposes:

1. To identify the levels of the lesions in different sensory pathways with an accurate and available methodology.
2. To disclose subclinical abnormalities that are often undetected in clinical examinations.
3. To avoid invasive neuroradiological procedures.
4. To observe the clinical development with a serial study of multimodal EPs.

MATERIALS AND METHODS

Subjects consisted of 30 patients (22 females and eight males) with multiple sclerosis (MS), aged from 18 to 47 years (mean value 30 ± 7); they were studied and compared to 52 control subjects without previous history of sensory disturbances. The age of the controls was the same as that of the patients. The diagnoses of the MS subjects, according to the McAlpine criteria, were definite (24 cases), probable (three cases), and possible (three cases).

Before the recording sessions, all subjects underwent examinations of visual field, fundus oculi, visual acuity, acoustic function, and neurological parameters (Kurtzke schedule and functional tests). The sessions were scheduled in a 24-month period during worsening attacks or at appearance of subjective symptoms.

Evoked Potentials

Tests were carried out in a dark, sound-proof room. The VEP was recorded monopolarly during a monocular pattern-reversal stimulation with checks of variable size (transient stimulation: 2 Hz, 64 replications, 7.5′, 15′, 30′, 60′ of arc; steady-state stimulation: 10, 20, 40 Hz, 256 replications, 15′ and 30′ of arc) (1,6).

Contrast depth modulation was 75 cd/m²; distance of the patients from the TV screen (25° × 21° radius) was 114 cm. The active electrode was located 4 cm above the inion on the midline, reference electrodes on the connected earlobes, ground electrode in C_z (International 10–20 System).

Refractory defects were corrected. The recording parameters were: gain, 10^4; HF filter, 32 Hz (time constant 5 msec, −6 db/octave); LF filter, 0.8 Hz (time constant 200 msec, −3 dB/octave). The latency of P100 (transient responses) and the amplitude and morphology of the sinusoidal curve (steady-state responses) were analyzed.

The BAEP was monopolarly recorded from the vertex during an acoustic stimulation (2,000–3,000 replications with a grounded earphone) with monaural clicks (0.1 msec, 10 Hz, 70 dB HSL). The reference electrodes were placed on the connected earlobes. The recording parameters were: gain, 5×10^4; HF filter, 3.2 kHz (−6 dB/octave); LF filter, 160 Hz (−3 dB/octave).

Positive (downward) peak latencies, interpeak times, and V/III, V/II, and III/II amplitude ratios were evaluated in the 10-msec period after the stimulus onset.

The scalp (7 cm lateral to C_z, contralateral to the stimulated nerve, and 1 cm behind the C_z–earlobe plane) and neck (seventh and third spinous processes) responses (SEP and electrospinogram, ESG) evoked by stimulation of the median nerve at the wrist sufficient to induce a slight thumb twitch (0.1 msec square pulses, 5 Hz) were also recorded.

The reference electrodes were on the linked earlobes. In the present study, we report only the data obtained during a 30-msec analysis time after 1,500 replications. The latency of N_9, N_{11}, N_{13} peaks recorded at the cervical electrodes and of the P_{14} and N_{20} (often bilobed in a N_{17}–N_{20} complex) were evaluated. The peripheral, cervical, and intracerebral propagation times were measured according to a technique fully described elsewhere (8). The parameters were filtered 32 to 3,200 Hz (−3 dB/octave); the electrode resistances were always below 5 kohms.

RESULTS

At the first observation, the clinical examinations revealed abnormalities in 93% of the patients in the pyramidal tract, in 83% in the cerebellar system, in 80% in the brainstem system, in 46% in the sensory pathways, and in 43% in the visual system. The abnormalities of the brainstem were distributed primarily in the pons at the middle (52%) and the high (15%) levels.

Brainstem Auditory Evoked Potentials

The percentage of patients with abnormal BAEPs was 57%. The percentages of patients with abnormally delayed or absent waves are illustrated in Tables 1 and 2.

The values for the patients were compared to the following control values: wave I, 1.62 ± 0.11 msec; wave II, 2.65 ± 0.19; wave III, 3.63 ± 0.21; wave IV, 4.68 ± 0.22; wave V, 5.55 ± 0.23; wave VI, 6.84 ± 0.42.

The amplitude ratios were altered more than 2 SD from the control mean in 35, 28, and 25% of the patients, respectively, for V/III, V/II, and III/II. The follow-up revealed an increase in the corresponding latencies (Fig. 1) in 6% of the patients for waves II, III, and V. No differences were observed in the analysis of the amplitudes. Some patients (five), on the other hand, showed a decrease in signal abnormalities, particularly for waves II, III, and V (Fig. 2).

Visual Evoked Potentials

The P100 peak latency of transient (2 Hz) VEPs was abnormally delayed in 78% of the patients (>2 SD from controls). The mean control values are reported in another section of this book (P. M. Rossini et al., *this volume*).

The percentages were distributed as reported in Table 3. In 5% of recordings, both visual and automatic (PDP 11/10) reading failed to recognize any major positive deflection even when the patient reported seeing the reversing pattern. Moreover, a noticeable shift was noted between the latencies of VEPs evoked by small and coarse checks (in controls not higher than 30–35 msec) (Fig. 3).

The steady-state VEP (Fig. 3) was altered because of a lack of synchronization or a phase lag in 66% of cases at the 40 Hz rate of stimulation, in 44% at 20 Hz, and in 11% at 10 Hz.

The follow-up showed an increase of percentages of patients with latencies

TABLE 1. *Percentages of altered responses (>2 SD control mean) in BAEPs*

	I	II	III	IV	V	VI
Delayed latency (msec)	9.2	14.1	13.4	10.5	24.6	5.5
Absent waves	4.2	4.5	4.5	16.0	10.2	33.0

TABLE 2. *Percentages of altered interpeak times (>2 SD control mean) in BAEPs*

	I–II	I–III	I–V	I–VI	II–III	II–V	III–V
Interpeak times (msec)	8.2	10.3	19.2	5.6	9.1	23.5	24.3

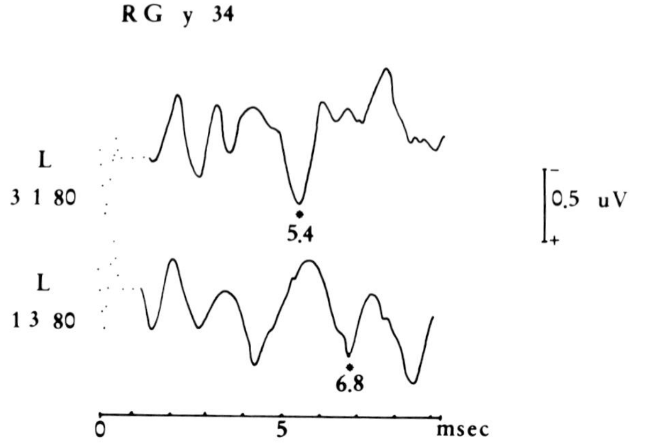

FIG. 1. Worsening of the BAEPs in a case of definite MS. In the first evoked responses, the wave V is at 5.4 msec (L, left side stimulation; trace 3-1-80); in the second evoked responses, the same wave fell at 6.8 msec.

more than 2 SD from normal in 6% of cases at the transient stimulation (VEP P100). The same percentage (6%) of patients was observed in the steady-state stimulations.

SEPs and ESGs

The control values of the peak at the C_7 and C_3 cervical electrodes were, respectively, 9.15 ± 0.67 msec (N_9), 11.65 ± 0.61 msec (N_{11}), 13.03 ± 0.46

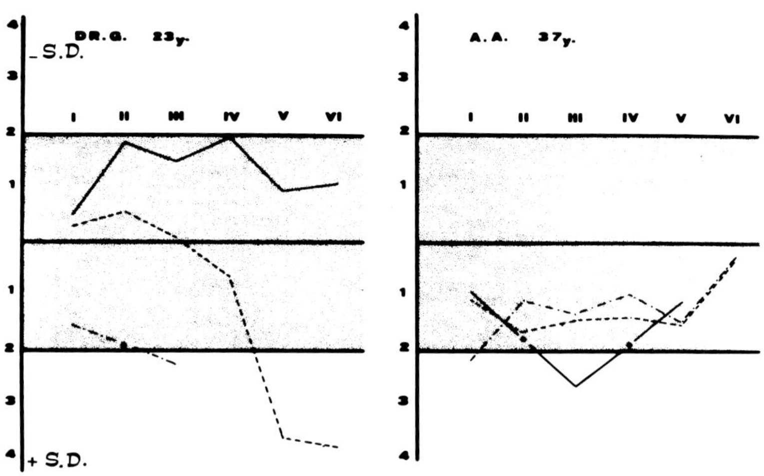

FIG. 2. Graph of the peak latencies of the six waves in two cases of MS in three different registrations. The *gray areas* between two parallel lines correspond to the mean control values ±2 SD. In Dr.G. (definite MS) on the **left,** worsening; in A.A. (definite MS) on the **right,** improvement.———, first registration; ------, second registration; -·-·-·, third registration.

TABLE 3. *Percentages of altered P100 latencies in VEPs*

	Contrast	7.5′	15′	30′	60′ arc
Left eye	20%	43.11	55.18	62.07	48.28
Left eye	50%	55.18	62.07	56.90	41.38
Right eye	20%	58.63	60.35	66.35	46.56
Right eye	50%	55.18	62.07	56.90	51.73

msec (N_{13}), and 9.56 ± 0.67 msec (N_9) 11.78 ± 0.86 msec (N_{11}), 13.33 ± 0.21 msec (N_{13}). From the scalp electrodes, a negative peak at 19.6 ± 0.3 msec was the sturdiest electric event utilized for the intracerebral propagation time measurement (pathologic threshold, 7.2 msec).

The SEPs showed an abnormally delayed N_{20} (>2 SD from the controls) in 61% of the cases. The intracerebral transmission time, measured between the N_{20} detected at the scalp and the N_{13} peak detected by the high cervical electrode, was altered in 13% and 47% of the patients, respectively, in stimulation from the left and right side. The neck recordings disclosed a delayed transmission of the sensory impulse along the cervical tract in 38% of the patients.

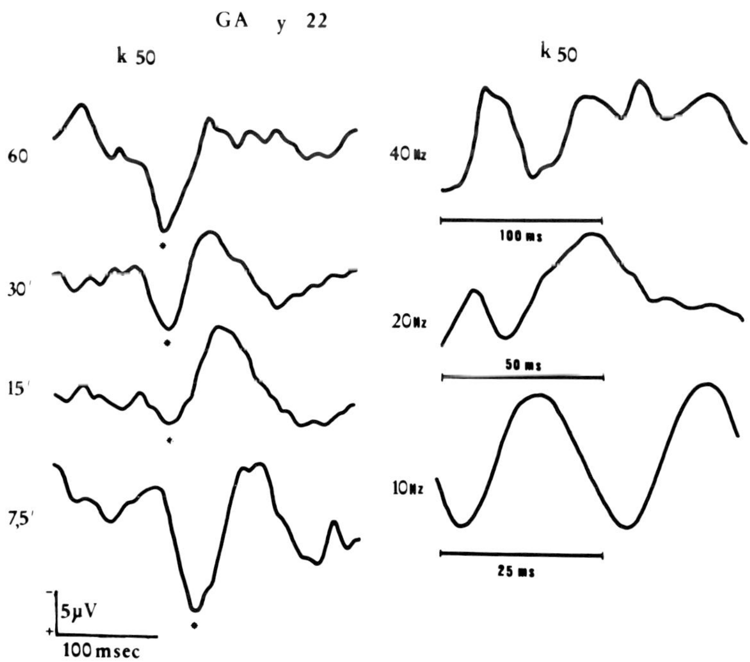

FIG. 3. The VEP in a subject with probable MS. Normal values for the P100 intrinsic time and latency shift of VEP at small checks (7.5′ of arc) **(left bottom)** in the transient response; lack of synchronization in the steady-state responses at 20 Hz and 40 Hz stimulations.

The peripheral nerve sensory conduction up to Erb's point was never altered. The follow-up revealed an increase in the intramedullary conduction velocity in 14% of the patients and in the intracerebral time in 4%.

COMMON DATA

Considering the whole group and the four responses studied (visual, acoustic, and neck and scalp somatosensory), 18% of the cases had altered responses to all of the evoking modalities, 27% were altered in three EP, and 30% were altered in at least two EPs.

In the three cases who passed from probable to definite MS during the follow-up period, the EPs were already altered at the first recording sessions, whereas in the three subjects who suffered from possible MS, only the EP testing the sensory pathway clinically involved was markedly altered.

Considering the clinical follow-up, in no cases did the EPs provide useful information about the onset of a new release, even if they always deteriorated according to the clinical course. In five subjects, we noted an amelioration of latency and morphology during an epoch with complete remission of the symptomatology.

CONCLUSIONS

Our findings confirm the importance of neurophysiological techniques (evoked potentials) in the early diagnosis of multiple sclerosis, even if the clinical symptoms are not clearly apparent. This multimodal approach, in fact, can test sensory pathways having clinically "silent" plaques that induce abnormal responses.

Regarding each evoked potential, the following can be emphasized.

1. The BAEP must be measured on both left and right sides because of frequent unilateral lesions which are not clearly seen in binaural stimulation. The waves with a highest percentage of lesions are peaks V (mesencephalon–pons levels), II, and III (pons levels). The interpeak latency, and particularly I–V, II–V, and III–V, can be useful in detecting slowing of impulse transmission when the latency of the wave is in the normal range; this was often the case during the early stages of the clinical history.

The percentage of altered BAEPs, regarding only acoustic pathways compared to those of the Kurtzke's schedule and including all brainstem lesions, supports this theory. The BAEP parameters worsen in the follow-up in a large number of cases but occasionally improve. This fact could indicate an amelioration of the conditions causing the impeded impulse transmission, possibly through reintegration of myelin sheets.

Experimental study (5) in chronic EAE has demonstrated the possibility of remyelination in the rabbit 12 months after onset. Another possibility is the variation of the biochemical environment surrounding the plaque which could account for the variable BAEP morphology.

2. The visual evoked potential by checkerboard pattern reversal is the most sensitive test among the ones we studied. The evaluation of the P100 latency proved to be a reliable index in the follow-up: 6% of the patients, in fact, showed an increase of this parameter, which illustrates the evolution of alterations in the myelin sheets of the optic nerve fibers. These lesions can sometimes be revealed by repetitive stimulation, during which the transmission of the impulses is impeded when a plaque is encountered.

3. Similar considerations can be made regarding the somesthetic evoked potentials. Concerning these, we can emphasize that the intramedullary conduction velocity is more significant than the intracerebral conduction velocity in the evaluation of the follow-up.

REFERENCES

1. Gambi, D., Rossini, P. M., Onofrj, M., and Marchionno, L. (1980): Visual evoked cortical potentials (V.E.C.P.) by television presentation of different patterned stimuli to patients with multiple sclerosis. *Ital. J. Neurol. Sci.,* 2:101–106.
2. Halliday, A. M., McDonald, W. I., and Muschin, J. (1973): Visual evoked response in the diagnosis of multiple sclerosis. *Br. Med. J.,* 4:661–664.
3. McAlpine, D., Lumsden, C. E., and Acheson, E. D. (1972): *Multiple Sclerosis: A Reappraisal.* Churchill Livingstone, Edinburgh.
4. Paty, J., Deliac, P., Gioux, M., and Franqui-Zannettacci, M. (1980): An approach to diagnosis of multiple sclerosis with cerebral evoked potentials (visual, auditory, somatosensory). In: *Evoked Potentials,* edited by C. Barber, pp. 593–603. MTP Press, Lancaster.
5. Raine, C. S. (1978): Pathology of the demyelination. In: *Physiology and Pathobiology of Axons,* edited by S. G. Waxman, pp. 283–311. Raven Press, New York.
6. Regan, D., Milner, B. A., and Heron, J. R. (1977): Rapid methods for refracting the eye and assessing the visual acuity in amblyopia using steady-state visual evoked potentials. In: *Visual Evoked Potentials in Man. New Developments,* edited by J. E. Desmedt, pp. 418–26. Clarendon Press, Oxford.
7. Rosén, J., Bynke, H., and Sandberg, M. (1980): Pattern reversal visual evoked potentials after unilateral optic neuritis. In: *Evoked Potentials,* edited by C. Barber, pp. 567–74. MTP Press, Lancaster.
8. Rossini, P. M., Sollazzo, D., Onofrj, M., David, P., and Tonali, P. (1979): Potenziali evocati del mildollo cervicale e onde precocissime del PES. *Priv. Ital. EEG Neurofisiol.,* II:591–593.

Clinical Applications of Evoked Potentials in Neurology,
edited by J. Courjon, F. Mauguiere, and M. Revol.
Raven Press, New York © 1982.

Variability on Serial Testing of Visual Evoked Potentials in Patients with Multiple Sclerosis

*Stanley N. Cohen, *Karl Syndulko, *Edward Hansch,
*Wallace W. Tourtellotte, and **Alfred R. Potvin

**Neurology and Research Services, VA Wadsworth Medical Center, Los Angeles, California, 90073 and Department of Neurology, University of California at Los Angeles School of Medicine, Los Angeles, California 90024; and **Biomedical Engineering Program, *University of Texas at Arlington, Arlington, Texas 76019*

Pattern reversal-evoked potentials (PVEP) and critical frequency of photic driving (CFPD) have been shown to be sensitive diagnostic aids in detecting abnormalities in patients with proven or suspected multiple sclerosis (MS) (1,2). Since the tests appear to be sensitive to subclinical abnormalities, there is the potential for PVEP to be used in monitoring progression of disease in the visual pathways and in the assessment of putative therapies in MS. For PVEP testing to be useful in serial evaluations, it is necessary to demonstrate that PVEP changes are related to clinical changes and that PVEP remains relaivety stable in the absence of clinical change. These factors have been examined for the brainstem auditory evoked potential (4,6), somatosensory evoked potential (5), and PVEP in patients with normal or near normal latencies (5).

The purpose of this study was to serially examine MS patients with abnormal PVEP, to evaluate the inter- and intrasession stability of PVEP and CFPD, and to determine whether clinical changes were correlated with changes in the PVEP.

METHODS

Patient Selection

Patients ($N = 10$) were selected from the MS research ward at VA Wadsworth Medical Center. Each patient had definite MS as defined by criteria of Rose et al. (7). A patient was tested on a minimum of four occasions over a period of 3 years, with the majority of testing sessions conducted over a 2-year period. Intervals between tests were variable, with the minimum interval being 1 week. Seven patients were clinically stable during the period of testing. Clinical stability was defined as an absence of subjective or objective change in symptoms relatable to MS. Evaluation included the patient's opinion of change and qualitative testing by the primary physician which was summarized in the Kurtzke score. Several of the patients received putative therapies during the serial testing. Tests performed during those dates were not considered when evaluating the stability of PVEP. Three patients had clinical exacerbations during the observation period.

The PVEP and CFPD were tested in each eye separately by methods described by Cohen et al. (3). The upper limit of normal latency for P100 was 117 msec (mean plus 2 SD). Normal CFPD was defined as the presence of averaged photic driving at flash stimulus rates of 41 Hz or higher.

RESULTS

The results of the serial PVEP testing are shown in Table 1. During the periods of clinical stability, only three eyes in two MS patients demonstrated intersession evoked potential stability. However, each of these eyes showed a consistent absence of a definable P100 component to pattern reversal stimulation. The remaining eyes that demonstrated a positive peak in the first 200 msec showed an intersession variability of 10 msec or greater on at least one occasion. The largest variability was seen in a patient who demonstrated an absence of a P100 in one session and a P100 latency of 104 msec in another. Another patient demonstrated a similar failure to have a major positive peak in the first 200 msec on at least one occasion and the presence of such a peak on another. More typical examples of intersession variabilities are shown in Figs. 1 and 2.

The MS patients showed intrasession variability as well. An example of intrasession variability is shown in Fig. 2. Eight of the 10 patients demonstrated

TABLE 1. *Variability of VEP in 10 MS patients*

Patient	Shortest latency		Longest latency		PVER maximum intrasession variance (msec)	PVER maximum variance (msec)	CFPD maximum variance (Hz)
	R	L	R	L			
ERd	113	115	134	136	16	21	40
WJ	111	118	128	129	11	17	40
WW	137	144	147	153	3	10	20
RM	[a]	159	[a]	178	16	19	20
JC	[a]	[a]	[a]	[a]	[a]	[a]	0
DR	138	162	163	[a]	25	25	30
JF	185	195	200	200	10	15	10
ERk	122	122	158	147	24	36	30
WP	110	140	180[b]	165[b]	[c]	[c]	40
LD	104	130	160[b]	146	[c]	[c]	50

[a] Absence of P100.
[b] At least one test with an absence of P100.
[c] Maximum variance includes a comparison of a trial with P100 of normal latency to a trial with an absence P100.

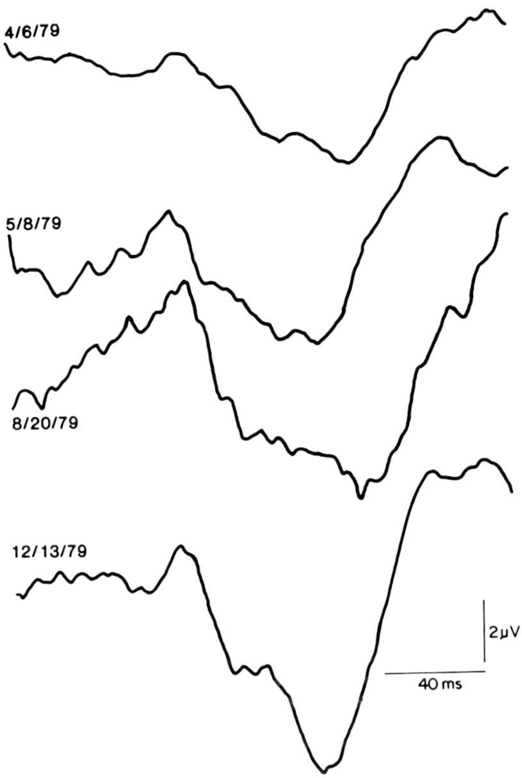

FIG. 1. Variability of PVEP latencies on serial testing in a patient with MS.

more than a 10-msec intrasession variability in at least one eye on at least one occasion. One of the remaining two demonstrated a failure to respond with either eye on all dates tested while clinically stable. The other had remarkable intrasession stability of response with a maximum latency difference of 3 msec over seven testing dates.

The MS patients showed intersession variability for CFPD similar to that for PVEP testing. Only one patient demonstrated stability. Each of the other patients had a minimum of a 10 Hz difference in at least one eye from his/her best performance to his/her worst. Intrasession variability could not be assessed for CFPD, since most frequencies were tested only once on any test date.

Three patients had exacerbations during the serial monitoring. One of these patients showed deterioration of visual acuity as a result of his exacerbation. This patient had a corresponding increase in latency and a decrease in photic driving (Fig. 3). Two others had no visual changes with their exacerbation. Both had no consistent change in PVEP and CFPD associated with the exacerbation.

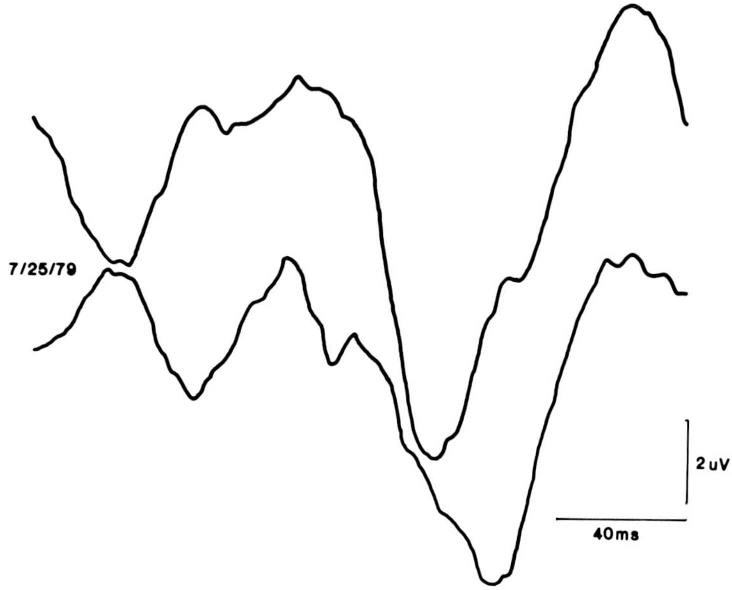

FIG. 2. Intrasession variability of PVEP in a patient with MS.

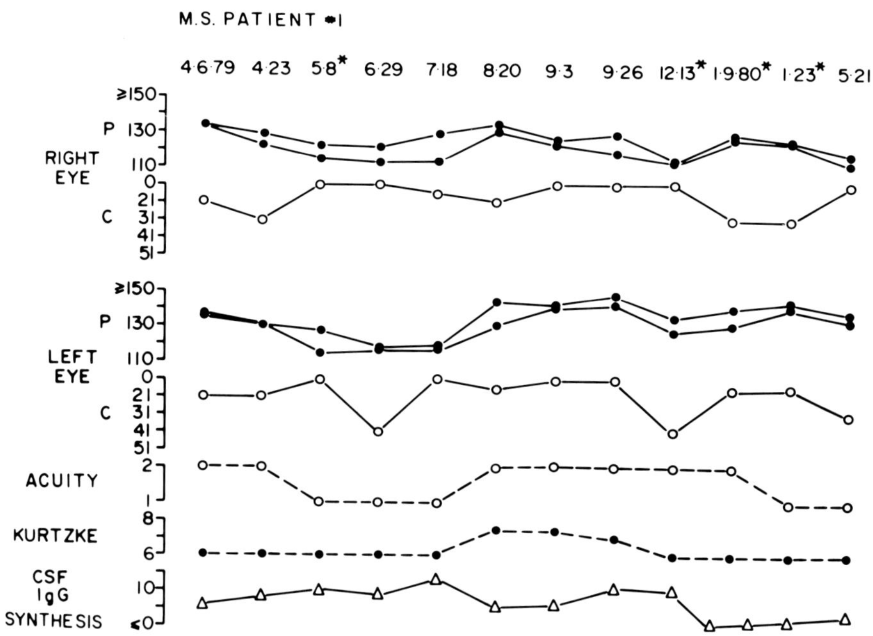

FIG. 3. Vairability of PVEP latencies and CFPD frequencies as compared to visual acuity, Kurtzke disability score, and CSF IgG synthesis measured on the same date. P, PVEP; C, CFPD; *dates patient was given a putative therapy.

In six normals tested on at least two occasions separated by 2 years, there were no eyes with an intersession difference greater than 10 msec (Fig. 4). Out of 40 normal patients tested in one session, intrasession variability was greater than 10 msec in one eye of only two subjects. In each case, the test–retest latency difference was less than 15 msec.

DISCUSSION

The combination of PVEP and CFPD has been shown to be a sensitive method of detecting abnormalities in the anterior optic pathways. Their utility as aids in the diagnosis of MS is established (1,2). The potential use of this test as an objective means of monitoring disease progression and/or evaluating putative therapies was assessed in the present study.

In our patients, the results indicate that patients with clinically definite MS can show P100 latency fluctuations of greater than 10 msec for both intersession and intrasession testing. The greatest intrasession change was from an absence of a P100 on one trial to a P100 with a normal latency on the next. Intersession fluctuations were also seen in CFPD.

A serial study of PVEP in MS was performed by Matthews and Small (5).

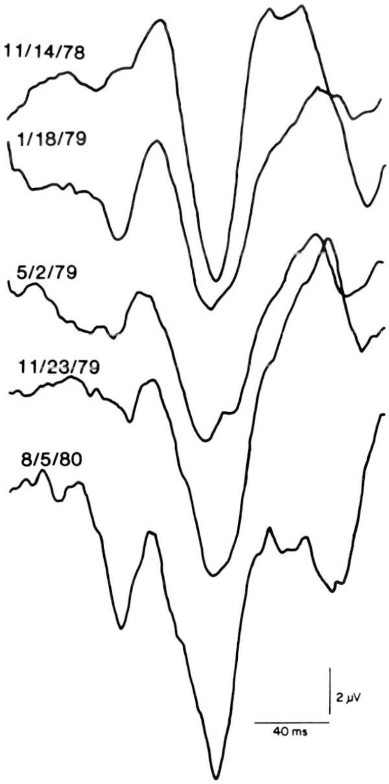

FIG. 4. Stability of PVEP latencies seen in a normal volunteer on serial testing.

In seven patients followed serially, they reported that increasing latency was associated with increased visual symptomatology. They also found relative stability of latency during clinically quiescent periods. In 51 patients tested on at least two occasions, 27 of 39 eyes had changes in latency and/or amplitude appropriate to changes in their visual symptoms, whereas 37 of 58 clinically stable eyes showed PVEP stability.

The study of Matthews and Small (5) and ours each indicate that PVEP latency tends to increase with relapses that include visual symptomatology. Furthermore, both studies indicate that relapses without visual symptomatology do not have obligatory increases in latency. The studies differ in that the patients studied serially by Matthews and Small had fairly stable latencies during clinical quiescence. Our study indicates variance in latency even during clinical stability. One possible explanation for the difference between study results is differences in the patient population. Matthews and Small indicated that their patients fluctuated within a few milliseconds of the upper limit of normal. All but one of our patients had latencies well out of the normal range at the start of the study. It is possible that with near-normal latencies and, thus, presumably with early disease, the size of plaques that would allow the latency to be normal or near normal would also allow for consistent transmission time. As plaques increase in number or size, not only would the latency increase, but the variability of speed of transmission might increase. Thus, the two studies may be offering complementary data on differing states of the disease.

Matthews and Small also included data on the variability of somatosensory evoked potentials (SEP) in MS patients. They found in three patients with active disease that there was variation independent of clinical relapse or remission. Kjaer (4) reported on the variability of brainstem auditory evoked potentials in MS patients. He found that changes in BAEP reflecting clinical state occur in some but not all MS patients. Robinson and Rudge (6) also reported on serial testing of BAEP in MS patients. In their 16 clinically unstable patients, seven had variations in BAEP without relationship to the sites of the clinical lesion. Ten of 11 clinically stable patients had stable BAEP.

Our data indicate that patients with proven abnormalities on PVEP and CFPD testing have variability on serial testing despite clinical stability. This variability may represent subclinical "relapses" and "remissions." It is also possible that this represents inherent variability of PVEP testing in the advanced MS patient. A third factor is the broad irregular waveform often seen in the abnormal PVEP of the MS patient. It is often difficult to determine the latency with precision in these cases. Hence, difficulty in precise interpretation might contribute to variability.

These findings require confirmation with a larger series of patients. A tentative hypothesis is that the degree of variation is positively related to the initial extent of abnormality on PVEP testing.

We concluded that unless the relevant variables contributing to PVEP variability can be specified and perhaps controlled, the evaluation of disease progression and the assessment of putative therapies cannot be reliably conducted with PVEP and CFPD in patients with an initially markedly abnormal base-line PVEP.

ACKNOWLEDGMENT

The authors would like to thank Ms. Karen Cohen for editorial assistance and Ms. Diane Guntrip and Ms. Diane Varnas for clerical assistance.

REFERENCES

1. Celesia, G. G., and Daly, R. F. (1977): Visual electroencephalographic computer analysis (VECA). *Neurology (Minneap.),* 27:637–641.
2. Cohen, S. N., Syndulko, K., Hansch, E. C., Tourtellotte, W. W., and Potvin, A. R. (1980): Use of a visual evoked potential battery in the evaluation of multiple sclerosis. *Ann. Neurol.,* 8:112.
3. Cohen, S. N., Syndulko, K., Tourtellotte, W. W., and Potvin, A. R. (1980): Critical frequency of photic driving in the diagnosis of multiple sclerosis. *Arch. Neurol.,* 37:80–83.
4. Kjaer, M. (1980): Variations of brain stem auditory evoked potentials correlated to duration and severity of multiple sclerosis. *Acta Neurol. Scand.,* 61:157–166.
5. Matthews, W. B., and Small, D. G. (1979): Serial recording of visual and somatosensory evoked potentials in multiple sclerosis. *J. Neurol. Sci.,* 40:11–21.
6. Robinson, K., and Rudge, P. (1978): The stability of the auditory evoked potentials in normal man and patients with multiple sclerosis. *J. Neurol. Sci.,* 36:147–156.
7. Rose, A. S., Ellison, G. W., Myers, L. W., and Tourtellotte, W. W. (1976): Criteria for the clinical diagnosis of multiple sclerosis. *Neurology (Minneap.),* 26:20–22.

Clinical Applications of Evoked Potentials in Neurology,
edited by J. Courjon, F. Mauguiere, and M. Revol.
Raven Press, New York © 1982.

The Value of Sequential Evoked Potential Recordings in Multiple Sclerosis Patients

Mogens Kjaer

Department of Neurology, Municipal Hospital, DK-8000 Aarhus C, Denmark

Repeated evoked potential (EP) recording reflecting changes in the clinical state of a few MS patients has led to the idea of monitoring the state or even the possible benefits of therapy in MS patients with serial EP recording (1,4,7). More restricted views of the value of this procedure have been expressed by various authors on the basis of larger numbers of patients (2,3,5,6).

In an attempt to reach a conclusion with respect to the value of repeated BAEP and VEP recording in MS patients, I should like to present my own results. The techniques, normal materials, and evaluating criteria have already been summarized in this symposium (M. Kjaer, *this volume, Chapter 61*).

BRAINSTEM AUDITORY EVOKED POTENTIALS

In 49 patients, BAEP examinations were repeated a total of 62 times at intervals ranging from 1 month to 2 years.

Thirteen patients were examined before and after having developed brainstem symptoms. In these patients, the first BAEP was normal in seven and changed to abnormal in three. Of six patients with an abnormal first BAEP, no change was observed in three; in the remaining three patients, a decrease in amplitudes by 50% or more or an increase in latencies appeared (Table 1).

Ten patients were followed after the brainstem symptoms had disappeared. Of five patients with a normal first recording, one showed a decrease in amplitudes. In five patients, the initial BAEP was abnormal. One of these changed to normal, one had an increase of amplitudes, and one an increase of latencies.

Thirty-nine patients were in a clinically stable or slowly progressive phase without recognized attacks. In 20 of these patients, no change was observed, whereas almost all possible combinations of increases and decreases of amplitudes and latencies were seen in the remaining 19, with a tendency for the amplitudes to decrease and for the latencies to increase. Two recordings changed from normal to abnormal and one from abnormal to normal; two of these alterations reflected a change in the latency of wave V, and one showed disappearance of the components following wave III.

TABLE 1. *Comparison of first and second BAEP recordings related to changes in the clinical state of MS patients (number of patients)*

Clinical state between recordings	First BAEP			Change in second BAEP			
	Total	Normality		No change	Within first classification	To	
						Normal	Abnormal
Brainstem	13	Normal	7	4	0		3
symptoms		Abnormal	6	3	3		
Improved	10	Normal	5	4	1		
		Abnormal	5	2	2	1	
Stable or		Normal	17	7	8		2
progressive	39	Abnormal	22	13	8	1	

VISUAL EVOKED POTENTIALS

Visual evoked potentials were repeated 22 times with recording intervals from 2 to 12 months. Eight patients had had visual symptoms probably caused by optic neuritis before the first recording. All 16 recordings were abnormal. No change of VEPs was seen in two patients; in six, various changes were shown in latencies and recognizability of P100.

Two developed visual disturbances that might be caused by optic neuritis in the recording interval. The first VEPs showed borderline delays of P100, which were increased by 4 to 21 msec in the second tests.

The remaining 12 patients did not have visual symptoms at any time. Five had normal first recordings, and two of these showed a change to abnormality. Seven patients had an abnormal first VEP, and one of these changed to normal. The changes in all three were in borderline latencies. The 24 P100 latencies were increased by a nonsignificant average of 1.4 msec.

CONCLUSION

Changes in EP recordings paralleling the clinical state of the patient undoubtedly occur, but the value of monitoring the clinical condition by EP recording is dubious, as recordings also show alterations in clinically stable patients. The tests show the neurophysiological state, and it seems illogical to seek to reflect the clinical state of a patient with techniques capable of showing subclinical lesions.

REFERENCES

1. Kjaer, M. (1979): Evaluation and graduation of brain stem auditory evoked potentials in patients with neurological diseases. *Acta Neurol. Scand.*, 60:231–242.
2. Kjaer, M. (1980): Variations of brain stem auditory evoked potentials correlated to duration and severity of multiple sclerosis. *Acta Neurol. Scand.*, 61:157–166.
3. Kjaer, M. (1982): Evoked potentials in multiple sclerosis with special reference to the diagnostic value. *Acta Neurol. Scand. (in press).*

4. Mogensen, F., and Kristensen, O. (1979): Auditory double click evoked potentials in multiple sclerosis. *Acta Neurol. Scand.,* 59:96–107.
5. Robinson, K., and Rudge, P. (1978): The stability of the auditory evoked potentials in normal man and patients with multiple sclerosis. *J. Neurol. Sci.,* 36:147–156.
6. Small, D. G., Matthews, W. B., and Small, M. (1978): The cervical somatosensory evoked potential (SEP) in the diagnosis of multiple sclerosis. *J. Neurol. Sci.,* 35:211–224.
7. Stockard, J. J., and Rossiter, V. S. (1977): Clinical and pathologic correlates of brain stem auditory response abnormalities. *Neurology (Minneap.),* 27:316–325.

Subject Index

Subject Index